Antibiotics

Volume V / Part 2

Mechanism of Action of Antieukaryotic and Antiviral Compounds

Edited by Fred E. Hahn

Springer-Verlag
Berlin Heidelberg New York 1979

Professor Fred E. Hahn, Ph.D.
Department of the Army
Walter Reed Army Institute of Research
Walter Reed Army Medical Center
Washington, D.C. 20012, USA

With 138 Figures

ISBN 3-540-09396-6 Springer-Verlag Berlin · Heidelberg · New York
ISBN 0-387-09396-6 Springer-Verlag New York · Heidelberg · Berlin

Library of Congress Cataloging in Publication Data. Main entry under title: Mechanism of actions of antieukaryotic and antiviral compounds. (Antibiotics; v. 5, pt. 2). Includes bibliographical references and index. 1. Antibiotics. 2. Antiviral agents. 3. Eukaryotic cells – Drug effects. I. Hahn, Fred Ernest, 1916– . II. Series. III. Title: Antieukaryotic and antiviral compounds. RM267.M42. 615'.329. 79-12228.

Typesetting, printing, and bookbinding: Universitätsdruckerei H. Stürtz AG, Würzburg
2131/3130-543210

Preface

When *Antibiotics I* was published in 1967, the teleological view was held by some that "antibiotics" were substances elaborated by certain microorganisms for the purpose of competing with other microorganisms for survival in mixed ecological environments. However, not only had J. EHRLICH and his associates shown 15 years earlier that chloramphenicol was produced by *Streptomyces venezuelae* in cultures of sterilized soils but not in parallel cultures of the same soils which were not sterilized, but operationally, the search for anticancer antibiotics was actively under way (*Antibiotics I* reporting on numerous such substances), although the concept of *antibiosis* could not logically justify such undertakings.

This editor hesitates to accept the use of the term "antibiotic" for antimicrobial agents of nonmicrobiological origins which is sometimes encountered, but neither does he subscribe to the view that antibiotics are in some fundamental manner different from chemotherapeutic substances of other origins. Modes and mechanisms of action of chemotherapeutic compounds are not systematic functions of their origins nor of the taxonomical position of the target organisms. Consequently, in the selection of topics for *Antibiotics III* (published in 1975), synthetic drugs and natural products of higher plants (alkaloids) were represented, along with antibiotics in the strict sense of the definition.

We now present *Antibiotics V*, for whose assembly the same selection criteria were applied as for *Antibiotics III*. The aggregate length of the contributions rendered it impractical to place the entire text between the covers of one book. *Antibiotics V* is, therefore, published in two volumes: Part 1, dealing with the actions of antibacterial compounds and Part 2, with the actions of antieukaryotic and antiviral substances. For antieukaryotic substances of natural origin, we present for the first time reviews of the actions of certain bacterial toxins, as well as of toxins from higher plants.

The separation of *Antibiotics V* into two volumes for practical reasons does not imply that there exist fundamental scientific differences between the contents of the two books. Many substances that inhibit molecular processes in eukaryotic cells also produce inhibitions in prokaryotes. The reverse statement can also be made, although the frequency of such instances is less. This is not surprising because antibacterial drugs are chosen according to their *selective toxicity* for bacteria. It is also of interest that certain antiviral drugs, for example, 5-iododeoxyuridine and ara-A were originally developed as potential anticancer substances before it was discovered that they possess valuable activities against virus infections. The fact remains that the partition of *Antibiotics V* into two separate volumes does not signify systematic scientific differences but rests essentially on a descriptive distinction.

Our book does not aspire to encyclopedic completeness. This editor did not select certain substances for review at this time, for example mefloquin, nifurtimox, interferons and their inducers, ara-C, or 9-(2-hydroxyethoxymethyl) guanine since he felt that knowledge of the mechanisms of action of these substances should be left to mature before reviews are necessary. Even at the time of publication of this book, it is apparent that new chemotherapeutic drugs and much new information on the actions of existing drugs continue to be discovered and reported. Within a few years still another volume of *Antibiotics* will be required to review these current and impending developments.

This should not detract from the usefulness of *Antibiotics V*. It presents a series of reviews of actions of substances which have been studied in sufficient detail and depth to yield bodies of scientific knowledge which are more easily accessible through review articles than through the retrieval and study of the source literature.

There remains the pleasant task of thanking my publisher, Dr. KONRAD F. SPRINGER, for his unwavering interest in, and support of, this undertaking and for having once again provided for the production of such a well-appointed and handsome book.

Washington, D.C., Spring 1979 FRED E. HAHN

Contents of Part 2

Contents of Part 1

Contributors

CASS, CAROL E., Cancer Research Laboratory (McEachern Laboratory), 5–75 Medical Sciences Building, Edmonton, Alberta T6G 2H7, Canada

CHANDRA, PRAKASH, Klinikum der Johann Wolfgang Goethe-Universität, Gustav-Embden-Zentrum der Biologischen Chemie, Abteilung für Molekularbiologie, Theodor-Stern-Kai 7, 6000 Frankfurt/Main 70, FRG

CHEN, M.S., Department of Pharmacology, Yale University School of Medicine, New Haven, CT 06510, USA

CHORĄŻY, MIECZYSŁAW, Department of Tumor Biology, Institute of Oncology, ul. Armii Czerwonej 15, 44–100 Gliwice, Poland

COLLIER, R. JOHN, Department of Microbiology, College of Letters and Science, University of California, Los Angeles, CA 90024, USA

CREASEY, WILLIAM A., Department of Pharmacology, University of Pennsylvania, School of Medicine, Philadelphia, PA 19104, USA

EARHART, CHARLES F., JR., Department of Microbiology, The University of Texas at Austin, Austin, TX 78712, USA

FESTY, BERNARD, 4, avenue de l'Observatoire, 75006-Paris, France

FILIPSKI, JAN, Department of Tumor Biology, Institute of Oncology, ul. Armii Czerwonej 15, 44–100 Gliwice, Poland

FISHER, T.H., Department of Pharmacology, Yale University School of Medicine, New Haven, CT 06510, USA

GLAUBIGER, DANIEL, Pedriatric Oncology Branch, National Cancer Institute, National Institutes of Health, Building 10, Room 3B04, Bethesda, MD 20014, USA

GNIAŹDOWSKI, MAREK, Department of General Chemistry, Institute of Physiology and Biochemistry, Medical School in Lódź, Lindleya 6, 90–131 Lódź, Poland

GOLDBERG, IRVING H., Department of Pharmacology, Harvard Medical School, 250 Longwood Avenue, Boston, MA 02115, USA

GRUNBERGER, DEZIDER, Cancer Center/Institute of Cancer Research, Columbia University, 701 West 168 Street, New York, NY 10032, USA

Grunberger, George, Department of Medicine, Case Western Reserve University, University Hospitals of Cleveland, 2074 Abington Road, Cleveland, OH 44106, USA

Hahn, Fred E., Department of the Army, Walter Reed Army Institute of Research, Walter Reed Army Medical Center, Washington, DC 20012, USA

Haidle, Charles W., The University of Texas System Cancer Center, M.D. Anderson Hospital and Tumor Institute, Houston, TX 77030, USA

Holz, Ronald W., Department of Pharmacology, University of Michigan Medical School, Ann Arbor, MI 48109, USA

Jiménez, Antonio, Centro de Biología Molecular, Instituto de Bioquímica de Macromoléculas, Universidad Autónoma de Madrid, Facultad de Ciencias, Canto Blanco, Madrid 34, Spain

Kohn, Kurt W., Laboratory of Molecular Pharmacology, Developmental Therapeutics Program, Division of Cancer Treatment, National Cancer Institute, National Institutes of Health, Building 37, Room 5D18, Bethesda, MD 20205, USA

Lin, T.S., Department of Pharmacology, Yale University School of Medicine, New Haven, CT 06510, USA

Lloyd, R. Stephen, Department of Biological Sciences, Stanford University, Stanford, CA 94305, USA

Mizuno, Nobuko S., 3628 Loma Way, San Diego, CA 92106, USA

Olenick, John G., Department of Applied Biochemistry, Division of Biochemistry, Walter Reed Army Institute of Research, Walter Reed Army Medical Center, Washington, DC 20012, USA

Prusoff, William H., Department of Pharmacology, Yale University School of Medicine, New Haven, CT 06510, USA

Roberts, John J., Institute of Cancer Research, Pollards Wood Research Station, Chalfont St. Giles, Bucks, Great Britain

Ross, Warren E., Medical Oncology, Medical Science Building, Room M433, University of Florida, Gainesville, FL 32601, USA

Roy-Burman, Sumitra, Department of Biochemistry, University of Southern California, School of Medicine, 2025 Zonal Avenue, Los Angeles, CA 90033, USA

Shiau, G.T., Department of Pharmacology, Yale University School of Medicine, New Haven, CT 06510, USA

Vázquez, David, Centro de Biología Molecular, Instituto de Bioquímica de Macromoléculas, Universidad Autónoma de Madrid, Canto Blanco, Facultat de Ciencias, Madrid 34, Spain

VISSER, DONALD W., Department of Biochemistry, University of Southern California, School of Medicine, Los Angeles, CA 90033, USA

WARING, MICHAEL J., Department of Pharmacology, Medical School, University of Cambridge, Hills Road, Cambridge CB2 2QD, Great Britain

WOLTERSDORF, M., Klinikum der Johann Wolfgang Goethe-Universität, Gustav-Embden-Zentrum der Biologischen Chemie, Abteilung für Molekularbiologie, Theodor-Stern-Kai 7, 6000 Frankfurt/Main 70, FRG

WRIGHT, GEORGE J., A.H. Robins Company, Inc., 1211 Sherwood Avenue, Richmond, VA 23220, USA

Anisomycin and Related Antibiotics

A. JIMÉNEZ and D. VÁZQUEZ

The antibiotic anisomycin was first isolated by SOBIN and TANNER (1954) from culture filtrates of two different species of *Streptomyces*, subsequently identified as *S. griseolus* and *S. roseochromogenes* (TANNER et al., 1955), and more recently the drug has also been isolated from *Streptomyces* sp. No. 638

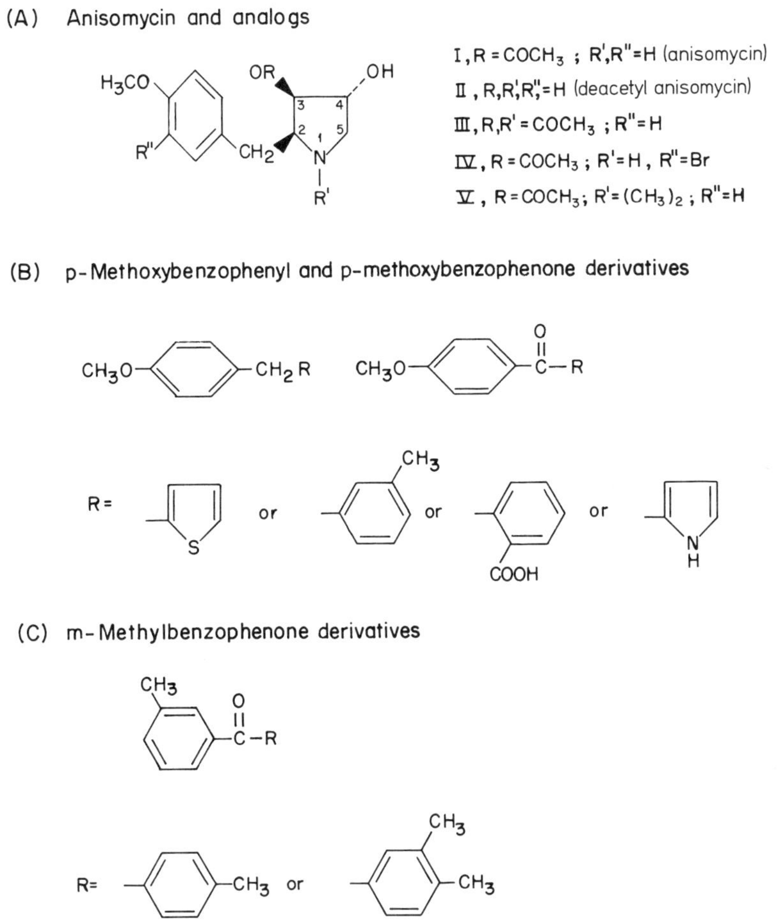

Fig. 1 A–C. Chemical structure of anisomycin and some structurally related compounds

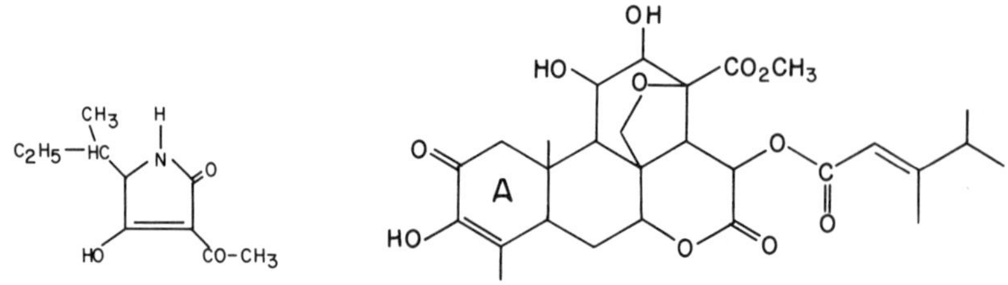

Tenuazonic acid Bruceantin

Fig. 2. Chemical structures of tenuazonic acid and bruceantin

by ISHIDA et al. (1974). Crystalline anisomycin is soluble in water, and aqueous solutions appear to be more stable at slightly acidic pH (pH 4 to 6) than at alkaline pH (TANNER et al., 1955; BARBACID and VÁZQUEZ, 1973). Both the chemical structure and the stereochemical configuration of the drug were established by BEEREBOOM et al. (1965) and BUTLER (1968) (Fig. 1), and its complete chemical synthesis has also been achieved (OIDA and OHKI, 1969; FELNER and SCHENKER, 1970).

Many antibiotics, alkaloids and other compounds of different chemical structures and origin apparently have modes of action very similar to that of anisomy-

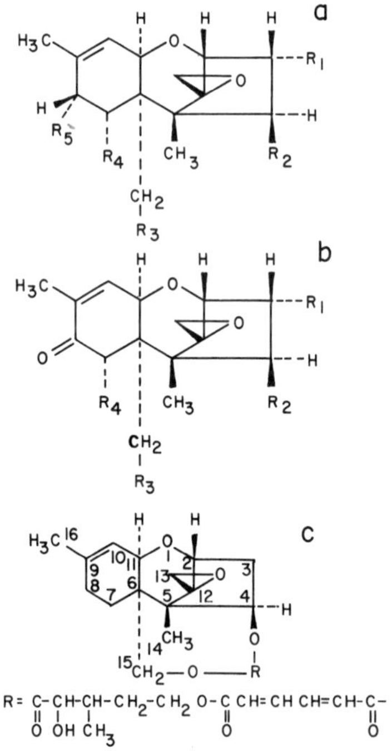

a	R_1	R_2	R_3	R_4	R_5
Scirpene	H	H	H	H	H
Trichodermol	H	OH	H	H	H
Trichodermin	H	OAc	H	H	H
Diacetoxyscirpenol	OH	OAc	OAc	H	H
Toxin T-2	OH	OAc	OAc	H	$OOCCH_2$-$CHMe_2$
Verrucarol	H	OH	OH	H	H
15-Desacetylcalonectrin	OAc	H	OH	H	H
Scirpenol	OH	OH	OH	H	H

b	R_1	R_2	R_3	R_4
Nivalenol	OH	OH	OH	OH
Trichothecin	H	OOCCH=CHMe	H	H
Fusarenon X	OH	OAc	OH	OH

c
Verrucarin A

Fig. 3a–c. Chemical structure of some trichothecene antibiotics

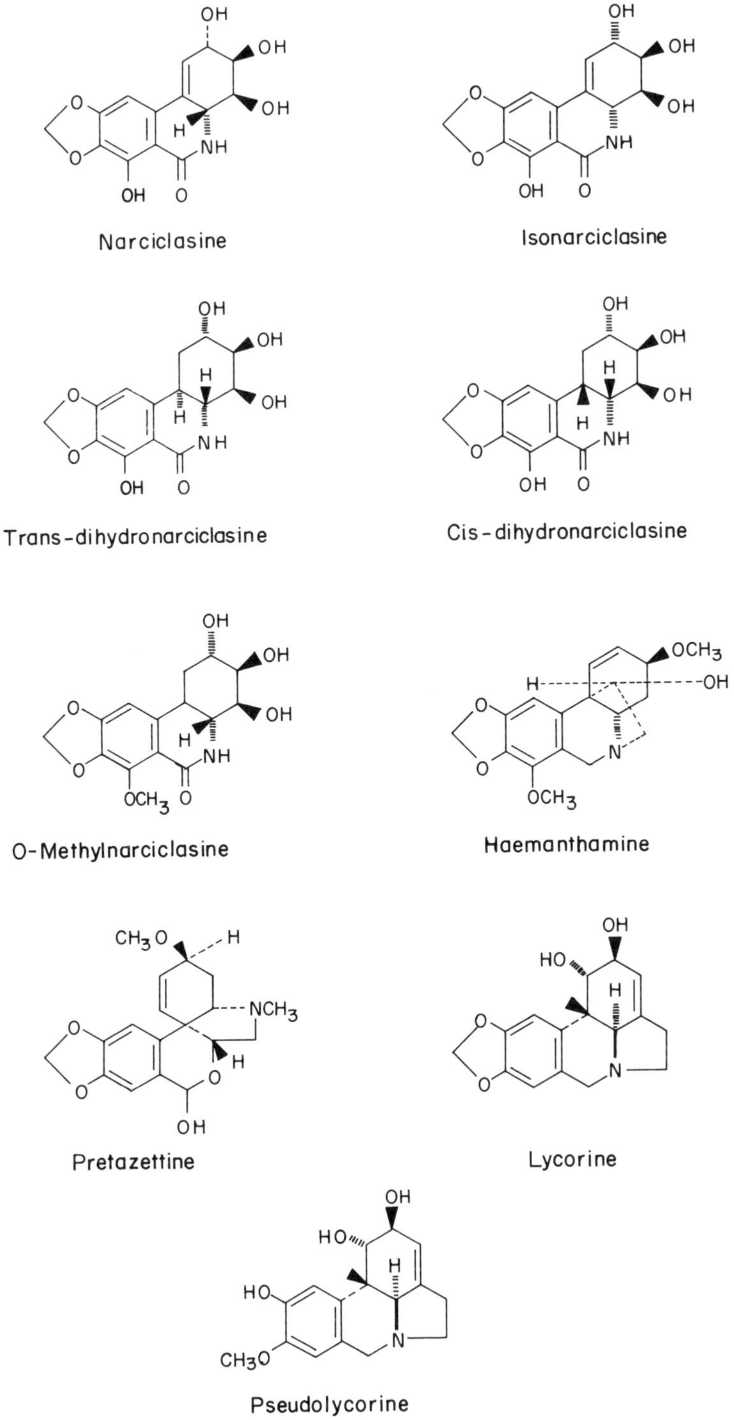

Fig. 4. Chemical structure of some active compounds of the Amaryllidaceae family

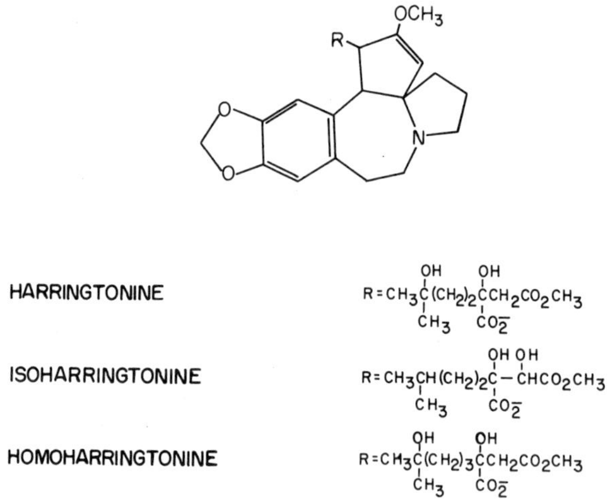

Fig. 5. Chemical structures of some *Cephalotaxus* alkaloids

Table 1. Producer species of anisomycin and related inhibitors

Antibiotic	Producer species	Reference
Anisomycin	*Streptomyces griseolus* *Streptomyces roseochromogenes* *Streptomyces* sp. No. 638	SOBIN and TANNER, 1954 TANNER et al., 1955 ISHIDA et al., 1974
Trichodermin	*Trichoderma viride*	GODFREDSEN and VANGEDAL, 1964
Trichodermol (synonym roridin C)	*Myrothecium roridum*	HARRI et al., 1962
Verrucarin A	*Myrothecium verrucaria* *Myrothecium roridum*	HARRI et al., 1962
Trichothecin	*Trichotherium roseum*	FREEMAN et al., 1947
Fusarenon X	*Fusarium nivale* Fn 2b	UENO et al., 1969
Crotocin (synonym antibiotic-T)	*Cephalosporium crotocinigenum*	GLAZ et al., 1959
Tenuazonic acid	*Alternaria tenuis*	ROSETT et al., 1957
Narciclasine Haemanthamine Pretazettine Lycorine Pseudolycorine	Bulbs of Amaryllidaceae	WILDMAN, 1968; FUGANTI, 1975
Harringtonine Homoharringtonine Isoharringtonine	Seeds of *Cephalotaxus harringtonia*	POWELL et al., 1972
Bruceantin	*Brucea antidysenterica*	LIAO et al., 1976b

cin. Examples include tenuazonic acid (Fig. 2), the trichothecene antibiotics [trichodermin, trichodermol, trichothecin, fusarenon X, diacetoxyscirpenol (synonym anguidine), T-2 toxin, nivalenol, and verrucarin A; Fig. 3] a number of Amaryllidaceae alkaloids and related compounds (narciclasine, isonarciclasine, trans- and cis-dihydronarciclasine, 0-methyl-narciclasine, haemanthamine, pretazettine, lycorine and pseudolycorine; Fig. 4), the *Cephalotaxus* alkaloids (harringtonine, homoharringtonine and isoharringtonine; Fig. 5) and bruceantin (Fig. 2), all these compounds having, also in common with anisomycin, little or no inhibitory activity towards bacteria, and affecting only certain eukaryotic organisms. Some of these compounds along with the organisms that produce them are listed in Table 1.

Biological Activity of Anisomycin on Living Organisms

The most sensitive organisms to the inhibitory action of anisomycin were found to be Protozoa, growth of *Trichomonas vaginalis, Trichomonas foetus*, and *Entamoeba histolytica* being inhibited by 1.5–3 μg/ml of the compound (LYNCH et al., 1954a). Several strains of *Candida albicans* and *Saccharomyces cerevisiae* were also found to be sensitive to the antibiotic (LYNCH et al., 1954a;

Table 2. Inhibitory spectra of anisomycin and related inhibitors

Inhibitor	Cells	Minimal growth inhibitory concentrations (M conc.)
Anisomycin	*Trichomonas vaginalis*[a]	1.2×10^{-5}
	Entamoeba histolytica[a]	6×10^{-6}
	Candida albicans[a]	6×10^{-6}
	Saccharomyces cerevisiae[b]	5×10^{-5}
	HeLa[b]	1.5×10^{-6}
Trichodermin	*Saccharomyces cerevisiae*[b]	5×10^{-6}
	HeLa[b]	2.5×10^{-6}
Fusarenon X	HeLa[c]	1.4×10^{-6}
Trichothecin	HeLa[c]	9×10^{-6}
Narciclasine	HeLa[d]	10^{-6}
	Saccharomyces cerevisiae[e]	2×10^{-4}
Haemanthamine	HeLa[d]	4×10^{-6}
	Saccharomyces cerevisiae[e]	4×10^{-3}
Lycorine	HeLa[d]	6×10^{-6}
	Saccharomyces cerevisiae[e]	2×10^{-4}
Pretazettine	HeLa[d]	10^{-6}
	Saccharomyces cerevisiae[e]	2×10^{-3}
Pseudolycorine	HeLa[d]	2.5×10^{-5}
	Saccharomyces cerevisiae[e]	4×10^{-3}

Data taken from [a] LYNCH et al., 1954a; [b] A. JIMÉNEZ and D. VÁZQUEZ, unpublished results; [c] SAITO and OTSHUBO, 1974; [d] JIMÉNEZ et al., 1976; [e] JIMÉNEZ et al., 1975c.

Tanner et al., 1955). Anisomycin has a moderate toxicity towards some experimental animals, the acute intravenous and oral LD_{50} in mice being 140 and 148 mg/kg body weight, respectively. However, monkeys can tolerate daily oral doses of anisomycin of 1–64 mg/kg of body weight over a period of more than six months (Gardocki et al., 1955). Mice, infected with *Trichomonas foetus*, were treated with doses of 25, 50, and 100 mg of anisomycin per kg body weight beginning either immediately or 24 h after infection. Even with the lowest doses, 95% of the mice, for which treatment commenced 24 h after infection, were cured by the drug (Lynch et al., 1954b). In addition anisomycin has been used with some success in clinical trials for the treatment of both amoebic dysentery and vaginitis caused by *Trichomonas vaginalis*. A comparison between the inhibitory spectra of anisomycin and some of the trichothecene antibiotics is presented in Table 2.

The Mode of Action of Anisomycin

Anisomycin halts protein synthesis specifically in eukaryotic organisms including HeLa cells and *Saccharomyces fragilis*. At concentrations of anisomycin causing 95% inhibition of protein synthesis (Grollman, 1967), synthesis of RNA is not affected, although synthesis of DNA is slowed down. This latter effect is probably a secondary result of the inhibition of protein synthesis, being frequently observed when eukaryotic cells are treated with protein synthesis inhibitors (Vázquez, 1974). However, with anisomycin, the effects on DNA and protein synthesis are reversible. Anisomycin inhibits synthesis of both polyphenylalanine and hemoglobin, starting from aminoacyl-tRNA, in reticulocyte cell-free extracts and synthesis of polyphenylalanine, starting from phenylalanyl-tRNA, in yeast extracts (Grollman, 1967; Battaner and Vázquez, 1971; Lodish et al., 1971) and the drug therefore blocks some step after formation of aminoacyl-tRNA. Since anisomycin is a specific inhibitor of eukaryotic protein synthesis (Grollman, 1967), it has no effect when added to extracts from *Escherichia coli*. The drug inhibits the puromycin-induced release of peptides from reticulocyte polysomes (Grollman, 1967; Grollman and Huang, 1973) and blocks formation of N-acetyl-(^{3}H)Leu-puromycin in both the "fragment reaction" (Vázquez et al., 1969; Neth et al., 1970; Battaner and Vázquez, 1971) and the puromycin reaction (Carrasco and Vázquez, 1972). Furthermore anisomycin stabilizes polyribosome profiles (Grollman, 1967) and inhibits the puromycin-induced release of peptides in intact HeLa cells (Cundliffe et al., 1974). These observations support the conclusion that the drug specifically blocks peptide bond formation on eukaryotic ribosomes.

Since peptide chain termination is catalyzed by the peptidyl transferase center on both prokaryotic and eukaryotic ribosomes (Vogel et al., 1969; Caskey and Beaudet, 1972) this reaction should be inhibited by anisomycin. The drug does, in fact, inhibit release of f-Met in a termination assay in the presence of release factor R (Beaudet and Caskey, 1971). However, in a simplified system where f-Met is released, in the absence of release factor R, but in the presence of 30% acetone, anisomycin considerably enhances the reaction (CASKEY et al., 1971) although under these experimental conditions the drug has a low binding affinity for ribosomes (BARBACID and VÁZQUEZ, 1974a). This system is, of course, artificial, but nevertheless the lack of inhibitory response may be meaningful (CASKEY et al., 1971) since a similar finding has also been observed in bacterial systems in the presence of the peptidyl transferase inhibitor lincomycin (CASKEY and BEAUDET, 1972).

Anisomycin (10^{-4} M) partially inhibits the binding of phenylalanyl-tRNA and N-Ac-phenylalanyl-tRNA to the ribosomal A and P sites respectively (CARRASCO and VÁZQUEZ, 1972) and the antibiotic also inhibits, albeit partially, interaction of the fragments CACCA-Leu-Ac and CACCA-Leu with the donor and acceptor sites respectively of 60S ribosomal subunits (BATTANER and VÁZQUEZ, 1971). Thus anisomycin might inhibit peptide bond formation by affecting the correct positioning of the 3′ termini of aminoacyl-tRNA and/or peptidyl-tRNA on the peptidyl transferase center (VÁZQUEZ, 1974), a theory compatible with the proposal that anisomycin competitively inhibits the puromycin reaction on eukaryotic polyribosomes (PESTKA et al., 1972). It should be noted, however, that puromycin inhibits binding of (^{3}H)anisomycin and (^{14}C)-trichodermin to ribosomes only poorly (BARBACID and VÁZQUEZ, 1974a, 1974c).

Binding of Anisomycin to Eukaryotic Ribosomes

Preparation of (^{3}H)anisomycin by tritium exchange (BARBACID and VÁZQUEZ, 1973) has enabled experiments to be carried out on the binding of the antibiotic to eukaryotic ribosomes. Only one molecule of (^{3}H)anisomycin can be bound per molecule of 60S or 80S ribosomal particles and the affinity of (^{3}H)anisomycin for eukaryotic ribosomes is decreased in the presence of some organic solvents (ethanol and acetone). Furthermore, binding of (^{3}H)anisomycin to yeast ribosomes is affected, although not drastically, by changes in the ionic conditions (BARBACID and VÁZQUEZ, 1974a). (^{3}H)-anisomycin binds to high salt-washed ribosomes from human tonsils and yeast with two different affinities. The higher affinity binding accounts for inhibition of peptide bond formation, since on the basis of this value the theoretical level calculated for inhibition of the puromycin reaction by anisomycin corresponds to the experimental value actually observed (BARBACID and VÁZQUEZ, 1974a). Furthermore both run-off ribosomes (obtained by treating yeast spheroplasts with 1 mM sodium azide or cooling them to 8° C) and in vitro released ribosomes (obtained by treatment of yeast polyribosomes with puromycin) bind anisomycin with a single type of affinity. Nevertheless if run-off ribosomes are washed in buffers containing high KCl or NH_4Cl concentrations, binding heterogeneity is again acquired (BARBACID and VÁZQUEZ, 1974a, 1975). Heterogeneity is associated with the 40S ribosomal subunits since 60S subunits bind (^{3}H)anisomycin with a single affinity, intermediate between the higher and the lower affinities characteristic of 80S ribosomes, heterogeneity being restored by reconstitution of 80S ribosomes from 60S and 40S subunits (BARBACID and VÁZQUEZ, 1974a; JIMÉNEZ and VÁZQUEZ, 1975). A similar situation has also been found for gougerotin, another inhibitor of the peptidyl-transferase center (BARBACID and VÁZQUEZ, 1974b), since (^{3}H)gougerotin binds to 80S ribosomes again with two different affinities.

The affinity of (^{3}H)anisomycin for its target site on 80S ribosomes is drastically affected by the different conformational states acquired by these particles during the various steps of the translation process. Thus by blocking translation with either puromycin, chlortetracycline, cycloheximide or diphtheria toxin, free ribosomes, ribosomes with peptidyl-tRNA bound to the P-site, ribosomes with peptidyl-tRNA bound to the A-site and ribosomes carrying both peptidyl-tRNA bound to the A-site and elongation factor EF-2 can be obtained respectively. Ribosomes with peptidyl-tRNA bound to the donor site have the highest affinity (Kd=0.8 μM) for (^{3}H)anisomycin (BARBACID and VÁZQUEZ, 1975), and it is precisely at this stage of translation (postranslocated ribosomes) that the antibiotic might be expected to bind and hence inhibit formation of the peptide bond. The lowest affinity for (^{3}H)anisomycin is found for ribosomes present in polyribosomes previously treated with either cycloheximide or diphtheria toxin. Such ribosomes have peptidyl-tRNA attached to the acceptor site (Kd=12 μM). Ribosomes treated with puromycin have an intermediate affinity (Kd=3.6 μM) for (^{3}H)anisomycin (BARBACID and VÁZQUEZ, 1975).

It will be apparent from the above considerations that studies on the quantitative binding of (^{3}H)anisomycin allows the detection of conformational changes that might take place on eukaryotic ribosomes during translation. Such studies can also be applied to calculate the percentage of peptidyl-tRNA bound to each ribosomal site for any given preparation of eukaryotic polyribosomes. Thus in yeast polyribosomes approximately 80% of the ribosomes bind (^{3}H)anisomycin with low affinity and therefore have peptidyl-tRNA bound to the A-site. The remaining 20% bind (^{3}H)anisomycin with the higher affinity and hence carry peptidyl-tRNA bound to the P-site (BARBACID et al., 1975). It was also observed by CANNON et al. (1976) that (^{14}C)trichodermin had a different affinity for free ribosomes compared with that for polyribosomes.

Mechanisms of Inhibition and Sites of Action of Trichothecene Antibiotics, Tenuazonic Acid, *Amaryllidaceae* and *Cephalotaxus* Alkaloids and Bruceantin

The trichothecene antibiotics are sesquiterpenes that strongly inhibit protein synthesis in both eukaryotic cells and cell-free systems (UENO et al., 1968; UENO et al., 1969; CARRASCO et al., 1973; STAFFORD and MCLAUGHLIN, 1973; TATE and CASKEY, 1973) and the chemistry of these compounds has recently been reviewed (BAMBURG, 1976). Of the trichothecenes tested trichodermin, trichodermol, trichothecin, verrucarin A, fusarenon X, nivalenol, diacetoxyscirpenol (synonym anguidine), and T-2 toxin actively block both the puromycin reaction

(UENO et al., 1968; UENO et al., 1969; CARRASCO et al., 1973; STAFFORD and McLAUGHLIN, 1973; TATE and CASKEY, 1973) and the "fragment reaction" (CARRASCO et al., 1973). The compounds are, therefore, inhibitors of both peptide bond formation (CARRASCO et al., 1973; TATE and CASKEY, 1973) and termination of protein synthesis (STAFFORD and McLAUGHLIN, 1973; TATE and CASKEY, 1973). However, on the basis of their effects on polyribosomes in either intact cells or cell-free systems, these trichothecene toxins have been classified into two groups (SCHINDLER, 1974). Thus trichodermin, trichodermol, crotocin, and trichothecin stabilize polyribosomes, prevent their reaction with puromycin and have therefore been regarded as inhibitors of peptide bond formation (CUNDLIFFE et al., 1974; SCHINDLER, 1974; LIAO et al., 1976a). In contrast verrucarin A, nivalenol, T-2 toxin, fusarenon X, and diacetoxyscirpenol (synonym anguidine) cause breakdown of polyribosomes and fail to inhibit their reaction with puromycin, and on these grounds were considered inhibitors of initiation (CUNDLIFFE et al., 1974; SCHINDLER, 1974; MIZUNO, 1975; LIAO et al., 1976a). Further work with the toxins has, however, clearly shown that they are all inhibitors of peptide bond formation (SMITH et al., 1975; CANNON et al., 1976). Apparently, trichodermin, trichodermol, crotocin and trichothecin interact with both polyribosomes and run-off ribosomes, whereas the affinity of verrucarin A, nivalenol, T-2 toxin, fusarenon X and diacetoxyscirpenol for polyribosomes is very low. The latter group of compounds is excluded from the ribosomal receptor site by nascent polypeptide chains above a certain minimal size (CANNON et al., 1976) and hence does not associate with polyribosomes. Certainly these compounds are not inhibitors of the initiation phase of protein synthesis (CANNON et al., 1976; FRESNO et al., 1976). One molecule of (^{14}C)trichodermin binds to each molecule of sensitive ribosomes (BARBACID and VÁZQUEZ, 1974c; WEI et al., 1974) and the binding site is located on the 60S subunit (BARBACID and VÁZQUEZ, 1974c). Binding of trichodermin to free ribosomes is prevented by the various active toxins (BARBACID and VÁZQUEZ, 1974c; WEI et al., 1974) and although (^{14}C)trichodermin binds to polyribosomes, it does so with a lower affinity than the one it has for ribosomes carrying no nascent peptide chains (CANNON et al., 1976). However, in contrast to the behavior of anisomycin, trichodermin binds with an equal affinity to ribosomes carrying peptidyl-tRNA either in the donor or the acceptor site (VÁZQUEZ et al., 1977). Binding of (^{14}C)trichodermin to polyribosomes is inhibited by those trichothecene antibiotics that stabilize polyribosomes, but binding is not affected by those toxins indicated above that allow polyribosome breakdown since these cannot interact with their receptor site (CANNON et al., 1976).

Tenuazonic acid inhibits protein synthesis in mammalian systems (SHIGEURA and GORDON, 1963) by preventing peptide bond formation (NETH et al., 1970; CARRASCO and VÁZQUEZ, 1972; CARRASCO and VÁZQUEZ, 1973). The target site for the antibiotic is on the 60S ribosomal subunit, and the drug prevents interaction of both (^{3}H)anisomycin (BARBACID and VÁZQUEZ, 1974a) and (^{14}C)trichodermin with these particles (BARBACID and VÁZQUEZ, 1974c). An important and unusual characteristic of tenuazonic acid is its preferential inhibition of mammalian systems. Thus studies on inhibition, by tenuazonic acid, of both protein synthesis (CARRASCO and VÁZQUEZ, 1973) and binding of (^{3}H)anisomycin to ribosomes (BARBACID and VÁZQUEZ, 1974a) have shown that the antibiotic is a relatively poor inhibitor of ribosomes from plants and green algae, and is inactive toward yeast ribosomes.

Narciclasine is a compound which accumulates in the bulbs of different species of *Narcissus*. It has antitumor activity and blocks the growth of eukaryotic cells (CERIOTTI, 1967). Narciclasine specifically inhibits protein synthesis in both intact cells (JIMÉNEZ et al., 1976) and in cell-free systems (CARRASCO et al., 1975) by preventing peptide bond formation as assayed in both the fragment and puromycin reactions catalysed by yeast and ascites ribosomes (CARRASCO et al., 1975; JIMÉNEZ et al., 1976). In addition, narciclasine blocks the puromycin reaction with polysomes and inhibits the sparsomycin-induced binding of UACCA-Leu-Ac to ribosomes (JIMÉNEZ et al., 1976). (^{3}H)Narciclasine interacts with 60S ribosomal subunits (BAEZ et al., 1977) and drastically inhibits binding of both (^{3}H)anisomycin and, to a lesser extent, (^{14}C)trichodermin to ribosomes (CARRASCO et al., 1975). Furthermore, anisomycin and trichodermin can themselves prevent the interaction of (^{3}H)narciclasine with ribosomes (BAEZ and VÁZQUEZ, 1978). These results clearly indicate that narciclasine inhibits the peptidyl transferase center of eukaryotic ribosomes by acting at a site closely connected to or overlapping the binding site(s) for anisomycin and trichodermin. A large number of compounds, whose chemical structures are closely related to that of narciclasine, have in fact been synthesised (MONDON and KROHN, 1975). Some of these compounds (isonarciclasine, trans- and cis-dihydronarciclasine and O-methyl-narciclasine) (Fig. 4) also inhibit eukaryotic protein synthesis and prevent binding of (^{3}H)narciclasine to ribosomes. Other related synthetic derivatives are, however, devoid of biological activity (BAEZ and VÁZQUEZ, 1978). The bulbs of the Amaryllidaceae are the source of more than one hundred alkaloids all structurally related to narciclasine (WILDMAN, 1968; FUGANTI, 1975). A number of these alkaloids including pretazettine, haemanthamine, lycorine and pseudolycorine (Fig. 4) block peptide bond formation (JIMÉNEZ et al., 1976) and they also prevent binding of (^{3}H)narciclasine to ribosomes (BAEZ and VÁZQUEZ, 1978). Although both pretazettine and narciclasine inhibit the peptidyl transferase center, pretazettine alone is very active against both lymphocytic choriomeningitis virus infections in mice (FURUSAWA and CUTTING, 1970) and rauscher leukemia (FURUSAWA et al., 1976). Furthermore pretazettine, present at high concentrations, has an inhibitory effect on reverse transcriptase (PAPAS et al., 1973).

The alkaloids harringtonine, isoharringtonine and homoharringtonine have antitumor activity (POWELL et al., 1972), and are very effective inhibitors of protein synthesis in both eukaryotic cells and cell-free systems (TSCHERNE and PESTKA, 1975; HUANG, 1976). These alkaloids were classed initially as inhibitors of initiation since they induce breakdown of polyribosomes in both intact cells and cell-free systems (TSCHERNE and PESTKA, 1975; HUANG, 1976). This effect results because the harringtonine alkaloids have a very low affinity for polyribosomes. In fact these compounds inhibit both peptide bond formation and the EF-1-dependent binding of aminoacyl-tRNA to ribosomes in the early rounds of elongation. Possibly these compounds are excluded from their ribosomal receptor site(s) when the growing nascent peptide has reached a certain critical length (e.g., certain of the trichothecenes). Certainly they have no effect on any of the steps of the initiation process (FRESNO et al., 1976).

The antitumor compound bruceantin inhibits protein synthesis both in eukaryotic cells and cell-free systems (LIAO et al., 1976b) and it has been postulated that the drug, at low concentrations, inhibits initiation since it induces breakdown of polyribosomes (LIAO et al., 1976b). However, bruceantin inhibits peptide bond formation by ribosomes and the drug also prevents interaction of both (^{3}H)anisomycin and (^{14}C)trichodermin with these particles (FRESNO et al., 1977b). Again bruceantin has a very low affinity for polyribosomes and can inhibit only the first rounds of peptide bond formation (FRESNO et al., 1977b). In many respects, therefore, it resembles many of the alkaloids and trichothecenes considered above.

Ribosomal Receptor Site(s) for Anisomycin and Related Inhibitors

A number of different anisomycin-resistant mutants of *Saccharomyces cerevisiae* have been studied. These strains were initially isolated as spontaneous mutants resistant to trichodermin and were shown to be cross resistant in vivo to anisomycin (SCHINDLER et al., 1974; JIMÉNEZ et al., 1975a). Detailed genetic studies by tetrad analysis presented strong evidence that the simultaneous resistance to anisomycin and trichodermin results from the expression of a single recessive mutation in a nuclear gene. In general, resistance in vivo to anisomycin is weaker than the resistance to trichodermin (JIMÉNEZ et al., 1975a; GRANT et al., 1976). The gene responsible for the pleiotropic phenotype has been mapped on the right arm of chromosome XV, 1.1 cM nearer the centromere than pet17 (GRANT et al., 1976). Studies of protein synthesis in vitro using cell-free extracts from both wild-type and mutant strains have shown that resistance to anisomycin is associated with the ribosomes of the mutant yeast strains at the level of peptide bond formation (Table 3). Moreover the alteration was located on the 60S ribosomal subunit (JIMÉNEZ et al., 1975a). This result is in agreement with previous findings which showed that anisomycin inhibits the peptidyl transferase center (VÁZQUEZ et al., 1969) and therefore binds to 60S ribosomal subunits (BARBACID and VÁZQUEZ, 1974a). The mutation to anisomycin resistance induces a complex phenotype since the mutant peptidyl transferase center is cross-resistant to a wide range of compounds as follows: (a) the trichothecene antibiotics trichodermin, trichothecin, trichodermol, fusarenon X, verrucarin A, nivalenol, and T-2 toxin (SCHINDER et al., 1974; JIMÉNEZ et al., 1975a); (b) the active Amaryllidaceae alkaloids and related compounds narciclasine, pretazettine, haemanthamine, isonarciclasine, trans- and cis-dihydronarciclasine and O-methyl-narciclasine (JIMÉNEZ et al., 1975b; JIMÉNEZ et al., 1976; BAEZ and VÁZQUEZ, 1978); (c) the *Cephalotaxus* alkaloids harringtonine, homoharringtonine and isoharringtonine (FRESNO et al., 1977a) and (d) bruceantin (FRESNO et al., 1977b). The results of these studies are summarized in Table 3. The ribosomal binding sites for all the above compounds are overlapping since

Table 3. Effects of anisomycin and related inhibitors on poly(U)-directed polyphenylalanine synthesis and peptide bond formation by wild-type and resistant yeast ribosomes

Inhibitor (M conc.)		Polyphenylalanine synthesis (% control)		Fragment reaction (% control)	
		Wild-type	Resistant	Wild-type	Resistant
Anisomycin	2×10^{-6}	33	80	59	91
	10^{-5}	20	53	30	51
Trichothecene antibiotics:					
Fusarenon X	2×10^{-5}	38	102	7	71
Trichothecin	2×10^{-5}	40	90	–	–
Trichodermin	2×10^{-4}	72	85	6	67
Cephalotaxus alkaloids:					
Harringtonine	2×10^{-5}	29	68	12	39
Homoharringtonine	2×10^{-5}	23	65	6	27
Isoharringtonine	2×10^{-5}	35	64	19	55
Amaryllidaceae compounds:					
Haemanthamine	10^{-3}	34	100	34	100
Lycorine	7×10^{-4}	100	100	61	50
Narciclasine	10^{-6}	58	99	5	48
Pretazettine	3×10^{-4}	5	87	50	100
Pseudolycorine	10^{-3}	38	32	34	10
Bruceantin	2×10^{-6}	13	47	7	–

Data taken from CARRASCO et al., 1973; JIMÉNEZ et al., 1975a, b, c; FRESNO et al., 1977a, b; A. JIMÉNEZ and D. VÁZQUEZ, unpublished results.

all the drugs totally inhibit the association of (^{3}H)anisomycin, (^{14}C)trichodermin and (^{3}H)-narciclasine with sensitive ribosomes (BARBACID and VÁZQUEZ, 1974a, c; BAEZ and VÁZQUEZ, 1978).

The alteration induced by the mutation to anisomycin resistance must be restricted to a well-defined area of the peptidyl transferase center, since sensitivity to other inhibitors of peptide bond formation, such as gougerotin and blasticidin S, is not impaired (JIMÉNEZ and VÁZQUEZ, 1975). Furthermore both the antibiotic sparsomycin and the Amaryllidaceae alkaloids lycorine and pseudolycorine, which themselves are specific inhibitors of peptide bond formation are more active against ribosomes from the anisomycin-resistant strain than against ribosomes from the sensitive strain (JIMÉNEZ and VÁZQUEZ, 1975; JIMÉNEZ et al., 1975c; Table 3). The most plausible explanation for this pleiotropic alteration of the mutant ribosomes is that the structural modification increases the affinity of a number of inhibitors such as lycorine, pseudolycorine and sparsomycin for their binding sites. These compounds clearly have a different receptor site from that of the compounds described above and, as predicted by this hypothesis, sparsomycin, gougerotin and blasticidin S do not significantly affect the interaction of (^{3}H)anisomycin, (^{14}C)trichodermin and (^{3}H)narciclasine with the 80S ribosomes (BARBACID and VÁZQUEZ, 1974a, c; BAEZ and VÁZQUEZ, 1977).

Binding of (^{3}H)Anisomycin and (^{14}C)-Trichodermin to Resistant Yeast Ribosomes: Effects of Peptidyl Transferase Inhibitors That Mutually Exclude Anisomycin

Scatchard plots obtained by studying binding of (^{3}H)-anisomycin to ribosomes from yeast cells either sensitive or resistant to the antibiotic are presented in Fig. 6. It is apparent that two types of interaction occur on washed ribosomes (BARBACID and VÁZQUEZ, 1974a; JIMÉNEZ and VÁZQUEZ, 1975). The drug has a high affinity binding, (Kd = 0.9 μM; n = 0.29), that is identical for both sensitive and resistant ribosomes. In addition a low affinity binding can be detected which again is practically identical for both sensitive (Kd = 7 μM, n = 0.89) and resistant (Kd = 6 μM, n = 0.89) ribosomes. These results agree with those previously reported by JIMÉNEZ and VÁZQUEZ (1975) and clearly indicate that mutant ribosomes are altered such that the binding affinity of anisomycin for its target site (the peptidyl transferase center) has not changed, despite the fact that the antibiotic does poorly inhibit these ribosomes. As expected from these results (^{3}H)anisomycin binds with a similar affinity to 60S ribosomal subunits derived from either sensitive or resistant ribosomes.

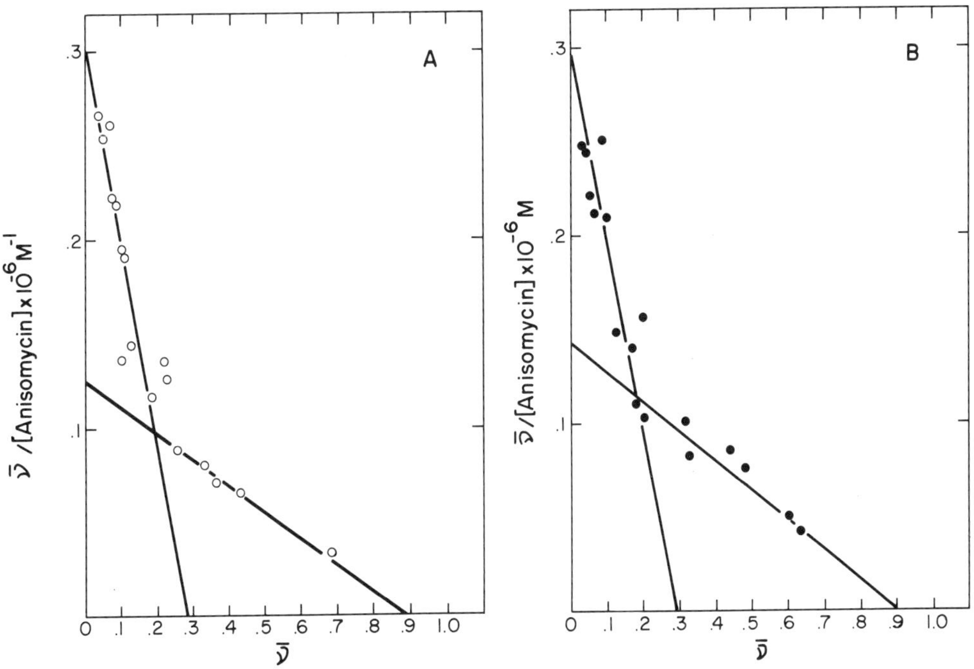

Fig. 6A and B. Scatchard plots of (^{3}H)anisomycin (251 mCi/mmol) binding to yeast ribosomes from wild-type and resistant strains. Data were obtained from binding experiments performed by sedimentation in the ultracentrifuge as previously described (JIMÉNEZ and VÁZQUEZ, 1975). **A** Wild-type ribosomes. **B** Anisomycin-resistant ribosomes. The ribosome concentration was 3 μM for (^{3}H)anisomycin concentrations ranging from 0.25 to 3 μM and 5.4 μM for a (^{3}H)anisomycin range of 3 to 30 μM

Table 4. Binding of (^{3}H)anisomycin to ribosomes. The effects of related inhibitors

Inhibitor (M conc.)		% Control binding to ribosomes from:		
		Saccharomyces cerevisiae		Human tonsils
		Wild-type	Resistant mutant	
Tenuazonic acid[a]	(10^{-4})	86	–	13
	(10^{-3})	68	–	3
Trichothecene antibiotics:				
Trichodermin[a]	(10^{-4})	22	61	4
	(10^{-3})	7	21	0
Trichodermol[a]	(10^{-4})	36	–	20
	(10^{-3})	14	–	0
Trichothecin[a]	(10^{-4})	8	54	0
	(10^{-3})	0	19	0
Fusarenon X[a]	(10^{-4})	16	36	18
	(10^{-3})	3	15	0
Verrucarin A[b]	(7×10^{-5})	26	45	–
	(7×10^{-4})	9	32	–
Cephalotaxus alkaloids:				
Harringtonine[b]	(2×10^{-4})	39	67	–
Homoharringtonine[b]	(2×10^{-4})	32	69	–
Isoharringtonine[b]	(2×10^{-4})	45	70	–
Bruceantin[b]	(10^{-4})	39	39	–
Amarillydaceae compounds:				
Narciclasine[a]	(10^{-6})	18	54	–
	(10^{-5})	11	18	–
Haemanthamine[a]	(5×10^{-5})	25	90	–
	(5×10^{-4})	9	57	–
Pretazettine[a]	(2×10^{-5})	21	82	–
	(2×10^{-4})	11	57	–
Lycorine[a]	(3.5×10^{-4})	66	43	–
	(3.5×10^{-3})	27	14	–
Pseudolycorine[a]	(5×10^{-4})	60	48	–
	(5×10^{-3})	31	20	–

[a] Binding to high-salt-washed ribosomes. [b] Binding to run-off ribosomes. Data taken from Barbacid and Vázquez, 1974a; Jiménez and Vázquez, 1975; Jiménez et al., 1975b, c; Fresno et al., 1977a; Fresno et al., 1977b; A. Jiménez and D. Vázquez, unpublished results.

The above observations are of particular interest since ribosomes resistant to anisomycin bind (^{14}C)trichodermin with an affinity at least 15 times lower than that found for sensitive ribosomes (Jiménez and Vázquez, 1975). Resistance to trichodermin can thus be explained in terms of this altered affinity, but clearly such considerations do not apply to anisomycin. Rather a conformational and/or structural change in the peptidyl transferase center of 60S ribosomal subunits may allow anisomycin to bind in low functional fashion. Anisomycin may of course bind at a site different than that of trichodermin (although both antibiotics mutually exclude each other from their ribosomal receptor sites; BARBACID and VÁZQUEZ, 1974a, c).

The binding of (^{3}H)anisomycin to sensitive and resistant ribosomes is affected differently by peptidyl transferase inhibitors that mutually exclude each other from their ribosomal receptor sites and the results of these studies are summarized in Table 4. The trichothecene antibiotics trichodermin, trichothecin, fusarenon X, and verrucarin A totally block the binding of (^{3}H)anisomycin to sensitive yeast ribosomes, whereas their effects on the binding of the radioactive antibiotic to resistant ribosomes are considerably diminished (BARBACID and VÁZQUEZ, 1974a; JIMÉNEZ and VÁZQUEZ, 1975; CANNON et al., 1976). As considered above for trichodermin, resistance to trichothecene antibiotics in anisomycin-resistant yeast strains results because these antibiotics have a low affinity for mutant ribosomes. However, verrucarin A inhibits binding of (^{3}H)anisomycin only to free ribosomes since it cannot associate with polyribosomes (CANNON et al., 1976) and a similar situation exists for the *Cephalotaxus* alkaloids harringtonine, homoharringtonine, and isoharringtonine (VÁZQUEZ et al., 1977). However, binding of (^{3}H)anisomycin is not completely blocked by these alkaloids, and their receptor site(s) may not correspond precisely with that for anisomycin. In fact the affinity of *Cephalotaxus* alkaloids for mutant ribosomes is lower than for wild-type ribosomes, and their binding site might be more related to that of trichodermin (FRESNO et al., 1977a). The Amaryllidaceae derivatives haemanthamine, narciclasine and pretazettine are potent inhibitors of (^{3}H)anisomycin binding. However, even these compounds may not associate precisely with the anisomycin binding site since once again mutant ribosomes have a reduced binding affinity for these alkaloids (JIMÉNEZ et al., 1975b; Table 4).

Bruceantin inhibits binding of (^{3}H)anisomycin to yeast run-off ribosomes and the antibiotic has no effect on the anisomycin-resistant strain either in vivo or in vitro (FRESNO et al., 1977b). The affinity of bruceantin is actually identical for both sensitive and resistant yeast ribosomes (Table 4), thus suggesting that resistance to bruceantin may be of the same type as that for anisomycin. This result implies that the binding sites for bruceantin and trichodermin might be different. However both inhibitors exclude each other competitively from their interaction with sensitive ribosomes (FRESNO et al., 1977b). In addition since bruceantin does not interact with polyribosomes, it hardly inhibits binding of either (^{3}H)anisomycin or (^{14}C)trichodermin to polyribosomes from sensitive strains.

Anisomycin Analogs: Structural Requirements for Anisomycin Action

The activities of several analogs of anisomycin (Fig. 1A) have been studied in cell-free protein-synthesizing systems from both rabbit reticulocytes and *Saccharomyces fragilis* (GROLLMAN, 1967). All the compounds tested had less than

1% of the activity of anisomycin, these results being in agreement with those obtained in intact cells (GROLLMAN, 1967). The basic pyrrolidin ring is important for the activity of the anisomycin molecule since either acetylation of the nitrogen atom, or deacetylation at the 3′ position renders the molecule inactive. Similar effects are produced by bromination of the p-methoxyphenyl moiety. The extremely low activity of these analogs may result from their low binding affinity for eukaryotic ribosomes. Deacetyl anisomycin, at high concentrations, does in fact competitively inhibit the binding of (^{3}H)anisomycin to yeast ribosomes and quantitative data of this inhibition, represented in a Klotz plot, shows that deacetyl anisomycin binds at the same ribosomal site as anisomycin but with an affinity 350 times lower (BARBACID and VÁZQUEZ, 1974a). This result agrees with the finding that deacetyl anisomycin is 300 times less active than anisomycin in inhibiting both the fragment reaction and the binding of substrates to either the donor or the acceptor sites of the peptidyl transferase center (BARBACID and VÁZQUEZ, 1974a). It is curious, however, that both deacetyl anisomycin and certain other compounds whose chemical structures are related to that of anisomycin (Fig. 1) are very active in preventing plant growth (ISHIDA et al., 1974). Nevertheless compounds of groups B and C (Fig. 1) have no activity against either poly(U)-directed polyphenylalanine synthesis or protein synthesis directed by endogenous mRNA in yeast cell-free extracts. Furthermore they do not affect binding of either (^{3}H)anisomycin or (^{14}C)trichodermin to yeast ribosomes (GONZÁLEZ, A., JIMÉNEZ, A. and VÁZQUEZ, D., unpublished results). Either there are important structural differences between the peptidyl-transferase centers of ribosomes from plants and yeast, or alternatively deacetyl anisomycin and the anisomycin analogs of ISHIDA et al. (1974) prevent plant growth by inhibiting a cell function other than protein synthesis.

References

Baez, A., Vázquez, D.: Binding of (^{3}H)narciclasine to eukaryotic ribosomes. A study on a structure-activity relationship. Biochim. Biophys. Acta *518*, 95–103 (1978)

Baez, A., Angoso, M., Alonso, G., Vázquez, D.: Labelling of narciclasine by tritium exchange. Biochimie *59*, 751–753 (1977)

Bamburg, J.R.: Chemical and biochemical studies of the trichothecene mycotoxins. In: Mycotoxins and other fungal related food products. Rodricks, J.V. (ed.), pp. 144–162. Washington D.C.: American Chemical Society 1976

Barbacid, M., Vázquez, D.: Preparation of pure (^{3}H)-anisomycin by tritium exchange labelling. Anal. Biochem. *56*, 16–25 (1973)

Barbacid, M., Vázquez, D.: (^{3}H)Anisomycin binding to eukaryotic ribosomes. J. Mol. Biol. *84*, 603–623 (1974a)

Barbacid, M., Vázquez, D.: (G-^{3}H)Gougerotin binding to ribosomes. Heterogeneity of eukaryotic ribosomes. Eur. J. Biochem. *44*, 445–453 (1974b)

Barbacid, M., Vázquez, D.: Binding of (acetyl-^{14}C)trichodermin to the peptidyl transferase centre of eukaryotic ribosomes. Eur. J. Biochem. *44*, 437–444 (1974c)

Barbacid, M., Vázquez, D.: Ribosome changes during translation. J. Mol. Biol. *93*, 449–463 (1975)

Barbacid, M., Fresno, M., Vázquez, D.: Inhibitors of polypeptide elongation on yeast polysomes. J. Antibiotics *28*, 453–462 (1975)

Battaner, E., Vázquez, D.: Inhibitors of protein synthesis by ribosomes of the 80S type. Biochim. Biophys. Acta *254*, 316–330 (1971)

Beaudet, A.L., Caskey, C.T.: Mammalian peptide chain terminations. II. Codon specificity and GTPase activity of release factor. Proc. Natl. Acad. Sci. U.S.A. *68*, 619–624 (1971)
Beereboom, J.J., Butler, K., Pennington, F., Solomons, I.: Anisomycin. I. Determination of the structure and stereochemistry of anisomycin. J. Org. Chem. *30*, 2334–2342 (1965)
Butler, K.: Anisomycin. III. Conformational studies of the pyrrolidine ring. J. Org. Chem. *33*, 2136–2141 (1968)
Cannon, M., Jiménez, A., Vázquez, D.: Competition between trichodermin and several other sesquiterpene antibiotics for binding to their receptor site(s) on eukaryotic ribosomes. Biochem. J. *160*, 137–145 (1976)
Carrasco, L., Vázquez, D.: Survey of inhibitors in different steps of protein synthesis by mammalian ribosomes. J. Antibiotics *25*, 732–737 (1972)
Carrasco, L., Vázquez, D.: Differences in eukaryotic ribosomes detected by the selective action of an antibiotic. Biochim. Biophys. Acta *319*, 209–215 (1973)
Carrasco, L., Barbacid, M., Vázquez, D.: The trichodermin group of antibiotics, inhibitors of peptide bond formation by eukaryotic ribosomes. Biochim. Biophys. Acta *312*, 368–376 (1973)
Carrasco, L., Fresno, M., Vázquez, D.: Narciclasine: an antitumour alkaloid which blocks peptide bond formation by eukaryotic ribosomes. FEBS Lett. *52*, 236–239 (1975)
Caskey, C., Beaudet, A.: Antibiotic inhibitors of peptide chain termination. In: Molecular mechanism of antibiotic action on protein biosynthesis and membranes. Muñoz, E., García-Ferrandiz, F., Vázquez, D. (eds.), pp. 326–336. Amsterdam, London, New York: Elsevier Scientific Publishing Company
Caskey, C., Beaudet, A., Scolnick, E.M., Rosman, M.: Hydrolysis of fMet-tRNA by peptidyl hydrolase. Proc. Natl. Acad. Sci. *68*, 3163–3167 (1971)
Ceriotti, G.: Narciclasine: an antimitotic substance from Narcissus bulbs. Nature (London) *213*, 595–596 (1967)
Cundliffe, E., Cannon, M., Davies, J.: Mechanism of inhibition of eukaryotic protein synthesis by trichothecene fungal toxins. Proc. Natl. Acad. Sci. *71*, 30–34 (1974)
Felner, I. von, Schenker, K.: Totalsynthese des antibioticums anisomycin. Helv. Chim. Acta *53*, 754–763 (1970)
Freeman, G.G., Morrison, R.I., Michael, S.E.: Metabolic products of Trichothecium roseum Link. Biochem. J. *45*, 191–199 (1949)
Fresno, M., Carrasco, L., Vázquez, D.: Initiation of the polypeptide chain by reticulocyte cell-free systems. Survey of different inhibitors of translation. Eur. J. Biochem. *68*, 355–364 (1976)
Fresno, M., Jiménez, A., Vázquez, D.: Inhibition of translation in eukaryotic systems by harringtonine. Eur. J. Biochem. *72*, 323–330 (1977a)
Fresno, M., González, A., Vázquez, D., Jiménez, A.: Bruceantin -a novel inhibitor of peptide bond formation. Biochim. Biophys. Acta (1977b)
Fuganti, C.: Alkaloids of the Amaryllidaceae. In: The alkaloids. Manske, R.H.F. (ed.), Vol. 15, Ch. 3, pp. 83–164. New York: Academic Press 1975
Furusawa, E., Cutting, W.: The higher plants with antiviral and anti-lethal activity on virus infections in mice. Ann. N.Y. Acad. Sci. *173*, 668–679 (1970)
Furusawa, E., Furusawa, S., Lee, J.Y.B., Patanavanich, S.: Therapeutic activity of pretazettine, a Narcissus alkaloid on rauscher leukemia: comparison with tazettine and streptonigrin. Proc. Soc. Exp. Biol. Med. *152*, 186–191 (1976)
Gardocki, J.F., Timmens, E., Wilson, L., Sodergren, J., Hettinger, B., P'an, S.: Acute and chronic toxicity of anisomycin in experimental animals. Antibiot. Chem. *9*, 490–495 (1955)
Glaz, E., Scheiber, E., Gyimesi, J., Horvath, I., Steezee, K., Szentirmai, A., Bohus, G.: A new trichothecin-like antifungal antibiotics. Nature (London) *184*, 908 (1959)
Godfredsen, W.O., Vangedal, S.: Trichodermin a new antibiotic, related to trichothecin. Proc. Chem. Soc. 188–189 (1964)
Grant, P., Schindler, D., Davies, J.: Mapping of trichodermin resistance in Saccharomyces cerevisiae: a genetic locus for a component of the 60S ribosomal subunit. Genetics *83*, 667–673 (1976)
Grollman, A.P.: Inhibitors of protein synthesis. II. Mode of action of anisomycin. J. Biol. Chem. *242*, 3226–3233 (1967)
Grollman, A.P., Huang, M.T.: Inhibitors of protein synthesis in eukaryotes: tools in cell research. Fed. Proc. *32*, 1673–1678 (1973)

Härri, E., Loefler, W., Sigg, H.P., Stähelin, H., Stoll, Ch., Tamm, Ch., Wiesinger, D.: Über die verrucarine and roridine, eine Gruppe von cytostatisch doch wirksamen Antibiotica aus *Myrothecium*-Arten. Helv. Chim. Acta *45*, 839–853 (1962)

Huang, M.T.: Harringtonine, an inhibitor of initiation of protein biosynthesis. Mol. Pharmacol. *11*, 511–519 (1976)

Ishida, S., Yamada, O., Futatsuya, F., Ito, K., Yamamoto, H., Munakata, K.: New herbicides derived from an antibiotic, anisomycin. Proc. First Int. Congress of IAMS *3*, 641 (1974)

Jiménez, A., Vázquez, D.: Quantitative binding of antibiotics to ribosomes from a yeast mutant altered on the peptidyltransferase center. Eur. J. Biochem. *54*, 483–492 (1975)

Jiménez, A., Sánchez, L., Vázquez, D.: Simultaneous ribosomal resistance to trichodermin and anisomycin in Saccharomyces cerevisiae mutants. Biochim. Biophys. Acta *383*, 427–434 (1975a)

Jiménez, A., Sánchez, L., Vázquez, D.: Location of resistance to the alkaloid narciclasine in the 60S ribosomal subunit. FEBS Lett. *55*, 53–56 (1975b)

Jiménez, A., Sánchez, L., Vázquez, D.: Yeast ribosomal sensitivity and resistance to the Amaryllidaceae alkaloids. FEBS Lett. *60*, 66–70 (1975c)

Jiménez, A., Santos, A., Alonso, G., Vázquez, D.: Inhibitors of protein synthesis in eukaryotic cells. Comparative effects of some Amaryllidaceae alkaloids. Biochim. Biophys. Acta *425*, 342–348 (1976)

Liao, L.L., Grollman, A.P., Horwitz, S.B.: Mechanism of action of the 12, 13 epoxytrichothecene, anguidine, an inhibitor of protein synthesis. Biochim. Biophys. Acta *454*, 273–284 (1976a)

Liao, L.L., Kupchan, S.M., Horwitz, S.B.: Mode of action of the antitumor compound bruceantin, an inhibitor of protein synthesis. Mol. Pharmacol. *12*, 167–176 (1976b)

Lodish, H.F., Houssman, D., Jacobsen, M.: Initiation of hemoglobin synthesis. Specific inhibition by antibiotics and bacteriophage ribonucleic acid. Biochemistry *10*, 2348–2356 (1971)

Lynch, J.E., English, A., Bauck, H., Deligianis, H.: Studies on the in vitro activity of anisomycin. Antibiot. Chemother. *4*, 844–848 (1954a)

Lynch, J.E., English, A.R., Morrison, J., Maven, I.: Protective action of anisomycin in mice infected with Trichomonas foetus. Antibiot. Chemother. *4*, 899–904 (1954b)

Menninger, J.R.: A simple assay for protein chain termination using natural peptidyl-tRNA. Biochim. Biophys. Acta *240*, 237–243 (1971)

Mizuno, S.: Mechanism of inhibition of protein synthesis initiation by diacetoxyscirpenol and fusarenon X in the reticulocyte lysate system. Biochim. Biophys. Acta *383*, 207–214 (1975)

Mondon, A., Krohn, K.: Zur Kenntnis des Narciclasine. Chem. Ber. *108*, 445–463 (1975)

Neth, R., Monro, R.E., Heller, C., Battaner, E., Vázquez, D.: Catalysis of peptidyl transfer by human ribosomes and effects of some antibiotics. FEBS Lett. *6*, 198–202 (1970)

Oida, S., Ohki, E.: Total synthesis of dl-anisomycin. Chem. Pharm. Bull. *17*, 1405–1421 (1969)

Papas, T.S., Sandhaus, L., Chirigos, M.A.: Inhibition of DNA polymerase of avian myeloblastosis virus by an alkaloid extract from Narcissus tazetta L. Biochem. Biophys. Res. Commun. *52*, 88–92 (1973)

Pestka, S., Rosenfeld, H., Harris, R., Hintikka, H.: Studies on transfer ribonucleic acid-ribosome complex. XXI. Effect of antibiotics on peptidyl-puromycin synthesis by mammalian polyribosomes. J. Biol. Chem. *247*, 6895–6900 (1972)

Powell, R.G., Weisleder, D., Smith, C.R.: Antitumor alkaloids from *Cephalotaxus harringtonia*: structure and activity. J. Pharm. Sci. *61*, 1227–1230 (1972)

Rosett, T., Sankhala, R.H., Stickngs, C.E., Taylor, M.E.U., Thomas, R.: Studies in the biochemistry of microorganisms. 103. Metabolites of Alternaria tenuis Auct: culture filtrate products. Biochem. J. *67*, 390–400 (1957)

Saito, M., Otshubo, K.: Trichothecene toxins of *Fusarium* species. In: Mycotoxins. Purchase, I.F.H. (ed.), pp. 263–281. Amsterdam, Oxford, New York: Elsevier Scientific Publishing Company 1974

Schindler, D.: Two classes of inhibitors of peptidyl transferase activity in eukaryotes. Nature (London) *249*, 38–41 (1974)

Schindler, D., Grant, P., Davies, J.: Trichodermin resistance-mutation affecting eukaryotic ribosomes. Nature (London) *248*, 535–536 (1974)

Shigeura, H.T., Gordon, C.N.: The biological activity of tenuazonic acid. Biochemistry *2*, 1132–1137 (1963)

Smith, K.E., Cannon, M., Cundliffe, E.: Inhibition at the initiation level of eukaryotic protein synthesis by T-2 toxin. FEBS Lett. *50*, 8–12 (1975)

Sobin, B.A., Tanner, F.W., Jr.: Anisomycin, a new antiprotozoan antibiotic. J. Am. Chem. Soc. *76*, 4053 (1954)

Stafford, M.E., McLaughlin, C.S.: Trichodermin, a possible inhibitor of the termination process of protein synthesis. J. Cell. Physiol. *82*, 121–128 (1973)

Tanner, F.W., Jr., Sobin, B.A., Gardocki, J.F.: Some chemical and biological properties of anisomycin. Antibiot. Ann. 809 (1954–55)

Tate, W.P., Caskey, C.T.: Peptidyl transferase inhibition by trichodermin. J. Biol. Chem. *248*, 7970–7972 (1973)

Tscherne, J.S., Pestka, S.: Inhibition of protein synthesis in intact HeLa cells. Antimicrob. Agents Chemother. *8*, 479–487 (1975)

Ueno, Y., Hosoya, M., Morita, Y., Ueno, I., Tatsuno, T.: Inhibition of the protein synthesis in rabbit reticulocyte by nivalenol a toxic principle isolated from Fusarium nivale growing rice. J. Biochem. *64*, 479–485 (1968)

Ueno, Y., Ueno, I., Tatsuno, T., Ohokubo, K., Tsunoda, H.: Fusarenon-X, a toxic principle of Fusarium nivale-culture filtrate. Experientia *25*, 1062 (1969)

Vázquez, D.: Inhibitors of protein synthesis. FEBS Lett. Suppl. *40*, S63–S84 (1974)

Vázquez, D., Battaner, E., Neth, R., Heller, G., Monro, R.E.: The function of 80S ribosomal subunits and effect of some inhibitors. Cold Spring Harbor Symp. Quant. Biol. *34*, 369–375 (1969)

Vázquez, D., Contreras, A., Fresno, M., Jiménez, A.: Interaction of translation inhibitors with ribosomes and polysomes. In: Proceedings of Symposium on Translation of Synthetic and Natural Polynucleotides. Legocki, A.B. (ed.), pp. 380–385. Poznan (Poland) (1977)

Vogel, Z., Zamir, A., Elson, D.: The possible involvement of peptidyl transferase in the termination step of protein biosynthesis. Biochemistry *8*, 5161–5168 (1969)

Wei, C.M., Campbell, I.M., McLaughlin, C.S., Vaughan, M.H.: Binding of trichodermin to mammalian ribosomes and its inhibition by other 12,13-epoxytrichothecenes. Mol. Gen. Biochem. *3*, 215–219 (1974)

Wildman, W.C.: Alkaloids of the Amaryllidaceae. In: The Alkaloids. Manske, R.H.F. (ed.), Vol. 11, Chap. 10, pp. 307–405. New York: Academic Press 1968

Antitumor Platinum Compounds

J.J. ROBERTS

I. Introduction

As a consequence of a classic case of serendipity in science a range of platinum coordination complexes were demonstrated to have potent antitumor action against Sarcoma 180 and Leukemia L1210 (ROSENBERG et al., 1969; ROSENBERG and VAN CAMP, 1970), a viral-induced reticulum cell sarcoma in mice (TALLEY, 1970), the Dunning ascitic leukemia, Walker 256 carcinosarcoma (KOCIBA et al., 1970), and a DMBA-induced mammary carcinoma (WELSH, 1971) in rats.

While this review will be concerned with the antitumor properties of these agents it should be noted that they have been shown to possess a broad range of biological activities including bacteriocidal, viricidal, immunosuppressive and anti-arthritic activities. The structures of some of the original square planar platinum compounds synthesized and investigated by ROSENBERG and his colleagues (1969) are shown in Fig. 1.

These compounds represented an entirely new class of antitumor compound, and since 1970 numerous laboratories have undertaken extensive programs to

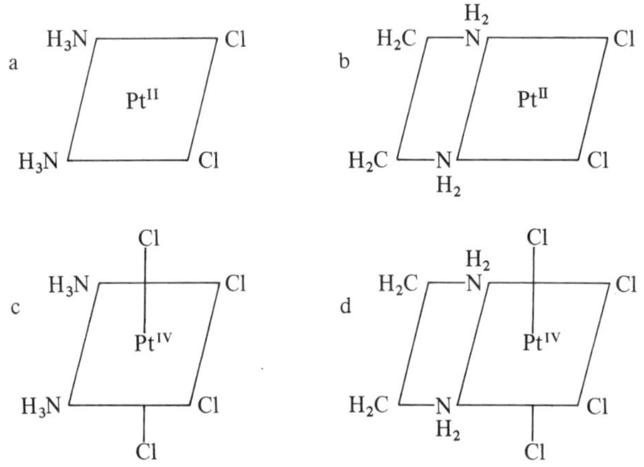

Fig. 1a–d. Structures of the original platinum complexes described by ROSENBERG et al. (1969). **a** cis Pt(II) diammine dichloride, cis Pt(II) $(NH_3)_2Cl_2$. **b** cis Pt(II) ethylenediamine dichloride, cis Pt(II) (en) Cl_2. **c** cis-platinum(IV)diammine tetrachloride, cis Pt(IV) $(NH_3)_2Cl_4$. **d** cis Pt(IV) ethylenediamine tetrachloride, cis Pt(IV) (en)Cl_4

synthesize a variety of metal transition complexes. Systematic replacement of the ligands has been carried out and this has led to some clear indications of structure-activity relationships. Parallel clinical studies with the platinum complexes, and cis dichlorodiammine platinum II [cis Pt(II)] in particular, has established that they are drugs with a permanent place in the armamentarium of clinical oncologists both in their own right and as drugs to be used effectively in combination with others. The initial problems of renal toxicity have largely been overcome and cis Pt(II) has been shown to have a broad spectrum of activity against human cancer.

The site of the primary lesion in cells which results in toxicity and hence tumor destruction is now generally agreed to be DNA in preference to other macromolecules such as RNA or protein. Modification of the DNA template results in the selective inhibition of DNA synthesis and, hence, unbalanced growth. The primary biochemical effect in treated cells thus resembles that induced by a number of other cytotoxic antitumor agents. The extent, therefore, to which such drugs elicit selective effects on cells may be a reflection of differences in their ability to handle damage to the DNA template. Much effort has therefore been applied to elucidating the nature of the chemical interaction of platinum compounds with DNA, mechanisms for circumventing such damage during DNA replication and mechanisms for eliminating the damage by specific DNA excision repair processes. Variations in the levels of such repair processes among cell populations could therefore provide a partial explanation for the evolution of drug-resistant cells during the chemotherapeutic treatment of tumors.

II. Antitumor Effects of Platinum Compounds

A. Animal Tumor Studies

1. General Features of Platinum Chemistry

In order to understand better some of the structural requirements for activity in a series of platinum complexes, it is worthwhile to consider some of the special features of the chemistry of these particular compounds. For a fuller discussion of this topic the reader is referred to reviews by Thomson et al. (1972), Thomson (1974) and Cleare (1977). Some of the key conclusions are summarized below.

Aqueous platinum centers involve two oxidation states namely 2+ and 4+ which exist with four or six nucleophilic groups (ligands) respectively, exhibiting square planar and octohedral geometry (Fig. 1). Interconversion between the two states is readily achieved but the commonest oxidation state is +2+. The nature of the ligands attached to platinum influences both the stability and the reactivity of the complexes. Stability is a thermodynamic property of the ground state and reactivity is a kinetic property involving transition states in a reaction path. In general, both oxidation states for platinum form their most stable complexes with the larger more polarisable donor atoms. The following order of stability usually holds.

$$S \sim C > I > Br > Cl > N > O > F.$$

Stability is also greatly enhanced if a ligand can bind to the metal in more than one site. This is called a multi-dentate ligand and this is referred to as the chelate effect.

The aqueous chemistry of Pt(II) is dominated by the effect of a ligand on the rate of substitution of the ligand opposite it in the coordination sphere i.e., the trans effect. Generally, strongly bound ligands have a strong trans influence and kinetically this effect can be very large with a factor of 10^6 or more between complexes containing a ligand high and low in the trans effect series. The affinities of various ligands for Pt(II) generally follow the trans effect with the exceptions of NH_3 and OH^-. The strong affinity of NH_3 and organic amines for Pt(II) dominates the chemistry of the Pt(II)A_2Cl_2 (A= amine) complexes overriding the trans effect, and results in such compounds containing two A groups which are difficult to replace and two relatively labile chloride groups.

2. Structure-Activity Relationships

a) Role of Configuration. Excellent reviews by CLEARE and HOESCHELE (1973a, b) and CLEARE (1977) have already appeared on this topic. An important point is that all substitution reactions proceed with complete retention of configuration: isomerisations are very rare and if present occur very slowly via a two step process. Trans compounds are more reactive than cis compounds the trans $Pt(NH_3)_2Cl_2$ aquating four times faster and ammonating some thirty times faster than the cis isomer. This means that trans compounds are likely to react faster and with a wider variety of body constituents than the cis isomers. Hence the unique activity of the cis isomers (Table 1) must reside in the particular reactions with target molecules which their configuration dictates. The results summarised in Table 1 clearly indicate that activity is confined to neutral complexes with cis leaving ligands (CONNORS et al., 1972; CLEARE and HOESCHELE, 1973a, b). A comparison of cis and trans compounds of the type (PtA_2X_2) show activity either (1) only for cis and not trans or (2) not in either cis or trans compounds. No example of activity in the trans but not in cis isomer has been found.

In general charged complexes show no activity even when they have cis leaving groups (particularly chlorides).

b) Role of Leaving Group (X in PtA_2X_2). Two main classes have been found to give active compounds, either (1) monodentate anionic ligands of intermediate leaving ability – mainly Cl^- but also Br^- (Table 2), and (2) bidentate ligands such as oxalate, malonate and sulfate (Table 3; Fig. 2). Various model studies have been carried out which indicate the leaving ability of certain monodentate ligands in particular structures (for discussion see CLEARE, 1977). The screening of analogues of cis Pt(II) and ethylenediamine complexes (Table 2) reflected this same general leaving order and showed that the optimum monodentate leaving groups were chloride and bromide (CONNORS et al., 1972). Less labile groups were inactive and relatively nontoxic, while labile groups gave extremely toxic compounds. Chloride has the further advantage of being compatible with the body fluid system. Variations in the leaving group can sometimes confer considerable increases in aqueous solubility. (N.B. the insolubility of many of these complexes has often limited their application in chemotherapeutic

Table 1. Comparison of activities of cis and trans isomers against Sarcoma 180 and ADJ/PC6 plasma cell tumor. For solid tumors the amount of inhibition is measured by a comparison of the weight of treated and untreated (control) tumors. This is expressed as a percentage and termed T/C. Values less than 50 are generally considered significant. Toxic level is the highest dose at which survivors are ≧83%. Dose in final column is that at which the T/C was obtained. Several dose levels of the drugs were given at 5-fold spacings and ranged from lethal to nontumor inhibitory allowing the calculation of LD_{50} (minimum dose required to kill 50% of the animals) and ID_{90} (minimum dose to cause 90% tumor regression) in the one experiment. The ratio of LD_{50}/ID_{90} is a therapeutic index and is a measure of the selectivity of a compound as an antitumor compound (CONNORS et al., 1972)

Sarcoma 180

Complex		Solvent	Dose range mg/kg	Dose response	Toxic level mg/kg	T/C	Dose mg/kg
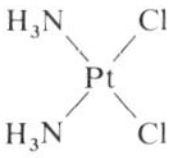	cis	S	0.5–20	+	9	1	8
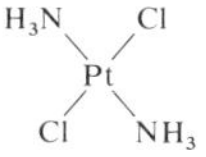	trans	S	2.5–40[b]	–	>40	85	2.5–40
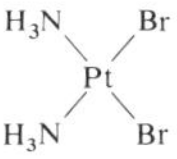	cis	B	5–20	+	15	30	14
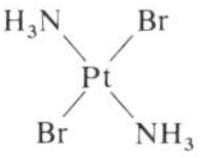	trans	B	10–40	–	>40	110	10–40
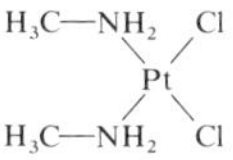	cis	S	10–30	+	12–20[c]	25	15[a]
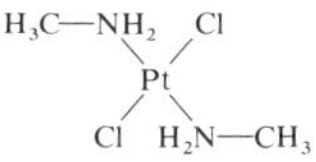	trans	S	5–100	–	25	100	5–20
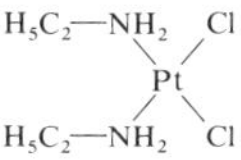	cis	S	5–50[b]	+	45	14	40
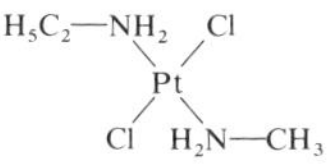	trans	SS	5–20	–	>20	105	5–20

Table 1 (continued)

ADJ/PC6 plasma cell tumour

Complex		Solvent	Dose range mg/kg	Dose response	LD_{50}	ID_{90}	TI
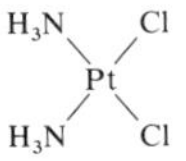	cis	A	0.1–40	+	13.0	1.6	8.1
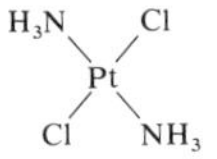	trans	A		–	27.0	>27.0	<1.0
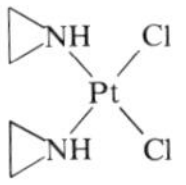	cis	A	2.5–160	+	56.5	2.6	21.7
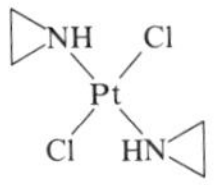	trans	A		–	18.0	>18.0	<1.0
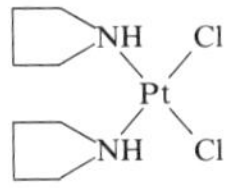	cis	A	6–800	+	240	17.5	13.7
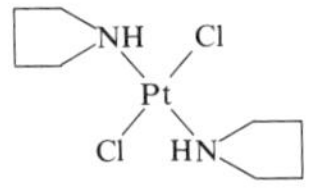	trans	A		–	72	>72	<1.0

[a] Only 66 per cent survivors. [b] Slurry at higher concentrations. [c] Sporadic toxicity over this range.

Abbreviations for Tables 1–3: The solvent is indicated by A = arachis oil; S = saline (0.15 M NaCl); SS = saline slurry; B = sodium bromide (0.04 M); BS = sodium bromide slurry; W = water.

studies). Of the bidentate structures the oxalate and malonate are not expected to be good leaving groups so some active mechanism of removal may be operating. On the other hand, the four-membered ring chelates, such as sulfates (Fig. 2) are likely to be less stable.

c) Role of the Nonlabile Ligand (A in PtA_2Cl_2*).* The nature of group A has a primary influence on the antitumor activity or more specifically the selectivity, by varying the toxicity (LD_{90}) of compounds. The activities of many such compounds against the Sarcoma 180 and ADJ/PC6 plasma cell tumor in mice have been reported by CONNORS et al. (1972), BRADDOCK et al. (1975) and TOBE and KOKHAR (1977). For the straight chain amines (Table 4), it is to be noted that potency increases to a maximum with the butylamine derivative, $n\text{-}C_4H_9NH_2$, while toxicity decreases markedly. Primary amines with an alicyclic substituent (Table 5) yielded two compounds, the cyclopentylamine and cyclohexylamine complexes with very high therapeutic indexes against the ADJ/PC 6 tumor. The cyclohexylamine complex was, however, inactive against all other

Table 2. Variation of X in cis Pt(II) $(NH_3)_2$ X_2 and activity against Sarcoma 180 (Cleare and Hoeschele, 1973)

X	Solvent	Dose range mg/kg	Dose response	Toxic level mg/kg	T.C.	Dose mg/kg
NO_3^-	W	6–12	–	7 [c]	54	6
NO_3^-	S	2.5–12	+	11	8	10
H_2O [d]	W	2–20	–	5 [c]	–	–
Cl^-	S	0.5–20	+	9	1	8
Br^-	B	5–20	+	15	30	14
Br^-	S	2–6 [b]	+	5–6 [b]	13	5
I^-	WS	10–25	–	>25	110	10–25
SCN^-	S	5–100 [a]	–	~50	70	20–35
NO_2^-	SS	5–100	–	>100	99	5–100

[a] Slurry at higher concentrations. [b] Daily injections for 9 days. [c] Highly toxic–convulsions. [d] Cationic complex ion (2+).

Abbreviations see Table 1.

tumors and the cyclopentylamine, while active against the Walker tumor and the L1210 leukemia, was found to be too insoluble for intravenous administration and therefore not particularly suitable for clinical use. Marked variation within a series of cyclic secondary amines was noted with the three-membered ring (aziridine) complex being the most active. Unfortunately again, the compound was inactive against other animal tumors. Considerable variation in activity also exists within the branched chain series (Table 6) of primary amines. The isopropylamine complex, in addition to being active against the PC 6 tumor, also had marked activity against the Walker tumor and L1210 leukemia and is likely to be one of the "second generation" clinically useful compounds. The introduction of a second branched chain however seems to remove the antitumor activity completely. Aromatic heterocyclic and alicyclic amine complexes have shown little or no activity at the levels at which they have been tested. Again the insertion of a small substituent like a methyl group into the cyclohexylamine ring can greatly modify both the toxic and tumor-inhibitory activity (Table 7). The same substituents inserted into the o-phenylene diamine moiety however can have quite opposite effects. The o-phenylene diamine ligand, it should be noted, is the only example of an aromatic amine that forms antitumor platinum complexes. The pyridine complex shows some activity against the Ehrlich ascites carcinoma (Gale et al., 1971). This compound possessed actions similar to the wholly inorganic parent compound, cis Pt(II) but was somewhat less potent. However the compound could be labeled with tritium which permitted a study of its absorption, binding, distribution, and excretion. By similar labeling studies it could be shown that the methylamine congener, cis dichlorobis (methylamine) platinum (II), while also lacking the potency of the parent compound, interacts with cells and molecules in a fashion similar to that of either the pyridine analogue or cis Pt(II) itself (Gale et al., 1973).

Of the bidentate amines the ethylene diamine showed a good response (Rosenberg et al., 1969) but the introduction of substituents again loses activity.

Table 3. Activity of various platinum amine complexes containing oxalate and malonate ligands against sarcoma 180 (Cleare and Hoeschele, 1973)

Sarcoma 180						
Complex	Solvent	Dose range mg/kg	Dose response	Toxic level mg/kg	T/C	Dose mg/kg
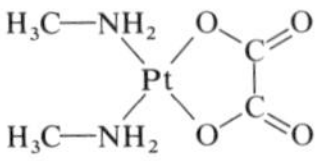 oxalatobis(methylamine) platinum(II)	W	5–80	+	20–30[b]	21	30
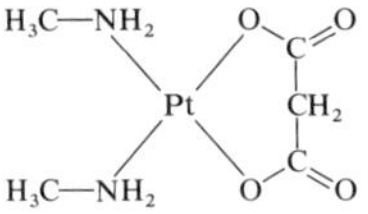 malonatobis(methylamine) platinum(II)	W	80–180	+	180	20	120–180
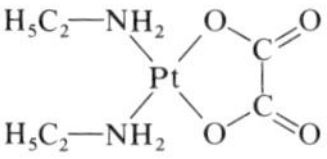 oxalatobis(ethylamine) platinum(II)	W	10–80	±	20–40	21	10
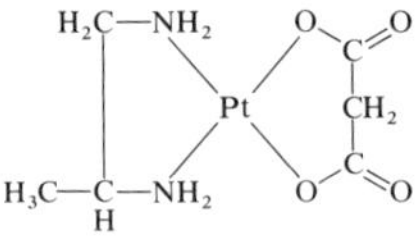 malonato-1,2-propylene-diamineplatinum(II)	W	45–90	+	65	9	60
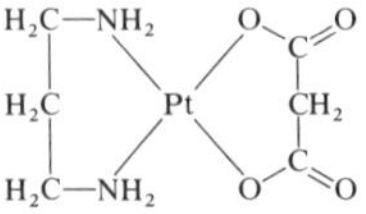 malonato-1,3-propylene-diamineplatinum(II)	W	20–80	+	90	28	60–80
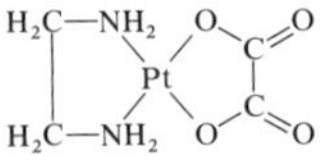 oxalatoethylenediamine-platinum(II)	W	0.25–16	–	3[a]	75	0.25–2
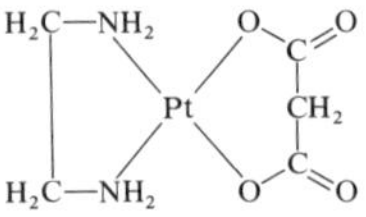 malonatoethylenediamine-platinum(II)	W	5–80	+	45–60	18	40

Table 3 (continued)

Sarcoma 180						
Complex	Solvent	Dose range mg/kg	Dose response	Toxic level mg/kg	T/C	Dose mg/kg
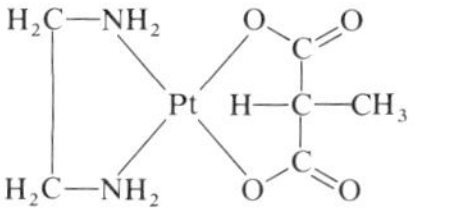 methylmalonatoethylene-diamineplatinum(II)	W	30–90	+	>90	4	90
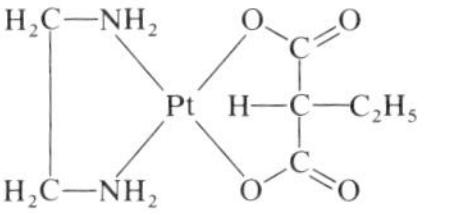 ethylmalonatoethylene-diamineplatinum(II)	WS	40–120	±	>120	51	90–120

[a] Highly toxic – convulsions. [b] Only 50 per cent survivors.

Abbreviations see Table 1.

Another bidentate organoplatinum congener of cis Pt(II), dichloro(1,2-diamino-cyclohexane)platinum (II) was highly effective against the L1210 leukemia in mice (GALE et al., 1974). Combination of the 1,2-diaminocyclohexane with the bidentate sulfato ligand (Fig. 2) has resulted in a most potent compound against murine L1210 leukemia (GALE et al., 1977; SPEER et al., 1977) and Shay tumor in rats, the Gardner lymphoma OG in mice (SPEER et al., 1977), and one which is currently being applied in the clinic as discussed later.

Dinitrato (1,2-diaminocyclohexane) platinum (II) is a non-cell cycle-dependent congener, active against murine myeloma and apparently requiring active transport (OGAWA, 1976).

The reasons for these major variations in biological activity with minor modifications to the amine structure are by no means obvious. Attempts have been made, without success, to explain them in terms of the kinetic, steric or solubility properties of the various platinum complexes (TOBE and KOKHAR, 1977). It does not seem as though kinetic effects alone can explain these differences and hydrogen bonding interactions between the amine ligands and biological macromolecules could play a role in stabilizing the receptor-drug complex. In an attempt to explain variations in activity on the basis of solubility, TOBE and KHOKHAR (1977) measured the solubility of various complexes in water and a lipid solvent. At one time it appeared as though there might be a relationship between the chloroform-water distribution coefficient and the effectiveness of the complexes toward the plasma cell tumor, with an optimum distribution coefficient of 1. The solubilities and distribution coefficients of the cis $[Pt(am)_2Cl_2]$ complexes however varied as dramatically with minor changes

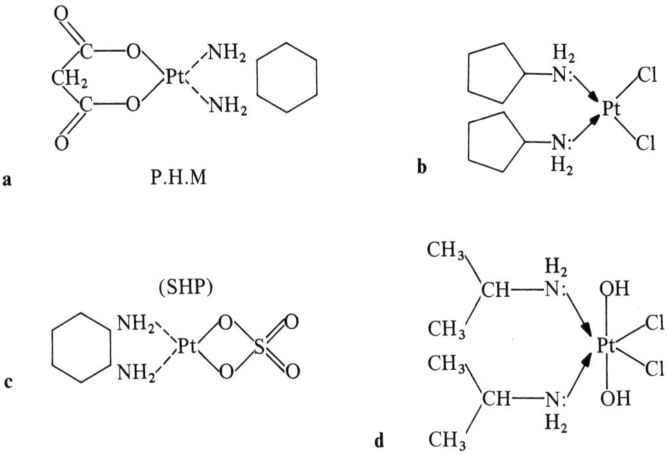

Fig. 2a–d. Structures of newer platinum complexes shown to have activity against experimental or human tumors. **a** Malonato 1,2-diaminocyclohexane platinum (II) (PHM). **b** Sulphato 1,2-diaminocyclohexane platinum (II) (SHP). **c** cis-dichloro bis (cyclopentylamine) platinum (II) (PAD). **d** cis-dichloro-bis (isopropylamine) trans dihydroxy platinum(IV) (CHIP)

Table 4. The effect of variations in the length of alkyl chain in di-n-alkylamine Pt(II)Cl_2 compounds against ADJ/PC6 plasmacytoma in mice

am	LD_{50}/mg kg^{-1}	ID_{90}/mg kg^{-1}	TI
NH_3	13.0	1.6	8.1
CH_3NH_2	18.5	12	—
n-$C_2H_5NH_2$	26.5	12	2.2
n-$C_3H_7NH_2$	26.5	12	2.2
n-$C_4H_9NH_2$	110	10	11
n-$C_5H_{11}NH_2$	92	37	2.5
n-$C_6H_{13}NH_2$	1000	1500	—
n-$C_7H_{15}NH_2$	900	900	—
n-$C_8H_{17}NH_2$	200	200	—

in the amine substituents as did the toxicities and the potencies; but the variation was not always in parallel. Clearly the solubilities of the complexes is only a partial explanation for their activities.

Of all the amines synthesized and tested by Tobe and Connors and their co-workers it appears that only the isopropylamine derivative stands out as being more effective than the original ammonia complex prepared by Rosenberg and his colleagues. Unlike so many of the other complexes, it proved to be effective against all three animal tumors investigated, the Walker tumor, the PC6 plasma cell tumor and the L1210 leukemia. No complexes in which the A ligands are non-N-donors have shown activity although relatively only few others have been tested. Alternative donor ligands could be oxygen or strongly labilizing neutral groups such as S-and P-.

Table 5. Antitumor activity against the ADJ/PC6 mouse plasmacytoma and aqueous and lipid solubility of cis $Pt(am)_2Cl_2$) where am is a primary amine with an alicyclic substituent (BRADDOCK et al., 1975)

	LD_{50} mg/kg	ID_{90} mg/kg	TI	Aqueous solubility		Distribution coefficient $CHCl_3/H_2O$
				μg/ml	mM	
NH_3	13.0[a]	1.6[a]	8.1[a]	2650	8.9	<0.008
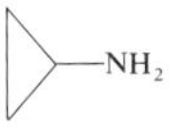	57[a]	2.3[a]	25[a]	610	1.6	<0.007
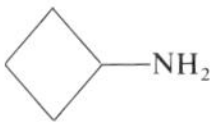	90[a]	2.9[a]	31[a]	87	0.21	0.05
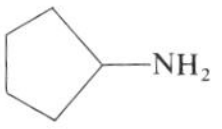	480	2.4	200	5.6	0.013	0.86
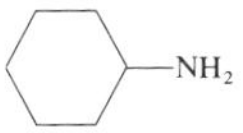	>3200[a]	12[a]	>267[a]	1.9	0.0040	4.3
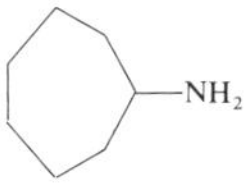	1000	7.7	130	0.71	0.0014	8.2
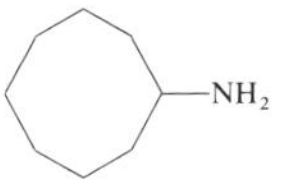	660	230	2.9	0.29	0.00056	16.7

[a] From CONNORS et al., 1972.

The fact that in these various studies toxicity could be shown to be unrelated to antitumor action leaves one optimistic that new agents may be found which are nontoxic but still possess antitumor activity.

d) Modifications Designed to Improve Water Solubility. Recent developments have involved attempts to produce complexes of increased solubility by means of either mixed amine complexes of the type cis-$[Pt(NH_3)ACl_2]$ or Pt(IV) complexes of the type cis $[Pt(A)_2Cl_4]$ or cis-trans-$[Pt(A_2)(OH)_2Cl_2]$ (TOBE and KHOKHAR, 1977). It was hoped that the lattice energy would be reduced by these modifications. While again no clear pattern emerged which related structure to solubility the compound cis-trans-$[Pt(NH_3)_2(OH)_2Cl_2]$ proved to be only one tenth as toxic as cis-$[Pt(NH_3)_2Cl_2]$ and with a higher therapeutic index. Other promising structures are likely to be the isopropylamine and cyclopentylamine congeners containing the trans hydroxy groups. Since it is believed that the Pt(IV) complexes are reduced to Pt(II) complexes in vivo by the loss of two axial ligands then the dihydroxy species is in effect a novel variant in the method of administering the corresponding Pt(II) complex.

e) Platinum Blues. The diaquo species of cis dichlorodiammine platinum (II) reacts with substituted pyrimidines to form very soluble deep-blue complexes (DAVIDSON et al. 1975; THOMPSON et al., 1977). The structures of the complexes are uncertain. Many of the complexes were found to show activity against

Table 6. The effect of branched chain substituents and the distance of the branch or ring from the–NH_2 group on the toxicity, antitumor activity (ADJ/PC6 plasmacytoma) and aqueous solubility of complexes of the type, cis ($Pt(am)_2Cl_2$) (Braddock et al., 1975)

	LD_{50} mg/kg	ID_{90} mg/kg	TI	Aqueous solubility	
				µg/ml	mM
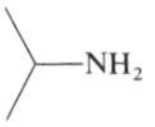	33.5	0.9	37	84	0.22
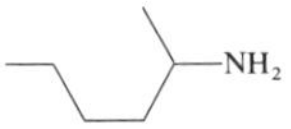	730	27.5	26.5	0.41	0.00087
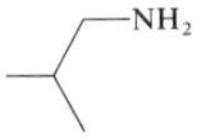	83	6.2	13.4	50	0.12
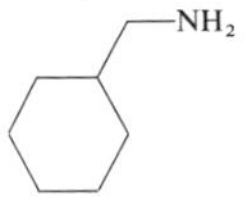	89	34	2.6	0.27	0.00056
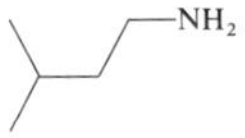	1150	5.8	198	0.56	0.0012
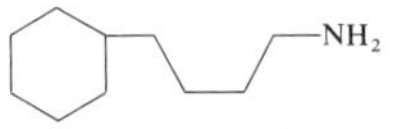	132	132	–	0.07	0.00012

Sarcoma 180 tumor in Swiss mice superior to that shown by cis Pt(II), as well as activity against the Rauscher leukemia, Ehrlich ascites and ADJ/PC6A tumor (Davidson et al., 1975). The uncertainty of some of these structures and irreproducibility of some of the biological activities, and hence their unknown mechanism of action, has limited progress in this initially promising area.

3. Combinations of Platinum Complexes with Other Drugs

An enhanced therapeutic effect of cis Pt(II) against early and advanced L1210 has been obtained when cis Pt(II) is used in combination with either cyclophosphamide (Walker and Gale, 1973; Woodman et al., 1973) or 1,2-bis(3,5-dioxopiperazine-1-yl)propane (ICRF 159); Woodman et al., 1973). Combinations of cis Pt(II) with many other antileukemic drugs showed some increase in life span in mice treated with early leukemia L1210 (Woodman et al., 1973). Similar promising results were obtained when cis Pt(II) was used in combination with other drugs against a variety of murine tumors (Page et al., 1977). Cis Pt(II) in combination with cyclophosphamide produced synergistic tumor cell kill in the BALBc mouse bearing a reticulum cell sarcoma (Fig. 3). The reticulum cell sarcoma used in this study has been called a Hodgkins type lesion (Stansly and Soule, 1962) because of the mixed pattern of normal and abnormal reticulum cells and the occasional Reed-Sternberg-like cell seen in histological sections. When combined with methotrexate, cis Pt(II) was greater

Table 7. The effect of ring substituents on the toxicity and antitumor activity of complexes of the cis ($Pt(LL)Cl_2$) or cis ($Pt(L)_2Cl_2$) against ADJ/PC6 mouse plasmacytoma (BRADDOCK et al., 1975)

L (or LL)	LD_{50} mg/kg	ID_{90} mg/kg	TI
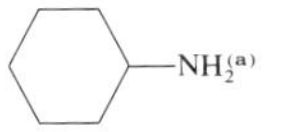	> 3200	12	> 267
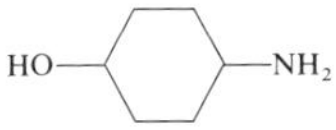	23	< 10	> 2.3
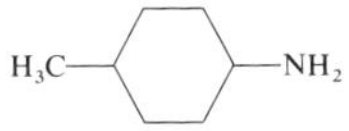	990	1180	–
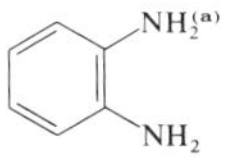	48	2.4	20
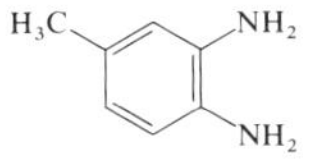	22.5	3.7	6.1
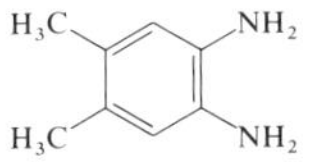	283	2.5	113
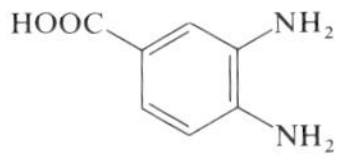	180	> 90	< 2

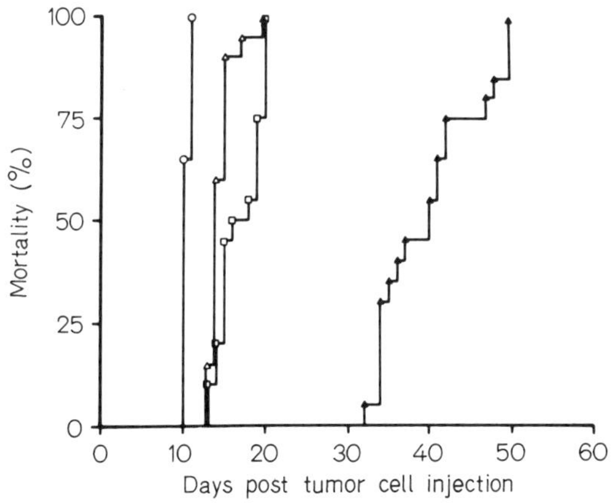

Fig. 3. Effect of cis Pt(II) and cyclophosphamide alone or in combination against reticulum cell sarcoma in BALBc mice tumored with 3×10^6 RCS cells (PAGE et al., 1977). ○—○ Control, △—△ cis diamminedichloroplatinum (II), 8 mg/kg, T 1, 8, 15, 22, □—□ cyclophosphamide, 50 mg/kg, T 1, 8, 15, 22, ▲—▲ Pt.-cyclophosphamide in combination

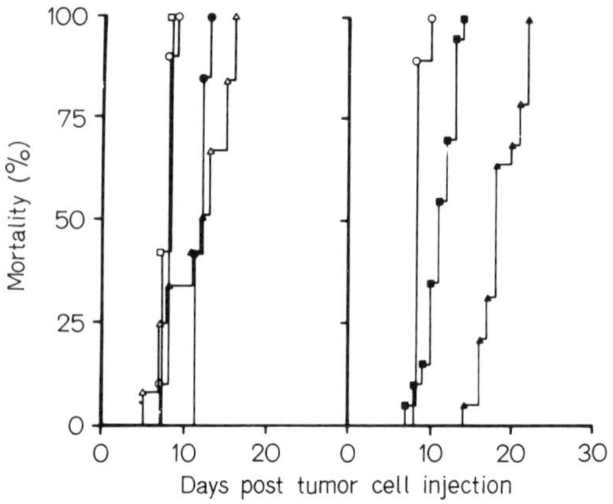

Fig. 4. Effect of cis Pt(II), cyclophosphamide and methotrexate alone or in combination against L1210 leukemia in DBA mice, tumored with 3×10^6 L-1210 leukemia cells. cis Pt(II) was more effective in combination with methotrexate than in combination with cyclophosphamide (PAGE et al., 1977). ○—○ Control, △—△ cis diamminedichloroplatinum (II), 8 mg/kg, days 1, 8, 15, 22, □—□ cyclophosphamide, 50 mg/kg, days 1, 8, 15, 22, ●—● methotrexate, 0.25 mg/kg, b.i.d. × 5, ■—■ combination of cis Pt. and cyclophosphamide, ▲—▲ combination of cis Pt. and methotrexate

than additive against the L1210 leukemia in DBA mice (Fig. 4) and combined with adriamycin it was additive against S180 sarcoma (Fig. 5).

4. Combinations of Platinum Complexes with Radiation: Radiation Sensitization

The discovery by RICHMOND and POWERS (1976) that cis Pt(II) could act as a radiation sensitizer in the *B. megaterium* bacterial spore, preferentially but not exclusively, in the absence of oxygen, and presumably by the sequestration of the hydrated electron which would prevent its reaction with a hydroxy radical, prompted studies on the effects of combined radiation and platinum treatment on mammalian tumor systems. Cis Pt(II) in combination with local X-irradiation was used against a transplantable mouse mammary adenocarcinoma (with a significant hypoxic fraction) and a well-vascularized rat brain tumor implanted intracerebrally (DOUPLE et al., 1977). Little evidence was obtained for cis Pt(II)-induced radiation sensitization of the mammary carcinoma possibly because the tumor contained only a small proportion of hypoxic cells. (Some equivocal evidence suggesting an effect of cis Pt(II) on the host's immune response was obtained from this study). In contrast to the lack of effect in the mammary tumor system a most pronounced synergistic effect of combined cis Pt(II) and radiation treatment was observed in the rat brain tumor system (Fig. 6). This is a somewhat surprising result in view of the reported low levels of cis Pt(II) in rat brain and the low hypoxic fraction in the well-vascularized brain tumor. DOUPLE et al. (1977) suggest, as alternative explanations for the observed synergism, that either radiation modifies the permeability of the so-

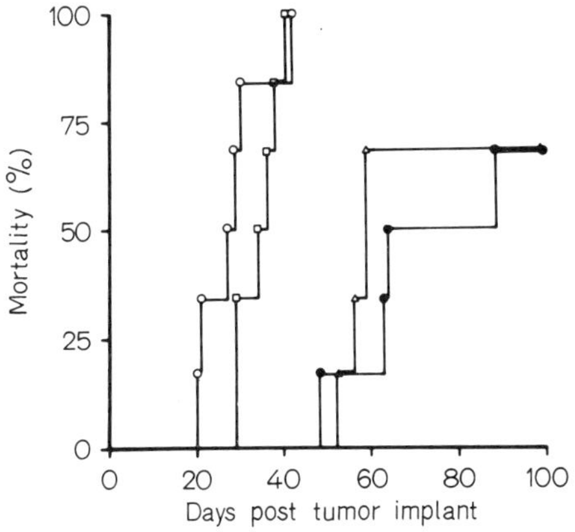

Fig. 5. Effect of cis Pt(II) and adriamycin alone or in combination against Sarcoma S-180 in BALBc mice tumored with Sarcoma S-180 (PAGE et al., 1977). ○——○ Control, △——△ cis diamminedichloroplatinum (II), 8 mg/kg, days 1, 8, 15, 22, □——□ adriamycin, 5 mg/kg, days 1, 15, ●——● combination of cis Pt. and adriamycin

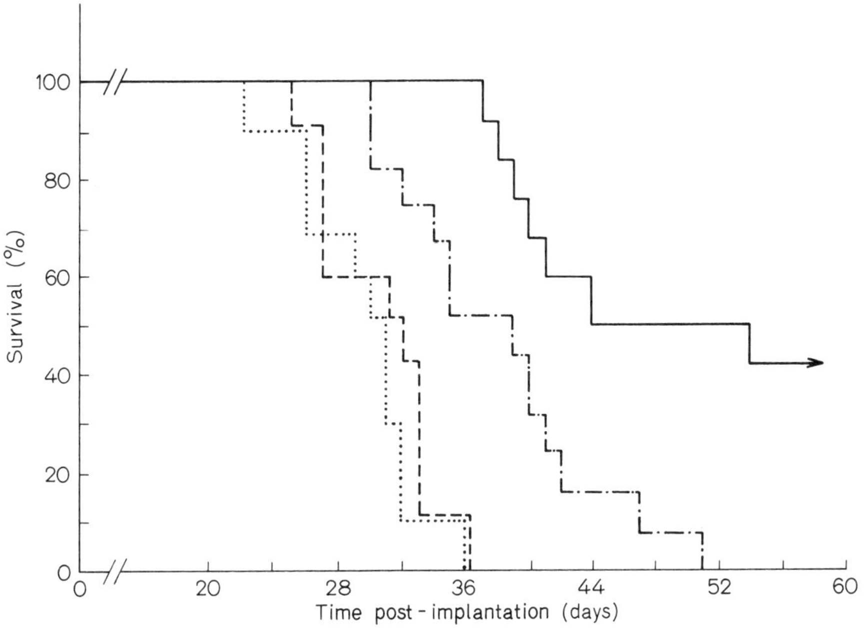

Fig. 6. Survival of rats containing intra cerebral brain tumours, either untreated (*dotted line*), treated with cis Pt(II) 4 mg/kg (*dashed line*), X-ray 1508 rad (*dashed-dotted line*) or cis Pt(II) followed by X-rays 24 h later (*solid line*) (DOUPLE et al., 1977)

called blood-brain barrier, or cis Pt(II) interferes with the processes which repair radiation damage.

It seems unlikely that the dose- and cell-cycle-dependent enhancement of the effects of radiation on Chinese hamster ovary cells in culture by either cis-dichlorobis (cyclopentylamine) platinum II (SZUMIEL and NIAS, 1976a) or the more soluble congener cis-dichlorobis(isopropylamine) trans dihydroxyplatinum (IV) (NIAS and SZUMIEL, 1977) is similarly due to the platinum drugs acting as radiation sensitizers.

Some antagonistic effects of cis Pt(II) on radiation damage had previously been reported. ZAK and DROBNIK (1971) found that cis Pt(II) administered prior to potentially lethal whole body irradiation could prolong survival, possibly by decreasing the proportion of cells in the bone marrow which would be in their most sensitive phase to irradiation. Administration of cis Pt(II) 24 h after irradiation on the other hand impaired survival.

B. Human Tumor Studies of Platinum Complexes

1. Clinical Studies with cis Platinum (II) Diammine Dichloride [cis Pt(II)]

Following the clear demonstration of activity against a broad spectrum of animal tumors, clinical trials were initiated on cis Pt(II) in many centers. A review of the clinical status of cis Pt(II) in cancer chemotherapy (GOTTLIEB and DREWINKO, 1975) of some early phase 1 clinical trials, generally on extremely advanced disease, indicated promising anticancer activity. The tumors most sensitive to cis Pt(II) were testicular carcinoma (WALLACE and HIGBY et al., 1974), head and neck cancer (KRAKOFF and LIPPMAN, 1974), squamous cell carcinoma, malignant lymphoma and endometrial carcinoma (HILL et al., 1974, 1975) and ovarian adenocarcinoma (WILTSHAW and CARR, 1974).

These early reports however stressed the limitations imposed by the severe toxicity to the kidney and bone marrow. Nausea and vomiting and sometimes audiotoxicity were also severe. However, subsequent studies showed that the renal toxicity of cis Pt(II) could be dramatically decreased without inhibiting the therapeutic effects of the drug by the induction of diuresis with mannitol (HAYES et al., 1976). Moreover, with further extended clinical trials of cis Pt(II) there has been confirmation of the early promise against ovarian carcinoma, either when used alone and not necessarily in high dose therapy (WILTSHAW and KRONER, 1976, BRUCKNER et al., 1977) or in combination with adriamycin and chlorambucil (BRUCKNER et al., 1977). Some instances of a complete response against advanced ovarian carcinoma (BRUCKNER et al., 1977) proven by second look surgery, have been produced by platinum alone and with the platinum–adriamycin combination. The initially observed extreme sensitivity of testicular tumors to cis Pt(II) has also been confirmed (HIGBY et al., 1974). When cis Pt(II) was used in combination with vinblastine and bleomycin, complete and overall response rates of 75% and 100% respectively, were obtained against this particular tumor (EINHORN et al., 1976). A summary of the cummulative response rate by tumor type (Table 8), compiled by ROZENCWEIG et al., (1977) for the Cancer Chemotherapy Evaluation program, notes the lack of effect of cis Pt(II) on all types of leukemias and colorectal tumors. It also emphasizes the need for further studies of the toxic effect of cis Pt(II) and for a continuing evaluation of its possible effect on tumors, such as head and neck, prostate, and lung where suggestions of activity had been noted earlier.

Table 8. Cumulative response rate by tumor type compiled by Cancer Therapy Evaluation programme National Cancer Institute (ROZENCWEIG et al., 1977). No response was obtained in cumulative series of less than 14 patients with the following tumor types: brain, breast, kidney, mesothelioma, myeloma, pancreas, stomach

Tumor type	No. of evaluable patients	No. of responding patients	Response Ra %
Testicle	89	54	61
Acute Leukemia	66	1	2
AML	2	0	–
ALL	24	0	–
Colorectum	39	0	0
Ovary	38	11	29
Head and Neck	31	5	16
Bladder	28	12	43
Lung[a]	27	2	7
Sarcoma[b]	21	4	–
Lymphoma[a]	14	3	–
Neuroblastoma	14	3	–
Melanoma	8	1	–
Prostate	6	2	–
Endometrium	2	2	–
Hepatoma	2	1	–
Thyroid[b]	1	1	–

[a] Insufficient information available regarding activity of cis Pt(II), by histologic sub-types.
[b] Includes reticulum cell sarcoma. Additional responses were reported but without mention of the total number of evaluable patients.

2. Other Platinum Compounds

Of the newer platinum complexes to be applied clinically, malonato 1:2-diaminocyclohexane platinum (II) exhibits little or no nephrotoxicity and has shown effectiveness in the treatment of acute leukemia (HILL et al., 1977) and limited activity against some solid tumors (LOEB et al., 1977). After extensive and promising animal experiments, sulfato 1,2-diaminocyclohexane platinum II (Fig. 2) has been subjected to phase 1 clinical trials (LOEB et al., 1977) but it is too early to make a proper appraisal of its potential value.

3. Nephrotoxicity of Platinum Complexes

Toxic effects on the kidneys of mice, rats and marmoset monkeys occur with daily doses of cis Pt(II) in excess of 2 mg/kg body wt. (LEONARD et al., 1971) and are manifested as degeneration and necrosis of the epithelium of the proximal convoluted tubule. The cis compound was found to be more toxic than the trans isomer. If, as seems likely from in vitro studies (PASCOE and ROBERTS, 1974a), both isomers bind to the same extent to tissue constituents then, as in the case of the antitumor action, the nephrotoxic properties depend on the specific configuration of the platinum drug. SLATER and his co-workers (1977) followed the course of kidney injury in rats over a period of 0–6 days by estimating urinary and serum components. The salts of many heavy metals are also capable of causing severe disturbances to kidney structure and function following their administration to various animal species and in general it is possible to reduce the extent of such damage by protective thiol reagents such as cysteine or penicillamine (ZBINDEN, 1969). The fact that it was not possible to similarly protect kidneys from the toxic effect of cis Pt(II) (SLATER et al., 1977) indicated that cis Pt(II) binds particularly firmly to proximal tubules.

The specific nature of the reaction of platinum compound with kidney membranes was shown by comparative studies with other membrane structures (SLATER et al., 1977). Thus the interaction of cis Pt(II) with the kidney mitochondrial membrane could be reversed by thiol agents, while the liver plasma membrane was relatively unaffected by these agents.

III. Biological Effects of Platinum Coordination Complexes Indicative of Reactions with DNA

A. Filament Formation in Bacteria

Probably the first observation of an effect of a platinum coordination complex in a biological system and one which gave a clear indication of its biochemical mode of action came during experiments to investigate the effect of an electric current on growing bacteria (ROSENBERG et al., 1965). It was noticed that when a low alternating current was passed through platinum electrodes to growing gram-negative bacteria in nutrient media that cell division was inhibited and the bacteria grew into long filaments. Subsequently it was discovered that some of the platinum dissolves under these conditions to give first of all the ionic species ammonium hexachloroplatinate. This compound can itself, at a high concentration, inhibit cell division, but aged solutions were found to be far more efficient in producing filaments but only if exposed to visible light. The photochemical change which occurred in a solution of hexachloroplatinate which gave rise to a more active agent was shown to involve the replacement of the chloride ligands by NH_3 with the loss of one negative charge per replacement to give finally a stable neutral species. The new species was shown convincingly to inhibit cell division but not growth, which was in contrast to the parent ionic species which was a bacteriocide and not a bacteriostat. The difference between the properties of the charged and uncharged platinum species are shown in Table 9 (ROSENBERG et al., 1967a). Salts of other group VIIIB metals such as rhodium and ruthenium have been shown similarly to produce filamental growth in *E. coli* but in all cases a much higher concentration was required than with platinum complexes (ROSENBERG et al., 1967b).

Table 9. Summary of effects of platinum complexes on *E. coli* growth (ROSENBERG et al., 1967)

Type of complex	Effects on cell growth	Effects on cell division
Doubly negative, $[PtCl_6]^{=}$	Inhibitory (bacteriocide) in low concentrations (>1 ppm)	No detectable effect
Singly negative, $[PtCl_5(NH_3)]^-$	No inhibition	Slight inhibition[a]
Neutral, $[PtCl_4(NH_3)_2]^0$	No effect at low concentrations (<4 ppm); slight inhibition at higher concentrations	Inhibitory (filamentous growth) in low concentrations (>2 ppm)
Singly positive, $[PtCl_3(NH_3)_3]^+$	Not tested in sufficient concentration	Not tested in sufficient concentration

[a] The slight inhibition observed may be due to lability of the complex.

Filamentous growth in bacteria is almost certainly indicative of the ability of an agent to react with DNA, leading to a selective inhibition of DNA synthesis with no accompanying effect on other biosynthetic pathways such as RNA or protein synthesis. A variety of agents, such as UV and X-irradiation and cytotoxic alkylating agents, can also elicit this response and as a result of their common ability to damage DNA. Other evidence which supported this mechanism for the formation of filamentous growth with the platinum complexes came from tracer studies. They compared the distribution of platinum ions within *E. coli* after the induction of filaments with cis $Pt(II)(NH_3)_2Cl_4$ and after growth inhibition with $PtCl_6^{2-}$ (RENSHAW and THOMSON, 1967). In the filamentous cells platinum ions were associated not only with the metabolic intermediates but also with cytoplasmic proteins and nucleic acids whcreas in the $PtCl_6^{2-}$ inhibited cells the platinum was combined only with the cytoplasmic proteins. The accumulation of areas of strikingly enhanced electron density within platinum induced filaments of *E. coli*, thought by HOWLE and GALE (1970) to be aggregates of ribonucleoprotein, which had lost its usual distribution pattern but retained some degree of biochemical integrity due to its unimpeded rate of synthesis, was therefore also consistent with this proposed biochemical mechanism of filament formation.

B. Induction of Lysogeny

Further important evidence for direct attack on DNA was provided by the results of RESLOVA (1971/2) who investigated the ability of platinum compounds to induce the growth of phage in lysogenic strains of *E. coli* bacteria. The release of the phage DNA to direct synthesis of new phage is normally a rare event. However, agents which react with DNA can cause the phage DNA and phage particles to be released with consequent cell lysis. RESLOVA (1971/2) was able to show that there exists an excellent correlation between the anti-tumor activity of platinum compounds and their ability to induce lysogenic *E. coli* to enter the lytic cycle.

The important question of whether viruses are similarly induced in mammalian cells by platinum compounds has not been fully resolved. Induction of viruses and subsequent cell lysis has been proposed as a possible explanation for the rapid disappearance of an S180 sarcoma following administration of cis Pt(II) (see ROSENBERG, 1975). Epstein Barr virus (EBV) can be demonstrated in cells of human lymphoblastoid origin either by electron microscopy or by the immunofluorescence test (IF-test). The proportion of such EBV positive cells, as detected by immunofluorescence, has been shown to increase after treatment with cis platinum (II) diammine dichloride (VONKA et al., 1972). It was not clear, however, whether virus particles or only virus-associated antigens were formed in positive cells. Subsequently electron microscopy studies (ANISIMOVA, 1974) revealed a fourfold increase in virus-like particles following treatment with the drug. The increase in particle count was however mainly due to the appearance of small particles and these were detected in cells which contained EB virus as well as in those in which electron microscopy failed to demonstrate EBV. As yet the nature of the small size particle has not been clarified. These particles were either immature forms of the virus or the product of aberrant cis Pt(II) influenced maturation. Alternatively, the small particles are unrelated to EBV and their number increased because of the effect of the platinum compound on the synthesis of a different virus. The further possibility exists that the positive human serum that was used in the IF-test also contained antibodies to this type of particle and that the increase in the percentage of IF-positive cells was a consequence of their reaction with their antigens.

C. Mutagenic Properties of Neutral Platinum Complexes

The radiomimetic nature of platinum compounds and the importance of the geometrical arrangement of ligands for biological effect also emerges from studies on the mutagenic properties of these agents in a number of systems, (TROSKO, 1974; BECK and BRUBAKER, 1975; MONTI-BRAGADIIN et al., 1975; LECOINTE, 1977). The cis derivatives were in all cases appreciably more mutagenic than the corresponding trans isomers.

D. Reaction with Viruses and Transforming DNA

The interactions of platinum compounds with viruses have further indicated the relatively greater importance of reactions with DNA as against those with protein in producing biological effects. KUTINOVA et al. (1972) demonstrated the inactivation of the infectious activity of extracellular papovavirus SV40 by cis Pt(II). An indication of the mechanism of inactivation was derived by following the capacity of the inactivated virus to induce either tumor or viral antigens. The capacity of the virus to induce the tumor antigen was found to be less sensitive to cis Pt(II) than the viral antigen formation or the infectivity of the virus. The slower rate of inactivation of the tumor antigen by cis Pt(II) thus corroborated studies in which SV40 or polyoma virus were inactivated by radiation or hydroxylamine. This revealed that the capacities to induce tumor antigen, thymidine kinase, or transplantation immunity, and the transformation activity of the virus were inactivated at a slower rate than the infectivity or viral antigen-inducing capacity (CARP et al., 1966; ALTSTEIN et al., 1967; LAJARJET et al., 1967; AARONSON, 1970). These findings indicate that the viral DNA and not the protein coat is the primary target for both radiation and the platinum compound.

The inactivation of *B. subtilis* transforming DNA by platinum compounds likewise indicated the effect of these agents on the biological function of DNA (RESLOVA et al., 1972). Moreover, by examining the changes in transformation frequency of three unlinked genetic markers, the positions of which on the *B. subtilis* chromosome were known, some indication of specificity in the reaction of the platinum complexes with regions of DNA or with individual DNA bases was obtained. The adenine marker, for example, is localized at the region close to the origin of replication and is rich in guanine-cytosine base pairs in DNA. This was found to be appreciably more sensitive than the methionine marker which is localized at the end of the *B. subtilis* chromosome. It is of interest that in this system it was found that the hydrolysis products of cis Pt(II) were more reactive than the parent compounds.

IV. Biochemical Effects of Platinum Complexes Indicative of Reactions with DNA

A. Inhibition of DNA Synthesis: the Primary Biochemical Lesion Induced by Platinum Complexes

The above clues as to the likely basis for the antitumor action of platinum complexes were soon confirmed by studies on cellular biosynthesis in mammalian cells. Simultaneously and independently it was found that cis Pt(II) selectively and persistently inhibited the rate of DNA synthesis as compared with effects on RNA and protein synthesis in human AV3 cells in culture (HARDER and ROSENBERG, 1970; Fig. 7) and in Ehrlich ascites cells in vivo (HOWLE and GALE, 1970). These observations were confirmed in HeLa cells in culture and extended to show that such selective inhibition of DNA synthesis occurs with low doses of drugs which produced only minimal cytotoxicity as measured by effects on colony-forming ability (ROBERTS and PASCOE, 1972; PASCOE and ROBERTS, 1974a, b). HARDER and ROSENBERG (1970) further showed that those compounds which had been found to be effective against Sarcoma 180 and which also caused filament formation, displayed similar effects whereas the inactive compounds showed no effects until very high dose levels were employed (Fig. 8). Selective inhibition of DNA synthesis has also been demonstrated in phytohemaglutin-stimulated human peripheral lymphocytes (HOWLE et al., 1971), in the folate-stimulated kidney, and intestinal mucosa of normal- and tumor-bearing rats (TAYLOR et al., 1976). Inhibition of DNA synthesis was also demonstrated in a novel manner by KARA et al. (1972) who showed that cis Pt(II) not only irreversibly blocked Rous sarcoma virus-stimulated DNA synthesis in infected chick embryo cells, but also inhibited their subsequent transformation.

The likely basis for this selective biochemical effect on DNA synthesis came from the observations that the inhibition of DNA synthesis was persistent and progressive with time after removal of the drug (Fig. 9). This latter effect was at first thought to reflect the possible conversion of the drug to other more reactive species. However it is now clear, particularly by comparison with analogous effects produced by direct reacting agents such as mustard gas (ROBERTS et al., 1971), that both effects are consistent with the view that the primary chemical lesion is in the DNA of the cell, which is then inhibited as a template for DNA replication. Thus modifications to the DNA template will block DNA replication but not affect transcription or translation. Under conditions of low cell killing the selective inhibition by platinum compounds of DNA synthesis but not of RNA or protein synthesis leads to the formation of giant cells, a feature observed in cells treated with a variety of agents also known to block DNA replication selectively. No marked variations in the sensitivity of

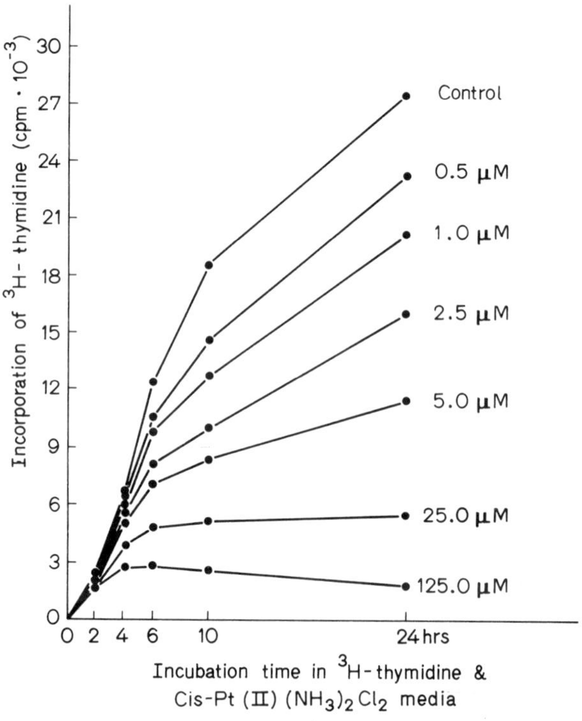

a

Fig. 7a–c. Effect of cis Pt(II) $(NH_3)_2Cl_2$ on: **a** DNA, **b** RNA or **c** protein synthesis in human AV3 cells as measured by the uptake of tritiated thymidine, uridine or leucine respectively. The radioactive precursors and the platinum compound were applied to the cells of zero time (HARDER and ROSENBERG, 1970)

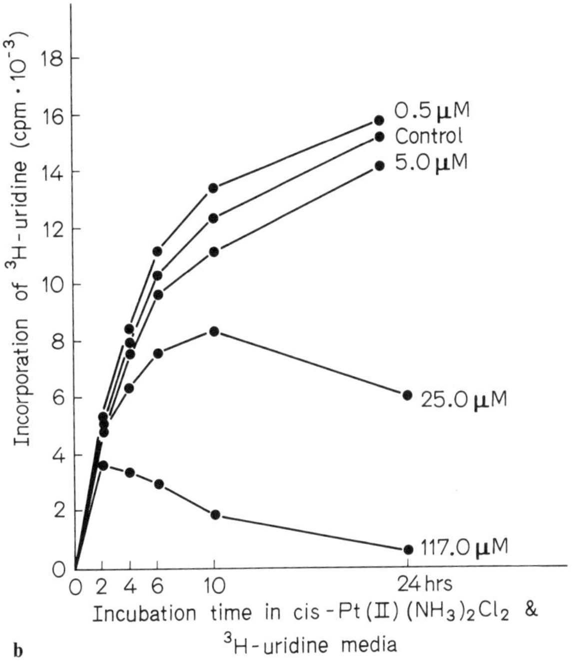

Incorporation of ^{3}H-uridine (cpm · 10^{-3})
0
2
4
6
8
10
12
14
16
18
0.5 µM
Control
5.0 µM
25.0 µM
117.0 µM
0 2 4 6 10 24 hrs
Incubation time in cis-Pt(II)(NH3)2Cl2 & ^{3}H-uridine media

b

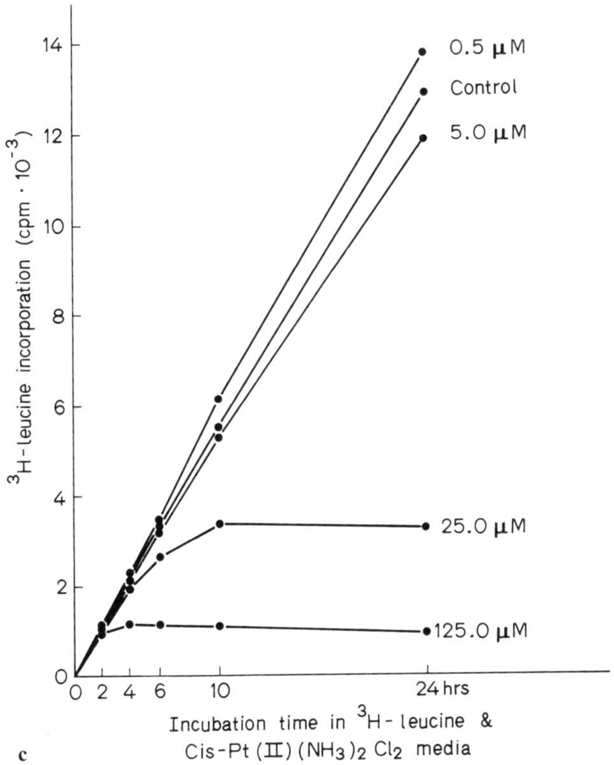

^{3}H-leucine incorporation (cpm · 10^{-3})
0
2
4
6
8
10
12
14
0.5 µM
Control
5.0 µM
25.0 µM
125.0 µM
0 2 4 6 10 24 hrs
Incubation time in ^{3}H-leucine & Cis-Pt(II)(NH3)2Cl2 media

c

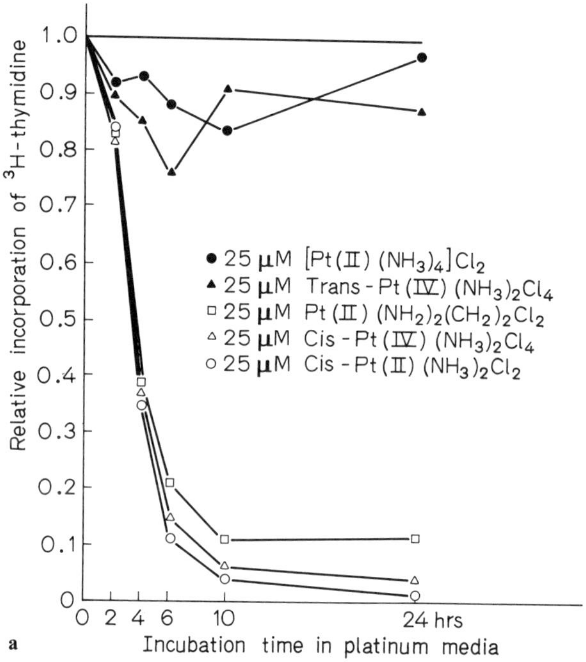

a

Fig. 8a–c. Effect of some active antitumor platinum compounds (see Fig. 1) and the inactive congeners Pt(II) $(NH_3)_4Cl_2$ and trans Pt(IV) $(NH_3)_2Cl_4$ on **a** DNA, **b** RNA and **c** protein synthesis in human AV3 cells (HARDER and ROSENBERG, 1970)

cells to platinum compounds throughout the cell cycle have been noted (Fig. 10; DREWINKO et al., 1975; OGAWA et al., 1976; SZUMIEL and NIAS, 1976a). The G_1 phase is, as with alkylating agents (ROBERTS et al., 1971), slightly more sensitive than other phases of the cell cycle. In this respect therefore, platinum compounds resemble other non cell cycle-specific drugs such as alkylating agents and other radiomimetic agents which also act by inactivating the DNA template for DNA replication. The effect of cis Pt(II) on the bone marrow has also been likened to other effects of X-irradiation (ZAK et al., 1972).

Convincing support for the proposed mechanism of action of platinum compounds has come from other studies on the extent of reaction with DNA and other macromolecules at measured levels of cell survival, discussed later in detail. The above studies on the inhibition of macromolecular synthesis in cultured cells were based on the rate of incorporation of labelled precursors into macromolecules. Other indications of effects on DNA synthesis based on the size of DNA synthesized at various times after treatment with cis Pt(II), are also discussed in detail later.

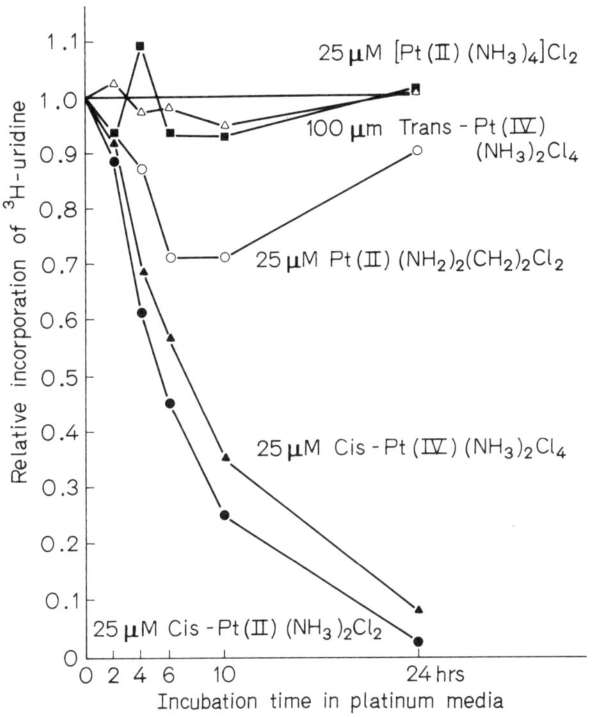

25 μM [Pt (II) (NH3)4]Cl2
100 μm Trans - Pt (IV) (NH3)2Cl4
25 μM Pt (II) (NH2)2(CH2)2Cl2
25 μM Cis - Pt (IV) (NH3)2Cl4
25 μM Cis - Pt (II) (NH3)2Cl2
Relative incorporation of 3H-uridine
Incubation time in platinum media
24 hrs

b

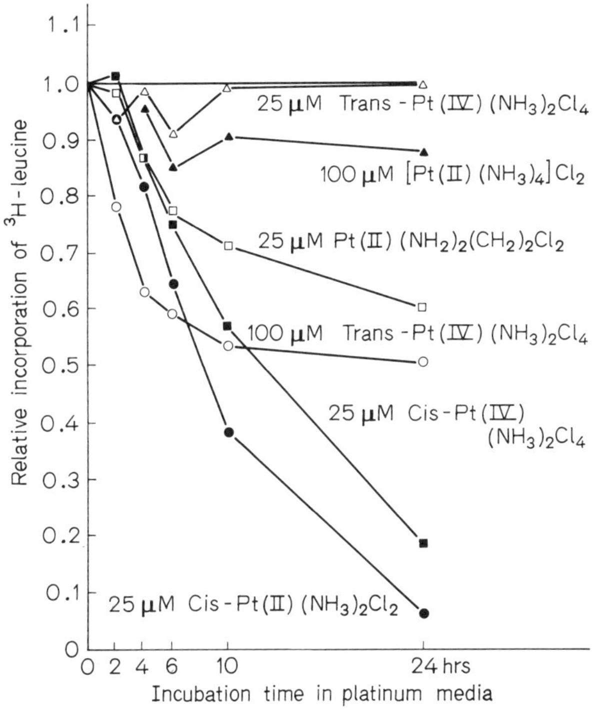

25 μM Trans - Pt (IV) (NH3)2Cl4
100 μM [Pt (II) (NH3)4] Cl2
25 μM Pt (II) (NH2)2(CH2)2Cl2
100 μM Trans - Pt (IV) (NH3)2Cl4
25 μM Cis - Pt (IV) (NH3)2Cl4
25 μM Cis - Pt (II) (NH3)2Cl2
Relative incorporation of 3H-leucine
Incubation time in platinum media
24 hrs

c

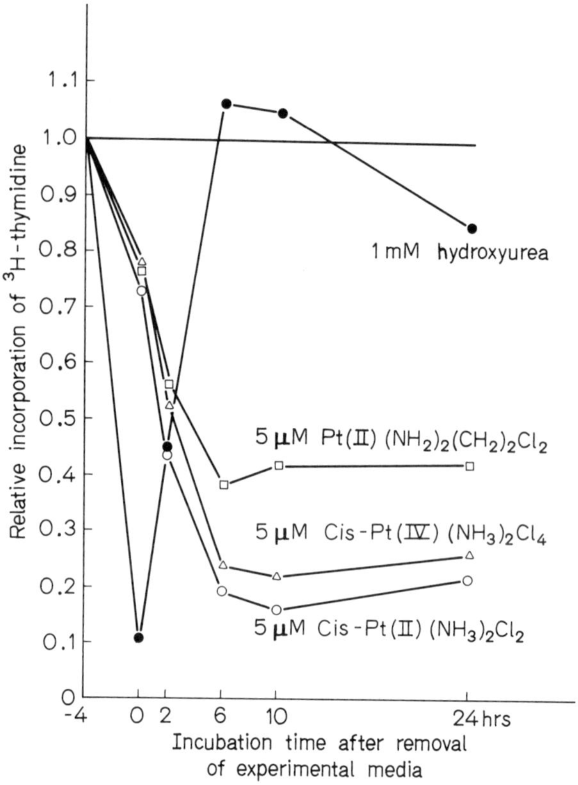

Fig. 9. The relative effect of a 4-h pretreatment of human AV3 cells with various platinum compounds or with 1 mM hydroxyurea on DNA synthesis as measured by uptake of [^{3}H] thymidine into DNA. Medium containing the various compounds was added at time −4 h and removed at zero time, and the cells washed before applying fresh medium. Cells were then labelled for only the last 2 h of incubation for each data point. The thymidine uptake into DNA is expressed as a fraction of that in control cells (HARDER and ROSENBERG, 1970)

B. Enzyme Studies

The alternative possibility that DNA synthesis is inhibited because of the inactivation of enzymes involved in DNA replication seems contraindicated not only by the failure of cis Pt(II) to block protein synthesis but also by its failure to inactivate DNA polymerase in vitro except with very high concentrations (HARDER et al., 1976). Other studies on the reversible interaction of cis and trans platinum coordination complexes with a variety of enzymes also make it unlikely that inhibition of enzymes is involved in the mechanism of action of these agents (FRIEDMAN and TEGGINS, 1974; TEGGINS and FRIEDMAN, 1974). The extent of binding to the enzyme by either cis or trans isomer was more dependent on the enzyme than on the configuration of the complex. However the recent proposal (FRIEDMAN and MELIUS, 1977) that some form

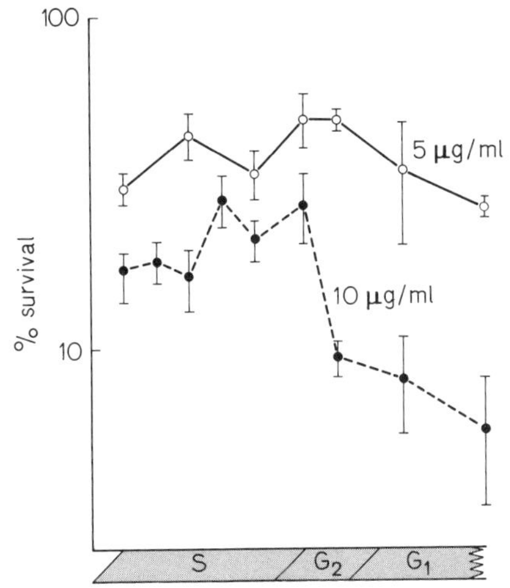

Fig. 10. Effect of cis Pt(II) $(NH_3)_2Cl_2$ on the survival of synchronised cultured human lymphoma cells. Cells were exposed to a single dose of 5 or 10 μg/ml of drug for 1 h at 2 h intervals throughout the cell cycle. Clearly cells are sensitive throughout the cell cycle although cells treated at the G_1/S boundary are slightly more sensitive than cells treated at other times of the cell cycle (DREWINKO et al., 1973)

of crosslinking between DNA and a DNA polymerase could account for the selective block to DNA replication possibly merits further consideration.

When platinum ethylenediamine dichloride-modified calf thymus DNA was used as a substrate for DNA or RNA polymerase, results at variance with those found in vivo were obtained, since both RNA and DNA synthesis were reduced similarly (GIRALDI and TAYLOR, 1974). On the other hand, an analogous study using salmon sperm DNA treated with cis and trans Pt(II) clearly suggested that the basis for the selectivity of the cis isomer may reside in its ability to react in a specific molecularly defined configuration with DNA (HARDER et al., 1976).

C. Other Proposed Mechanisms of Actions

1. Modification of the Immune Response

A main objective of this review has been to analyze the evidence which implicates DNA as the vital target for platinum compounds in mammalian cells. Thus studies of their extent of reaction with cellular DNA, their effects on DNA synthesis, and their effects on cells which differ in DNA repair capacity (see later), all indicated that cell killing occurred as a result of a selective block to DNA replication. However ROSENBERG (1975) felt that such a conclusion could not adequately explain a number of other "facts" and particularly the disappearance of large solid tumors in many systems following treatment with dose levels which were not apparently cytotoxic to the tumor. Nor did such a mechanism of action explain the apparent selective killing of certain tumor cells, and ROSENBERG therefore argued that specificity is inherent in the immune response of the host animals and is a dominant component in the selective destruction of tumor cells. On the other hand, it is equally not easy to envisage how the platinum compounds can stimulate a specific immune attack upon the tumor when almost all antitumor agents, in general, and certain of the platinum compounds, in particular, have themselves been shown to be immunosuppressors. A possible resolution of this apparent conflict was afforded by the observation that certain platinum blues stained the membrane of tumorogenic cells more readily than nontumorogenic cells (AGGARWAL et al., 1975). Further studies suggested that the stained patches could be DNA bound to the surface of cells through association with neuraminic acid (AGGARWAL et al., 1975). Transformed cells produce new antigens at the cell surface which can generate a host immune reaction and result in the destruction of cells. ROSENBERG (1975) proposed that in some transformed cells these "strong" antigens are masked by the relatively much "weaker" antigens such as nucleic acids. He therefore further proposed that the reaction of platinum drugs with the surface DNA leads to disruption of what he called the "antigen masking" action of the DNA in tumor cells and consequently leads to the exposure of the strong antigens on the cell surface to give the enhanced antigenicity discussed above. This appealing and highly original concept does not, however, seem to have been supported by subsequent studies. On examination of many more cell types, both normal and malignant, the initially observed correlation between tumorogenicity and cell surface associated nucleic acid does not appear to hold (MCALLISTER et al., 1977). However it is still conceivable that the mitotically inhibited enlarged cell is more antigenic than a normal cell.

2. Mutation as a Mechanism of Cell Death

The possible involvement of the extranuclear O^6-position of guanine as a site of reaction in DNA for the platinum compounds (MILLARD et al., 1975) (see later Fig. 19), and the known mispairing which can occur on bases alkylated in this position during DNA replication (LOVELESS, 1969; GERCHMAN and LUDLUM, 1973) led to yet another proposal for the mechanism of action of platinum compounds.

Reactions on the O^6-position of guanine could produce multiple mutations in DNA and these, it is proposed (ROSENBERG, 1977), would eventually lead to the death of the cell. Such a mechanism would offer an explanation for the apparent considerable delay in cell killing by these agents in some systems (ROSENBERG, 1977). Again, it is not immediately obvious how to reconcile this proposal with the wealth of evidence discussed above and later, which indicates that an effect on the rate of synthesis of DNA is critically important in determining toxicity. Certainly all lesions in DNA including those promutagenic lesions on the O^6-position (see PLANT and ROBERTS, 1971a, b) are likely to interfere with DNA replication. Moreover it has been found previously that one round of replication of DNA on a N-methyl-N-nitrosourea damaged template which would contain some O^6-methylguanine adducts amplifies that damage into lesions which are a block to further DNA replication. Such a process if it occurred in response to platinum damage (see later) would clearly contribute to some of the apparent delayed cell killing by these agents.

V. Interaction of Platinum Compounds with DNA

A. In vivo Studies Indicative of DNA as the Target Molecule

1. Quantitative Aspects of Reactions with Macromolecules

The biological and biochemical studies discussed so far clearly suggest that a modification of the DNA template by platinum compounds leads to its inactivation for DNA replication. They further indicated that an enhanced inactivation by a specific type of reaction occurs in the case of the cis isomers. Confirmation of these notions was convincingly obtained from a comparison of the effects of cis and trans Pt(II) on the survival of HeLa cells in vitro and their ability to bind to macromolecules.

The marked difference in the effect of the two isomers on tumors is similarly reflected in their effect on cells in culture (Fig. 11) indicating that this in vitro system is a valid model for mechanistic studies. Differences in concentrations of cis and trans Pt(II) required to produce equivalent effects in HeLa cell survival need not necessarily be indicative of the true amount of reaction occur-

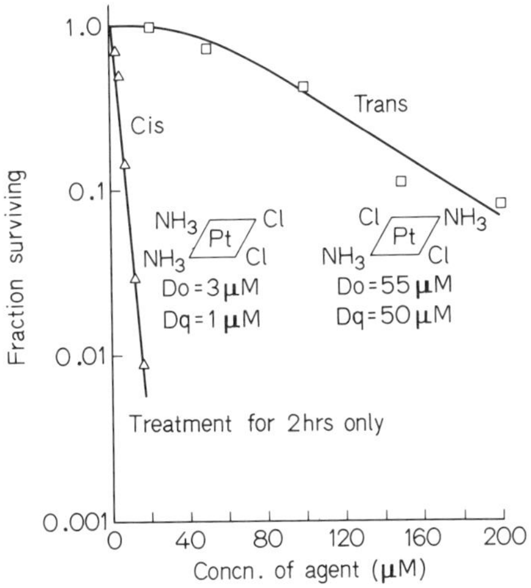

Fig. 11. The effect of cis and trans Pt(II) $(NH_3)_2Cl_2$ on the survival of HeLa cells. Various concentrations of the platinum compounds were applied to HeLa cells in DMSO for a period of 2 h, and survival determined by the ability of the cells to form colonies within 14 days (PASCOE and ROBERTS, 1974a)

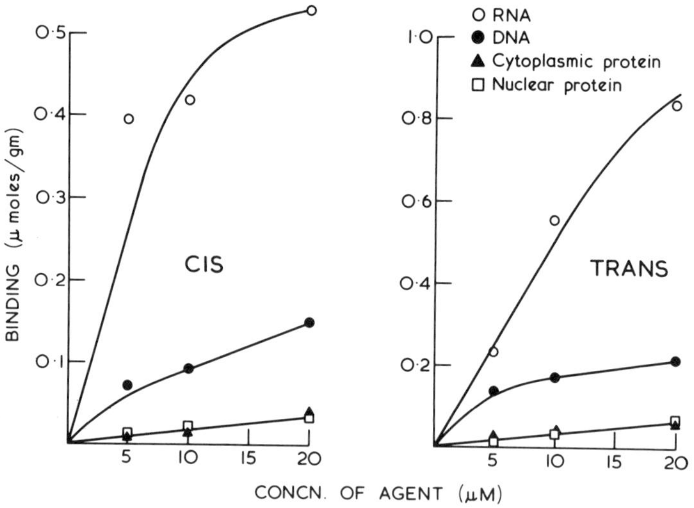

Fig. 12. Binding of cis and trans Pt(II) $(NH_3)_2Cl_2$ to HeLa cell macromolecules. Cells were treated for 2 h with the platinum compounds before isolation of DNA, RNA and protein components. Essentially the same binding to cellular components occurs with both isomers (Pascoe and Roberts, 1974a)

ring with cell constituents but could merely reflect differences in the relative ease of penetration of the two isomers into cells. However, Pascoe and Roberts (1974a) showed that the trans isomer bound to cell macromolecules quite as effectively as the cis isomer (Fig. 12).

To assess the possible importance of DNA, RNA and protein as primary targets for platinum II compounds these binding data (expressed as mol/gm of macromolecule) were used to construct curves of log survival against the amount of drug bound to each type of macromolecule. The resulting graphs were then characterized in a similar way to a curve of log cell survival versus dose of drug given to the cells. The shoulder width of the binding curve was given the value B_q and slope of the straight line portion by B_o. The binding coefficients B_q and B_o for the binding of each isomer to DNA, RNA and protein are given in Table 10. For both cis and trans Pt(II) the binding coefficients were higher for RNA than DNA. However the true significance of these binding coefficients can only be appreciated if account is taken of the molecular weights of the molecules concerned. If one assumes no selectivity in the binding to any particular RNA or protein molecule, and there is no evidence for such selectivity in any study with these agents, then it is possible to calculate the number of platinum molecules bound to each macromolecule at a given toxic dose. Table 11 shows the approximate molecular weights of DNA, RNA, and protein and the results of such a calculation performed at the concentration which reduced the surviving fraction from f to 0.37f. This is theoretically the concentration just required to kill one cell. There are strikingly more molecules bound to DNA than to either RNA or protein at this concentration of cis or trans-Pt(II), clearly indicating that DNA is the most sensitive cellular target for both cis- and trans-dichlordiammine Pt(II).

Table 10. Binding coefficients obtained from curves resulting from a combination of the lethal effects of various doses of cis and trans Pt(II) (Fig. 11) and the expected binding to DNA at these doses obtained from separate studies relating binding to DNA and the dose of platinum compound (Fig. 12). B_o represents the slope of the straight portion of the curves i.e., the binding to DNA associated with a reduction in survival from f to 0.37f while B_q represents the bindings to DNA when this portion of the curve is extrapolated to 100% (PASCOE and ROBERTS, 1974a). More recent data in which the binding to DNA was obtained at the same time as the measurement of cell survival have given lower B_O and B_Q values (FRAVAL and ROBERTS, 1979)

Compound	Binding to macromolecules					
	B_Q (μmol/gm (shoulder width)			B_O (μmol/gm) (slope of curve)		
	DNA	RNA	Protein	DNA	RNA	Protein
cis Pt(II) $(NH_3)_2Cl_2$	0.045	0.300	0.002	0.0225	0.030	0.00675
trans Pt(II) $(NH_3)_2Cl_2$	0.170	0.300	–	0.125	0.650	–

Table 11. Table giving the extent of reaction with DNA, RNA and protein on a molar basis at the B_O and B_Q levels of binding as obtained from Table 10 (PASCOE and ROBERTS, 1974a, b)

Molecule	Approx. mol wt.	*cis* Pt(II) $(NH_3)_2Cl_2$		*trans* Pt(II) $(NH_3)_2Cl_2$	
		B_O μmol/gm	No. Pt mol bound when surviving fraction reduced from *f* to 0.37 *f*	B_O μmol/gm	No. Pt mol bound when surviving fraction reduced from *f* to 0.37 *f*
DNA	1×10^9	0.0225	22 Pt/DNA mol	0.125	125 Pt/DNA mol
mRNA	4×10^6		1 Pt/8 mRNA mol		2.5 Pt/mRNA mol
rRNA	$0.5–1 \times 10^6$	0.030	1 Pt/30 rRNA mol	0.650	1 Pt/2 rRNA mol
tRNA	2.5×10^4		1 Pt/1500 tRNA mol		1 Pt/70 tRNA mol
Protein	1×10^5	0.00675	1 Pt/1500 protein mol	–	–

The binding data shown in Table 11 further indicate that only one molecule of protein out of 1,500 molecules will have received one platination reaction. Unless there is considerable specificity in the reaction of platinum drugs with a particular protein enzyme molecule then this level would be too low to inactivate enzyme activity. Moreover, the level of reaction with rRNA or tRNA or mRNA would not be expected, again in the absence of any selectivity of reaction, to inactivate all such molecules and lead to interference with protein synthesis.

2. Role of Crosslinking Reactions

a) Mammalian Cells. The structural requirement for difunctionality and the principal biochemical effects of the platinum compounds, as discussed above, soon suggested a parallel between the platinum drugs and the classical bifunctional alkylating agents such as the nitrogen mustards. The latter compounds have been thought for some time to produce an inhibtion of DNA synthesis by their ability to introduce crosslinks into the DNA of mammalian cells. It has however been a matter of contention as to whether the principal lesion is a crosslink between strands of the DNA helix or crosslinks between bases on one strand of DNA or possibly even between DNA and protein (see ROSENBERG, 1973). It soon became a matter of some interest to determine whether platinum compounds were similarly able to introduce crosslinks into cellular DNA and whether such reactions contributed to cell killing.

That the two types of agents act by a similar mechanism was indicated by the fact that a Walker Carcinoma with an acquired resistance to Melphalan, an aromatic nitrogen mustard, is cross-resistant to cis Pt(II). PASCOE and ROBERTS therefore asked the questions, does cis Pt(II) form interstrand crosslinks in DNA in vivo and are the number of crosslinks in the DNA of HeLa cells at a measured level of cell survival comparable to the number of sulfur mustard-induced crosslinks present in the genome after treatment with an equitoxic dose of sulfur mustard (BALL and ROBERTS, 1970). In order to estimate crosslinks in the DNA, one strand of DNA was given a density and radioactivity label by growing cells in the presence of [^{3}H] BUdR. Crosslinking between a "labeled heavy" strand and a "light unlabeled" strand produced a "labeled hybrid" species, and these species could be separated in an alkaline cesium chloride gradient (Fig. 13). Not only was crosslinking of DNA by cis Pt(II) demonstrated by this technique (Fig. 14) but it could also be calculated, from a knowledge of the overall extent of platination of DNA at a dose which produced a measured number of crosslinks in the DNA of estimated molecular weight, that DNA interstrand crosslinking was a relatively rare event compared with mustard induced crosslinks. Thus whereas approximately one in eight sulfur mustard reactions gave rise to a crosslink in DNA, in the case of cis Pt(II) treated DNA the figure approximated to one crosslink in 400 platination reactions. This calculation assumed that the DNAs isolated after the two treatments have the same molecular weight.

A further indication of the possible role of the crosslinking reaction in determining the cytotoxic action of platinum drugs was obtained from a study aimed at answering the question: does the extent of interstrand crosslinking of DNA correlate with the cytotoxic activity of a range of platinum compounds? (PASCOE and ROBERTS, 1974a, b). The relative toxicities of the cis and trans isomers of the platinum (II) and platinum (IV) neutral complexes can be defined by the slopes of the survival curves (D_o) obtained by treating HeLa cells in culture (Table 12). The relative abilities of the various compounds to induce crosslinking in vivo or in vitro is also given in Table 12. Comparison of these two sets of values initially suggested that the relative abilities of cis and trans Pt(II) compounds to crosslink DNA in vivo (but not in vitro) was related to their cytotoxic action. Thus the relative ability of cis and trans Pt(II) to kill cells, measured either on the basis of dose [$D_o^{trans}/D_o^{cis}=18$] or DNA binding (Table 10) [$B_o^{trans}/B_o^{cis}=5.6$] is of the same order as the 12-fold difference in the doses required to produce equal amounts of crosslinking with the two compounds. However in the case of the platinum (IV) compounds despite an

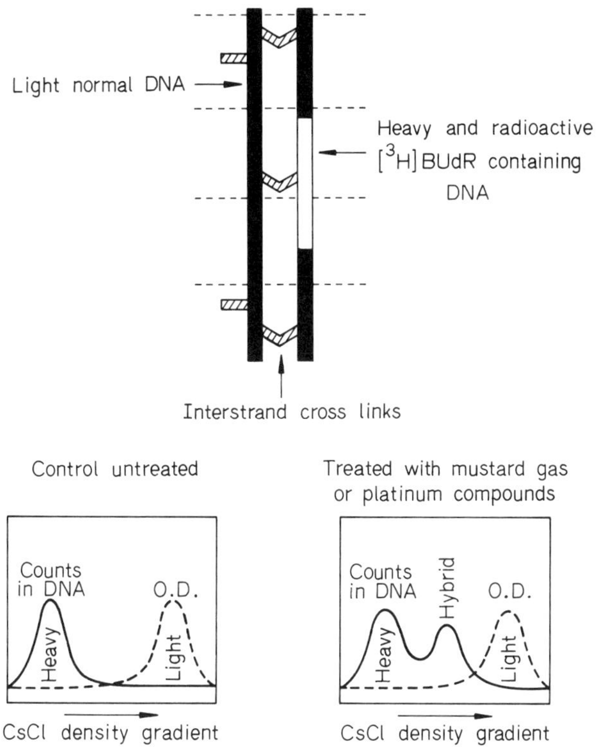

Fig. 13. Method used for quantitating the percentage of cellular DNA which has been crosslinked by cis Pt(II) $(NH_3)_2Cl_2$ in vivo. Cells were grown for a period of 3 h in medium containing BUdR and [^{3}H] thymidine to produce a proportion of labeled hybrid DNA. Following treatment with platinum compounds the isolated DNA was separated into single-stranded heavy, cross-linked hybrid, and single-stranded light DNAs by means of isopycnic alkaline caesium chloride gradient centrifugation. The proportion of the single stranded heavy DNA present as the hybrid species gives a measure of the amount of crosslinking (BALL and ROBERTS, 1971/2; ROBERTS and PASCOE, 1972)

even greater difference in the relative toxicities of the cis and trans compounds [$D_0^{trans}/D_0^{cis}=43$] there was very little difference in their capacities to induce crosslinks in DNA either in vitro or in whole cells. It would seem therefore that interstrand crosslinking is not an important cytotoxic event in the case of the platinum complexes (see also HARDER, 1975). Other evidence which supports this conclusion was obtained from studies on bacteriophage (see below).

b) Bacteriophage. A study by SHOOTER et al. (1972) on the inactivation of bacteriophage also indicated that DNA interstrand crosslinking reactions are unlikely to be important cytotoxic events. These authors compared cis- and trans-platinum (II) diammine dichloride and cis platinum (II) ethylenediamine dichloride for their ability to inactivate T7 bacteriophage. They also carried out parallel studies on the extent of interstrand crosslinking of phage DNA with all agents (Figs. 15, 16) and the extent of overall reaction of the ^{14}C-labeled ethylene diamine derivative with double stranded T7 phage DNA. It was thus

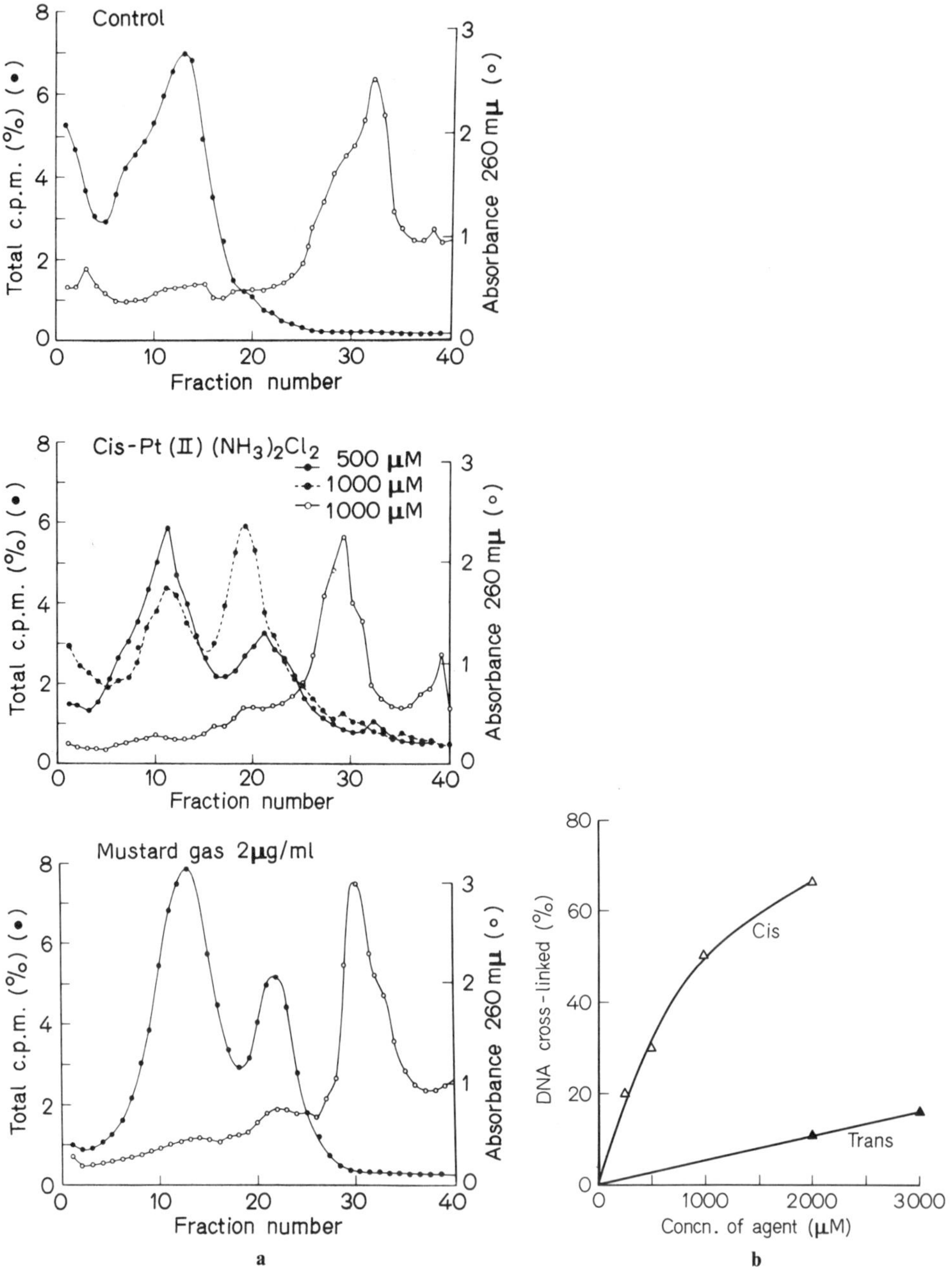

Fig. 14. a Formation of crosslinked DNA in HeLa cells following treatment with mustard gas or cis Pt(II) $(NH_3)_2Cl_2$ (Roberts and Pascoe, 1972). **b** Quantitation of crosslinking of HeLa cell DNA by cis and trans Pt(II) $(NH_3)_2Cl_2$ (Pascoe and Roberts, 1974a)

Table 12. Relationship between the concentrations of platinum compounds required to produce measured effects on cell survival and those required to produce 10% crosslinking of complementary strands of DNA either in vitro or in vivo (PASCOE and ROBERTS, 1974a, b)

Compound	$D_o(\mu M)$	$D_Q(\mu M)$	Dose required to produce 10% crosslinking in vitro (μM)	Dose required to produce 10% crosslinking in vivo (μM)
cis-Pt(II) $(NH_3)_2Cl_2$	3.0	1.0	0.5	150
trans Pt(II) $(NH_3)_2Cl_2$	55.0	50.0	1.0	1,900
cis Pt(IV) $(NH_3)_2Cl_4$	1.5	1.0	33.7	420
trans Pt(IV) $(NH_3)_2Cl_4$	65.0	37.5	67.0	570

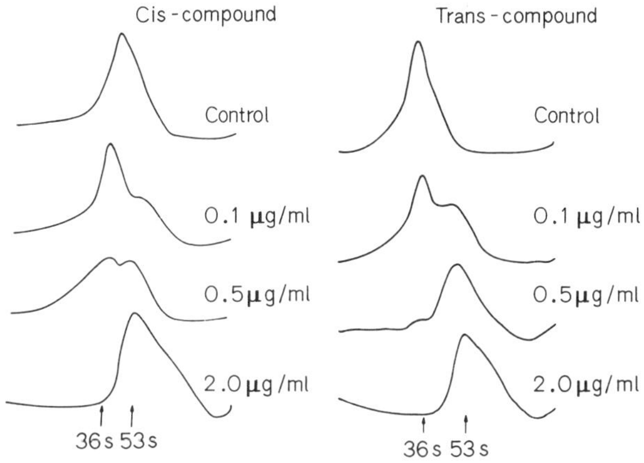

Fig. 15. Band sedimentation profiles of denatured T7 DNA observed after incubating native DNA in phosphate buffer at 37° C for 2 h with cis or trans Pt(II) $(NH_3)_2Cl_2$. Under these conditions the sedimentation coefficient of single chains of DNA is 36s and of the crosslinked chains 53s. From measurements under the areas of the two peaks the proportion of crosslinked DNA molecules can be calculated. These values were plotted against dose of platinum compounds to give the relationships shown in Fig. 16 from which were calculated the concentrations required to give on average one crosslink in phage DNA with cis Pt(II) $(NH_3)_2Cl_2$ (△), trans Pt(II) $(NH_3)_2Cl_2$(○), and cis Pt(II) ethylenediamine dichloride (□)

possible to calculate that at the dose of labeled drug which reduces survival to 37% (i.e. the mean lethal dose, D_o) there are five molecules bound to each T7 phage particle. However it could be shown that at a dose which induces on average one crosslink into the phage DNA there were 35 molecules of platinum drug bound to the phage. Crosslinking is, therefore, a relatively rare event under these conditions of treatment. Moreover, since there were only five platination reactions with the phage particle at the mean lethal dose, four of which were with the nucleic acid, it follows that the crosslinking reaction could not be an inactivating event. In other words when one has a level of reaction which would inactivate all phages only a small proportion of them would contain a crosslink in their DNA.

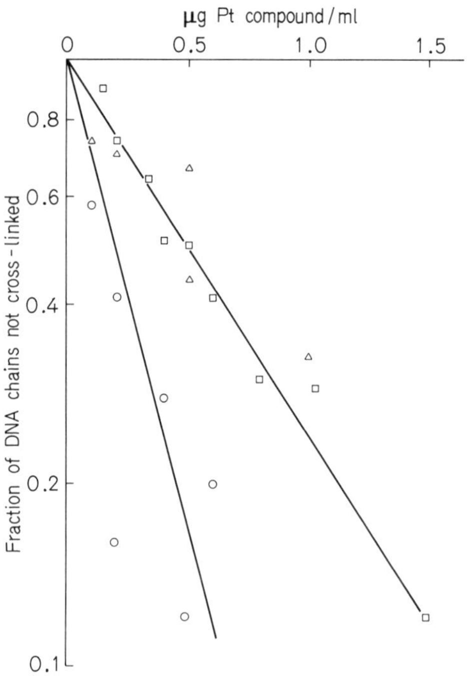

Fig. 16. Relationships between crosslinking of bacteriophage T7 and concentrations of ethylenediamine Pt(II) dichloride (□); cis (△) and trans (○) platinum (II) diammine dichloride. The slopes of these curves give the concentrations required to give on average one crosslink in phage DNA. These values were appreciably higher than the mean lethal doses for inactivation of bacteriophage T7 suggesting that crosslinking of the DNA is not a major inactivating reaction (SHOOTER et al., 1972)

A further indication of the lack of importance of a DNA interstrand crosslink as an inactivating event came from the finding that while the two cis platinum compounds were appreciably more effective than the trans isomer in inactivating the bacteriophage nevertheless all three compounds crosslink DNA with approximately equal efficiency (Figs. 15 and 16).

Analogous reasoning to that described above indicated that crosslinking of DNA to protein also contributed little to the inactivating process.

On the other hand an indication of what was likely to be an inactivating event in this system and for the inactivation of the single-stranded RNA phages, R17 and µ2, was gained from a comparison of the inactivation of phages by platinum compounds with their inactivation by mono- and di-functional alkylating agents (LAWLEY et al., 1969; SHOOTER et al., 1971). The extent of binding of the [^{14}C]ethylenediamine platinum (II) dichloride and its sensitivity towards the T7 and R17 phages are more comparable of those of the di-functional alkylating agent than they are to those of the mono-functional alkylating agent: this would indicate that a bi-functional attack on the DNA or RNA by either type of agent is biologically more effective than a mono-functional one. Calculations of the numbers of reactions which occur with the phage nucleic acids at the mean lethal doses of the mono- and di-functional alkylating agents combined with a knowledge of the extent of crosslinking with the bi-functional compound and of the products of reaction with DNA indicated that, as with the platinum compounds, interstrand crosslinking was not likely to be the major inactivating event with di-functional alkylating agents. However since both single (R17 and μ2) and double stranded (T7) phage molecules were inactivated more readily by di-functional than by mono-functional alkylating agents it was suggested that the main contribution to inactivation came from crosslinking of neighboring bases on the same nucleic acid chain, a reaction which is known to occur with the di-functional alkylating agents. It would therefore appear from these comparative studies between alkylating agents and platinum compounds that some form of crosslinking on one strand of the nucleic acid molecule is responsible for the inactivation of both single and double stranded phage molecules by the platinum II compounds.

B. In vitro Reactions of Neutral Platinum Complexes with Nucleic Acid Components

1. Reaction with Bases

Changes in the ultraviolet absorption spectrum of salmon sperm DNA after reaction with either cis or trans $Pt(II)(NH_3)_2Cl_2$ provided conclusive evidence that both platinum compounds bind to the organic bases of DNA (Fig. 17; HORACEK and DROBNIK, 1971; MANSY et al., 1973). Spectrophotometric studies further confirmed that the three bases guanine, adenine and cytosine would all react with both isomers, the rate of reaction with guanine being faster than with the other two bases (MANSY et al., 1973). The ^{14}C labeled platinum (II) ethylenediamine dichloride similarly reacted preferentially with guanosine as compared with adenosine and cytosine (ROBBINS, 1973). A very slow reaction occurs with thymine (MANSY et al., 1973) while substituted thymines react to

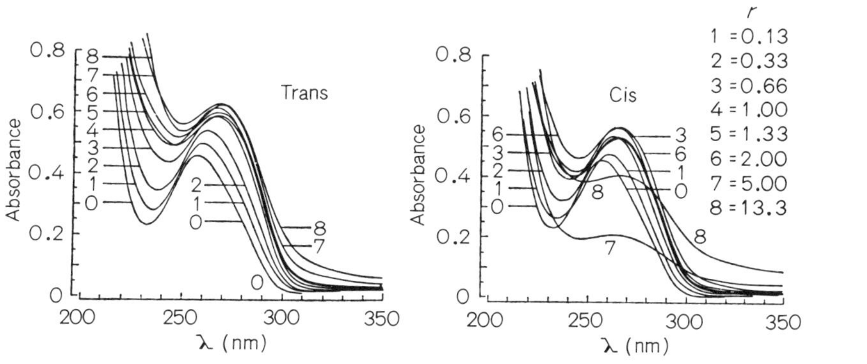

Fig. 17. The absorption spectra (1 cm path) of solutions of salmon sperm DNA in 0.1 M $NaClO_4$ in the presence of cis and trans Pt(II) $(NH_3)_2Cl_2$ after equilibrium had been achieved (r = Pt:P ratio), which indicate reactions with bases in DNA by both isomers (HORACEK and DROBNIK, 1971; MANSEY et al., 1973)

give blue colored unidentified complexes (THOMPSON et al., 1977). The above indication that guanine is the base in DNA with which reaction is most likely to occur preferentially was supported by studies on the extent of reaction of cis Pt(II) to DNAs of varying GC/AT ratios (STONE et al., 1974), and by the ratio of the binding of a radioactively labeled platinum compound to the purine bases in DNA (MUNCHAUSEN and RAHN, 1975).

2. Sites of Reaction on Bases

By blocking the various possible binding sites in the purine bases by either methylation or protonation, MANSY et al. (1973) defined the sites most likely to be involved in reaction with either cis or trans Pt(II). They concluded that the cis isomer forms a bidentate chelate with either 6-NH_2 and N-7, or 6-NH_2 and N-1 of adenosine, and 4-NH_2 and N-3 of cytidine. The trans isomer on the other hand interacts monofunctionally at N-7 and N-1 of adenosine and N-3 of cytidine. Both isomers were found to react monofunctionally with N-7 of guanosine and inosine. ROBBINS (1973) used a similar approach and blocked the N-7, N-9 or both positions of guanine or its derivatives and concluded that the N-7 position of guanine is a primary point of attack for cis Pt(II) but that reaction probably also occurs at a second site.

Recent X-diffraction studies of the complexes formed between either cis $Pt(NH_3)_2I_2$ and inosine (GOODGAME et al., 1975) or cis Pt(II) and guanosine (GELLERT and BAU, 1975; CRAMER and DAHLSTROM, 1977) also indicated that binding occurs at the N-7 positions of these bases.

3. Crosslinking Reactions

As discussed elsewhere cis Pt(II) has been shown to be able to induce the formation of X-links into DNA in vivo (ROBERTS and PASCOE, 1972). There is however no direct in vitro evidence indicating which of the many possible binding sites discussed above are involved in such a reaction. A possibility suggested from an examination of a model of DNA is that crosslinking could occur between the 6-amino groups of adenines in opposing strands of DNA in an ApT sequence (THOMSON, 1974). These groups would be 3.5 Å apart which approximates to 3 Å, the distance between the cis leaving groups in cis Pt(II). Evidence has been obtained that cis Pt(II) can link two NH_2 groups in this way in a simple nucleotide (ROOS et al., 1974; KLEINWÄCHTER and ZALUDOVA, 1977).

The affinity of platinum compounds for the N-7 position of guanine, the preferential drug binding by GpG sequences of DNA (STONE et al., 1976) and various other findings led KELMAN et al. (1977) to argue strongly in favor of a crosslinking reaction between neighboring guanine bases in DNA. For such a reaction to occur, local perturbation of the double helix must occur and evidence for such distortion is available (MUNCHAUSEN and RAHN, 1975; BUTOUR and MACQUET, 1977; TAMBURRO et al., 1977). The platinum guanine

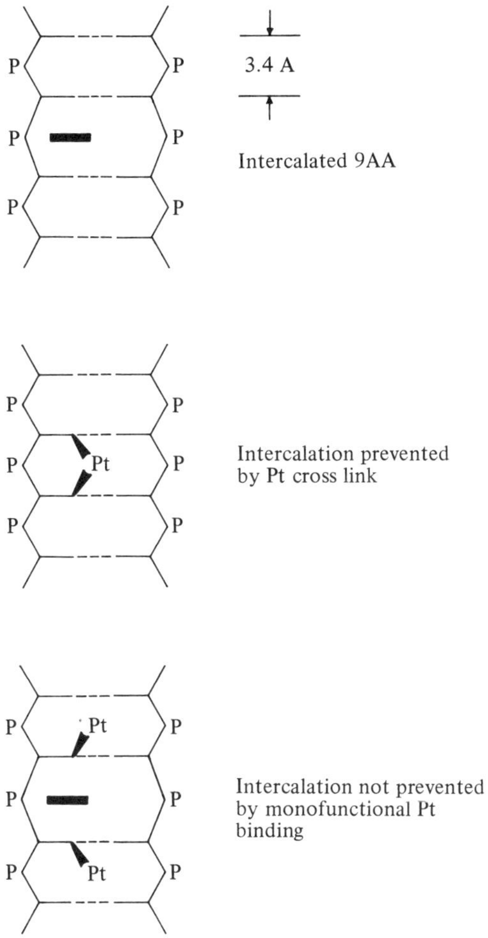

Fig. 18. Scheme showing how intercalation of DNA by a dye can be prevented by platinum-induced crosslinks (Roos, 1977)

N(7) binding weakens G-C base pair hydrogen bonding which, it is proposed, makes the N1 position of guanine available for further reaction (Kelman et al., 1977)

Another method of investigating platinum drug-induced DNA crosslinks is illustrated in Fig. 18 (Roos, 1977; Roos and Arnold, 1977). 9-Aminoacridine and other planar aromatic molecules intercalate into DNA and in doing so increase the interplanar base separation from 3.4 Å to 6.7 Å at the intercalation site. The introduction of crosslinks into DNA will therefore prevent the intercalation of 9-aminoacridine. Roos and Arnold (1977) studied this inhibition of binding as a function of G-C content or base sequence of DNAs or co-polymers. It was concluded from such studies that the binding of $Pt(en)Cl_2$ is both monofunctional and bifunctional. The extent of crosslinking, both inter and intra strand, is about 30% for *E. coli* DNA and the crosslinking increases with G-C

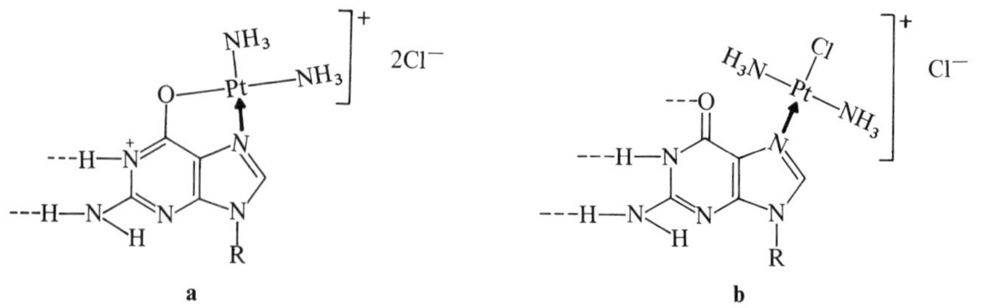

Fig. 19a and b. Proposed structures formed by reaction of cis (**a**) and trans (**b**) Pt(II) $(NH_3)_2Cl_2$ with guanine residues in DNA (GOODGAME et al., 1975; MILLARD et al., 1975)

content of the DNA. The A-T sequence is also a crosslinking site but not the A-A (ROOS and ARNOLD, 1977), a finding consistent with the earlier chemical evidence which favored crosslinking between the $6\text{-}NH_2$ groups of adenine (MANSY et al., 1973).

A crosslinking reaction which would satisfactorily explain the unique properties of the cis isomer was suggested from electronic binding energies using electron spectroscopy for chemical analysis. Chelation between the N-7 position and O^6 position of the same guanine moiety has been claimed for the cis but not the trans isomer (MACQUET and THEOPHANIDES, 1975; MILLARD et al., 1975; Fig. 19a, b).

GOODGAME et al. (1975) similarly argued that the crosslinking of guanine moieties via the N-7 position would require considerable distortion of the DNA structures and therefore be unlikely to occur in vivo. They therefore proposed that a firm binding at N-7 of guanine would initially be formed with possibly a second weaker bond with the O^6 position in the same guanine molecule. During DNA replication, however, which would involve separation of the strands of DNA, it could be envisaged that the weak link to the O^6 position could be broken and a new one established with the N-7 position of another guanine moiety. Similar reasoning led GOODGAME et al. (1975) to consider that the crosslinked species present in the DNA of cells treated in vivo with cis Pt(II) (ROBERTS and PASCOE, 1972), and visualized by isopycnic gradient centrifugation of alkali-denatured DNA, could possibly have been formed during the denaturing process. If however this were the mechanism for the observed in vivo and in vitro crosslinking then cis and trans compounds should be equally effective.

4. Reactions with Sugar Molecules

Reactions of platinum compounds with other components of nucleic acids, such as the deoxyribose moiety, must now also be considered following the formation of complexes between D-mannitol and cis Pt(II) (ESHAQUE et al., 1977). A yellow and a green complex were isolated and both shown to have a Pt:mannitol ratio of 2:1. ^{13}C NMR studies showed that the platinum binds with the three nonequivalent carbons in D-mannitol and one of the proposed

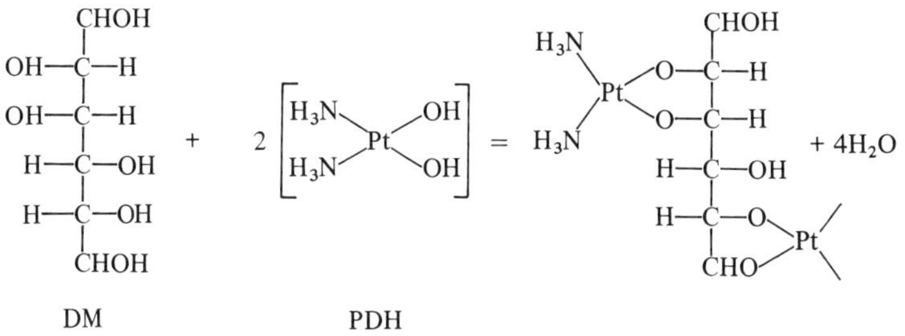

Fig. 20. Proposed reaction between cis platinum (II) diammine dihydroxy and D-mannitol (Eshaque et al., 1977)

structures is shown in Fig. 20. This reaction is of particular interest in view of its possible relevance to the protective action of D-mannitol against cis Pt(II) induced renal toxicity. It is of further interest in view of the contention regarding the ease of formation and stability of platinum–oxygen bonds in DNA as, for example, on the O^6-position of guanine (see earlier).

VI. Repair of DNA Damage Induced by Platinum Compounds

A. General Comments

Some cells are known to be able to remove or circumvent damage to their DNA that has been introduced by diverse agents, using various cellular repair processes. This is an area of high current interest and may well be important for understanding further aspects of drug action. The fact that cells can acquire resistance to drugs is an important limitation to their clinical usefulness. It is now necessary to ask whether tumor cells develop this resistance to platinum compounds by use of a DNA repair mechanism(s). Model studies using prokaryotic and eukaryotic cells in vitro do indicate that this is indeed a possibility and these findings strongly support the notion that DNA is indeed the target for these cytotoxic agents.

Investigations of the modifying influence of cellular repair processes on the lethal effects of radiation and chemically-induced damage in both microbial and mammalian cells have revealed basically two different repair mechanisms. In one of these the DNA bound adducts are recognized and removed by one of two excision processes. If, however, the damage to the DNA is not excised before the DNA is used as a template for DNA replication it now appears that the cell can circumvent the damage either by a mechanism involving recombination, or by a process called post replication repair (or replication repair). Both excision and post replication repair processes facilitate the recovery of cells from DNA damage introduced by a variety of physical and chemical agents. These processes have been studied extensively in UV-irradiated cells (for review see Cleaver, 1974).

B. Excision Repair

1. Bacterial Studies

The main photoproduct in the DNA of UV-irradiated *E. coli* or mammalian cells is a pyrimidine dimer. The distortion created in the DNA by the dimer is thought to be recognized by an endonuclease which inserts a nick in the DNA adjacent to the dimer. Subsequent steps in this excision repair process involve removal of the dimer attached to an oligonucleotide and resynthesis of the removed section of the DNA. The contribution which this excision repair process makes to the ultimate survival of bacterial cells treated with various agents can be assessed by determining the sensitivities of strains of *E. coli* carrying mutations in genes known to code for steps in this repair pathway. It was concluded from such studies that damage introduced into DNA by certain bi-functional agents, such as nitrogen mustards, mitomycin C and psoralen-plus-visible light, as well as the damage introduced by certain bulky monofunctional carcinogenic agents such as 4-nitroquinoline-1-oxide and 7-bromomethylbenz(a)anthracene was also eliminated by enzymes coded by genes known to code for the enzymes required for the repair of UV-induced thymine dimers. From analogous studies on the sensitivities of such DNA repair deficient *E. coli* mutants to cis platinum (II) diammine dichloride it was similarly concluded that excision repair process(es) contribute only a small extent to the recovery of strains of *E. coli* from the DNA damaging effects of this agent (DROBNIK et al., 1973; BECK and BRUBAKER, 1973). Thus DROBNIK et al., 1973 studied the effects of cis Pt(II) on the colony-forming abilities of strains of *E. coli* mutated at the fil, exr and hcr loci and compared their different sensitivities with their known abilities to survive X- or UV-irradiation or treatment with an alkylating agent. An approximate sensitivity-increasing factor attributed to mutations at various loci is given in Table 13. The results indicated that the effects of mutations to the individual loci for the survival of colony forming ability is different after treatment with cis Pt(II) from that for treatment with *N*-methyl-N′-nitro-*N*-nitrosoguanidine or for UV- or X-irradiation. Mutation at the fil marker had a pronounced effect on the growing culture when it affected both filament formation and the preservation of colony forming ability. Some kinds of damage to the DNA of T-odd bacteriophage can be repaired by the enzymatic excision repair system of the host bacterium (host cell repair). The role played by the hcr locus is important for the survival of cells after UV irradiation but not after treatment with MNNG and only minimally so after treatment with cis Pt(II). This relatively minor importance of the hcr locus for the inactivation of *E. coli* by cis Pt(II) was confirmed by the observation that the bacteriophages T3 or T4 BOL after treatment with cis Pt(II) gives the same inactivation curves in both Hcr^+ and Hcr^- strains of the indicator bacteria (DROBNIK et al., 1975). Similarly it was found that platinum-treated transforming DNA does not appear to be more sensitive when assayed in a strain of *H. influenzae* which carries the uvrl mutation and hence lacks the activity of the specific UV endonuclease which incises UV-irradiated DNA (MUNCHAUSEN, 1974).

Table 13. The effect of mutation in individual loci on the relative sensitivity of colony forming ability to UV, X-irradiation, or cis Pt(II) and *N*-methyl-*N'*-nitro-*N*-nitrosoguanidine (NG). (Compiled by DROBNIK et al., 1973)

Phenotype tested	Other phenotypes	Inactivating treatment	Sensitivity increase factor	Reference
Fil^-/Fil^+	$Hcr^- Exr^+$	UV	11–12	2
	$Hcr^+ Exr^+$	UV	8–12	2
	$Hcr^+ Exr^+$	UV	4.0	1
	$Hcr^- Exr^+$	NG	3.1	2
	$Hcr^+ Exr^+$	cis Pt(II)	1.0	1
Exr^+/Exr^-	$Fil^- Hcr^+$	UV	2.7–4.5	2
	$Fil^+ Hcr^+$	UV	3.0	2
	$Fil^+ Hcr^+$	UV	6–(18.3)[a]	1
	$Fil^+ Hcr^+$	NG	3.0	2
	$Fil^+ Hcr^-$	NG	3.6	2
		X	1.65–1.93	3
	$Fil^+ Hcr^+$	cis Pt(II)	13.5	1
	$Fil^+ Hcr^+$	cis Pt(II)	23.0	1
Hcr^+/Hcr^-	$Fil^- Exr^+$	UV	8–15	2
	$Fil^- Exr^+$	UV	16.6	1
	$Fil^+ Exr^-$	UV	(1.4)[a]–4.3	1
	$Fil^- Exr^+$	NG	1.0	2
	$Fil^+ Exr^+$	NG	1.0	2
	$Fil^+ Exr^-$	NG	1.2	2
	$Fil^+ Exr^-$	cis Pt(II)	1.9	1
	$Fil^+ Exr^-$	cis Pt(II)	1.8	1
	$Fil^- Exr^+$	cis Pt(II)	5.0	1

Abbreviations: NG = *N*-methyl-*N'*-nitro-*N*-nitrosoguanidine.
[a] Taken from initial steep part of the curve.
References: (1) DROBNIK et al., 1973; (2) WITKIN, 1968; (3) RÖRSCH et al., 1966.

The role of the exr locus in determining the sensitivity of *E. coli* to various agents (Table 13) will be dicussed later in connection with other pathways of DNA repair.

Recently evidence has accumulated for the existence of a second excision repair process in both bacterial and mammalian cells, which is able to remove alkyl groups from DNA (possibly those on sites involved in hydrogen bonding (KIRTIKAR and GOLDTHWAIT, 1974)), as well as abnormal bases in DNA like uracil (LINDAHL, 1976). The first step involves the removal of a free base by the action of a *N*-glycosylase. The apurinic or apyrimidinic acid so produced is then a substrate for a specific apurinic acid or apyrimidinic acid endonuclease which incises the DNA. Subsequent steps in this excision process are possibly the same as those for the excision process previously described, namely degradation of a section of the DNA, followed by resynthesis and resealing to the original DNA strand. As a consequence of these various steps in either of the excision processes it could be envisaged that DNA which has been modified by physical and chemical agents will be reduced in size by the action of the

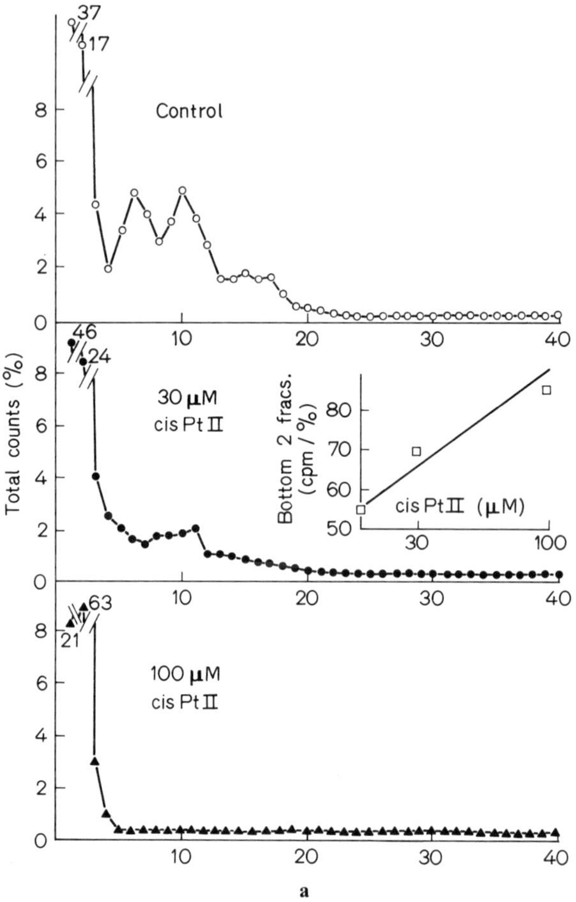

Fig. 21a and b. Alkaline sucrose gradient sedimentation profiles of [^{14}C]thymidine-labeled DNA from Chinese hamster cells, **a** immediately after a 2-h treatment with cis Pt(II). Inset the relationship between dose of cis Pt(II) and proportion of radioactivity recovered in fractions 1 and 2 ("700 s" region), **b** 21-h after a 2-h treatment. Greater than 92% recovery of applied radioactivity was observed in all gradients (van den Berg and Roberts, 1975a)

various endonucleases, and then after completion of the other steps in the repair process(es) be restored to its original size. Possibly, depending on the rates and extent of these various processes such changes could lead to a modification of the molecular weight of cellular DNA and be visualised by physicochemical techniques.

2. Mammalian Cell Studies

Alkaline sucrose gradient sedimentation of prelabelled cellular DNA following treatment of cells with cis platinum (II) diammine dichloride did not reveal any accumulation of low molecular weight DNA (van den Berg and Roberts,

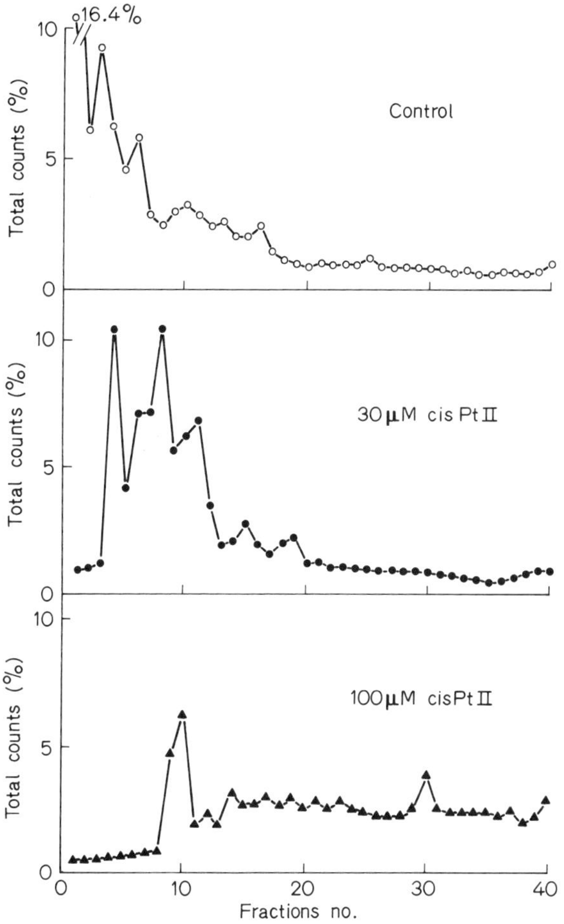

Fig. 21 b

1975). From a knowledge of the extent of reaction of the platinum compound with DNA at the concentration employed it could be concluded either that lesions were not generally recognized by an endonuclease which inserted "nicks" into DNA, or, alternatively, if the lesions were recognized by an endonuclease then completion of the later stages of the excision repair process(es) leads to the rapid restoration of high molecular weight DNA. Moreover, since any apurinic sites in DNA would be converted into DNA single strand breaks under these alkaline conditions there was no obvious evidence from these studies for the removal of substituted purines by means of a *N*-glycosylase. On the other hand, the time-dependent changes in the sedimentation profiles of fully labeled DNA which were observed following a pulse treatment of Chinese hamster cells with cis Pt(II) could be interpreted as being due to the initial formation of DNA interstrand or DNA-protein crosslinks that were subsequently removed during several hours, presumably by a DNA excision repair process (van den Berg and Roberts, 1975). In these experiments, mammalian cells were lysed under conditions which released labeled DNA which sedimented to positions in an alkaline sucrose gradient corresponding to sedimentation coefficients of 700 s and (a lesser proportion) 400–650 s (Fig. 21 a). Prior treatment with cis Pt(II) consistently resulted in a dose-dependent increase in the proportion of counts recovered in the 700 s region of the gradient at the expense of the DNA sedimenting in the 400–650 s region of the gradient (Fig. 21 a). Hence treatment of cells with these concentrations of cis Pt(II) hinders the release of DNA from the 700 s "complex".

It is probable that this effect is a consequence of crosslinking of complementary strands of DNA or of crosslinking DNA to protein which hinders its denaturation under alkaline conditions. cis Pt(II) has been found to increase the amount of protein cosedimenting with DNA and to inhibit the deproteination of DNA by phenol and its extraction into p-aminosalicyclic acid (Pascoe and Roberts, unpublished results). The subsequent changes in this sedimentation profile which occurred by 24 h after treatment, when the s value of the DNA (or complex) was reduced from 700 to 350, may reflect the enzymatic production of breaks in the DNA at platinum-damaged sites (Fig. 21). While these results cannot be fully interpreted at present because structures with such high s values are not fully defined, they do indicate that changes in the molecular weight of DNA or a DNA-protein complex do occur under physiological conditions which are compatable with the concept that platinum-induced damage in DNA can be repaired. Whether these changes contribute to the recovery of cells from the toxic action of the drug is still not clear. Cellular studies did not indicate any rapid recovery from the damaging effect of cis Pt(II) comparable to the classic split dose radiation recovery experiment normally regarded an indicative of repair. In fact lymphoma cells when exposed to a second dose of cis Pt(II) after an equal "priming" dose suffered more killing than that produced by the double dose given at one time (Drewinko and Gottlieb, 1975). Synergism was also noted when cis Pt(II) was given with camptothecin or BCNU but it is also not known if these agents can act at the molecular level to inhibit a cellular repair process in platinum-treated cells.

The rare skin condition *Xeroderma pigmentosum* (XP) is characterised by extreme sensitivity to sunlight and a predisposition to skin cancer. Cells taken from persons suffering from this condition are more sensitive to UV-irradiation than normal cells and are deficient in excision repair of UV-induced damage. These same cells are also sensitive to other DNA damaging agents such as hydrocarbon epoxides, 4-nitroquinoline-1-oxide and 7-bromomethylbenz(a)-anthracene and sensitivity is again associated with decreased levels of various manifestations of DNA excision repair (for review see Roberts, 1976). Moreover these findings were originally thought to indicate that the repair system which excises thymine dimers is also able to excise certain types of chemical damage. It has now been found that these repair deficient XP cells are also more sensitive than normal fetal lung cells to cis platinum (II) diammine dichloride, when the lethal effects of the drug are expressed as a function of reaction with DNA rather than as a function of dose of reagent. It could therefore be reasoned that this increased sensitivity of XP cells is similarly due to their decreased ability to excise cis Pt(II)-induced DNA damage (FRAVAL et al., 1978). If this conclusion is correct then the additional finding that an extract from *Micrococcus luteus* which can incise UV-irradiated DNA does not similarly incise cis Pt(II)-treated DNA would, however, indicate that different mechanisms are likely to be involved for the repair of the two types of damage.

C. Post Replication Repair (Replication Repair)

1. Bacterial Studies

From the previous discussion it would appear that the majority of DNA-platinum products, those involving one strand of a double helix, are chemically stable and refractory to enzymatic removal. If this is indeed so, then it could be supposed that persistent lesions in DNA are circumvented during DNA replication by an alternative repair process and one which is analogous to that which facilitates the survival of excision defective bacteria after UV-irradiation. Evidence has been adduced for the existence of processes which permit DNA replication to proceed on a radiation or chemically damaged DNA template in both microbial and mammalian cells. DNA which is synthesised on a template containing unexcised UV induced thymine dimers has been shown to be of smaller molecular weight than that synthesized in control cells. During the subsequent incubation of treated cells the newly-synthesized DNA increases in size and eventually attains the size of the DNA in control cells. Evidence has been adduced that gaps are initially left in the daughter DNA opposite thymine dimers in the template strand of DNA (RUPP and HOWARD-FLANDERS, 1968) and these gaps are subsequently filled by a process involving recombination which is controlled by the rec genes (RUPP et al., 1971) and/or de novo DNA synthesis which is probably controlled by the exr (now called lex) gene. It can be seen in Table 13 that mutation of Exr^+ to Exr^- resulted in an increase of 3–6 times in the sensitivity of *E. coli* toward UV and MNNG and less than a 2-fold increase in the sensitivity to the X-irradiation. On the other hand, the increase in sensitivity of colony forming ability to cis Pt(II) due to this mutation is 13–23 times. BECK and BRUBAKER (1973) reached a similar conclusion with regard to the important role of this particular repair pathway from a comparison of the effect of treatment with UV light and cis Pt(II) on cell survival and filamentation in recombination repair deficient mutants of *E. coli* K-12. The recombination repair deficient mutant *recA13* and the double mutant uvrA6 lex1 which is known to undergo extensive autodegradation of DNA after treatment with UV-irradiation were particularly sensitive to cis Pt(II). Additional evidence implicating attack on DNA by platinum compounds therefore came from the observation that degradation of DNA in *recA* mutants occurs following either UV-irradiation or treatment with cis Pt(II). The platinum compound also promoted the release of trichloracetic acid-insoluble fragments of DNA from growing cells. The nature of these products is not known but they may be analogous to the repair products which arise after treatment of bacteria with UV and certain radiomimetic chemicals.

2. Mammalian Cell Studies

a) General Comments. It now seems certain that mammalian cells also possess varying capacities to replicate their DNA on a template containing unexcised damage, which may be regarded as indicative of different levels of some form of so-called post-replication repair capacity. It is also apparent, however, that the mechanism of any such repair process differs from that which is thought to occur in bacteria. Newly synthesized DNA in some UV-irradiated mammalian cells is initially smaller than that in control cells and it has been proposed that gaps are left in new DNA opposite thymine dimers. The subsequent increase in the molecular weight of nascent DNA during post treatment incubation of cells (and defined operationally as post-replication repair) was, as for bacteria, thought to involve sealing of gaps. However, no evidence for recombinational exchanges was initially forthcoming. Instead it was proposed that so-called gaps are filled by de novo DNA synthesis (LEHMANN, 1972). [Some unconfirmed recent findings do however suggest that recombinational exchanges may also occur in irradiated mammalian cells to a limited extent (MENEGHINI, 1976; MENEGHINI and HANAWALT, 1976)].

On the other hand, others have argued that gaps are not formed in newly synthesized DNA but that there is simply a delay in the rate of synthesis at the site of each lesion (PAINTER, 1974). Thus it was found that the newly synthesized DNA in cis Pt(II) treated cells attained the same size as that in control cells if the post treatment incubation time was extended to allow for the same amount of overall DNA synthesis in treated and control cells (see later). It has further been proposed that the lesion can be circumvented during DNA replication by a mechanism involving strand displacement (FUJIWARA and TATSUMI, 1976; HIGGINS et al., 1976). However, irrespective of the mechanism involved in synthesizing past radiation or chemically induced lesions in DNA, it has been found that in some cells the process is amenable to inhibition by the trimethylxanthine, caffeine. Thus it has been shown that the rate of ligation of newly synthesized DNA in UV-irradiated (CLEAVER and THOMAS, 1969) and in *N*-acetoxy-2-acetylaminofluorene (TROSKO et al., 1973) *N*-methyl-*N*-nitrosourea (ROBERTS, 1975) or 7-bromomethylbenz(a)anthracene (ROBERTS et al., 1977) treated cells was dramatically impaired in the presence of caffeine. As a consequence of this inhibition, many cell lines, competent in this replicative by pass repair, are rendered extremely sensitive to the lethal effects of either UV-irradiation (RAUTH, 1967) or chemical damage (RAUTH et al., 1970; WALKER and REID, 1971; ROBERTS and WARD, 1973; ROBERTS et al., 1974; ROBERTS et al., 1977) by post treatment incubation in the presence of nontoxic concentrations of caffeine.

There is now ample evidence which indicates that UV- or X-irradiation or chemically induced cell death is a function of the amount of chromosome damage which can be observed at the first or second mitosis after treatment (GROTE and REVELL, 1972; SCOTT et al., 1974). Post treatment incubation in the presence of caffeine enhances dramatically the chromosome damaging effects of UV-irradiation and chemicals in both plant and animal cells (ROBERTS and STURROCK, 1973; KIHLMAN et al., 1974). Further evidence that the potentiating

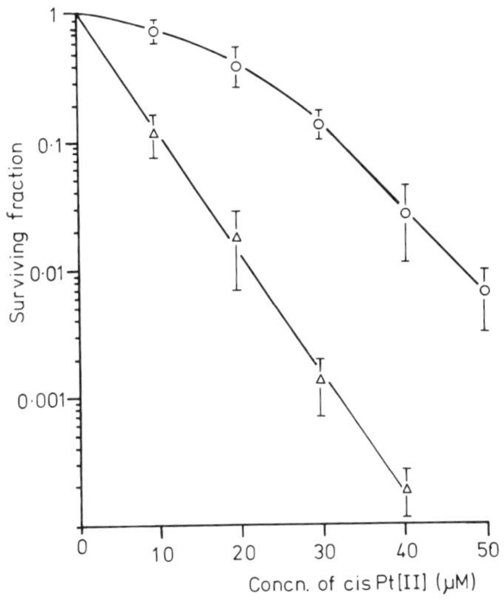

Fig. 22. Survival curves (based on colony forming ability) for treatment of Chinese hamster V79-379A cells in suspension culture with cis Pt(II) alone (○) or cis Pt(II) followed by growth in the presence of 0.75 mM caffeine (△). Cells were exposed to cis Pt(II) for 2 h at 37° C (VAN DEN BERG and ROBERTS, 1975b)

effects of caffeine are the result of inhibition of the above replicative by pass process by inhibiting ligation of newly synthesized DNA came from the S-phase specificity of these caffeine effects (DOMON and RAUTH, 1969; ROBERTS and WARD, 1973)

b) Effects of Caffeine on cis Pt(II)-Induced Cell Death and Chromosome Damage. The various cellular effects of cis Pt(II) and their modification by caffeine suggests that lesions are introduced onto DNA by platinum compounds which are also circumvented by a caffeine-sensitive repair process.

The effect of a 2 h treatment with cis Pt(II) and the potentiation of this effect by caffeine is shown in Fig. 22. It can be seen that the shoulder on the survival curve is completely abolished by post-treatment incubation in a nontoxic concentration of caffeine (VAN DEN BERG and ROBERTS, 1975). The potentiating effect of caffeine on cis Pt(II) induced lethality persists for approximately 12 h in asynchronously growing Chinese hamster cells and during the first S phase only after treatment during the G_1 phase of synchronously growing Chinese hamster cells (FRAVAL and ROBERTS, 1977a). In this respect, therefore, the response of cis Pt(II)-treated cells resembles that of UV-irradiated (DOMON and RAUTH, 1969) or sulfur mustard-treated cells (ROBERTS and WARD, 1973).

Cytological studies were made on Chinese hamster cells at various times after treatment with either cis Pt(II) alone or in combination with post treatment in a nontoxic concentration of caffeine, conditions which reduced ultimate cell survival to 50% and 4% respectively. Four hours after treatment with 15 μM cis Pt(II), the number of metaphases containing visible chromosomal abnormalities was not significantly above control level, and this proportion was unaffected

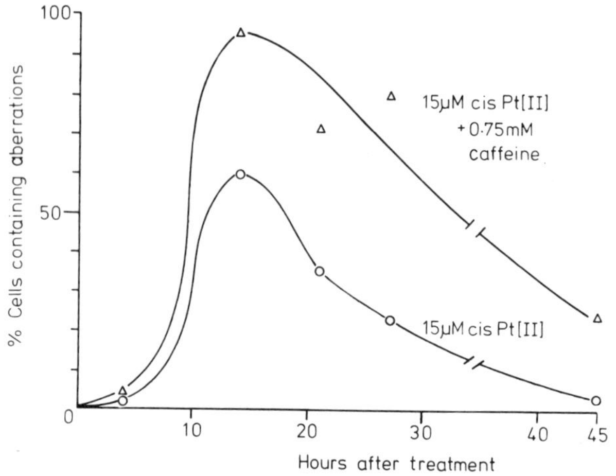

Fig. 23. Relationship between appearance of chromosomal aberrations and time after treatment with 15 µM cis (o—o) or 15 µM cis Pt(II) followed by growth in the presence of 0.75 mM caffeine (△—△). Cells were exposed to cis Pt(II) for 2 h at 37° C (VAN DEN BERG and ROBERTS, 1975b)

by caffeine (Fig. 23). By 14 h after treatment 60% of platinum-only treated cells contained chromosomal aberrations and this proportion declined to less than 5% by 45 h after treatment. Post-treatment incubation of cells in medium containing 0.75 m*M* caffeine dramatically increased the number of cells containing chromosome damage with only 4% of the metaphases being classified as normal by 14 h after treatment. Less than 1% of cells exposed to caffeine alone exhibited any chromosome abnormalities during the course of the experiment. Caffeine not only increases the number of cis Pt(II)-treated cells containing chromosomal aberrations, but it also enhances the severity of the damage observed. The most dramatic effect was a marked increase in the number of cells containing shattered chromosomes and those with numerous chromatid deletions and exchanges. The delayed appearance of chromosome abnormalities after cis Pt(II) treatment also suggests that DNA replication is necessary for their formation and in this respect cis Pt(II) resembles UV-irradiation and alkylating agents rather than X-irradiation.

The proposal has therefore been made that inadequate replication of DNA on a DNA-damaged template is responsible for both cell death and chromosome damage. The post-treatment incubation of cells in medium containing caffeine enhances the latter two effects of DNA damage by inhibiting a process which would permit replication to proceed past lesions. Support for this notion has come from studies on both the rate of DNA synthesis and the size of DNA synthesized in both asynchronous and synchronized populations of cis Pt(II) treated cells in the presence and absence of caffeine. A study of chromosome damage in Chinese ovary cells treated with another platinum drug revealed that gaps and breaks are found in the first mitosis after treatment while chromatid exchanges are present only in cells at the second mitosis (SZUMIEL and NIAS, 1976b), a response which according to BENDER et al. (1974), is characteris-

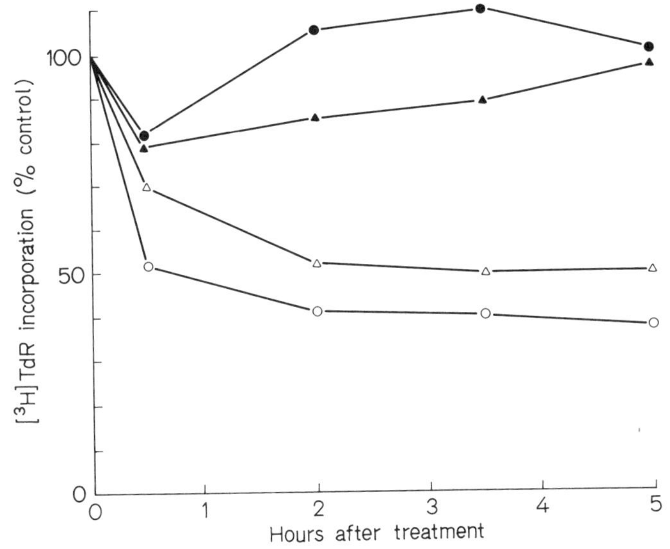

Fig. 24. The effect of cis Pt(II) on DNA synthesis in Chinese hamster V79–379A cells and the modifying influence of caffeine. After a 2 h treatment with 30 μM (△) or 50 μM (○) cis Pt(II), cells were resuspended in fresh medium in the absence (*open symbols*) or presence (*closed symbols*) of caffeine (0.75 mM), and DNA synthesis measured at the times shown by the incorporation of [^{3}H]TdR during 20′ into acid insoluble material (VAN DEN BERG and ROBERTS, 1976)

tic of compounds which produce lesions repaired by a post replication repair mechanism.

c) Effects of Caffeine on the Rate of DNA Synthesis in cis Pt(II)-Treated Asynchronous and Synchronous Cells. The dose-dependent depression in rate of synthesis in cis Pt(II) treated asynchronous Chinese hamster cells (Fig. 24 and see earlier) can be seen as a dose-dependent delay in the peak rate of DNA synthesis (mid-S) in G_1-treated synchronous populations of cells (Fig. 25) (FRAVAL and ROBERTS, 1978a). As a consequence of the dose-dependent extension of the time for passage through the S phase, cells were corresponding delayed in the time at which they underwent cell division. The overall amounts of DNA synthesized after treatment with three different doses of cis Pt(II), which resulted in a wide range of cell survivals, were not markedly different (i.e., the *areas* under the S phase peaks were similar).

However the amount of DNA synthesized in treated cultures at much later times after treatment (~20 h) was very much less than that in control cultures, being decreased in a dose-dependent manner. Part of the decreased amount of DNA synthesis was due to a decrease in the proportion of treated cells undergoing cell division and passage into the DNA synthetic phase of the following cell cycle as compared to untreated control cells. In addition, it appears that those cells which did pass into the next DNA synthetic phase in the following cell cycle synthesized DNA at a reduced rate relative to that in control cells. A possible explanation for this observation is that the DNA which had

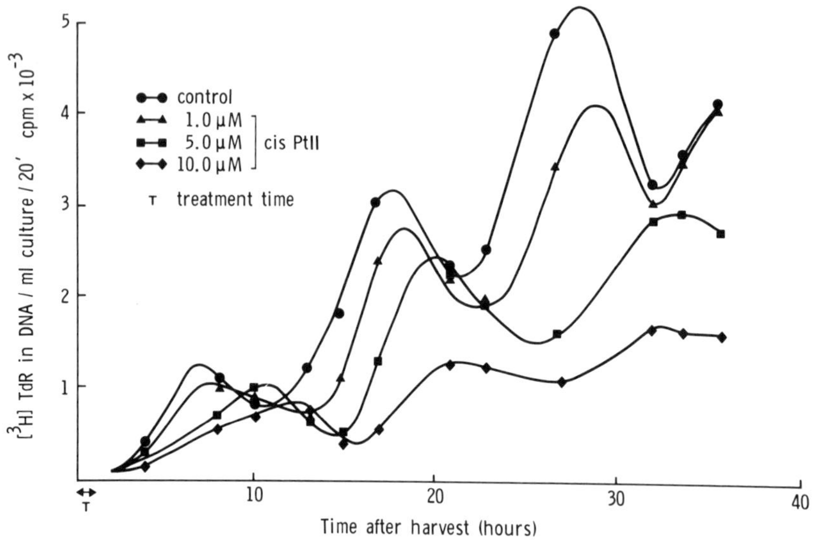

Fig. 25. The effect of treatment with cis Pt(II) during 1 h of the early G_1 phase of the Chinese hamster cell cycle on subsequent DNA synthesis (measured as in Fig. 24) (FRAVAL and ROBERTS, 1978a)

been synthesized on a damaged template during the first cell cycle was an inadequate template for further DNA replication in the succeeding cell cycle.

The apparent impaired $G_1 \rightarrow S$ transition reported to occur in Chinese hamster ovary cells treated with cis-dichlorobisdicyclopentylamine platinum (II) (SZUMIEL and NIAS, 1976b) may well be a manifestation of this depressed rate of DNA synthesis as discussed above.

It has been found that post treatment incubation in medium containing a nontoxic concentration of caffeine rapidly reverses the cis Pt(II) induced inhibition of DNA synthesis in asynchronous populations of cells and this reversal was most rapid in cells previously treated with the higher dose of the platinum compound (Fig. 24) (VAN DEN BERG and ROBERTS, 1976). Post-treatment incubation in the presence of caffeine of G_1-treated cells therefore leads to a reversal of the cis Pt(II) induced delay in the peak rate of DNA synthesis (Fig. 26). Under these conditions of cis Pt(II) and caffeine treatment the peak rate of synthesis now approximates in time of appearance to that in the control cells.

d) Effects of Caffeine on the Size of Newly Synthesized (Nascent) DNA in cis Pt(II)-Treated Cells. The immediate, dose-dependent selective and persistent inhibition of DNA synthesis induced in cis Pt(II) treated Chinese hamster cells as measured by the decreased uptake of (^{3}H)TdR, into DNA and as discussed above (Fig. 24) can also be visualized as a dose-dependent decrease in the size of pulse-labeled newly synthesized DNA in treated cells (VAN DEN BERG and ROBERTS, 1976). If, however, compensation is made for the reduction in the *rate* of DNA synthesis by increasing the labeling period in cis Pt(II)-treated cells then the alkaline sucrose gradient sedimentation profile of labeled DNA

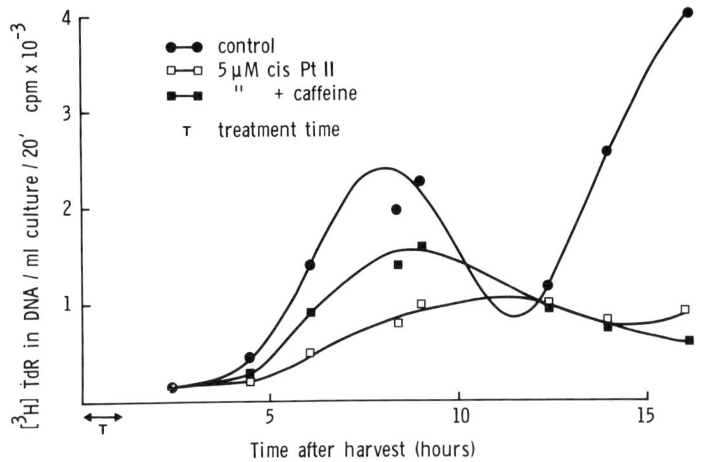

Fig. 26. The effect of treatment during 1 h of the G_1 phase of the cell cycle with cis Pt(II) alone (□——□), and following post treatment incubation in the presence of caffeine (■——■) on subsequent DNA synthesis (measured as in Fig. 24) (FRAVAL and ROBERTS, 1978a)

in treated cells is very similar to that of DNA in control untreated cells. It was concluded from such studies that the replicating machinery is delayed at the site of platinum-induced lesions in the template strand, but given sufficient time it can circumvent the lesions without forming discontinuities (gaps) in the newly synthesized DNA. Alternatively, if gaps are first formed opposite platinum reaction sites in DNA, then they must be rapidly filled and are too transitory for detection. In this respect, therefore, replication of DNA in cis platinum II diammine dichloride treated cells differs from that in some UV-irradiated cells (LEHMANN, 1972) in which so-called "gaps" can be detected (see earlier) but resembles that in *N*-acetoxy-2-acetylaminofluorene- (TROSKO et al., 1973) or 7-bromomethylbenz(a)anthracene-treated (ROBERTS et al., 1977) cells; in these latter studies no evidence was adduced for the presence of discontinuities (so-called gaps) in newly synthesized DNA.

The size of newly synthesized DNA in cis Pt(II)-treated cells may be contrasted with the size of such DNA in cells treated similarly with cis Pt(II) and labeled with (^{3}H)TdR in the presence of a non-toxic concentration of caffeine. Under these conditions the size of nascent DNA was markedly reduced as compared with that in untreated control or cis Pt(II)-only treated cells. The decrease in size of DNA was not the result of a decrease in overall rate of DNA synthesis since, as indicated earlier, the rate of DNA synthesis in cis Pt(II)-treated cells is faster in the presence of caffeine than in its absence. The size of the DNA synthesized during 4 h in the presence of caffeine in cis Pt(II)-treated cells was dependent on the initial dose of cis Pt(II) (Fig. 27). It thus appears that caffeine, in some as yet inexplicable manner, interferes with the mechanism by which the cell replicates DNA past lesions on the DNA template. Some support for this notion was obtained from a comparison of the distance between platinum-induced lesions on the template strand of

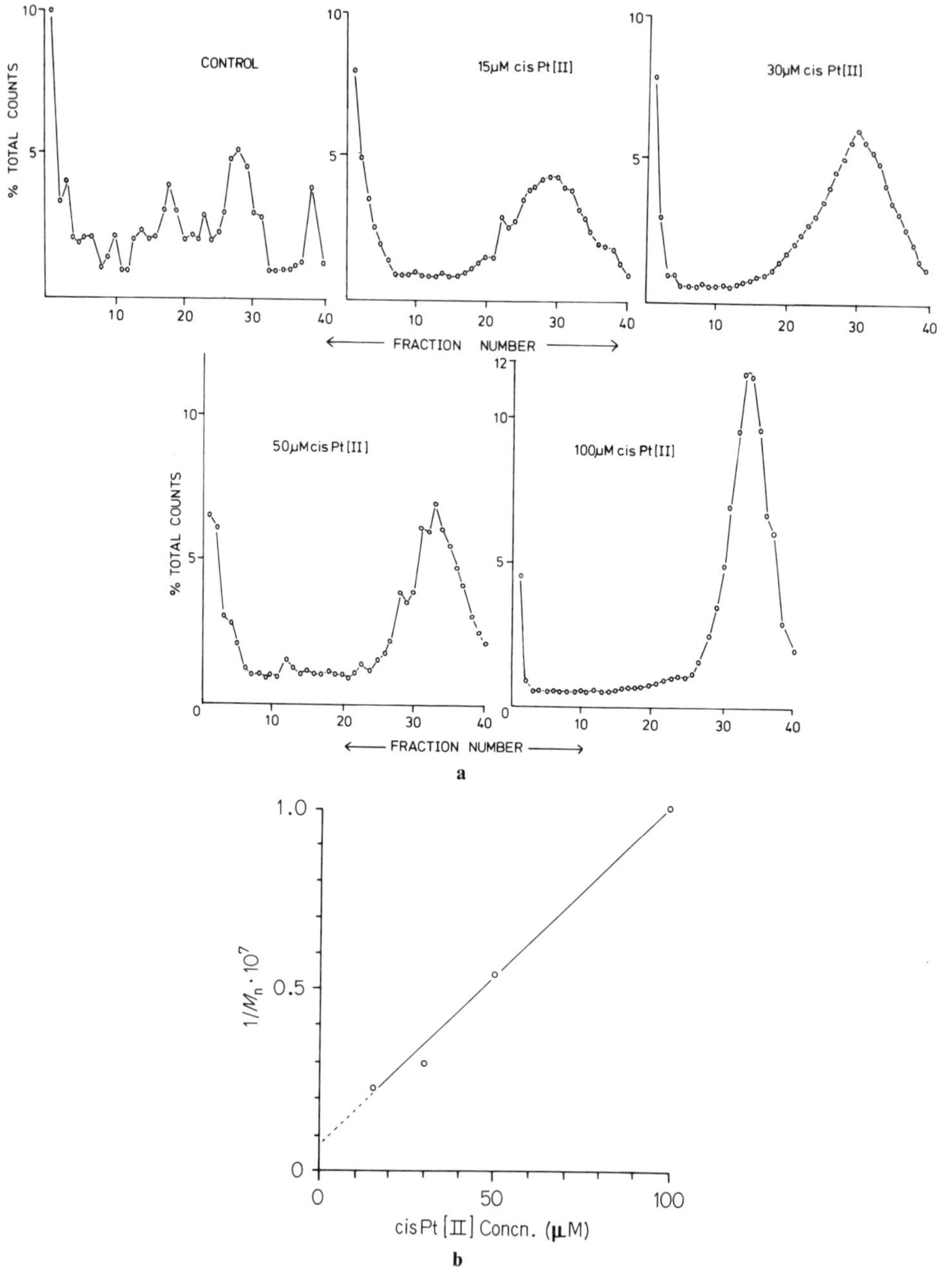

Fig. 27. a Alkaline sucrose gradient sedimentation profiles of DNA synthesized during a 2 h period in the presence of 0.75 mM caffeine in Chinese hamster cells treated for 2 h with various concentrations of cis Pt(II). Sedimentation analyses were performed after a 30 min incubation period in the absence of labelled precursor but in the presence of 0.75 mM caffeine. Sedimentation is from right to left. **b** Relationship between number average molecular weight (Mn) of DNA synthesized in the presence of 0.75 mM caffeine in Chinese hamster V79–379A cells treated with cis Pt(II) and the initial dose of cis Pt(II). The Mn values were derived from the sedimentation profiles shown in **a** (van den Berg and Roberts, 1976)

Table 14. Relationship between dose of cis Pt(II), level of binding to DNA, and molecular weight of DNA synthesized in the presence of 0.75 mM caffeine (VAN DEN BERG and ROBERTS, 1976). Figures in parenthesis were the previously published estimates of distance between platinations, which assumed smaller and variable molecular weights for DNA at the different doses of cis Pt(II) and which therefore allowed for an "end" platination. Revised estimates based on infinite length of DNA

Dose of *cis* Pt(II) (μ*M*)	Binding to DNA (μmol/g)	Calculated spacing between DNA platinations (daltons) × 10^{-7}	Mn of DNA synthesized (daltons) × 10^{-7}
30	0.040	5 (4.3)	3.5
50	0.076	2.6 (2.3)	1.85
100	0.111	1.8 (1.55)	0.95

DNA and the size of the newly synthesized DNA in cells treated with various doses of cis Pt(II) and post-incubated in the presence of caffeine. The distance between platinum atoms on one strand of DNA was calculated from atomic absorption measurements of the platinum bound to DNA isolated from cis Pt(II) treated cells and this was found to correspond closely to the size of the newly synthesized DNA (Table 14). It was concluded therefore that all platination reactions are normally circumvented during DNA replication by a caffeine-sensitive so-called DNA repair process. A model which depicts the effect of platinum lesions in DNA on the size and rate of synthesis of nascent DNA is shown in Fig. 28.

In hamster cells it is envisaged that DNA synthesis is delayed at the site of DNA-platinum adducts in DNA. If prior to sedimentation analysis of newly synthesized DNA this delay is compensated for by increasing the length of the labeling period, then, after treatment with low doses of cis Pt(II) no discontinuities are detectable in the daughter DNA. The absence of detectable gaps in the daughter DNA of cells exposed to concentrations of cis Pt(II) allowing some degree of cell survival suggests that either gaps are not formed at all, or that they are too transitory for detection. The absence of gaps under the above conditions is interpreted as representing the successful operation of a post replication repair system which allows the synthesis of a continuous daughter DNA molecule on a template containing unexcized damage. Caffeine inhibits this process by an as yet unknown mechanism. In so doing it causes the DNA replication machinery to proceed at a faster rate but to leave gaps in the newly synthesized DNA. These gaps seem to occur opposite lesions in the template strand of DNA (Table 14).

It has been proposed that the cellular process(es) which synthesize(s) high molecular weight DNA on a DNA template damaged by UV-irradiation or N-acetoxy-2-acetylaminofluorene (acetoxy-AAF) (D'AMBROSIO and SETLOW, 1976) may be inducible. The ability to ligate newly synthesized DNA in Chinese hamster cells treated with UV (CLEAVER and THOMAS, 1969) or N-acetoxy-2-acetylamino-fluorene (TROSKO et al., 1973) is also inhibited in the presence of caffeine. Conceivably therefore, caffeine could inhibit the induction of DNA replication enzymes required for this postulated inducible process.

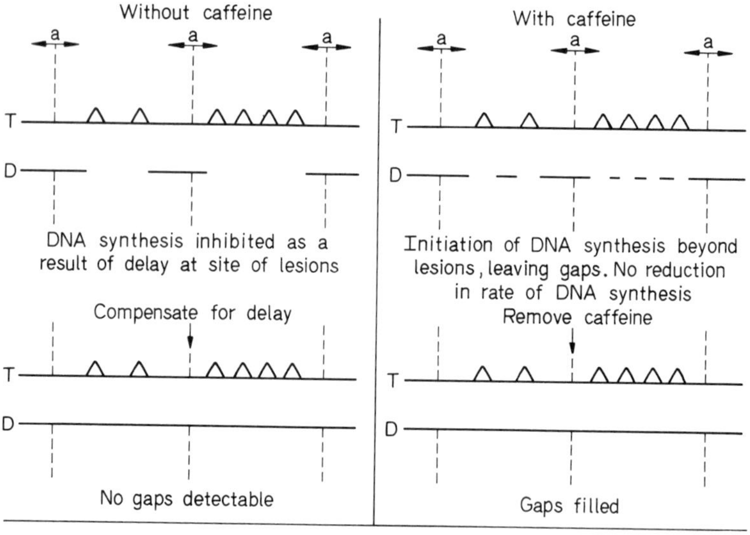

Fig. 28. DNA strand elongation in Chinese hamster cells treated with cis Pt(II) and the effects of caffeine. In the absence of caffeine (*left hand panel*) DNA synthesis is delayed at the site of DNA-platinum products (△). If the delay is compensated for, prior to sedimentation analyses by increasing the length of the labelling period, then no discontinuities in the daughter DNA strand are detectable. In the presence of caffeine (*right hand panel*) the DNA replicating machinery is no longer delayed at the site of DNA-platinum products (Figs. 24 and 25) but DNA synthesis is reinitiated beyond them with the formation of gaps presumably opposite the DNA-platinum products (Table 14). Whilst caffeine is present these gaps persist, but they are sealed on removal of caffeine from the incubation mixture

e) Comparisons Between HeLa and Chinese Hamster Cells. A comparison of the concentrations of cis Pt(II) which were required to achieve equal killing of HeLa and Chinese hamster cells (Pascoe and Roberts, 1974a; van den Berg and Roberts, 1975b; Fraval and Roberts, 1978a, b) indicated that HeLa cells were approximately three times as sensitive as hamster cells. A recent re-examination of the survival of these cells accompanying measured levels of binding of platinum to their DNA confirmed the greater sensitivity of Hella cells by a factor of nearly two on the basis of binding to their DNA rather than on the basis of dose of agent administered to the cells under equitoxic conditions (Fraval and Roberts, 1979). Previous studies using these two cell lines revealed no indications of major differences in their abilities to excise products from their DNA (Roberts et al., 1971; Roberts and Ward, 1973) and it was proposed that hamster cells possess a caffeine-sensitive replication repair process which was either not present in HeLa cells or if present, then only at a reduced level and then not amenable to inhibition by caffeine (Roberts et al., 1974). A comparison of the effect of a number of agents including cis Pt(II) on DNA synthesis in synchronized populations of HeLa and hamster cells appear to support this conclusion (Roberts et al., 1974). It can be seen in Fig. 29 that following the treatment of G_1 phase synchronous HeLa cells

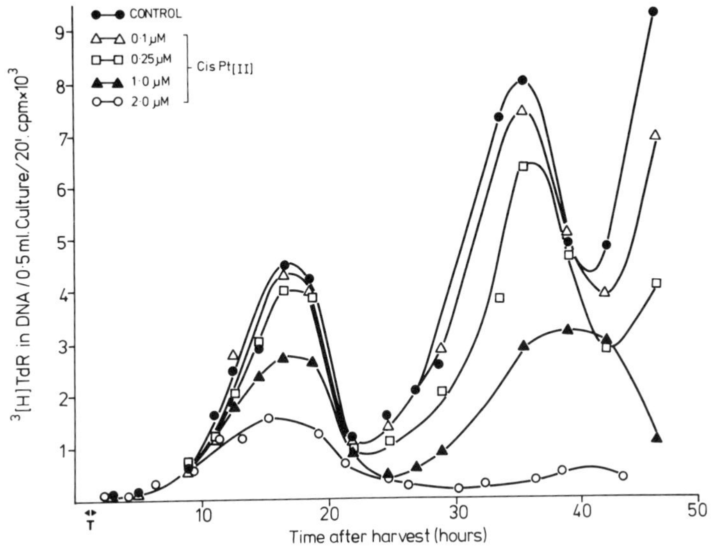

Fig. 29. The effect of treatment during the G_1 phase of synchronized HeLa cells on subsequent DNA synthesis. There is no delay in the time of appearance of the peak rate of DNA synthesis relative to that in the control culture (as in hamster cells, Fig. 25) but nevertheless a marked dose-dependent effect on overall DNA synthesis (FRAVAL and ROBERTS, 1978b)

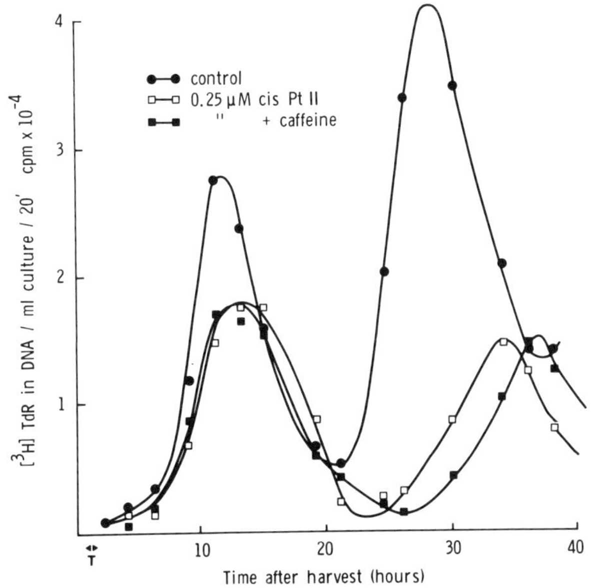

Fig. 30. The effect of treatment with cis Pt(II) (0.25 μM) with (■——■) and without (□——□) post treatment incubation in the presence of caffeine on DNA synthesis in synchronous HeLa cells (FRAVAL and ROBERTS, 1978b)

with cis Pt(II) the subsequent rate of DNA synthesis is reduced in a dose-dependent manner relative to that in control cells, but there is no delay in the time of appearance of the peak rate of DNA synthesis as was observed in similarly treated Chinese hamster cells (Fig. 26).

The delay in peak rate of DNA synthesis in chemically treated Chinese hamster cells had previously been interpreted as a reflection of the operation of some form of replication repair process which circumvents lesions in the template DNA. Delays in the peak rate of DNA synthesis have been noted following treatment of synchronous Chinese hamster cells with other agents which produced less lethality in Chinese hamster cells as compared with HeLa cells. The partial reversal by caffeine of this chemically induced delay in DNA synthesis was correspondingly interpreted as a manifestation of its ability to inhibit this particular repair process (ROBERTS and WARD, 1973; ROBERTS et al., 1977). Possibly, owing to the speeding up of the rate of DNA replication in the presence of caffeine, insufficient time is permitted for the replication machinery to circumvent lesions in the template strand – with the result that unligated or "gap containing" nascent DNA molecules are produced. Caffeine failed to modify DNA synthesis in cis Pt(II)-treated HeLa cells in the same manner as in Chinese hamster cells as would be expected on the above interpretation of its effects (Fig. 30).

Consistent with these observations was the failure of caffeine to potentiate the lethal effects of cis Pt(II) in HeLa cells.

VII. Concluding Remarks

This review has compiled a wealth of evidence which clearly indicates that DNA is the principal target molecule for neutral platinum complexes in a variety of biological systems. Currently the most convincing mechanism for the cytotoxic action of these agents on cells in culture is that reactions with DNA impair its function as a template for further DNA replication. Alternative mechanisms which have been proposed have not been supported by subsequent studies. A variety of reactions with DNA have now been described but it is not yet known whether all, or only some, of these are important in inactivating the DNA template. Only a proportion of these lesions seem to be recognized by a DNA excision repair process, but in Chinese hamster cells all seem to be recognized by a caffeine-sensitive process which facilitates the ability of the replicating machinery to synthesize past them. Inability to synthesize past lesions is associated with mitotic delay, chromosome damage and, eventually, cell death. It remains to be determined whether all other cytotoxic platinum compounds act by a similar mechanism.

The finding that cells can differ in their response to platinum compounds, due either to a decreased ability to excise lesions, as in the case of Xeroderma pigmentosum cells, or to a decreased ability to circumvent lesions during DNA replication by some form of replication repair as in the case of HeLa cells, leaves one hopeful that selective attack on tumor cells is feasible.

It has been found that caffeine can potentiate the antitumor activity of cyclophosphamide and nitrogen mustard in mice (GAUDIN and YIELDING, 1969) probably as a consequence of inhibition of the above replication repair system. Conceivably therefore, caffeine could be used in humans to achieve selective sensitization of tumor cells to the neutral platinum compounds.

With the discovery that enforced diuresis can dramatically decrease the kidney toxicity induced by these agents, one of the initial obstacles to their clinical application seems to have been overcome. On the basis of their present clinical status these agents clearly have a permanent place in the armamentarium of the clinician. Finally, the structure-activity relationships discussed in this review indicated that platinum complexes superior to those initially described are now available for clinical trials. Moreover the nature of these molecules allows considerable scope for the ingenuity of chemists to modify the structure to achieve compounds with possibly optimum solubility characteristics for achieving even greater selectivity.

Acknowledgments. I should like to record my appreciation of the acumen and foresight of the late Professor Sir Alexander Haddow who, when Director of Chester Beatty Research Institute, early recognized the importance of Prof. Barnett Rosenberg's elegant discoveries and inspired and encouraged many of us at the Institute to become similarly interested in the platinum compounds as cytotoxic agents. I am also most grateful to the Rustenberg Platinum Mines Ltd. who provided me with generous financial support to work with the compounds and to my post doctoral colleagues, Drs. Janet Pascoe, Hendric van den Berg and Hadrian Fraval who provided so many of their skills and much of their enthusiasm to produce the results with which I have personally been associated.

References

Aaronson, S.A.: Effect of ultraviolet irradiation on the survival of simian virus 40 functions in human and mouse cells. J. Virol. *6*, 393–399 (1970)

Aggarwal, S.K., Wagner, R.W., McAllister, P.K., Rosenberg, B.: Cell surface-associated nucleic acid in tumourogenic cells made visible with platinum-pyrimidine complexes by electron microscopy. Proc. Natl. Acad. Sci. *72*, 928–932 (1975)

Altstein, A.D., Deichman, G.I., Sarycheva, O.F., Dodonova, N.N., Tsetlin, E.M., Vassilieva, N.N.: Oncogenic and transforming activity of hydroxylamine inactivated SV 40 virus. Virology *33*, 746–748 (1967)

Anisimová, E., Roubal, J., Vlčková, I., Kutinová, L., Vonka, V.: Electron microscopic findings in EB-3 lymphoblastoid cell line exposed to *cis*-dichlorodiammine platinum (II). Acta Virol. *18*, 203–209 (1974)

Ball, C.R., Roberts, J.J.: DNA repair after mustard gas alkylation by sensitive and resistant Yoshida Sarcoma cells *in vitro*. Chem. Biol. Interact. *2*, 321–329 (1970)

Ball, C.R., Roberts, J.J.: Estimation of interstrand DNA cross linking resulting from mustard gas alkylation of HeLa cells. Chem. Biol. Interact. *4*, 297–303 (1971/2)

Beck, D.J., Brubaker, R.R.: Effect of *cis* platinum (II) diammine dichloride on wild type and deoxyribonucleic acid repair-deficient mutants of *Escherichia coli*. J. Bacteriol. *116*, 1247–1252 (1973)

Beck, D.J., Brubaker, R.R.: Mutagenic properties of *cis*-platinum (II) diammine-dichloride in *Escherichia coli*. Mutat. Res. *27*, 181–189 (1975)

Bender, M.A., Griggs, H.G., Bedford, J.C.: Mechanisms of chromosomal aberration production. III Chemicals and ionising radiation. Mutat. Res. *23*, 197–212 (1974)

Berg, van den, H.W., Roberts, J.J.: Investigations into the mechanism of action of anti tumour platinum compounds: time and dose-dependent changes in the alkaline sucrose gradient sedimentation profiles of DNA from hamster cells treated with *cis* platinum (II) diammine dichloride. Chem. Biol. Interact. *11*, 493–499 (1975a)

Berg, van den, H.W., Roberts, J.J.: Post replication repair of DNA in Chinese hamster cells treated with *cis* platinum (II) diammine dichloride. Enhancement of toxicity and chromosome damage. Mutat. Res. *33*, 279–284 (1975b

Berg, van den, H.W., Roberts, J.J.: Inhibition by caffeine of post replication repair in Chinese hamster cells treated with *cis* platinum (II) diammine dichloride: the extent of platinum binding to template DNA in relation to the size of low molecular weight nascent DNA. Chem. Biol. Interact. *12*, 375–390 (1976)

Braddock, P.D., Connors, T.A., Jones, M., Khokhar, A.R., Melzack, D.H., Tobe, M.L.: Structure and activity relationships of platinum compounds with anti-tumour activity. Chem. Biol. Interact. *11*, 145–161 (1975)

Bruckner, H.W., Cohen, C.C., Deppe, G., Kabakow, B., Wallach, R.C., Greenspan, E.M., Gusberg, S.B., Holland, J.F.: Chemotherapy of gynecological tumours with platinum II. J. Clin. Hematol. Oncol. *7*, 619–630 (1977)

Butour, J.-L., Macquet, J.-P.: Differentiation of DNA platinum complexes by fluorescence: the use of an intercalative dye as a probe. J. Clin. Hematol. Oncol. *7*, 469–486 (1977)

Carp, R.I., Kit, S., Melnick, J.L.: The effect of ultraviolet light on the infectivity and enzyme-inducing capacity of papovavirus SV40. Virology *29*, 503–509 (1966)

Cleare, M.J.: Some aspects of platinum complex chemistry and their relation to anti-tumour activity. J. Clin. Hematol. Oncol. *7*, 1–25 (1977)

Cleare, M.J., Hoeschele, J.D.: Studies on the anti-tumour activity of Group VIII transition metal complexes. Part I platinum (II) complexes. Bioinorg. Chem. *2*, 187–210 (1973a)

Cleare, M.J., Hoeschele, J.D.: Anti tumour platinum compounds. Relationships between structure and activity. Platinum Met. Rev. *17*, 1–13 (1973b)

Cleaver, J.E.: Repair replication of mammalian cell DNA: effects of compounds that inhibit DNA synthesis or dark repair. Radiat. Res. *37*, 428–435 (1969)

Cleaver, J.E.: Repair processes for photochemical damage in mammalian cells. In: Advances in radiation biology. Lett, J.T., Adler, H., Zelle, M. (eds.), Vol. 4, pp. 1–75. New York: Academic Press 1974

Cleaver, J.E., Thomas, G.H.: Single strand interruptions in DNA and the effects of caffeine in Chinese hamster cells irradiated with ultraviolet light. Biochem. Biophys. Res. Commun. *36*, 203–208 (1969)

Connors, T.A., Jones, M., Ross, W.C.J., Braddock, P.D., Khokhar, A.R., Tobe, M.L.: New platinum complexes with anti-tumour activity. Chem. Biol. Interact. *5*, 415–424 (1972)

Cramer, R.E., Dahlstrom, M.S.: The crystal and molecular structure of *cis* $[Pt(NH_3)_2(Guo)_2Cl_{3/2}$ $(ClO_4)_{1/2}7HO_2O$. J. Clin. Hematol. Oncol. *7*, 330–336 (1977)

D'Ambrosio, S.M., Setlow, R.B.: Enhancement of post replication repair in Chinese hamster cells. Proc. Natl. Acad. Sci. USA *73*, 2396–2400 (1976)

Davidson, J.P., Faber, P.J., Fischer, Jr., R.S., Mansy, S., Peresie, H.J., Rosenberg, B., Van Camp, L.: "Platinum Pyrimidine Blues" and related complexes: a new class of potent anti-tumour agents. Cancer Chemother. Rep. *59*, 287–300 (1975)

Domon, M., Rauth, A.R.: Ultraviolet light irradiation of mouse L-cells: effects on cells in the DNA synthesis phase. Radiat. Res. *40*, 414–429 (1969)

Douple, E.B., Richmond, R.C., Logan, M.E.: Therapeutic potentiation in a mouse mammary tumour and an intracerebral rat brain tumour by combined treatment with *cis* dichlorodiammine platinum (II) and radiation. J. Clin. Hematol. Oncol. *7*, 585–600 (1977)

Drewinko, B., Gottlieb, J.A.: Action of *cis*-dichlorodiammine platinum (II) (NSC 119875) at the cellular level. Cancer Chemother. Rep. *59*, 665–673 (1975)

Drewinko, B., Brown, B.W., Gottlieb, J.A.: The effect of *cis*-diamminedichloro platinum (II) on cultured human lymphoma cells and its therapeutic implications. Cancer Res. *33*, 3091–3095 (1973)

Drobnik, J., Urbánková, M., Krekulová, A.: The effect of *cis* dichlorodiammine platinum (II) on *Escherichia coli* B. Mutat. Res. *17*, 13–20 (1973)

Drobnik, J., Blahušková, A., Vasiluková, S., Krekulová, A.: Inactivation of bacteriophages with *cis*-platinum (II) diammine dichloride. Chem. Biol. Interact. *11*, 365–375 (1975)

Einhorn, L.H., Furnas, B.E., Powell, N.: Combination chemotherapy of disseminated testicular

carcinoma with *cis* platinum (II) diammine dichloride (CPDD) vinblastine (VLB) and bleomycin (Bleo). Proc. Am. Soc. Clin. Oncol. *17*, 240 (1976)
Epstein, M.A., Achong, B.G.: Specific immunoflorescence test for herpes-type EB virus of Burkitts lymphoblasts, authenticated by electron microscopy. J. Natl. Cancer Inst. *40*, 593–607 (1968)
Eshaque, M., McKay, M.J., Theophanides, T.: D-Mannitol platinum complexes. J. Clin. Hematol. Oncol. *7*, 338–345 (1977)
Fraval, H.N.A., Roberts, J.J.: The effect of *cis* platinum (II) diammine dichloride on survival and the rate of DNA synthesis in synchronously growing Chinese hamster V79-379A cells in the absence and presence of caffeine inhibited post replication repair. Evidence for an inducible repair mechanism. Chem. Biol. Interactions *23*, 99–110 (1978a)
Fraval, H.N.A., Roberts, J.J.: The effect of *cis* platinum (II) diammine dichloride on survival and rate of synthesis in synchronously growing HeLa cells in the absence and presence of caffeine Chem. Biol. Interactions *23*, 111–119 (1978b)
Fraval, H.N.A., Roberts, J.J.: G_1 phase Chinese hamster V79-379A and HeLa cells are inherently more sensitive to platinum bound to their DNA than mid S phase or asynchronously treated cells. Biochem. Pharmacol, in press (1979)
Fraval, H.N.A., Rawlings, C.J., Roberts, J.J.: Increased sensitivity of UV repair-deficient human cells to DNA-bound platinum products which unlike thymine diners are not recognized by an endonuclease extracted from *Micrococcus luteus*. Mutat. Res. *51*, 121–132 (1978)
Friedman, M.E., Melius, P.: Interactions of platinum (II) complexes with several oxido-reductases in the presence and absence of nucleic acids. J. Clin. Hematol. Oncol. *7*, 503–505 (1977)
Friedman, M.E., Teggins, J.E.: The reactivities of isomers of dichlorodiammine platinum (II) with dehydrogenase enzymes: evidence for inhibition via cross-linkage. Biochim. Biophys. Acta *350*, 263–272 (1974)
Fujiwara, Y., Tatsumi, M.: Replicative by pass repair of ultraviolet damage to DNA of mammalian cells: caffeine sensitive and caffeine resistant mechanisms. Mutat. Res. *37*, 91–116 (1976)
Gale, G.R., Howle, J.A., Walker, Jr. E.M.: Antitumour and antimitogenic properties of *cis* dichloro (dipyridine) platinum (II). Cancer Res. *31*, 950–952 (1971)
Gale, G.R., Rosenblum, M.G., Atkins, L.M., Walker, Jr. E.M., Smith, A.B., Meischen, S.J.: Antitumor action of *cis* dichloro bis(methylamine) platinum (II). J. Natl. Cancer Inst. *51*, 1227–1234 (1973)
Gale, G.R., Walker, Jr. E.M., Atkins, L.M., Smith, A.B., Meischen, S.J.: Antileukemic properties of dichloro(1,2-diaminocyclohexane) platinum (II). Res. Commun. Chem. Pathol. Pharmacol. *7*, 529–538 (1974)
Gale, G.R., Atkins, L.M., Meischen, S.J., Smith, A.B., Walker, E.M.: Combination therapy of L1210 leukemia with platinum compounds and cyclophosphamide plus selected other neoplastic agents. J. Natl. Cancer Inst. *57*, 1363–1366 (1976)
Gaudin, D., Yielding, K.L.: Response of 'resistant' plasmocytoma to alkylating agents and X-rays in combination with the excision repair inhibitors caffeine and chloroquine. Proc. Soc. Exp. Biol. Med. *131*, 1413–1416 (1969)
Gellert, R.W., Bau, R.: The structure of the platinum (ethylenediamine)-(guanosine)$_2$)$^{2+}$ cation. J. Am. Chem. Soc. *97*, 7379–7380 (1975)
Gerchman, L.L., Ludlum, D.B.: The properties of O^6-methylguanine in templates for RNA polymerase. Biochim. Biophys. Acta *308*, 310–316 (1973)
Giraldi, T., Taylor, D.M.: The effects of platinum ethylenediamine dichloride on the template activity of DNA. Biochem. Pharmacol. *23*, 1659–1661 (1974)
Goodgame, D.M.L., Jeeves, I., Phillips, F.L., Skapski, A.C.: Possible mode of action of anti-tumour platinum drugs: x-ray evidence for *cis* binding by platinum of two inosine 5'-monophosphates molecules via the N_7 positions. Biochim. Biophys. Acta *378*, 153–157 (1975)
Gottlieb, J.A., Drewinko, B.: Review of current clinical status of platinum coordination examples in Cancer Chemotherapy. Cancer Chemother. Rep. *59*, 621–628 (1975)
Grote, S.J., Revell, S.H.: Mitotic delay in Syrian hamster cells in relation to chromosome aberrations. Current Top. Radiat. Res. Q. *7*, 334–335 (1972)
Harder, H.C.: Renaturation effects of *cis* and *trans* platinum II and IV compounds on calf thymus deoxyribonucleic acid. Chem. Biol. Interact. *10*, 27–39 (1975)
Harder, H.C., Rosenberg, B.: Inhibitory effects of anti-tumour platinum compounds on DNA, RNA and protein synthesis in mammalian cells *in vitro*. Int. J. Cancer *6*, 207–216 (1970)

Harder, H.C., Smith, R.G., Leroy, A.F.: Template primer inactivation by *cis* and *trans* dichlorodiammine platinum for human DNA polymerase α, β and Rauscher murine leukemia virus reverse transcriptase, as a mechanism of cytotoxicity. Cancer Res. *36*, 3821–3829 (1976)

Hayes, D., Cvitkovic, E., Golbey, R., Scheiner, E., Krakoff, I.H.: Amelioration of renal toxicity of high dose *cis*-platinum (II) diammine dichloride (CPDD) by mannitol induced diuresis. Proc. Am. Ass. Cancer Res. *17*, 169 (1976)

Higby, D.J., Wallace, Jr. H.J., Albert, D.J., Holland, J.F.: Diaminochloroplatinum: a phase I study showing responses in testicular and other tumours. Cancer *33*, 1219–1225 (1974)

Higgins, N.P., Kato, K., Strauss, B.: A model for replication repair in mammalian cells. J. Mol. Biol. *101*, 417–425 (1976)

Hill, J.M., Loeb, E., Maclellan, A.S., Hill, N.O., Khan, A., Kogler, J.: Further clinical experience with *cis* platinum (II) diammine dichloride. Platinum coordination complexes in cancer chemotherapy. In: Recent results in cancer research. Connors, T.A., Roberts, J.J. (eds.), pp. 145–152. Berlin, Heidelberg, New York: Springer 1974

Hill, J.M., Loeb, E., Maclellan, A.S., Hill, N.O., Khan, A., King, J.J.: Clinical studies of platinum coordination compounds in the treatment of various malignant disease. Cancer Chemother. Rep. *59*, 647–659 (1975)

Hill, J.M., Loeb, E., Pardue, A.S., Khan, A., Hill, N.O., King, J.J., Hill, R.W.: Platinum coordination compounds in the treatment of acute leukemia and other malignant diseases with particular reference to malonato-1,2-diaminocyclohexane platinum (II). J. Clin. Hematol. Oncol. *7*, 681–698 (1977)

Horáček, P., Drobnik, J.: Interaction of *cis*-dichlorodiammine platinum II with DNA. Biochim. Biophys. Acta *254*, 341–347 (1971)

Howle, J.A., Gale, G.R.: *cis* Dichlorodiammine platinum (II): cytological changes induced in *Escherichia coli*. J. Bacteriol. *103*, 259–260 (1970a)

Howle, J.A., Gale, G.R.: *Cis*-dichlorodiammine platinum (II) persistent and selective inhibition of deoxyribonucleic acid synthesis *in vivo*. Biochem. Pharmacol. *19*, 2757–2762 (1970b)

Howle, J.A., Thompson, H.S., Stone, A.E., Gale, G.R.: *cis*-dichlorodiammine platinum (II). Inhibition of nucleic acid synthesis in lymphocytes stimulated with phytohemagglutinin. Proc. Soc. Exp. Biol. Med. *137*, 820–825 (1971)

Kara, J., Svoboda, J., Drobnik, J.: *Cis*-dichlorodiammine platinum (II): irreversible inhibition of DNA synthesis and cell growth in tissue culture and inhibition of chick embryo cell transformation by Rous sarcoma virus. Advances in antimicrobial and antineoplastic chemotherapy. Proc. VIIth Int. Congr. Chemother. Abstract, 1972

Kelman, A.D., Peresie, H.J., Stone, P.J.: An analysis of the models of binding of antitumour platinum complexes to DNA. J. Clin. Hematol. Oncol. *7*, 440–451 (1977)

Kihlman, B.A., Sturelid, S., Hartley-Asp, B., Nilsson, K.: The enhancement by caffeine of the frequencies of chromosomal aberrations induced in plant and animal cells by chemical and physical agents. Mutat. Res. *26*, 105–122 (1974)

Kirtikar, D.M., Goldthwait, D.A.: The enzymatic release of O^6-methylguanine and 3-methyladenine from DNA reacted with the carcinogen *N*-methyl *N*-nitrosourea. Proc. Natl. Acad. Sci. USA *71*, 2022–2026 (1974)

Kleinwächter, V., Zăludová, R.: Reactions of *cis* and *trans* isomers of platinum (II) diammine dichloride with purine, adenine and its derivatives in dilute solution. Chem. Biol. Interact. *16*, 207–222 (1977)

Kociba, R.J., Sleight, S.D., Rosenberg, B.: Inhibition of Dunning ascitic leukemia and Walker 256 carcinosarcoma with *cis*-diammine dichloride platinum (II). Cancer Chemother. Rep. *54*, 325–328 (1970)

Krakoff, I.H., Lippman, A.J.: Clinical trial of *cis* platinum (II) diammine chichloride in patients with advanced cancer. Platinum coordination complexes in cancer chemotherapy. In: Recent results in cancer research. Connors, T.A., Roberts, J.J. (eds.), pp. 183–190. Berlin, Heidelberg, New York: Springer 1974

Kutinová, L., Vonka, V., Drobnik, J.: Inactivation of papovavirus SV 40 by *cis*-dichlorodiammine platinum (II). Neoplasma *19*, 453–458 (1972)

Lajarjet, R., Cramer, R., Montagnier, L.: Inactivation by UV, X and gamma radiations of the infecting and transforming capacities of polyoma virus. Virology *33*, 104–111 (1967)

Lawley, P.D., Lethbridge, J.H., Edwards, P.A., Shooter, K.V.: Inactivation of bacteriophage T7 by mono- and difunctional sulphur mustards in relation to cross-linking and depurination of bacteriophage DNA. J. Mol. Biol. *39*, 181–189 (1969)

Lecointe, P., Macquet, J.-P., Butour, J.-L., Paoletti, C.: Relative efficiencies of a series of square planar platinum (II) compounds on salmonella mutagenesis. Mutat. Res. *48*, 139–144 (1977)

Lehmann, A.R.: Post replication repair of DNA in ultraviolet-irradiated mammalian cells. J. Mol. Biol. *66*, 319–337 (1972)

Leonard, B.J., Eccleston, E., Jones, D., Todd, P., Walpole, A.: Antileukemic and nephrotoxic properties of platinum compounds. Nature (London) *234*, 43–45 (1971)

Lindahl, T.: New class of enzymes acting on damaged DNA. Nature (London) *259*, 64–66 (1976)

Loeb, E., Hill, J.M., Pardue, A.S., Hill, N.O., Khan, A., King, J.J.: Solid tumour experience with newer platinum coordination compounds. J. Clin. Hematol. Oncol. *7*, 701–709 (1977)

Loveless, A.: Possible relevance of 0–6 alkylation of deoxyguanosine to the mutagenicity and carcinogenicity of nitrosamines and nitrosamides. Nature (London) *223*, 206–207 (1969)

Macquet, J.P., Theophanides, T.: DNA-platinum interactions *in vitro* with *trans* and *cis* $Pt(NH_3)_2Cl_2$. Bioinorg. Chem. *5*, 59–66 (1975)

Mansy, S., Rosenberg, R., Thomson, A.J.: Binding of *cis* and *trans*-dichlorodiammine platinum (II) to nucleosides I, location of binding sites. J. Amer. Chem. Soc. *95*, 1633–1640 (1973)

McAllister, P.K., Rosenberg, B., Aggarwal, S.K., Wagner, R.W.: Electron microscope studies of mammalian cells stained with platinum pyrimidine blues. J. Clin. Hematol. Oncol. *7*, 717–724 (1977)

Meneghini, R.: Gaps in DNA synthesised by ultraviolet light irradiated W138 human cells. Biochim. Biophys. Acta *425*, 419–427 (1976)

Meneghini, R., Hanawalt, P.: T4-endonuclease V sensitive sites in DNA from ultraviolet-irradiated human cells. Biochim. Biophys. Acta *425*, 428–437 (1976)

Millard, M.M., Macquet, J.P., Theophanides, T.: X-ray photoelectron spectroscopy of DNA-Pt complexes. Evidence of O^6 (Gua)-N_7(Gua) chelation of DNA with *cis*-dichlorodiammine platinum (II). Biochim. Biophys. Acta *402*, 166–170 (1975)

Monti-Bragadin, C., Tamaro, M., Banfi, E.: Mutagenic activity of platinum and ruthenium complexes. Chem. Biol. Interact. *11*, 469–472 (1975)

Munchausen, L.L.: The chemical and biological effects of *cis* dichlorodiammine platinum (II), an antitumour agent, on DNA. Proc. Natl. Acad. Sci. USA *71*, 4519–4522 (1974)

Munchausen, L.L., Rahn, R.O.: Physical studies on the binding of *cis*-dichlorodiammine platinum (II) to DNA and homopolynucleotides. Biochim. Biophys. Acta *414*, 242–255 (1975)

Nias, A.H.W., Szumiel, I.I.: The effects of *cis*-dichlorobiscyclopentylamine platinum (II) (PAD) and *cis*-dichlorobisisopropylamine *trans*-dihydroxy platinum (IV) (CHIP) and radiation on CHO cells. J. Clin. Hematol. Oncol. *7*, 562–566 (1977)

Ogawa, M., Gale, R.G., Meischen, S.J., Cooke, V.A.: Effects of dinitrato(1,2-diaminohexane) platinum on murine myeloma and hemopoietic precursor cells. Cancer Res. *36*, 3185–3188 (1976)

Page, R.H., Talley, R.W., Buhagiar, J.: The enhanced anti-tumour activity of *cis* diamminedichloro platinum (II) against murine tumours when combined with other agents. J. Clin. Hematol. Oncol. *7*, 96–102 (1977)

Painter, R.B.: DNA damage and repair in eukaryotic cells. Genetics *78*, 139–148 (1974)

Pascoe, J.M., Roberts, J.J.: Interactions between mammalian cell DNA and inorganic platinum compounds. I DNA interstrand cross-linking and cytotoxic properties of platinum (II) compounds. Biochem. Pharmacol. *23*, 1345–1357 (1974a)

Pascoe, J.M., Roberts, J.J.: Interactions between mammalian cell DNA and inorganic platinum compounds II. Interstrand cross-linking of isolated and cellular DNA by platinum (IV) compounds. Biochem. Pharmacol. *23*, 1359–1365 (1974b)

Plant, J.E., Roberts, J.J.: A novel mechanism for the inhibition of DNA synthesis following methylation. The effect of *N*-methyl-*N*-nitrosourea on HeLa cells. Chem. Biol. Interactions *3*, 337–342 (1971a)

Plant, J.E., Roberts, J.J.: Extention of the pre-DNA synthetic phase of the cell cycle as a consequence of DNA alkylation in Chinese hamster cells: A possible mechanism of DNA repair. Chem. Biol. Interact. *3*, 343–351 (1971b)

Rauth, A.M.: Evidence for dark reactivation of ultraviolet light damaged DNA in mouse L cells. Radiat. Res. *31*, 121–128 (1967)

Rauth, A.M., Barton, B., Lee, C.P.Y.: Effects of caffeine on L cells exposed to mitomycin C. Cancer Res. *30*, 2724–2729 (1970)

Renshaw, E., Thomson, A.J.: Tracer studies to locate the site of platinum ions within filamentous and inhibited cells of *Escherichia coli*. J. Bacteriol. *94*, 1915–1918 (1967)

Reslova, S.: Induction of lysogenic strains of *Escherichia coli* by *cis*-dichlorodiammine platinum (II). Chem. Biol. Interact. *4*, 66–70 (1971/2)

Reslova, S., Srogl, M., Drobnik, J.: The transforming activity of *B. subtilis* DNA treated with *cis* Pt II complexes. Advances in antimicrobial and antineoplastic chemotherapy. Vol. II, p. 209. Baltimore: Univ. Park Press 1972

Richmond, R.C., Powers, E.L.: Radiation sensitization of bacterial spores by *cis* dichlorodiammine platinum (II). Radiat. Res. *68*, 251–257 (1976)

Robbins, A.B.: The reaction of ^{14}C-labelled platinum ethylenediamine dichloride with nucleic acid constituents. Chem. Biol. Interact. *6*, 35–45 (1973)

Roberts, J.J.: Repair of alkylated DNA. In: Molecular mechanism for repair of DNA, part B. Hanwalt, P.C., Setlow, R.B. (eds.), pp. 611–615. New York: Plenum Publishing Corp. 1975

Roberts, J.J.: DNA repair and carcinogenesis. In: Scientific foundation of oncology. Symington, T., Carter, R.L. (eds.), pp. 319–333. London: Heinmann Medical Books Ltd. 1976

Roberts, J.J., Pascoe, J.M.: Cross linking of complementary strands of DNA in mammalian cells by anti tumour platinum compounds. Nature (London) *235*, 282–284 (1972)

Roberts, J.J., Sturrock, J.E.: Enhancement by caffeine of *N*-methyl-*N*-nitrosourea induced mutations and chromosome aberrations in Chinese hamster cells. Mutat. Res. *20*, 243–255 (1973)

Roberts, J.J., Ward, K.N.: Inhibition of post replication repair of alkylated DNA by caffeine in Chinese hamster cells but not HeLa cells. Chem. Biol. Interact. *7*, 241–264 (1973)

Roberts, J.J., Brent, T.P., Crathorn, A.R.: Evidence for the inactivation and repair of the mammalian DNA template after alkylation by mustard gas and half mustard gas. Eur. J. Cancer *7*, 515–524 (1971)

Roberts, J.J., Sturrock, J.E., Ward, K.N.: The enhancement by caffeine of alkylation induced cell death, mutations and chromosomal aberrations in Chinese hamster cells as a result of inhibition of post replication DNA repair. Mutat. Res. *26*, 129–143 (1974)

Roberts, J.J., Friedlos, F., Van den Berg, H.W., Kirkland, D.J.: Inhibiton by caffeine of post replication repair in Chinese hamster cells treated with 7-bromomethylbenz(*a*)anthracene: enhancement of toxicity, chromosome damage and inhibition of ligation of newly-synthesised DNA. Chem. Biol. Interact. *17*, 265–290 (1977)

Roos, I.A.G.: The interaction of an anti-tumour platinum complex with DNA. Chem. Biol. Interact. *16*, 39–55 (1977)

Roos, I.A.G., Arnold, M.C.: Interaction of anti-tumour active platinum complex with DNA. J. Clin. Hematol. Oncol. *7*, 374–388 (1977)

Roos, I.A.G., Thomson, A.J., Mansy, S.: Inter-action of platinum compounds with dinucleotides. J. Am. Chem. Soc. *96*, 6484–6091 (1974)

Rorsch, A., Van de Putte, P., Mattern, I.E., Zwenk, H.: Genetic and enzymatic control of radiation sensitivity in *Escherichia coli* – genetic aspects of radiosensitivity; mechanism of repair, p. 105–129. Vienna: Int. At. Energy Agency 1966

Rosenberg, B.: Platinum coordination complexes in cancer chemotherapy. Naturwissenschaften *60*, 399–406 (1973)

Rosenberg, B.: Possible mechanisms for the anti-tumour activity of platinum coordination complexes. Cancer Chemother. Rep. *59*, 589–598 (1975)

Rosenberg, B.: On the mechanisms of action of platinum complexes as anti cancer agents. J. Clin. Hematol. Oncol. *7*, 817–823 (1977)

Rosenberg, B., Van Camp, L.: The successful regression of large solid sarcoma 180 tumours by platinum compounds. Cancer Res. *30*, 1799–1802 (1970)

Rosenberg, B., Van Camp, L., Krigas, T.: Inhibition of cell division in *Escherichia coli* by electrolysis products from a platinum electrode. Nature (London) *203*, 698–699 (1965)

Rosenberg, B., Van Camp, L., Grimley, E.B., Thomson, A.J.: The inhibition of growth and cell division in *Escherichia coli* by different ionic species of platinum (IV) complexes. J. Biol. Chem. *242*, 1347–1352 (1967a)

Rosenberg, B., Renshaw, E., Van Camp, L., Hartwick, J., Drobnik, J.: Platinum-induced filamentous growth in *Escherichia coli*. J. Bacteriol. *93*, 1347–1352 (1967b)

Rosenberg, B., Van Camp, L., Trosko, J.E., Mansour, V.H.: Platinum compounds: a new class of potent anti tumour agents. Nature (London) *222*, 385–386 (1969)

Rozencweig, M., Von Hoff, D.D., Penta, J.S., Muggia, F.M.: Clinical status of *cis* diammine dichloroplatinum II. J. Clin. Hematol. Oncol. *7*, 672–680 (1977)

Rupp, W.D., Howard-Flanders, P.: Discontinuities in the DNA synthesised in an excision defective strain of *E. coli* following ultraviolet irradiation. J. Mol. Biol. *31*, 291–304 (1968)

Rupp, W.D., Wilde III, C.E., Reno, D.L., Howard-Flanders, P.: Exchanges between DNA strands in ultraviolet-irradiated *E. coli*. J. Mol. Biol. *61*, 25–44 (1971)

Scott, D., Fox, M., Fox, B.W.: The relationship between chromosomal aberrations, survival and DNA repair in tumour cell lines of different sensitivity to X-rays and sulphur mustard. Mutat. Res. *22*, 207–221 (1974)

Shooter, K.V., Edwards, P.A., Lawley, P.D.: The action of mono- and difunctional sulphur mustards on the ribonucleic acid-containing bacteriophage μ2. Biochem. J. *125*, 829–840 (1971)

Shooter, K.V., Howse, R., Merrifield, R.K., Robbins, A.B.: The interaction of platinum II compounds with bacteriophages T7 and R17. Chem. Biol. Interact. *5*, 289–307 (1972)

Slater, T.F., Ahmed, M., Ibrahim, S.A.: Studies of the nephrotoxicity of *cis*-dichlorodiammine platinum^{2+} and related substances. J. Clin. Hematol. Oncol. *7*, 534–546 (1977)

Speer, R.J., Ridgeway, H., Stewart, D.P., Hall, L.M., Zapata, A., Hill, J.M.: Sulphato 1,2-diaminocyclohexane-platinum (II): a potential new anti-tumour agent. J. Clin. Hematol. Oncol. *7*, 210–219 (1977)

Stansly, P.G., Soule. H.D.: Transplantation and cell free transmission of a reticulum-cell sarcoma in BALB/c mice. J. Natl. Cancer Inst. *29*, 1083–1105 (1962)

Stone, P.J., Kelman, A.D., Sinex, F.M.: Specific binding of anti tumour drug *cis* $Pt(NH_3)_2Cl_2$ to DNA rich in guanine and cytosine. Nature (London) *251*, 736–737 (1974)

Stone, P.J., Kelman, A.D., Sinex, F.M., Bhargava, M.M., Halvorson, H.O.: Resolution of α, β and γ DNA of *saccharomyces cerevisiae* with the antitumour drug *cis* $Pt(NH_3)_2Cl_2$. Evidence for preferential drug binding by GpG sequences of DNA. J. Mol. Biol. *104*, 793–801 (1976)

Szumiel, I.I., Nias, N.H.W.: The effect of combined treatment with a platinum complex and ionizing radiation on Chinese hamster ovary cells in vitro. Br. J. Cancer *33*, 450–458 (1976a)

Szumiel, I.I., Nias, A.H.W.: Action of a platinum complex [*cis*-dichlorobis-(cyclopentylamine)]-platinum (II) on Chinese hamster cells in vitro. Chem. Biol. Interact. *14*, 217–232 (1976b)

Talley, R.W.: Chemotherapy of a mouse reticulum cell sarcoma with platinum salts. Proc. Am. Assoc. Cancer Res. *11*, 78 (1970)

Tamburro, A.M., Celotti, L., Furlan, D., Guantieri, V.: Interaction of Pt(II) complexes with DNA: from various sources, a circular dichroism study. Chem. Biol. Interact. *16*, 1–4 (1977)

Taylor, D.M., Tew, K.D., Jones, J.D.: Effects of *cis*-dichlorodiammine platinum (II) on DNA synthesis in kidney and other tissues of normal and tumour-bearing rats. Eur. J. Cancer *12*, 249–254 (1976)

Teggins, J.E., Friedman, M.E.: The inhibition of malate dehydrogenase by chloroammine-platinum complexes. Biochim. Biophys. Acta *350*, 273–276 (1974)

Thomson, A.J.: The interaction of platinum compounds with biological molecules. Platinum coordination complexes in cancer chemotherapy. In: Recent results in cancer research. Connors, T.A., Roberts, J.J. (eds.), pp. 38–62. Berlin, Heidelberg, New York: Springer 1974

Thomson, A.J., Williams, R.J.P., Reslova, S.: The chemistry of complexes related to *cis* $Pt(NH_3)_2Cl_2$ an anti tumour drug. Struct. Bonding (Berlin) *11*, 1–46 (1972)

Thomson, A.J., Roos, I.A.G., Graham, R.D.: The nature of a purple platinum complex. J. Clin. Hematol. Oncol. *7*, 242–256 (1977)

Tobe, M.L., Khokhar, A.R.: Structure activity, reactivity and solubility relationships of platinum diamine complexes. J. Clin. Hematol. Oncol. *7*, 114–136 (1977)

Trosko, J.E.: Mutagenicity of *cis* platinum II diammine dichloride in Chinese hamster cells. Platinum coordination complex in cancer chemotherapy. In: Recent results in cancer research. Connors, T.A., Roberts, J.J. (eds.), p. 108. Berlin, Heidelberg, New York: Springer 1974

Trosko, J.E., Frank, P., Chu, E.H.Y., Becker, J.E.: Caffeine inhibition of post replication repair of *N*-acetoxy-2-acetylaminofluorene-damaged DNA in Chinese hamster cells. Cancer Res. *33*, 2444–2449 (1973)

Vonka, V., Kutinová, L., Drobnik, J., Bräuerová, J.: Increase of Epstein-Barr virus positive cells in EB-3 cultures after treatment with *cis* dichlorodiammine platinum (II). J. Natl. Cancer Inst. *48*, 1277–1281 (1972)

Walker, E.M. Jr., Gale, G.R.: Anti-leukemic synergism between cyclophosphamide and an anti-tumour platinum compound. Research Commun. Chem. Pathol. Pharmacol. *6*, 419–423 (1973)

Walker, I.G., Reid, B.D.: Caffeine potentiation of the lethal effects of alkylating agent on L cells. Mutat. Res. *12*, 101–104 (1971)

Wallace, H.J., Higby, D.J.: Phase I evaluation of *cis*-platinum diammine dichloride (PDD) and a combination of PDD plus adriamycin. Platinum coordination complexes in cancer chemotherapy. In: Recent results in cancer research. Connors, T.A., Roberts, J.J. (eds.), pp. 167–177. Berlin, Heidelberg, New York: Springer 1974

Welsh, C.W.: Growth inhibition of rat mammary carcinoma induced by *cis*-platinum diammino-dichloride II. J. Natl. Cancer Inst. *47*, 1071–1078 (1971)

Wiltshaw, E., Carr, B.: *Cis*-platinum diammine dichloride: clinical experience at the Royal Marsden Hospital, London. Platinum coordination complexes in cancer chemotherapy. In: Recent results in cancer research. Connors, T.A., Roberts, J.J. (eds.), pp. 178–182. Berlin, Heidelberg, New York: Springer 1974

Wiltshaw, E., Kroner, T.: Phase II study of *cis* dichloro diammine platinum (II) in advanced adenocarcinoma of the ovary. Cancer Treat. Rep. *60*, 55–60 (1976)

Witkin, E.M.: Mutation-proof and mutation-prone modes of survival in derivatives of *Escherichia coli* B differing in sensitivity to ultraviolet light. Brookhaven Symp. Biol. *20*, 17 (1968)

Woodman, R.J., Sirica, A.E., Gang, M., Kline, I., Venditti, J.M.: The enhanced therapeutic effect of *cis*-platinum (II) diamminodichloride against L1210 leukemia when combined with cyclophosphamide or 1,3 bis(13,5-dioxopiperazine-1-yl) propane or several other anti tumour agents. Chemotherapy *18*, 169–183 (1973)

Žák, M., Drobnik, J.: Effect of *cis* dichlorodiammine platinum (II) on the post-irradiation lethality in mice after irradiation with X-rays. Strahlentherapie *142*, 112–115 (1971)

Žák, M., Drobnik, J., Režný, Z.: The effect of *cis* platinum (II) diamminodichloride on bone marrow. Cancer Res. *32*, 595–599 (1972)

Zbiden, G.: In: The kidney, Chap. 6. Rouiller, C., Muller, A.F. (eds.), Vol. 2. New York: Academic Press 1969

9-β-D-Arabinofuranosyladenine (AraA)

C.E. Cass

Introduction

AraA (9-β-D-arabinofuranosyladenine; vidarabine; NSC-404241) was first synthesized as a potential antitumor agent in 1960 (Lee et al.) and later isolated by Parke, Davis and Company (British Patent No. 1,159,290) as an antibiotic produced by *Streptomyces antibioticus*. Chemical synthesis, initially achieved through the conversion of a xylonucleoside to araA (Lee et al., 1960; Reist et al., 1962), was subsequently accomplished on a larger scale by the condensation of 2,3,5-tri-O-benzyl-D-arabinofuranosyl chloride with N-benzoyladenine (Glaudemans and Fletcher, 1963; Reist et al., 1964). Detailed discussions of the synthetic procedures and chemical properties of araA and certain other D-arabinosyl nucleosides may be found in the comprehensive reviews by Cohen (1966) and Suhadolnik (1970).

The chemical structure of araA is illustrated in Fig. 1. AraA is relatively insoluble in water[1] (Lee et al., 1960) and has the following properties: mp 257–257.5 °C; λ_{max} 257.5 nm ($\varepsilon = 12.7 \times 10^3$) at pH 1; λ_{max} 259 nm ($\varepsilon = 13.4 \times 10^3$) at pH 7; λ_{max} 259 nm ($\varepsilon = 14 \times 10^3$) at pH 13 (Lee et al., 1960; Reist et al., 1962).

1 0.0018 M, 0.5 mg/ml (Repta et al., 1975).

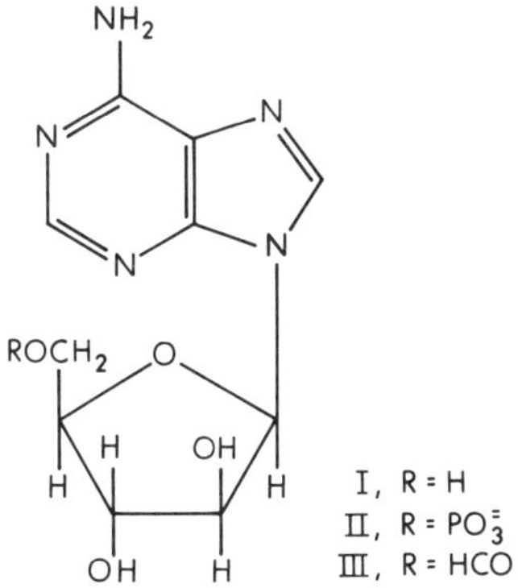

Fig. 1. Chemical structure of araA and araA derivatives. *I*, 9-β-D-arabinofuranosyladenine (araA); *II*, 9-β-D-arabinofuranosyladenine 5′-monophosphate (araAMP); *III*, 9-β-D-arabinofuranosyladenine 5′-formate (araA formate)

Biologic activity of araA was first demonstrated in studies with a purine-deficient strain of *Escherichia coli* (HUBERT-HABART and COHEN, 1962) in which an important biochemical effect was specific inhibition of DNA synthesis. Shortly thereafter, araA was shown to have activity against several transplantable tumors in mice (BRINK and LEPAGE, 1964) and against cultured mouse fibroblasts (DOERING et al., 1966); however, low solubility and rapid inactivation of araA by enzymatic conversion to 9-β-D-arabinofuranosylhypoxanthine (araH) seriously limited its effectiveness in these systems (BRINK and LEPAGE, 1965; COHEN, 1966; DOERING et al., 1966). Renewed interest in araA as an antitumor agent has recently occurred with the availability of more soluble, less rapidly inactivated derivatives of araA (LEE et al., 1971; HUGHES and KIMBALL, 1972; LEPAGE et al., 1972; ORTIZ et al., 1972; REPTA et al., 1975) and of potent inhibitors of araA deamination (SAWA et al., 1967; NAKAMURA et al., 1974; SCHAEFFER and SCHWENDER, 1974; WOO et al., 1974) which enhance the efficacy of araA against certain experimental tumors and cultured cells (PLUNKETT and COHEN, 1975b; CASS and AH-YEUNG, 1976; LEPAGE et al., 1976).

AraA has been shown to possess activity against a number of DNA viruses in cultured cells and experimental animals (for reviews, see SCHABEL, 1968; CH'IEN et al., 1973; PAVAN-LANGSTON et al., 1975), and a number of uncontrolled clinical studies have suggested usefulness in the therapy of certain of the herpes infections (PAVAN-LANGSTON et al., 1975). Recent results from multi-institutional, controlled trials of araA therapy of herpes zoster in immunosuppressed patients have been especially encouraging (CH'IEN et al., 1976; WHITLEY et al., 1976). Controlled clinical trials of araA therapy of herpes simplex encephalitis have demonstrated successful systemic therapy when araA was administered early in the course of the disease (WHITLEY et al., 1977).

Biochemical Effects of AraA

Since studies of the biochemical properties of araA have been reviewed previously, consideration here of work published up through 1969 is limited; the reader is referred to the review articles by COHEN (1966) and SUHADOLNIK (1970) for more detailed discussions. This section reviews in depth biochemical and metabolic studies of araA, and certain of its derivatives, which have appeared during the period 1970–1977.

From studies conducted with intact or cell-free material obtained from a variety of systems, including *Escherichia coli*, cultured mammalian cells and transplantable murine tumors, it is apparent that araA has two major biochemical fates, phosphorylation to the triphosphate level (araATP) and conversion by deamination to araH (COHEN, 1966; SUHADOLNIK, 1970; LEPAGE, 1975). It is generally accepted that the deamination product, araH, has relatively little biologic activity [2] per se; the biologically active form of araA is araATP, which inhibits or participates in various reactions associated with DNA replication.

2 Possible antiviral activity of araH will be discussed in the section concerned with viral chemotherapy.

That araA is phosphorylated to araA nucleotides by animal tissues was suggested from analysis of acid-soluble fractions of tissues obtained from tumor-bearing mice treated with [8-^{14}C]araA (BRINK and LEPAGE, 1964a;) and subsequently established in studies with cell-free tissue extracts and suspensions of intact TA3 ascites cells (YORK and LEPAGE, 1966b; LEPAGE, 1970). More recently PLUNKERT and COHEN (1975a) have shown that cultured mouse fibroblasts phosphorylate a small, but significant, proportion of exogenously added [2-^{3}H]araA to arabinosyl nucleotides. In these experiments quantitation of radioactivity present in cellular arabinosyl nucleotides was based on methods which separated the latter from other radioactive adenine-containing nucleotides, thereby avoiding misinterpretations arising from re-utilization of radioactive hypoxanthine produced by cleavage of the deamination product, araH. In addition, BROCKMAN et al. (1976, 1977) and ROSE and BROCKMAN (1977), utilizing high pressure liquid chromatography to separate araATP from ATP, have quantitated araATP levels in mouse leukemia L1210 and P388 cells under a variety of conditions.

It is not clear which enzyme(s) are involved in the phosphorylation of araA. It has been suggested (LEPAGE, 1975) that deoxyadenosine kinase (EC 2.7.1.76) phosphorylates araA, however the data available are inconclusive; whereas partially purified deoxyadenosine kinase of calf thymus (KRYGIER and MOMPARLER, 1971) apparently did not phosphorylate araA, crude extracts of that tissue were capable of phosphorylating araA (unpublished results cited in the review article by LEPAGE, 1975). A partially purified preparation of deoxycytidine kinase from calf thymus, free of detectable adenosine kinase (EC 2.7.1.20) activity, accepted deoxyadenosine (K_m, 0.33 mM) and araA (K_m, 1.0 mM) as substrates (KRENITSKY et al., 1976); the substrate efficiencies (expressed as the ratio of apparent V_{max} values over K_m values) of deoxycytidine, deoxyadenosine and araA were, respectively, 1000, 88 and 5. Conflicting results concerning acceptability of araA as substrate have also been reported for adenosine kinase. LINDBERG et al. (1967) found that partially purified preparations of adenosine kinase from rabbit liver phosphorylated araA and deoxyadenosine, although to a much lesser extent than adenosine; in contrast, there was no detectable activity toward araA or deoxyadenosine in preparations from cultured human HEp-2 cells (SCHNEBLI et al., 1967). In a more recent publication the latter authors have postulated that adenosine kinase requires, for substrate activity, nucleosides with a 2′-hydroxyl group trans to the purine moiety (BENNETT and HILL, 1975) and have suggested that the apparent activity reported for adenosine kinase toward araA and deoxyadenosine may be due to small amounts of contaminating deoxyadenosine kinase. Further study will be required to determine which cellular kinases are primarily responsible for phosphorylation of araA.

The phosphorylation of araAMP and araADP is presumably catalyzed, respectively, by adenylate kinase (EC 2.7.4.3) and nucleoside-diphosphate kinase (EC 2.7.4.6), however, there have been apparently no detailed studies of production of araA nucleotides with the purified enzymes (COHEN, 1976).

Many animal tissues and cells rapidly convert araA to araH through the action of adenosine deaminase (adenosine aminohydrolase, EC 3.5.4.4), and, as will be discussed below, rapid inactivation of araA has significantly hindered attempts to use araA as an antitumor agent. In the initial studies of araA toxicity, conducted with *Escherichia coli* (HUBERT-HABART and COHEN, 1962), araA added to exponentially growing cultures was rapidly, and almost completely, converted to araH. Similarly, when [8-^{14}C]araA was administered to mice, 35% of administered radioactivity was recovered as araH in urine within 1 h, and the capacity of cell-free extracts of various mouse tissues to deaminate araA was substantial (BRINK and LEPAGE, 1964). There have since been numerous additional studies in which the araA-deaminating capacity of serum, intact cells, and cell-free extracts from a variety of sources has been examined.

Substantial differences in araA-deamination rates were obtained when intact erythrocytes from several species were compared, with increasing levels of activity exhibited by rat, human, mouse, and monkey erythrocytes (KOSHIURA and LEPAGE, 1968; LEPAGE, 1969). Lysates from human erythrocytes deaminated araA much more rapidly than did those from rat erythrocytes (DRACH et al., 1974). In addition to species-specific differences, large tissue and tumor-specific differences in araA-deamination capacity have been observed in crude extracts from a variety of mouse tissues and transplantable tumors; of the latter, the mouse leukemia L1210 exhibited the highest levels of araA-deaminating activity (KOSHIURA and LEPAGE, 1968; LEPAGE, 1969; CHAO and KIMBALL, 1972; LEPAGE, 1973). In humans, large variations in araA-deamination rates by particular tissues (e.g., crude homogenates of normal bone marrows) have also been observed between individuals (LEPAGE, 1973).

Rates of deamination of araA in various types of animal sera used to supplement cell culture growth media have been compared in a study which also reported heating conditions sufficient to inactivate adenosine deaminase activity (SCHWARTZ et al., 1974). Horse serum had no detectable deaminase activity (see also ISHII and GREEN, 1973), whereas fetal calf, newborn calf and calf serum exhibited substantial deaminase activity, which appeared to vary significantly between commercial preparations. Using heat-inactivated fetal calf serum as a growth supplement, PLUNKETT and COHEN (1975a) found that, after a 4 h incubation with 0.1 mM [2-^{3}H]araA, suspension cultures of mouse L cells had deaminated almost half of the araA in the medium.

In kinetic studies of the structural requirements of adenosine deaminase for substrate activity, araA compared favorably with adenosine as a substrate for preparations partially purified from calf intestinal mucosa (CORY and SUHADOLNIK, 1965; FREDERIKSEN, 1966; YORK and LEPAGE, 1966b; BLOCH et al., 1967) and purified 3000-fold from human erythrocytes (AGARWAL et al., 1975). The apparent K_m values for the erythrocytic and intestinal enzymes were, respectively, for araA 100 and 77–140 μM, and for adenosine 25 and 35 μM; expressing the V_{max} value for adenosine deamination as 100, the relative values for araA deamination by the erythrocytic and intestinal enzymes were, respectively, 47 and 18–25 (AGARWAL et al., 1975).

Recently several potent inhibitors of adenosine deaminase have become available, thereby permitting the study of araA metabolism in absence of deamination, and, as will be discussed below, have substantially enhanced the growth inhibitory activity of araA.

Two of the most potent of these inhibitors are coformycin, originally isolated from culture filtrates of *Nocardia interforma* and *Streptomyces kaniharaensis* (SAWA et al., 1967; NAKAMURA et al., 1974) and subsequently prepared by organic synthesis (OHNO et al., 1974), and deoxycoformycin (covidarabine, NSC 218321), a fermentation product of *Streptomyces antibioticus* (WOO et al., 1974; DION et al., 1977). The structures of these inhibitors have been elucidated and defined chemically (Fig. 2) as (R)-3-(β-D-*erythro*-pentafuranosyl)-3,6,7,8-tetrahydroimidazo[4,5-*d*][1,3]diazepin-8-ol and the 2′-deoxyribosyl homologue (NAKAMURA et al., 1974; WOO et al., 1974). Deoxycoformycin is very soluble in water and aqueous alcohols and has the following properties (WOO et al., 1974; DION et al., 1977): MW 268.27; mp 220–225° C; λ_{max} 282 nm ($\varepsilon = 8 \times 10^3$) at pH 7; λ_{max} 283 nm ($\varepsilon = 7.97 \times 10^3$) at pH 11. Deoxycoformycin is chemically unstable at acid pH; at room temperature inhibitory activity against adenosine deaminase was completely lost after 24 h at pH 1 and was reduced by 28% after 192 h at pH 5.2 (DION et al., 1977).

Two additional, somewhat less potent, inhibitors of adenosine deaminase obtained by organic synthesis are *erythro*-9-(2-hydroxy-3-nonyl)adenine (EHNA, NSC 263164) (SCHAEFFER and SCHWENDER, 1974) and 1,6-dihydro-6-hydroxymethyl purine ribonucleoside (EVANS and WOLFENDEN, 1970). The structure of EHNA is presented in Fig. 3.

Apparent K_i values, using adenosine as substrate, for inhibition of adenosine deaminase from human erythrocytes (AGARWAL et al., 1975) were deoxycoformycin, 2.5×10^{-12}M; coformycin, $1–10 \times 10^{-11}$M; EHNA, 1.6×10^{-9}M; and 1,6-dihydro-6-hydroxymethyl purine ribonucleoside, 1.3×10^{-6}M (CHA et al., 1975; AGARAWAL and PARKS, 1977); the K_i for inhibition of adenosine deaminase from calf intestine by coformycin was $0.7–3.7 \times 10^{-10}$M (CHA, 1976). Coformycin and deoxycoformycin have also been reported to inhibit 5′-AMP deaminase (5′-AMP aminohydrolase, EC 3.5.4.6) obtained from rabbit muscle with apparent K_i values, respectively, of about 5×10^{-8}M and 2.5×10^{-6}M (AGARWAL and PARKS, 1977).

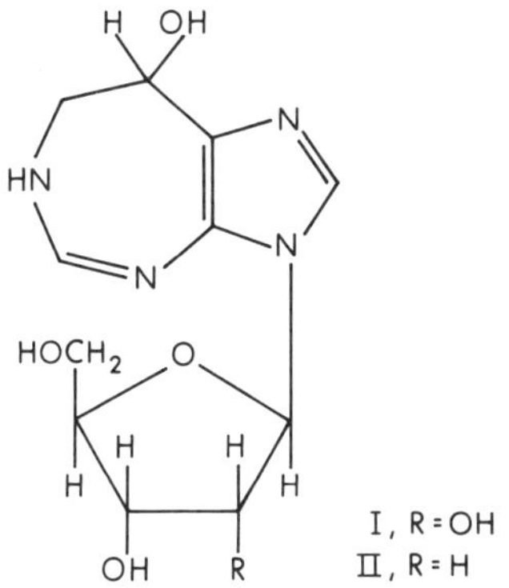

Fig. 2. Chemical structure of coformycin (*I*) and 2′-deoxycoformycin (*II*)

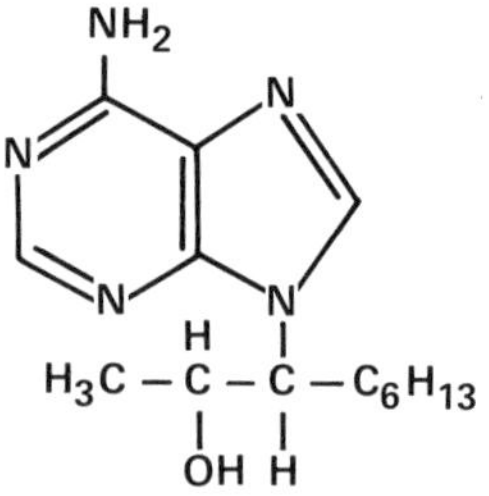

Fig. 3. Chemical structure of EHNA

With respect to adenosine deaminase, coformycin and deoxycoformycin are tight-binding inhibitors of the type described in a series of publications concerned with kinetic analysis of interaction of a tight-binding inhibitor with enzyme (CHA, 1975, 1976; CHA et al., 1975). With such "pseudo-irreversible" inhibitors, both the association and dissociation of enzyme-inhibitor complex are slow processes, and under usual experimental conditions the classical steady-state equations for inhibition kinetics are inadequate (CHA, 1975).

Deoxycoformycin and EHNA have received the greatest attention as inhibitors of adenosine deaminase which might enhance the therapeutic activity of araA; coformycin, although a highly potent inhibitor, has not been available in sufficient quantity for consideration in chemotherapy studies.

Inhibition of araA deamination was first reported for EHNA in studies with homogenates of mouse L cells and Ehrlich ascites tumor cells (PLUNKETT and COHEN, 1975b). Inhibition of adenosine deaminase by deoxycoformycin was reported shortly thereafter from studies conducted with suspensions of intact L1210 cells (LEPAGE et al., 1976; KIMBALL et al., 1976).

Using araA as substrate, the apparent K_i for inhibition by deoxycoformycin of adenosine deaminase from mouse brain was estimated to be 2×10^{-11}M (CARON et al., 1977; KIMBALL et al., 1977; LEE et al., 1977); the latter value was obtained by application of the methods of CHA (1976) and is similar to values obtained with the erythrocytic and intestinal adenosine deaminase preparations (AGARWAL and PARKS, 1977). That deoxycoformycin, like coformycin, behaves as a "pseudo-irreversible" inhibitor, binding tightly to adenosine deaminase with a very slow rate of dissociation, was further suggested by the duration of inhibition of araA deamination observed in homogenates of mouse tissues after single i.p. doses of 1.25–1.0 mg/kg deoxycoformycin (KIMBALL et al., 1976; LEPAGE et al., 1976; LEE et al., 1977); almost complete inhibition was obtained in a variety of tissues up to 24 h after injection, and partial inhibitions were observed 72 h after injection.

The effect of deoxycoformycin and EHNA on cellular utilization of araA is a greatly decreased rate of araA deamination, thereby permitting greater accumulation of araA nucleotides in those cells which possess the appropriate kinase(s). When tumor-bearing mice were treated with either deoxycoformycin or EHNA in combination with araA, the cellular content of araATP was significantly higher in mouse leukemia L1210 cells and in P388 cells than in cells obtained from mice treated with araA alone (BROCKMAN et al., 1976, 1977;

ROSE and BROCKMAN, 1977); in these experiments, after i.p. injections of drugs, acid-soluble extracts of leukemia cells were analyzed using a high pressure liquid chromatography system which separated araATP from ATP.

In experiments with mouse L cells in culture, PLUNKETT and COHEN (1977) observed significant increases in cellular content of arabinosyl nucleotides in the presence of EHNA. Analysis of acid-soluble fractions of cells incubated with 100 μM araA in presence or absence of 10 μM EHNA indicated a twofold difference in the amount of arabinosyl nucleotides recovered from EHNA-treated and untreated cells, with estimated intracellular araATP concentrations of 43 μM and 24 μM, respectively.

The effect of deoxycoformycin on araA utilization is illustrated for human tissues by the results obtained when [2-^{3}H]araA was added at a final concentration of 10 μg/ml (37 μM) to freshly collected whole blood after a 1 h incubation with deoxycoformycin at 5 μg/ml (19 μM) (CHANG and GLAZKO, 1976). In absence of deoxycoformycin all of the radioactivity recovered in the plasma fraction was converted to araH within 30 min, whereas in presence of inhibitor all of the plasma radioactivity was recovered as araA, with none present as araH after a 3 h incubation at 37° C. There was a five-fold increase in total cellular radioactivity and a marked shift in the distribution of radioactivity among araA metabolites after exposure to deoxycoformycin. From untreated cells the major radioactive metabolite was the 5′-monophosphate of araH, araIMP, with small amounts of ribosylnucleotides and trace amounts of arabinosylnucleotides present. In contrast, radioactivity in deoxycoformycin-treated cells was evenly distributed between araAMP, araADP and araATP, with only traces in araIMP. Thus, deoxycoformycin not only protected araA deamination by human blood, but also significantly increased the accumulation of araA nucleotides in erythrocytes.

Cellular uptake[3] of araA is a process that begins with a membrane-dependent step, which, in human erythrocytes (CASS and PATERSON, 1973, 1975), appears to be catalyzed by the "uridine-thymidine" transport mechanism (OLIVER and PATERSON, 1971; CASS and PATERSON, 1972). The efflux of uridine from human erythrocytes was accelerated similarly by addition of araA and adenosine to extracellular medium, indicating their acceptability as substrates for the erythrocyte nucleoside transport mechanism (CASS and PATERSON, 1973). Treatment of intact human and mouse erythrocytes with nitrobenzylthioinosine (6-[(4-nitrobenzyl)thio]-9-β-D-ribofuranosylpurine), a potent inhibitor of nucleoside transport which binds with high affinity to transport-inhibitory sites in the erythrocyte membrane (CASS et al., 1974; Cass and PATERSON, 1976), reduced formation of metabolites from extracellular araA, adenosine, and deoxyadenosine, but had no effect on metabolite formation by sonicated erythrocytes (CASS and PATERSON, 1975). AraA inhibited binding of ^{14}C-nitrobenzylthioinosine to the transport-inhibitory sites of erythrocytes (CASS and PATERSON, 1976), a further indication that araA is a substrate for the erythrocyte nucleoside transport mechanism. Very little is known about araA transport in other cell types; araA was a competitive inhibitor of ^{3}H-labeled adenosine uptake by rabbit

3 In the uptake of nucleosides by animal cells the "uptake process" has been described as a process that includes both transport and metabolic events (PATERSON et al., 1977a, b).

polymorphonuclear leukocytes (TAUBE und BERLIN, 1972). Adenosine uptake by monolayer cultures of HeLa cells was more sensitive to inhibition by the arabinosyl homologue of nitrobenzylthioinosine than to nitrobenzylthioinosine (PATERSON et al., 1977), and binding studies with radioactive 6-[(4-nitrobenzyl)-thio]-9-β-D-arabinofuranosylpurine have shown that the arabinosyl homolog binds to the transport inhibitory sites of HeLa cells with an affinity comparable to that of nitrobenzylthioinosine (PATERSON, A.R.P., LAU, E.Y., CASS, C.E., unpublished results).

The most notable biochemical effects of araA nucleotides are inhibition of reactions required for cellular and viral DNA synthesis, in particular the inhibition by araATP of DNA polymerase(s) (EC 2.7.7.7; YORK and LEPAGE, 1966a; FURTH and COHEN, 1967, 1968) and ribonucleoside-diphosphate reductase (EC 1.17.4.1) (YORK and LEPAGE, 1966a; MOORE and COHEN, 1967).

Investigations of araATP inhibition of DNA synthesis in animal cells began with the observation that araA treatment of mice bearing TA3 and C3HED ascites tumors resulted in a marked reduction in DNA synthesis by tumor cells (BRINK and LEPAGE, 1964a, b, 1965). Subsequently, araATP was shown to inhibit DNA synthesis, apparently noncompetitively, in crude extracts of TA3 cells with a K_i of 90 μM (YORK and LEPAGE, 1966a). AraATP also inhibited DNA polymerase activity in crude extracts of bovine lymphosarcoma (FURTH and COHEN, 1967) and calf thymus (FURTH and COHEN, 1968); in the latter study, araATP appeared to inhibit dATP incorporation into DNA competitively with a K_i of 1.3 μM. AraATP did not inhibit DNA synthesis in crude extracts obtained from *Escherichia coli* (FURTH and COHEN, 1967).

It now appears that animal cells contain at least three separate, major species of DNA polymerase, termed α, β and γ (WEISSBACH et al., 1975), which are readily distinguished from each other by their molecular weights, chromatographic properties, and template requirements. There are also a number of unique virus-induced DNA polymerases. The specific functions of the DNA polymerases in DNA replication in animal cells is, as yet, unknown. For recent reviews of the general properties of eukaryotic and viral DNA polymerases

Table 1. AraATP inhibition of cellular and viral DNA polymerases

Polymerase	Source	Km(μM) dATP	Ki(μM) araATP	Ki/Km
Cellular DNA-dependent DNA polymerase:				
α	Rabbit kidney cells[b]	7.9	8.8	1.11
α	Quail oviduct[a]	7.4	8.9	1.20
β	Rabit kidney cells[b]	7.4	8.9	1.20
β	Quail oviduct[a]	9.7	4.7	0.48
Viral DNA-dependent DNA polymerase:	*Herpesvirus hominis*[b]	13.7	0.14	0.01
	Rous sarcoma virus[a]	4.9	9.1	1.86
Viral RNA-dependent DNA polymerase:	Rous sarcoma virus[a]	7.3	42.9	5.88

[a] MÜLLER et al., 1975. [b] MÜLLER et al., 1977b.

from a variety of sources, the reader is referred to the articles by LOEB (1974), BOLLUM (1975) and WEISSBACH (1975, 1977).

The early studies of araATP inhibition of DNA synthesis (YORK and LEPAGE, 1966a; FURTH and COHEN, 1967, 1968) were conducted with crude preparations, containing mixtures of the various species of DNA polymerase. Recently MÜLLER et al. (1975, 1977b) have reported results, summarized in Table 1, from kinetic studies of araATP inhibition of several of the DNA-synthesizing enzymes; the inhibitions obtained with each of the DNA polymerases of Table 1 were competitive with respect to dATP. Using the ratio of K_i value over K_m value as a basis for assessing relative affinities of enzyme for inhibitor and substrate in competitive inhibition, as suggested by WEBB (1963), the herpes-induced enzyme appeared to be most sensitive, and the RNA-dependent DNA polymerase from Rous sarcoma virus least sensitive to araATP inhibition (MÜLLER et al., 1975, 1977b). The cellular polymerases, α and β, were similar in their sensitivities to araATP inhibitions, exhibiting K_i values somewhat higher than the value reported previously for the unfractionated preparation from calf thymus (K_i, 1.3 μM; K_m (dATP), 2.5 μM; K_i/K_m, 0.5). (FURTH and COHEN, 1968).

Of interest is the apparent difference in sensitivities of cellular and herpes-induced DNA polymerases to araATP inhibition since araA is a highly promising chemotherapeutic agent against herpetic infections in man. After infection of cultured KB cells with herpes simplex virus, viral DNA synthesis was inhibited to a greater extent than cellular DNA synthesis when araA, alone or in presence of coformycin, was added to culture media (SCHWARTZ et al., 1976; SHIPMAN et al., 1976; DRACH and SHIPMAN, 1977). Similarly, when K_i/K_m ratios were used as a basis for comparison, the herpes-induced polymerase appeared to be 39-fold more sensitive to araATP than DNA polymerase β, and 116-fold more sensitive than DNA polymerase α, from rabbit kidney cells (MÜLLER et al., 1977b). In an earlier study there were no differences in sensitivity to araATP inhibition between the polymerases from herpes-infected and uninfected HEp-2 cells (BENNETT et al., 1975); however, these experiments were conducted with crude, unfractionated preparations which, in the case of infected cells, probably contained mixtures of cellular and viral-induced enzymes. Although it is not known whether the herpes-induced DNA-dependent polymerase catalyzes synthesis of DNA in intact cells, the observation of greater araATP sensitivity of this enzyme, relative to cellular polymerase, suggests a possible explanation for the apparent selectivity of araA for herpetic infections (MÜLLER et al., 1977b).

Although inhibition of DNA polymerase activity is the most readily apparent biochemical effect of araATP, incorporation of araA nucleotides into DNA of cellular and viral origin has been reported (WAQAR et al., 1971; PLUNKETT et al., 1974; MÜLLER et al., 1975, 1977b; PLUNKETT and COHEN, 1975). "Nearest-neighbor" analysis (JOSSE et al., 1961) of DNA synthesized by preparations of nuclei isolated from rat liver and thymus in the presence of [α-^{32}P]araATP indicated incorporation of arabinosyl nucleotides into DNA (WAQAR et al., 1971); the results obtained under conditions of limited primer availability raised the possibility that araATP functions as a chain terminator. There have since been at least three studies (PLUNKETT et al., 1974; MÜLLER et al., 1975; PLUNKETT and COHEN, 1975a) which demonstrated incorporation of araA, primarily into internucleotide linkages of DNA, suggesting relatively low levels of chain-terminating activity of araA.

In araA-incorporation experiments with mouse L cells small amounts of araA nucleotides were detected in DNA after a 4 h exposure of logarithmically proliferating cells to 0.1 mM [^{3}H]-labeled araAMP (PLUNKETT et al., 1974) or araA (PLUNKETT and COHEN, 1975a); for identification of arabinosyl nucleotides in DNA, 3′- or 5′-mononucleotides resulting from sequential enzymatic degradation of DNA were separated by high pressure liquid chromatography or, in some experiments, the mononucleotides were dephosphorylated and the resulting deoxyribosyl and arabinosyl nucleosides were separated using thin layer chromatography. In similar experiments with mouse L5178Y lymphoma cells which were incubated with [8-^{3}H]araA at 0.1 μg/ml (0.37 μM) for 72 h, MÜLLER et al. (1975) reported incorporation of araA into cellular DNA with an estimated molar ratio of deoxyadenosine to araA of about 8,000 to 1. In both this and the preceeding studies with mouse L cells, incorporation was shown to be primarily into internucleotide linkages of DNA, with little indication of terminal incorporation. Incorporation of araA into viral-specific, as well as cellular, DNA was demonstrated in experiments in which herpes virus-infected rabbit kidney cells were incubated with [8-^{3}H]araA during the period of DNA synthesis (MÜLLER et al., 1977b).

In addition to inhibition of DNA polymerases, araATP is an inhibitor of ribonucleoside-diphosphate reductase of bacteria (FOLLMANN and HOGENKAMP, 1971) and animal cells (YORK and LEPAGE, 1966a; MOORE and COHEN, 1967). AraATP inhibited reduction of the common ribonucleoside diphosphates, in a manner similar to that of dATP, when tested in a partially purified enzyme system obtained from Novikoff ascites tumor cells of rats (MOORE and COHEN, 1967); in these experiments concentrations of araATP of 30–110 μM were required to achieve 50% inhibitions of reduction of the various nucleoside diphosphates. Since, in absence of an exogenous supply of deoxyribosyl nucleosides, the activity of ribonucleoside-diphosphate reductase is required for provision of deoxyribosylnucleotides for DNA synthesis, significant inhibition of this enzyme by araATP would, indirectly, result in an inhibition of cellular DNA synthesis.

From early studies of araA effects on transplantable tumors of mice (BRINK and LEPAGE, 1964) and cultured mouse cells (DOERING et al., 1966) and from more recent studies of araATP effects in cell-free systems (MÜLLER et al., 1975), it is apparent that araA nucleotides do not significantly inhibit synthesis of RNA or protein.

Antitumor Activity of AraA

AraA, originally synthesized as a potential antitumor agent (REIST and GOODMAN, 1964; LEE et al., 1971), was tested soon after it became available for chemotherapeutic activity against a variety of transplantable murine tumors (BRINK and LEPAGE, 1964a, 1965). Those tumors with the lowest adenosine deaminase activities (e.g., 6C3HED) exhibited the greatest sensitivity to araA, while those with high levels of adenosine deaminase activity (e.g., L1210 leukemia, Sarcoma 180) were completely unresponsive (BRINK and LEPAGE, 1964a, 1965; KOSHIURA and LEPAGE, 1968). From these studies it was apparent that araA could be effective only against tumors with low levels of adenosine deaminase, or if protected against deamination either by administration in combination with inhibitors of adenosine deaminase or in a form not susceptible to rapid deamination (e.g., as araAMP).

Although attempts were made to identify deaminase inhibitors which would prolong the existence of araA in cellular and tissue fluids and thereby enhance its therapeutic activity (KOSHIURA and LEPAGE, 1968), significant success was not achieved until the compounds EHNA (SCHAEFFER and SCHWENDER, 1974) and deoxycoformycin (WOO et al., 1974) became available. The feasibility of enhancing tumor lethality of araA by inhibiting its deamination was suggested by the greater survival times of mice bearing the Ehrlich ascites carcinoma when treated with EHNA plus araA, relative to those of mice treated with araA alone (PLUNKETT and COHEN, 1975).

A number of investigators have recently demonstrated significant increases in therapeutic activity of araA against the L1210 and P388 mouse leukemias when used in combination with EHNA or deoxycoformycin (CASS, 1976; CASS and AH-YEUNG, 1976; KIMBALL et al., 1976, 1977; LEPAGE et al., 1976; SCHABEL et al., 1976; CARON et al., 1977; LEE et al., 1977, PLUNKETT et al., 1977). The L1210 leukemia, unresponsive to araA therapy alone because of high levels of adenosine deaminase, was highly sensitive, in both intracerebral and ascites form, to combination therapy with araA (or araA derivatives) and deoxycoformycin (LEPAGE et al., 1976; LEE et al., 1977). The most effective treatment regimen resembled the dosage scheduling employed by SKIPPER et al. (1967) for araC (1-β-D-arabinofuranosylcytosine) therapy of the L1210 leukemia; beginning 24 h after tumor implantation, mice were treated at 3 or 4 day intervals with a single dose of deoxycoformycin followed by 8 doses of araA, administered at 3 h intervals (LEPAGE et al., 1976; KIMBALL et al., 1976; SCHABEL et al., 1976; LEE et al., 1977). In all of the studies reported thus far treatment of tumor-bearing mice with either EHNA or deoxycoformycin alone had no demonstrable effect on host survival times.

That the deaminase inhibitors increased the anti-tumor activity of araA by prolongation of effective intracellular levels of araA nucleotides is suggested by the in vivo studies reported recently (BROCKMAN et al., 1976, 1977; ROSE and BROCKMAN, 1977). AraATP levels in P388 and L1210 leukemia cells were higher, for longer periods of time, after treatment of mice with EHNA or deoxycoformycin, than after treatment with araA alone. Consistent with these observations, prolonged inhibition of DNA synthesis was observed in L1210 and P388 leukemia cells after treatment of tumor-bearing mice with deaminase inhibitor and araA, or araA derivatives (LEPAGE et al., 1976; PLUNKETT et al., 1977). Comparison of the two inhibitors indicated a longer-lasting effect on cellular araATP levels after in vivo treatment with deoxycoformycin than with EHNA, suggesting a greater reversibility of deaminase inhibition by the latter compound (BROCKMAN et al., 1977; ROSE and BROCKMAN, 1977).

Enhancement of araA activity by deaminase inhibitors has also been demonstrated in cultured cells. In the initial studies effectiveness of araA was severely limited by rapid deamination; araA concentrations in excess of 200 μM were required to obtain significant growth inhibitions (Doering et al., 1966). Using the same line of cultured mouse cells, Plunkett and Cohen (1975b, 1977) demonstrated a marked increase in araA toxicity in the presence of EHNA; 20 μM araA, which alone had no growth inhibitory effect, significantly decreased cell viability, as determined by assay of cloning efficiencies after drug exposures, when combined with 10 μM EHNA. Increased araA lethality after EHNA treatment appeared to be related to increased levels of cellular araATP since acid-soluble fractions of EHNA-treated cells contained about twice as much araATP as untreated cells (Plunkett and Cohen, 1977).

Deoxycoformycin also markedly enhanced araA toxicity to cultured cells (Cass, 1976; Cass and Ah-Yeung, 1976). A cultured line of mouse leukemia L1210 cells with in vivo growth properties like those of the parental transplantable tumor was used to assess drug effects on cellular proliferation, viability, and tumorigenicity. In absence of deoxycoformycin araA concentrations of 100 μM were required to obtain maximal inhibition of growth, whereas in presence of deoxycoformycin (0.02–2 μM) araA was growth inhibitory at 10 μM. Cell kill and loss of tumorigenicity were significantly greater when araA exposures were conducted in presence of deoxycoformycin; in these experiments, the degree of cell kill achieved was highly dependent on the length of exposure to drug. Continuous exposure of L1210 cells to araA and deoxycoformycin induced a prolonged inhibition of proliferation and DNA synthesis, while RNA and protein synthesis continued and cells became progressively larger, suggesting that an imbalance of macromolecular synthetic rates contributed to araA toxicity (Cass and Ah-Yeung, 1976).

AraA-induced lethality, in absence of deaminase inhibitors, has been studied in synchronous cultures of a cell line characterized by low levels of adenosine deaminase activity (Müller et al., 1977a). Mouse lymphoma L5178Y cells, synchronized by double thymidine blockade, were exposed at different points during the cell cycle to araA and assayed for cellular araATP and dATP content, DNA polymerase α and β activities, and RNA polymerase activities. Although DNA synthesis was inhibited completely upon addition of araA (93 μM) to culture fluids, cycle-dependent fluctuations in dATP levels and DNA polymerase activities were unchanged, relative to untreated cells; the capacity of cells to accumulate araATP increased 41% as cells progressed through S phase. Incubation of asynchronous, exponentially proliferating L5178Y cells with nontoxic levels of deoxyadenosine (32 μM) increased cellular dATP levels and reduced the growth-inhibitory effects of araA (39 μM). On the basis of these results and considerations of kinetics of araATP inhibition of cellular polymerases, these authors have suggested that araATP inhibition of DNA polymerase α, competitive with respect to dATP, was responsible for growth inhibition of L5178Y cells.

It is not possible from data currently available to evaluate the relative significance of araATP inhibition of DNA synthesis and incorporation into DNA in the lethal action of the drug. Both effects may contribute importantly to araA toxicity. The reader is referred to a recent review article (COZZARELLI, 1977) in which there is considerable discussion of mechanisms of araATP and araCTP inhibition of DNA synthesis in cell-free and intact bacterial systems.

A number of derivatives of araA, in particular araAMP, cyclic araAMP (cyclic 9-β-D-arabinofuranosyladenine 3′,5′-monophosphate), and araA formate (9-β-D-arabinofuranosyladenine 5′-formate), have been tested for activity against experimental tumors in mice (HUGHES and KIMBALL, 1972; LEPAGE and HERSH, 1972; LEPAGE et al., 1972, 1976; KIMBALL et al., 1976; CARON et al., 1977) and against cultured cells (ORTIZ et al., 1972; PLUNKETT et al., 1974; PLUNKETT and COHEN 1975b; COHEN, 1975, 1976; CASS, 1976; CASS and AH-YEUNG, 1976). The apparent advantages of these compounds, relative to araA, are greater solubility in aqueous solution and a reduced susceptibility to deamination; the major disadvantage, in the case of araAMP and cyclic araAMP, has generally been thought to be poor penetrability of nucleotides, as such, into cells.

AraA formate, synthesized in an effort to obtain a highly water-soluble "prodrug" of araA (REPTA et al., 1975), had antiproliferative activity comparable to that of araA against the L1210 leukemia in mice (KIMBALL et al., 1976; LEPAGE et al., 1976) and in cell culture (CASS, 1976; CASS and AH-YEUNG, 1976). It was apparent from studies of chemical stability in aqueous solution at pH 7.4 (half-life, 4.5 h at 25° C) and in whole blood (half-life, 6–8 min at 37° C) that araA formate was rapidly converted, by chemical and enzymatic hydrolysis, respectively, to araA REPTA et al., 1975).

AraAMP has been tested for activity against transplantable mouse tumors and cultured cells. In mice, because of rapid enzymatic dephosphorylation in tissues of the kidney, araAMP behaved as though it were araA, the only advantage being its greater solubility (LEPAGE et al., 1972, 1976). Against cultured mouse L cells araAMP was more effective than araA alone, when used in absence of deaminase inhibitors (ORTIZ et al., 1972; COHEN and PLUNKETT, 1975b). Metabolic studies with doubly-labeled [^{3}H, ^{32}P]-araAMP indicated that small amounts of araAMP penetrated cells without degradation, thereby giving rise to intracellular araA nucleotides (PLUNKETT et al., 1974; COHEN and PLUNKETT, 1975a). These results are of interest since it has generally been assumed that nucleotides do not readily cross the cell membrane (for discussion, see COHEN, 1975; COHEN, 1976).

Cyclic araAMP, originally synthesized by LEE et al. (1971) and by MIAN et al. (1974), also had greater activity than araA against the mouse leukemia L1210 in therapy tests in vivo and in short-term in vitro assays of effects on DNA synthesis (HUGHES and KIMBALL, 1972; LEPAGE and HERSH, 1972). Cyclic araAMP was as toxic to cultured L cells as araAMP (PLUNKETT and COHEN, 1975b), suggesting that it, too, may slowly penetrate cells without first being dephosphorylated.

Toxicology and Metabolic Disposition of AraA

A major advantage of araA as a therapeutic agent is its low toxicity to normal host tissues. Administration of araA i.p. to normal mice at a dose level of 240 mg/kg per day for 6 days resulted in a 25% loss of body weight, which was regained within 2–3 weeks, and there was no repressive effect on the hemopoietic system; the drug was rapidly cleared from the blood or excreted in the urine as araH (BRINK and LEPAGE, 1964b).

Tests of araA toxicity have been conducted by Parke, Davis and Company in mice, rats, monkeys, and rabbits (KURTZ et al., 1969; KURTZ, 1975). In mice the i.p. LD_{50} dose was 4677 mg/kg, with morbidity and mortality apparently related to trauma and peritonitis. When araA was fed to mice orally in daily doses of 177 to 1532 mg/kg for 4 weeks, the major effect was weight loss; no mortality occurred at the highest single dose (7950 mg/kg) given orally. When a variety of suspensions and ointments containing araA were applied daily for 5 days to conjunctival sacs or to the skin of rabbits, there was little evidence of local irritation and no signs of systemic toxicity.

Comparative toxicologic studies of araA and araAMP in rodents, rabbits, and dogs indicated that the 5′-monophosphate of araA is no more toxic, and in some aspects less toxic, than araA (KURTZ et al., 1977). In acute toxicity studies in rats the LD_{50} doses for i.p. administration of single doses of araA and araAMP were, respectively, 2300 mg/kg and 1700 mg/kg, and the i.v. LD_{50} for a single dose of araAMP was 1200 mg/kg (KURTZ et al., 1977). In mice urinary excretion rates after administration of single i.p. doses of araA (25 mg/kg) and araAMP (32.5 mg/kg) were comparable; araAMP was rapidly dephosphorylated, primarily in the kidney, and excreted at the same rate and in the same form as araA (LEPAGE et al., 1972).

Perhaps the most important finding of toxicology studies with araA and araAMP is the absence of toxicity to hematopoietic tissues, indicating that araA, in contrast to many other nucleoside drugs, is not immunosuppressive (BRINK and LEPAGE, 1964b; KURTZ et al., 1969, 1977). Studies of effects of araA treatment on humoral immunity in rabbits and cellular immunity in guinea pigs have shown that araA, administered s.c. daily for 14 days at relatively high dosages (250 mg/kg), was not immunosuppressive (ZAM et al., 1976). Similarly, in vitro studies of araA effects on the blastogenic responses of human lymphocytes to mitogens, and the blastogenic and cytotoxic responses of human cell cultures to herpes virus infections, indicated a lack of depression of immune responses by araA (STEELE et al., 1975); in comparable experiments with araC there was significant inhibition of these immune responses. Lymphocytes removed from patients before, during, and after treatment with araA exhibited similar blastogenic responses to mitogen exposure, indicating that in vivo treatment did not alter these in vitro measures of the immune response (STEELE et al., 1975).

AraA and araAMP have been tested in experimental animals for teratogenic effects (ADLARD et al., 1975; FISHAUT et al., 1975; GASSET and AKABOSHI, 1976; KURTZ et al., 1977). Prenatal or postnatal treatment of rats with araA had negligible effects on brain growth and development, whereas similar treatment with much lower doses of araC severely impaired brain growth and development (ADLARD et al., 1975; FISHAUT et al., 1975). When pregnant rabbits were treated i.p. with 20 mg/kg daily of araA from day 6 to day 18 of gestation, there were no detectable teratogenic or embryocidal effects in fetuses collected on day 29 of gestation (GASSET and AKABOSHI, 1976). In contrast, araA was teratogenic in rabbits at 5 mg/kg and higher when given intramuscularly during days 6–18 of pregnancy, with multiple gross anomalies at birth, including skeletal abnormalities and cleft palate; rats were somewhat less sensitive to teratogenic effects of araA, requiring doses of 150 mg/kg on days 6 through 15 (KURTZ et al., 1977). In comparable tests with araAMP there were no teratogenic effects at birth in rabbits (25 mg/kg, daily, days 6–18) or rats (200 mg/kg, daily, days 6–15) (KURTZ et al., 1977).

Although experiments were not reported in detail, araA and araAMP were reported to be negative in bacterial mutagenesis assays (KURTZ, 1975; KURTZ et al., 1977). Induction of chromosome breaks in human leukocytes after short-term (24 h) in vitro culture with araA (100 μM) has been described (NICHOLS, 1964), suggesting the possibility of genetic damage after severe exposures to araA.

Only limited toxicologic and pharmacologic studies have been conducted with araA or araAMP in humans. AraA toxicity in patients who received total daily doses of 20 and 30 mg/kg (continuous i.v. infusion) for 7 days consisted of nausea, weight loss, weakness, tremors, and megaloblastosis in the erythroid series in bone marrow; adverse side effects in patients receiving daily doses of 10 mg/kg were much less severe (ROSS et al., 1976). KEENEY (1975) has summarized adverse experiences encountered in administration of araA to 143 patients with viral infections and has also concluded that araA is relatively nontoxic to humans.

Substantial variations in plasma levels and urinary excretion rates were observed after administration of ^{3}H-araA to humans by several different routes (LEPAGE et al., 1972, 1973); cumulative urinary excretion, primarily as araH, during the first 24 h was 88%–97% after fast i.v. infusion, 33%–41% during slow continuous i.v. infusion, and 2%–7% after i.m. injection (LEPAGE et al., 1973). When araA was administered by slow i.v. infusion in daily doses of 10–20 mg/kg, plasma levels of araA (barely detectable) were significantly lower than those of araH; radioactivity excreted in urine represented 42%–53% of daily doses and was recovered as araH (KINKEL and BUCHANAN, 1975). Metabolism and excretion of ^{3}H-labeled araA (i.v. infusion) and araAMP (i.v. injection) have been compared in humans (LEPAGE et al., 1972, 1975); araA plasma levels were significantly higher, and urinary excretion of araH was slower[4], after administration of araAMP, suggesting that araAMP may have advantages over araA in treatment of human disease.

In a comparative study of the metabolic disposition of araA after i.v. and i.m. administration of [2-^{3}H]araA to a variety of species, including humans, GLASKO et al. (1975) also reported rapid urinary excretion of radioactivity in the form of araH. In the animal studies tissue accumulation of radioactivity (araA or araA metabolites) was highest in the kidneys, with progressively lower concentrations in the spleen, liver, heart, skeletal muscle, lungs, brain, and blood plasma. Assays for cerebrospinal fluid levels of araA-derived radioactivity

4 Humans dephosphorylate araAMP more slowly than do mice, hence the apparent difference in plasma clearance and urinary excretion of araA metabolites between humans and mice (LEPAGE et al., 1972, 1975).

in human subjects indicated ready passage of araA or its metabolites into the central nervous system.

There are, at present, limited data on toxicity and metabolism of the deaminase inhibitors, alone or in combination, with araA or its derivatives. When toxicity testing of deoxycoformycin was conducted in normal female mice, single doses of 10 mg/kg and daily doses of 0.5 mg/kg for 6 days were tolerated with little effect; however, doses of 0.5 mg/kg or greater given two times daily for 6 days resulted in significant weight loss and death of most of the treated animals (LEPAGE et al., 1976). In mice, after daily treatment with 1 mg/kg deoxycoformycin for 5 days, at a time when significant toxicity (convulsions, severe spasticity, collapse) was apparent, there was no detectable impairment of immune function, as measured in vitro by the response of mouse thymocytes to stimulation by concanavalin A, or of spleen cells to irradiated heterologous spleen cells (BURRIDGE et al., 1977). In these experiments adenosine deaminase in mouse thymus, spleen, lymph nodes, and a number of other tissues was inhibited almost completely. The explanation for the severe toxicity induced by deoxycoformycin is, as yet, unknown; association of toxicity with inhibition of adenosine deaminase, as suggested by the debilitating symptoms in patients with an hereditary absence of this enzyme (MEUWISSEN et al., 1975), has not been established.

Results from preliminary studies of the metabolic disposition of deoxycoformycin in experimental animals have recently become available. Deoxycoformycin, assayed indirectly by biologic and enzymatic techniques (CHASSIN et al., 1977; MCCONNELL, 1977; SULING et al., 1977) and directly by radiochemical techniques (BORONDY et al., 1977) was rapidly cleared from plasma, with a half-life of about 20 min in mice (MCCONNELL, 1977; SULING et al., 1977), 75–120 min in dogs (CHASSIN et al., 1977), and 1.5–3.7 h in rats (BORONDY et al., 1977). Most of the administered drug was recovered in urine unchanged within a few hours after treatment.

Antiviral Effects of AraA

There is currently considerable interest in araA as a clinically useful antiviral agent, particularly against herpes simplex virus, cytomegalovirus, and varicella-zoster virus infections in humans. The literature concerning antiviral effects of araA has been reviewed through 1968 (SCHABEL, 1968), and 1973 (CH'IEN et al., 1973), and a comprehensive collection of reports of preclinical and clinical studies with araA and araA derivatives are available in two recent monographs (PAVAN-LANGSTON et al., 1975; HERRMANN, 1977).

The antiviral activity of araA was first observed by two different groups of investigators. DE RUDDER and PRIVAT DE GARILHE (1965) reported activity of araA against herpes simplex virus and vaccinia virus in cell cultures, and an antibiotic concentrate, obtained by workers at Parke, Davis and Company from *Streptomyces antibioticus* and subsequently identified as araA, had activity in vitro against herpes simplex virus, cytomegalovirus, and vaccinia virus (SCHABEL, 1968; MILLER et al., 1969). From many additional studies, conducted in vitro and in vivo, araA currently appears to have broad spectrum activity against certain of the DNA-containing viruses, in particular herpesviruses and poxviruses, with limited activity against adenoviruses, and no apparent activity against papovaviruses (SHANNON, 1977a). AraA is also active against a number of RNA tumor viruses, but not against the non oncogenic RNA viruses (SCHABEL, 1968; MILLER et al., 1969; SHANNON, 1975, 1977b). Detailed listings of the reported in vitro activities of araA against DNA- and RNA-containing viruses are presented in the recent review articles by SHANNON (1975) and CONNOR et al. (1975).

Since most in vitro studies of araA antiviral activity have been conducted in the absence of inhibitors of adenosine deaminase, assay systems have contained undefined mixtures of araA and araH, depending on the deaminase activity of indicator cell lines and growth media. Recently a number of investigators have reported significant enhancement of araA activity against certain DNA-containing viruses and an RNA-containing tumor virus in the presence of deoxycoformycin (BRYSON et al., 1974; CONNOR et al., 1974, 1975; WILLIAMS et al., 1975; SLOAN et al., 1977). In these studies low levels of deoxycoformycin (1 μg/ml or less) increased the antiviral efficacy of araA against herpes simplex virus (types 1 and 2), varicella-zoster virus, vaccinia virus, and Rauscher murine leukemia virus 10- to 50-fold over that of araA alone; when combined with deoxycoformycin, concentrations of araA resulting in 50% reduction of plaque formation on indicator cell cultures were 0.1–2.0 μg/ml.

The araA-deamination product, araH, has also been shown to exhibit in vitro antiviral activity, although to a lesser extent than araA (MILLER et al., 1969; CONNOR et al., 1974; 1975; SHANNON, 1975; SLOAN et al., 1977). The difference in activity between the two compounds now appears to be greater than originally proposed. Whereas early studies, conducted without deaminase inhibitors, had suggested that araA was about ten fold more active than araH (MILLER et al., 1969), more recent studies, conducted under conditions of complete inhibition of araA deamination, have suggested a 50-fold difference in activity (CONNOR et al., 1974, 1975; SLOAN et al., 1977). At least 25 μg/ml araH was required to suppress plaque formation in herpes simplex or vaccinia virus-infected cultures, as compared to 0.5 μg/ml araA when combined with deoxycoformycin (SLOAN et al., 1977). An apparent enhancement of araH antiviral activity by deoxycoformycin in these studies was attributed to the presence of 4.8% araA as a contaminant in araH preparations.

The significance of the antiviral activity of araH in cell culture systems is not clear. It is now apparent that many of the earlier in vitro studies of araA activity were assays of antiviral effects of araH, since araA was rapidly degraded by cellular and serum deaminases. In the extreme case plaque formation on a high-deaminase line of monkey kidney cells infected with vaccinia virus was equally sensitive to araA and araH (CONNOR et al., 1975); subsequent studies with this in vitro system have shown that araA, when combined with deoxycoformycin, was at least 50-fold more active than araH (SLOAN et al., 1977). The biochemical basis of the antiviral activity of araH is unknown. DRACH and SHIPMAN (1977) have reported selective inhibition of viral DNA synthesis after araH exposure of KB cells infected with herpes simplex virus; however, dosage levels were high, relative to similarly effective levels of araA in combination with the deaminase inhibitor. Additional studies are needed to assess the importance of araH as an antiviral agent in itself, and in the manifestation of antiviral activity attributed to araA.

Deoxycoformycin does not have in vitro antiviral activity at the concentrations generally employed to inhibit effectively adenosine deaminase (0.05–1 μg/ml). At relatively high concentrations (145 μg/ml) deoxycoformycin was somewhat inhibitory to infectious herpesvirus in HEp-2 cell cultures; at lower concentrations (15–50 μg/ml) deoxycoformycin was inactive (SLOAN et al., 1977). Concentrations of deoxycoformycin (about 1 μg/ml), sufficient to enhance araA activity against herpes simplex, vaccinia, and varicella-zoster virus infections of cultured cells, were themselves inactive (CONNOR et al., 1975). Under conditions comparable to those for assay of antiviral activity deoxycoformycin completely inhibited deamination of araA in uninfected cull cultures (SWEETMAN et al., 1975).

AraAMP and cyclic AMP exhibited activities comparable to that of araA when tested in vitro against a variety of DNA-containing viruses, including herpes simplex virus, cytomegalovirus, and vaccinia virus (SIDWELL et al., 1973). Similarly araAMP and araA were equally inhibitory when assayed, in absence of deaminase inhibitors, in herpes-infected cell cultures (TROBE et al., 1976; HASKELL, 1977). When plaque-inhibitory activities of araA and araAMP were compared in the presence of deoxycoformycin (0.83 μg/ml), 50% inhibitions in cells infected with herpes simplex virus were obtained with araA and araAMP, respectively, at 0.14 and 0.22 μM (BRYSON and KRONENBERG, 1977).

AraA has been tested extensively for antiviral activity in a variety of animal systems; a recent review of chemotherapy studies in virus-infected animals is available in the monograph edited by PAVAN-LANGSTON et al. (see SLOAN, 1975). AraA had significant activity against experimental herpes and vaccinial keratitis, herpes (types 1 and 2) and vaccinial encephalitis, and herpes and vaccinial skin lesions. Therapeutic activity was obtained when araA was administered intraperitoneally, subcutaneously, perorally, percutaneously, intravenously, subconjunctivally, intracerebrally, and by topical application. Results from animal studies with araA have been sufficiently encouraging to warrant clinical evaluation of araA against a number of viral infections in humans.

Since araH also exhibited activity in animal chemotherapy studies (SCHABEL, 1968; SLOAN et al., 1969; SLOAN, 1975), consideration of its role in araA therapy is of interest. From numerous metabolic studies with araA it is evident that animals treated with araA or, to a lesser extent, araAMP quickly convert most of the drug to araH. In one of the earliest studies araA and araH had comparable activities in therapy of intracerebral herpes simplex virus infections in mice (SLOAN et al., 1969); more recently, results from therapy of similarly infected mice with araA and deoxycoformycin suggested that inhibition of deamination markedly improved araA activity (SLOAN, 1975; SLOAN et al., 1977). Using a different animal model, herpes simplex keratis in the rabbit cornea, FALCON and JONES (1977a, b) have demonstrated enhancement of antiviral activity of araA, but not of araH or araAMP, by deoxycoformycin. In these studies araAMP was most active and araH least active, and deoxycoformycin increased the efficacy of araA to near that of araAMP. Thus it appeared that araA, if protected from deamination in vivo, was a more effective antiviral agent than araH. Additional studies will be required with these and other animal models to establish the relative activities of araA and its deamination product in viral chemotherapy.

There are now many reports in the medical literature of araA therapy of viral infections in humans. Comprehensive summaris of results from clinical studies conducted before 1974 of araA therapy of herpes simplex virus, cytomegalovirus, and varicella-zoster virus infections are available in a recent monograph (PAVAN-LANGSTON et al., 1975); results from these and other uncontrolled Phase II clinical studies suggested clinical usefulness for certain of the herpetic infections, particularly herpes simplex virus and varicella-zoster virus. Phase III studies conducted with araA have provided further encouragement for the future of araA as an antiviral agent (CH'IEN et al., 1976; WHITLEY et al., 1976, 1977). Immunosuppressed patients with herpes zoster infections who received araA therapy early in the course of their disease recovered more quickly than those who were treated with placebo (saline). In controlled studies of patients with biopsy-proved herpes simplex encephalitis, treatment with araA (12 h i.v. infusions of 15 mg/kg, daily for 10 days) reduced mortality from 70% to 28%, and over half of the survivors were free of serious neurologic disorders (WHITLEY et al., 1977). The greatest success was achieved in those patients treated early in the course of their disease, before the advent of coma, and there was no evidence of serious drug toxicity. Future controlled studies will include definition of optimal doses of araA for therapy and testing of araA derivatives of greater solubility, such as araAMP.

References

Adlard, B.P.F., Dobbing, J., Sands, J.: A comparison of the effects of cytosine arabinoside and adenine arabinoside on some aspects of brain growth and development in the rat. Br. J. Pharmacol. *54*, 33–39 (1975)

Agarwal, R.P., Parks, R.E., Jr.: Potent inhibition of muscle 5′-AMP deaminase by the nucleoside antibiotics coformycin and deoxycoformycin. Biochem. Pharmacol. *26*, 663–666 (1977)

Agarwal, R.P., Sagar, S.M., Parks, R.E., Jr.: Adenosine deaminase from human erythrocytes: purification and effects of adenosine analogs. Biochem. Pharmacol. *24*, 693–701 (1975)

Bennett, L.L., Jr., Hill, D.L.: Structural requirements for activity of nucleosides as substrates for adenosine kinase: orientation of substituents on the pentofuranosyl ring. Mol. Pharmacol. *11*, 803–808 (1975)

Bennett, L.L., Jr., Shannon, W.M., Allan, P.W., Arnett, G.: Studies on the biochemical basis for the antiviral activities of some nucleoside analogs. Ann. N.Y. Acad. Sci. *255*, 342–357 (1975)

Bloch, A., Robins, M.J., McCarthy, J.R., Jr.: The role of the 5′-hydroxyl group of adenosine in determining substrate specificity for adenosine deaminase. J. Med. Chem. *10*, 908–912 (1967)

Bollum, F.J.: Mammalian DNA polymerases. Prog. Nucleic Acid Res. Mol. Biol. *15*, 109–144 (1975)

Borondy, P.E., Chang, T., Maschewske, E., Glazko, A.J.: Inhibition of adenosine deaminase by co-vidarabine and its effect on the metabolic disposition of adenine arabinoside (vidarabine). Ann. N.Y. Acad. Sci. *284*, 9–20 (1977)

Brink, J.J., LePage, G.A.: Metabolic effects of 9-D-arabinosylpurines in ascites tumor cells. Cancer Res. *24*, 312–318 (1964a)

Brink, J.J., LePage, G.A.: Metabolism and distribution of 9-β-D-arabinofuranosyladenine in mouse tissues. Cancer Res. *24*, 1042–1049 (1964b)

Brink, J.J., LePage, G.A.: 9-β-D-Arabinofuranosyladenine as an inhibitor of metabolism in normal and neoplastic cells. Can. J. Biochem. *43*, 1–15 (1965)

Bryson, Y.J., Kronenberg, L.H.: Combined antiviral effects of interferon, adenine arabinoside, hypoxanthine arabinoside, and adenine arabinoside-5′-monophosphate in human fibroblast cultures. Antimicrob. Agents Chemother. *11*, 299–306 (1977)

Bryson, Y., Connor, J.O., Sweetman, L., Carey, S., Stuckey, M., Buchanan, R.: Determination of plaque inhibitory activity of adenosine arabinoside (9-β-D-arabinofuranosyladenine) for herpesviruses using an adenosine deaminase inhibitor. Antimicrob. Agents Chemother. *6*, 98–101 (1974)

Brockman, R.W., Shaddix, S.C., Rose, L.M., Carpenter, J.: Increased araATP levels and inhibition of DNA synthesis in leukemia cells treated with a combination of 9-β-D-arabinosyladenine (araA) and an adenosine deaminase inhibitor. Proc. Am. Assoc. Cancer Res. *17*, 52 (1976)

Brockman, R.W., Rose, L.M., Schabel, F.M., Jr., Laster, W.R., Jr.: Effects of adenosine deaminase inhibitors in combination with araA on araATP levels and chemotherapeutic response in L1210 leukemia. Proc. Am. Assoc. Cancer Res. *18*, 48 (1977)

Burridge, P.W., Paetkau, V., Henderson, J.F.: Studies of the relationship between adenosine deaminase and immune function. J. Immunol. *119*, 675–678 (1977)

Caron, N., Lee, S.H., Kimball, A.P.: Effects of 2′-deoxycoformycin, 9-β-D-arabinosyladenine 5′-phosphate, and 1-β-D-arabinosylcytosine triple combination therapy on intracerebral leukemia L1210. Cancer Res. *37*, 3274–3279 (1977)

Cass, C.E.: The enhancement of 9-β-D-arabinofuranosyladenine toxicity to mouse leukemia L1210 by an inhibitor of adenosine deaminase. Proc. Am. Assoc. Cancer Res. *17*, 24 (1976)

Cass, C.E., Ah-Yeung, T.H.: Enhancement of 9-β-D-arabinofuranosyladenine cytotoxicity to mouse leukemia L1210 *in vitro* by 2′-deoxycoformycin. Cancer Res. *36*, 1486–1491 (1976)

Cass, C.E., Paterson, A.R.P.: Mediated transport of nucleosides in human erythrocytes. Kinetics of exchange diffusion of uridine and thymidine and specificity toward pyrimidine nucleosides as permeants. J. Biol. Chem. *247*, 3314–3320 (1972)

Cass, C.E., Paterson, A.R.P.: Mediated transport of nucleosides in human erythrocytes. Specificity toward purine nucleosides as permeants. Biochim. Biophys. Acta *291*, 734–746 (1973)

Cass, C.E., Paterson, A.R.P.: Inhibition by nitrobenzylthioinosine of uptake of adenosine, 2′-deoxyadenosine and 9-β-D-arabinofuranosyladenine by human and mouse erythrocytes. Biochem. Pharmacol. *24*, 1989–1993 (1975)

Cass, C.E., Paterson, A.R.P.: Nitrobenzylthioinosine binding sites in the erythrocyte membrane. Biochim. Biophys. Acta *419*, 285–294 (1976)

Cass, C.E., Gaudette, L.A., Paterson, A.R.P.: Mediated transport of nucleosides in human erythrocytes. Specific binding of the inhibitor nitrobenzylthioinosine to nucleoside transport sites in the erythrocyte membrane. Biochim. Biophys. Acta *345*, 1–10 (1974)

Cha, S.: Tight-binding inhibitors – I. Kinetic behavior. Biochem. Pharmacol. *24*, 2187–2197 (1975)

Cha, S.: Tight-binding inhibitors – III. A new approach for the determination of competition between tight-binding inhibitors and substrate-inhibition of adenosine deaminase by conformycin. Biochem. Pharmacol. *25*, 2695–2702 (1976)

Cha, S., Agarwal, R.P., Parks, R.E., Jr.: Tight-binding inhibitors. II. Non-steady state nature of inhibition of milk xanthine oxidase by allopurinal and alloxanthine and of human erythrocytic adenosine deaminase by coformycin. Biochem. Pharmacol. *24*, 2187–2197 (1975)

Chang, T., Glazko, A.J.: Effect of an adenosine deaminase inhibitor on the uptake and metabolism of arabinosyl adenine (vidarabine) by intact erythrocytes. Res. Commun. Chem. Pathol. Pharmacol. *14*, 127–140 (1976)

Chao, D.L.-S., Kimball, A.P.: Deamination of arabinosyladenine by adenosine deaminase and inhibition by arabinosyl-6-mercaptopurine. Cancer Res. *32*, 1721–1724 (1972)

Chassin, M.M., Adamson, R.H., Johns, D.G.: An enzyme inhibition titration assay for 2′-deoxycoformycin and its application to the study of the pharmacokinetics of the drug. Proc. Am. Assoc. Cancer Res. *18*, 147 (1977)

Ch'ien, L.T., Schabel, F.M., Jr., Alford, C.A., Jr.: Arabinosyl nucleosides and nucleotides. In: Selective inhibitors of viral functions, pp. 227–256. Cleveland, Ohio: CRC Press 1973

Ch'ien, L.T., Whitley, R.J., Alford, C.A., Jr., Galasso, G.J.: Adenine arabinoside for therapy

of herpes zoster in immunosuppressed patients: preliminary results of a collaborative study. J. Infect. Dis. (Suppl.) *133*, A184–A191 (1976)
Cohen, S.S.: Introduction to the biochemistry of D-arabinosyl nucleosides. Prog. Nucleic Acid Res. Mol. Biol. *5*, 1–88 (1966)
Cohen, S.S.: Commentary on the therapeutic use of nucleosides and the penetrability of phosphorylated compounds. Biochem. Pharmacol. *24*, 1929–1932 (1975)
Cohen, S.S.: The lethality of aranucleotides. Med. Biol. *54*, 299–326 (1976)
Cohen, S.S., Plunkett, W.: The utilization of nucleotides by animal cells. Ann. N.Y. Acad. Sci. *255*, 269–284 (1975)
Connor, J.D., Sweetman, L., Carey, S., Stuckey, M.A., Buchanan, R.: Effect of adenosine deaminase upon the antiviral activity *in vitro* of adenine arabinoside for vaccinia virus. Antimicrob. Agents Chemother. *6*, 630–636 (1974)
Connor, J.D., Sweetman, L., Carey, S., Stuckey, M.A., Buchanan, R.: Susceptibility *in vitro* of several large DNA viruses to the antiviral activity of adenine arabinoside: relation to human pharmacology. In: Adenine arabinoside: an antiviral agent. Pavan-Langston, D., Buchanan, R.A., Alford, C.A., Jr. (eds.), pp. 177–196. New York: Raven Press 1975
Cory, J.G., Suhadolnik, R.J.: Structural requirements of nucleosides for binding by adenosine deaminase. Biochemistry *4*, 1729–1732 (1965)
Cozzarelli, N.R.: The mechanisms of action of inhibitors of DNA synthesis. Ann u. Rev. Biochem. *46*, 641–668 (1977)
De Rudder, J., Privat de Garilhe, M.: Inhibitory effect of some nucleosides on the growth of various human viruses in tissue culture. Antimicrob. Agents. Chemother. 578–584 (1965)
Dion, H.D., Woo, P.W.K., Ryder, A.: Isolation and properties of a vidarabine deaminase inhibitor, co-vidarabine. Ann. N.Y. Acad. Sci. *284*, 21–29 (1977)
Doering, A., Keller, J., Cohen, S.S.: Some effects of D-arabinosyl nucleosides on polymer synthesis in mouse fibroblasts. Cancer Res. *26*, 2444–2450 (1966)
Drach, J.C., Shipman, C., Jr.: The selective inhibition of viral DNA synthesis by chemotherapeutic agents: an indicator of clinical usefulness? Ann. N.Y. Acad. Sci. *284*, 296–409 (1977)
Drach, J.C., Bus, J.S., Schultz, S.K., Sandberg, J.N.: Biotransformation of 9-β-D-arabinofuranosyladenine by rat and human erythrocytes. Biochem. Pharmacol. *23*, 2761–2767 (1974)
Evans, B., Wolfenden, R.: A potential transition state analog for adenosine deaminase. J. Am. Chem. Soc. *92*, 4751–4752 (1970)
Falcon, M.G., Jones, B.R.: Antiviral activity in the rabbit cornea of adenine arabinoside, ara-A 5'-monophosphate, and hypoxanthine arabinoside; and interactions with adenosine deaminase inhibitor. J. Gen. Virol. *36*, 199–202 (1977a)
Falcon, M.G., Jones, B.R.: Herpes simplex keratitis: animal models to guide the selection and optimal delivery of antiviral chemotherapy. J. Antimicrob. Chemother. (Suppl. A), *3*, 83–89 (1977b)
Fishaut, J.M., Connor, J.D., Lampert, P.W.: Comparative effects of arabinosyl nucleosides on the postnatal growth and development of the rat. In: Adenine arabinoside: an antiviral agent. Pavan-Langston, D., Buchanan, R.A., Alford, C.A., Jr. (eds.), pp. 159–170. New York: Ravan Press 1975
Follmann, H., Hogenkamp, H.P.C.: Interaction of ribonucleotide reductase with ribonucleotide analogs. Biochemistry *10*, 186–191 (1971)
Frederiksen, S.: Specificity of adenosine deaminase toward adenosine and 2'-deoxyadenosine analogues. Arch. Biochem. Biophys. *113*, 383–388 (1966)
Furth, J.J., Cohen, S.S.: Inhibition of mammalian DNA polymerase by the 5'-triphosphate of 9-β-D-arabinofuranosyladenine. Cancer Res. *27*, 1528–1533 (1967)
Furth, J.J., Cohen, S.S.: Inhibition of mammalian DNA polymerases by the 5'-triphosphate of 1-β-D-arabinofuranosylcytosine and the 5'-triphosphate of 9-β-D-arabinofuranosyladenine. Cancer Res. *28*, 2061–2067 (1968)
Gasset, A.R., Akaboshi, T.: Teratogenicity of adenine arabinoside. Invest. Opthalmol. *15*, 556–557 (1976)
Glaudemans, C.P.J., Fletcher, H.G., Jr.: Synthesis with partially benzylated sugars. III. A single pathway to a "cis-nucleoside," 9-β-D-arabinofuranosyladenine (spongo-adenosine). J. Org. Chem. *28*, 3004–3006 (1963)
Glazko, A.J., Chang, T., Drach, J.C., Mourer, D.R., Borondy, P.E., Schneider, H., Croskey,

L., Maschewski, E., Species differences in the metabolic disposition of adenine arabinoside. In: Adenine arabinoside: an antiviral agent. Pavan-Langston, D., Buchanan, R.A., Alford, C.A., Jr. (eds.), pp. 111–133. New York: Raven Press 1975

Haskell, T.H.: Relationship of structure and antiviral activity of 9-β-D-arabinofuranosyladenine analogs. Ann. N.Y. Acad. Sci. *284*, 81–90 (1977)

Herrmann, E.C., Jr. (ed.): Third Conference on Antiviral Substances. Ann. N.Y. Acad. Sci. *284* (1977)

Hubert-Habart, M., Cohen, S.S.: The toxicity of 9-β-D-arabinofuranosyladenine to purine-requiring *Escherichia coli*. Biochem. Biophys. Acta *59*, 468–471 (1962)

Hughes, R.G., Jr., Kimball, A.P.: Metabolic effects of cyclic 9-β-D-arabinofuranosyladenine 3′, 5′-monophosphate in L1210 cells. Cancer Res. *32*, 1791–1794 (1972)

Ishii, K., Green, H.: Lethality of adenosine for cultured mammalian cells by interference with pyrimidine biosynthesis. J. Cell Sci. *13*, 429–439 (1973)

Josse, J., Kaiser, A.D., Kornberg, A.: Enzymatic synthesis of deoxyribonucleic acid. VIII. Frequencies of nearest neighbor base sequences in deoxyribonucleic acid. J. Biol. Chem. *236*, 864–875 (1961)

Keeney, R.E.: Human tolerance of adenine arabinoside. In: Adenine arabinoside: an antiviral agent. Pavan-Langston, D., Buchanan, R.A., Alford, C.A., Jr. (eds.), pp. 265–273. New York: Raven Press 1975

Kimball, A.P., LePage, G.A., Worth, L.S., Lee, S.H.: Enhancement of the antileukemic activity of adenine arabinoside (ara-A) by deoxycoformycin (2′-dCF). Proc. Am. Assoc. Cancer Res. *17*, 168 (1976)

Kimball, A.P., Lee, S.H., Caron, N.: Deoxycoformycin, arabinosyladenine, arabinosylcytosine combination therapy of intracerebral leukemia L1210. Proc. Am. Assoc. Cancer Res. *18*, 125 (1977)

Kinkel, A.W., Buchanan, R.A.: Human pharmacology. In: Adenine arabinoside: an antiviral agent. Pavan-Langston, D., Buchanan, R.A., Alford, C.A., Jr. (eds.), pp. 197–204. New York: Raven Press 1975

Koshiura, R., LePage, G.A.: Some inhibitors of deamination of 9-β-D-arabinofuranosyladenine and 9-β-D-xylofuranosyladenine by blood and neoplasms of experimental animals and humans. Cancer Res. *28*, 1014–1020 (1968)

Krenitsky, T.A., Tuttle, J.V., Koszalka, G.W., Chen, I.S., Beachan, L.M., III, Rideout, J.L., Elion, G.B.: Deoxycytidine kinase from calf thymus. Substrate and inhibitor specificity. J. Biol. Chem. *251*, 4055–4061 (1976)

Krygier, V., Momparler, R.L.: Mammalian deoxynucleoside kinases. II. Deoxyadenosine kinase: purification and properties. J. Biol. Chem. *246*, 2745–2751 (1971)

Kurtz, S.M.: Toxicology of adenine arabinoside. In: Adenine arabinoside: an antiviral agent. Pavan-Langston, D., Buchanan, R.A., Alford, C.A., Jr. (eds.), pp. 145–157. New York: Raven Press 1975

Kurtz, S.M., Fisken, R.A., Kaump, D.H., Schardein, J.L.: Toxicity of 9-β-D-arabinofuranosyladenine in mice and rabbits. In: Antimicrob. agents chemother. Hobby, G.L. (ed.), pp. 180–189. Bethesda, Maryland: Am. Soc. Microbiol. 1969

Kurtz, S.M., Fitzgerald, J.E., Schardein, J.L.: Comparative animal toxicology of vidarabine and its 5′-monophosphate. Ann. N.Y. Acad. Sci. *284*, 6–8 (1977)

Lee, S.H., Caron, N., Kimball, A.P.: Therapeutic effects of 9-β-D-arabinofuranosyladenine and 2′-deoxycoformycin combinations on intracerebral leukemia L1210. Cancer Res. *37*, 1953–1955 (1977)

Lee, W.W., Benitez, A., Goodman, L., Baker, B.R.: Potential anticancer agents. XL. Synthesis of the β-anomer of 9-(D-arabinofuranosyl)-adenine. J. Am. Chem. Soc. *82*, 2648–2649 (1960)

Lee, W.W., Fisher, L.V., Goodman, L.: 9-(β-D-Arabinofuranosyl) adenine 3′,5′-cyclic phosphate (1). J. Heterocycl. Chem. *8*, 179–180 (1971)

LePage, G.A.: Alterations in enzyme activity in tumors and the implications for chemotherapy. Adv. Enzyme Regul. *8*, 323–332 (1969)

LePage, G.A.: Arabinosyladenine and arabinosylhypoxanthine metabolism in murine tumor cells. Can. J. Biochem. *48*, 75–78 (1970)

LePage, G.A.: Recent advances in the biochemical pharmacology of specific chemical agents. Purines and purine nucleoside antagonists. Transplant. Proc. *V*, 1157–1160 (1973)

LePage, G.A.: Purine arabinosides, xylosides, and lyxosides. In: Handbook of experimental pharmacology. New Series. Sartorelli, A.C., Johns, D.G. (eds.), Vol. XXXVIII/2, pp. 426–433. Berlin-Heidelberg, New York: Springer 1975
LePage, G.A., Hersh, E.M.: Cyclic nucleotide analogs as carcinostatic agents. Biochem. Biophys. Res. Commun. *46*, 1918–1922 (1972)
LePage, G.A., Lin, T.-T., Orth, R.E., Gottlieb, J.A.: 5′-Nucleotides as potential formulations for administering nucleoside analogs in man. Cancer Res. *32*, 2441–2444 (1972)
LePage, G.A., Khalig, A., Gottlieb, J.A.: Studies of 9-β-D-arabinofuranosyladenine in man. Drug Metab. Dispos. *1*, 756–759 (1973)
LePage, G.A., Naik, S.R., Katakkar, S.B., Kahliq, A.: 9-β-D-arabinofuranosyladenine 5′-phosphate metabolism and excretion in humans. Cancer Res. *35*, 3036–3040 (1975)
LePage, G.A., Worth, L.S., Kimball, A.P.: Enhancement of the antitumor activity of arabinofuranosyladenine by 2′-deoxycoformycin. Cancer Res. *36*, 1481–1485 (1976)
Lindberg, B., Klenow, H., Hansen, K.: Some properties of partially purified mammalian adenosine kinase. J. Biol. Chem. *242*, 350–356 (1967)
Loeb, L.A.: Eukaryotic DNA polymerases. In: The enzymes. Boyer, P.D. (ed.), Vol. 10, pp. 173–209. New York: Academic Press 1974
McConnell, W.R.: Development of an assay to determine the biological distribution of 2′-deoxycoformycin (NSC-218321). Proc. Am. Assoc. Cancer Res. *18*, 42 (1977)
Meuwissen, H.J., Pickering, R.J., Pollara, B., Porter, I.H.: Combined immunodeficiency disease and adenosine deaminase deficiency – a molecular defect. New York: Academic Press Inc. 1975
Mian, A.M., Harris, R., Sidwell, R.W., Robins, R.K., Khwaja, T.A.: Synthesis and biological activity of 9-β-D-arabinofuranosyladenine cyclic 3′,5′-phosphate and 9-β-D-arabinofuranosylguanine cyclic 3′,5′-phosphate. J. Med. Chem. *17*, 259–263 (1974)
Miller, F.A., Dixon, G.J., Ehrlich, J., Sloan, B.J., McLean, I.W., Jr.: Antiviral activity of 9-β-D-arabinofuranosyladenine. I. Cell culture studies. In: Antimicrob. agents chemother. Hobbs, G.L. (ed.), pp. 136–147. Bethesda, Maryland: Am. Soc. Microbiol. 1969
Moore, E.C., Cohen, S.S.: Effects of arabinonucleotides on ribonucleotide reduction by an enzyme system from rat tumor. J. Biol. Chem. *9*, 2116–2118 (1967)
Müller, W.E.G., Rohde, H.J., Beyer, R., Maidhof, A., Lachmann, M., Taschner, H.: Mode of action of 9-β-D-arabinofuranosyladenine on the synthesis of DNA, RNA, and protein *in vivo* and *in vitro*. Cancer Res. *35*, 2160–2168 (1975)
Müller, W.E.G., Maidhof, A., Zahn, R.K., Shannon, W.M.: Effect of 9-β-D-arabinofuranosyladenine on DNA synthesis *in vivo*. Cancer Res. *37*, 2282–2290 (1977a)
Müller, W.E.G., Zahn, R.K., Bittlingmaier, K., Falke, D.: Inhibition of herpesvirus DNA Synthesis by 9-β-D-arabinofuranosyladenine in cellular and cell-free systems. Ann. N.Y. Acad. Sci. *284*, 34–48 (1977b)
Nakamura, H., Koyama, G., Iitaka, Y., Ohno, M., Yagisawa, N., Kondo, S., Maeda, K., Umezawa, H.: Structure of coformycin, an unusual nucleoside of microbial origin. J. Am. Chem. Soc. *96*, 4327–4328 (1974)
Nichols, W.W.: *In vitro* chromosome breakage induced by arabinosyladenine in human leukocytes. Cancer Res. *24*, 1502–1505 (1964)
Ohno, M., Yakisawa, N., Shibahara, S., Kondo, S., Maeda, K., Umezawa, H.: Synthesis of coformycin. J. Am. Chem. Soc. *96*, 4326 (1974)
Oliver, J.M., Paterson, A.R.P.: Nucleoside transport. I. A mediated process in human erythrocytes. Can. J. Biochem. *49*, 262–270 (1971)
Ortiz, P.J., Manduka, M.J., Cohen, S.S.: The lethality of some D-arabinosyl nucleotides to mouse fibroblasts. Cancer Res. *32*, 1512–1517 (1972)
Pavan-Langston, D., Buchanan, R.A., Alford, C.A., Jr.: Adenine arabinoside: an antiviral agent. New York: Raven Press Publishers 1975
Paterson, A.R.P., Babb, L.R., Paran, J.H., Cass, C.E.: Inhibition by nitrobenzylthioinosine of adenosine uptake by asynchronous HeLa cells. Mol. Pharmacol. *13*, 1147–1158 (1977a)
Paterson, A.R.P., Naik, S.R., Cass, C.E.: Inhibition of uridine transport in HeLa cells by nitrobenzylthioinosine and related compounds. Mol. Pharmacol. *13*, 1014–1023 (1977b)
Plunkett, W., Cohen, S.S.: Metabolism of 9-β-D-arabinosyladenine by mouse fibroblasts. Cancer Res. *35*, 415–422 (1975a)

Plunkett, W., Cohen, S.S.: Two approaches that increase the activity of analogs of adenine nucleosides in animal cells. Cancer Res. *35*, 1547–1554 (1975b)
Plunkett, W., Cohen, S.S.: Increased toxicity of 9-β-D-arabinofuranosyladenine in the presence of an inhibitor of adenosine deaminase. Ann. N.Y. Acad. Sci. *284*, 91–105 (1977)
Plunkett, W., Lapi, L., Ortiz, P.J., Cohen, S.S.: Penetration of mouse fibroblasts by the 5′-phosphate of 9-β-D-arabinofuranosyladenine and incorporation of the nucleotide into DNA. Proc. Natl. Acad. Sci. *71*, 73–77 (1974)
Plunkett, W., Alexander, L., Loo, T.L.: Biochemical basis of the increased arabinofuranosyladenine (ara-A) activity in the presence of adenosine deaminase inhibitors (ADI). Proc. Am. Assoc. Cancer Res. *18*, 58 (1977)
Reist, E.J., Benitez, A., Goodman, L., Baker, B.R., Lee, W.W.: Potential anticancer agents. LXXVI. Synthesis of purine nucleosides of β-D-arabinofuranose. J. Org. Chem. *27*, 3274–3279 (1962)
Reist, E.J., Bartuska, V.J., Goodman, L.: Sodium-liquid ammonia debenzylations in nucleoside synthesis. J. Org. Chem. *29*, 3725–3726 (1964)
Repta, A.J., Rawson, B.J., Shatter, R.D., Sloan, K.R., Bodor, N., Higuchi, T.: Rational development of a soluble prodrug of a cytotoxic nucleoside: preparation and properties of arabinosyladenine 5′-formate, J. Pharm. Sci. *64*, 392–396 (1975)
Rose, L.M., Brockman, B.W.: Analysis by high-pressure liquid chromatography of 9-β-D-arabinofuranosyladenine 5′-triphosphate levels in murine leukemia cells. J. Chromatogr. *133*, 335–343 (1977)
Ross, A.H., Julia, A., Balakrishnan, C.: Toxicity of adenine arabinoside in humans. J. Infect. Dis. *133*, S, A192–A198 (1978)
Sawa, T., Fukagawa, Y., Homma, I., Takeuchi, T., Umezawa, H.: Mode of inhibition of coformycin on adenosine deaminase. J. Antibiot. Ser. A *20*, 227–231 (1967)
Schabel, F.M., Jr.: The antiviral activity of 9-β-D-arabinofuranosyladenine (ara-A). Chemotherapy *13*, 321–338 (1968)
Schabel, F.M., Jr., Trader, M.W., Laster, W.R., Jr.: Increased therapeutic activity of 9-β-D-arabinofuranosyladenine (ara-A) against leukemia P388 and L1210 by an adenosine deaminase inhibitor. Proc. Am. Assoc. Cancer Res. *17*, 46 (1976)
Schaeffer, H.J., Schwender, C.F.: Enzyme inhibitions. 26. Bridging hydrophobic regions on adenosine deaminase with some 9-(2-hydroxy-3-alky)adenines. J. Med. Chem. *17*, 6–8 (1974)
Schnebli, H.P., Hill, D.L., Bennett, L.L., Jr.: Purification and properties of adenosine kinase from human tumor cells of Type H. Ep. No. 2. J. Biol. Chem. *242*, 1997–2004 (1967)
Schwartz, P.M., Shipman, C., Jr., Carlson, R.H., Drach, J.C.: Thermal inactivation as a means of inhibiting the serum-associated deamination of 9-β-D-arabinofuranosyladenine in tissue culture media. Antimicrob. Agents Chemother. *5*, 337–343 (1974)
Schwartz, P.M., Shipman, C., Jr., Drach, J.C.: Antiviral activity of arabinosyladenine and arabinosylhypoxanthine in herpes simplex virus-infected KB cells. II. Selective inhibition of DNA synthesis in the presence of an adenosine deaminase inhibitor. Antimicrob. Agents Chemother. *10*, 64–74 (1976)
Shannon, W.M.: Adenine arabinoside: antiviral activity *in vitro*. In: Adenine arabinoside: an antiviral agent. Pavan-Langston, D., Buchanan, R.A., Alford, C.A., Jr. (eds.), pp. 1–43. New York: Raven Press 1975
Shannon, W.M.: Introductory remarks on adenine arabinoside. Ann. N.Y. Acad. Sci. *284*, 3–5 (1977a)
Shannon, W.M.: Selective inhibition of RNA tumor virus replication *in vitro* and evaluation of candidate antiviral agents *in vivo*. Ann. N.Y. Acad. Sci. *284*, 475–507 (1977b)
Shipman, C., Jr., Smith, S.H., Carlson, R.H., Drach, J.C.: Antiviral activity of arabinosyladenine and arabinosylhypoxanthine in herpes simplex virus-infected KB cells: selective inhibition of viral deoxyribonucleic acid synthesis in synchronized suspension cultures. Antimicrob. Agents Chemother. *9*, 120–127 (1976)
Sidwell, R.W., Allen, L.B., Huffman, J.H., Khwaja, T.A., Tolman, R.L., Robins, R.K.: Anti-DNA virus activity of the 5′-nucleotide and 3′,5′-cyclic nucleotide of 9-β-D-arabinofuranosyladenine. Chemotherapy *19*, 325–340 (1973)
Skipper, H., Schabel, F.M., Jr., Wilcox, W.: Experimental evaluation of potential anticancer agents. XXI. Scheduling of arabinocytosine to take advantage of its S-phase specificity against leukemic cells. Cancer Chemother. Rep. *51*, 125–141 (1967)

Sloan, B.J.: Adenine arabinoside: chemotherapy studies in animals. In: Adenine arabinoside: an antiviral agent. Pavan-Langston, D., Buchanan, R.A., Alford, C.A., Jr. (eds.), pp. 45–94. New York: Raven Press 1975

Sloan, B.J., Miller, F.A., Ehrlich, J., McLean, I.W., Machamer, H.E.: Antiviral activity of 9-β-D-arabinofuranosyladenine. IV. Activity against intracerebral herpes simplex virus infections in mice. In: Antimicrob. agents chemother. Hobby, G.L. (ed.), pp. 161–171. Bethesda, Maryland: Am. Soc. Microbiol. 1969

Sloan, B.J., Kielty, J.K., Miller, F.A.: Effect of a novel adenosine deaminase inhibitor (co-vidarabine, co-V) upon the antiviral activity *in vitro* and *in vivo* of vidarabine (vira-A) for DNA virus replication. Ann. N.Y. Acad. Sci. *284*, 60–80 (1977)

Steele, R.W., Chapa, I.A., Vincent, M.M., Hensen, S.A., Keeney, R.E.: Effects of adenine arabinoside on cellular immune mechanisms in humans. Antimicrob. Agents Chemother. *7*, 203–207 (1975)

Suhadolnik, R.M.: Nucleoside antibiotics, pp. 123–169. New York: Wiley Interscience 1970

Suhling, W.J., Rice, L.S., Shannon, W.M.: The quantitation of 2′-deoxycoformycin in animal fluids and tissues by microbiological assay. Proc. Am. Assoc. Cancer Res. *18*, 42 (1977)

Sweetman, L., Connor, J.D., Seshamani, R., Stuckey, M.A., Carey, S., Buchanan, R.: Deamination of adenine arabinoside in cell cultures used for *in vitro* viral inhibition studies. In: adenine arabinoside: an antiviral agent. Pavan-Langston, D., Buchanan, R.A., Alford, C.A., Jr. (eds.), pp. 135–144. New York: Raven Press 1975

Taube, R.A., Berlin, R.D.: Membrane transport in rabbit polymorphonuclear leukocytes. Biochim. Biophys. Acta *255*, 6–18 (1972)

Trobe, J.D., Centifanto, Z., Zam, S., Varnell, E., Kaufman, H.E.: Anti-herpes activity of adenine arabinoside. Invest. Opthalmol. *15*, 196–199 (1976)

Waqar, M.A., Burgoyne, L.A., Atkinson, M.R.: Deoxyribonucleic acid synthesis in mammalian nuclei. Incorporation of deoxyribonucleotides and chain-terminating nucleotide analogues. Biochem. J. *121*, 803–809 (1971)

Webb, J.L.: Enzyme and metabolic inhibitors. Vol. I, pp. 104–105. New York: Academic Press 1963

Weissbach, A.: Vertebrate DNA polymerases. Cell *5*, 101–108 (1975)

Weissbach, A.: Eukaryotic DNA polymerases. Annu. Rev. Biochem. *46*, 25–47 (1977)

Weissbach, A., Hong, S., Aucke, J., Müller, R.: Characterization of *Herpes simplex* virus-induced deoxyribonucleic acid polymerase. J. Biol. Chem. *248*, 6270–6277 (1973)

Weissbach, A., Baltimore, D., Bollum, F.J., Gallo, R.C., Korn, D.: Nomenclature of eukaryotic DNA polymerases. Science *190*, 401–402 (1975)

Whitley, R.J., Ch'ien, L.T., Dolin, R., Galasso, G.J., Alford, C.A., Jr.: Adenine arabinoside therapy of herpes zoster in the immunosuppressed. N. Engl. J. Med. *294*, 1193–1199 (1975)

Whitley, R.J., Ch'ien, L.T., Dolin, R., Galasso, G.J., Alford, C.A.: Adenine arabinoside therapy of herpes zoster in the immunosuppressed. N. Engl. J. Med. *294*, 1193–1199 (1976)

Whitley, R.J., Soong, S.-J., Dolin, R., Galasso, G.J., Ch'ien, L.T., Alford, C.A.: Adenine arabinoside therapy of biopsy-proved herpes simplex encephalitis. N. Engl. J. Med. *297*, 289–294 (1977)

Williams, B.B., Lerner, A.M.: Antiviral activity of an adenosine deaminase inhibitor: decreased replication of herpes simplex virus. J. Infect. Dis. *131*, 673–677 (1975)

Woo, P.W.K., Dion, H.W., Lange, S.M., Dahl, L.F., Durham, L.J.: A novel adenosine and ara-A deaminase inhibitor (R)-3-(2-Deoxy-β-D-*erythro*-pentofuranosyl)-3,6,7,8-tetrahydroimidazo-[4,5*d*] [1,3]diazepin-8-ol. J. Heterocyl. Chem. *11*, 641–643 (1974)

York, J.L., LePage, G.A.: A proposed mechanism for the action of 9-β-D-arabinofuranosyladenine as an inhibitor of the growth of some ascites cells. Can. J. Biochem. *44*, 19–26 (1966a)

York, J.L., LePage, G.A.: A kinetic study of the deamination of some adenosine analogues. Substrate specificity of adenosine deaminase. Can. J. Biochem. *44*, 331–337 (1966b)

Zam, Z.S., Centifanto, Y.M., Kaufman, H.E.: Failure of systemically administered adenine arabinoside to affect humoral and cell-mediated immunity. Am. J. Opthalmol. *81*, 502–505 (1976)

8-Azaguanine

D. GRUNBERGER and G. GRUNBERGER

I. History

ROBLIN et al. in 1945 observed that an inclusion of 8-azaguanine in the bacterial medium inhibited the growth of *Escherichia coli*. Addition of guanine to the medium reversed this inhibition. In 1949 KIDDER and DEWEY confirmed these findings when the analog inhibited multiplication of *Tetrahymena geleii*. Subsequently, several investigators proved 8-azaguanine to be an inhibitor of the chick embryo (YOUNGER et al., 1950), the Lucerne mosaic virus (MATTHEWS, 1952), the *Psittacosis* virus (MORGAN, 1952), human glioblastomas (PETERSON and MURRAY, 1953), and tobacco mosaic virus (MATTHEWS, 1954). Inhibition of growth of some transplanted mouse tumors was also shown (KIDDER et al., 1949). The analog was effective against a variety of murine carcinomas and certain leukemias (BURCHENAL et al., 1949). It was possible to reverse the inhibition in several of these by simultaneous addition of guanine (LAW, 1950; KIDDER et al., 1951). HIRSCHBERG et al. (1952) found that antimetabolite-resistant tumors had high azaguanine deaminase activity, while the activity in the susceptible tumors was low or negligible. The 8-azaguanine was enzymatically deaminated to 8-azaxanthine, which had no carcinostatic activity. Interference with this deamination led to a potentiation of the toxic and carcinostatic actions of the analog. Despite exhaustive research, however, no useful role has been found for 8-azaguanine in cancer chemotherapy.

II. Chemical and Crystal Structure

8-Azaguanine can be derived from guanine by the substitution of a nitrogen atom for the CH group in position-8 (Fig. 1). MACINTYRE et al. (1965) demonstrated the crystal structure of 8-azaguanine monohydrate. The azaguanine molecules are stacked on top of one another with the perpendicular distance between successive molecular planes of 3.25 Å, which is shorter than the van der Waals approach normally seen in aromatic molecules. The short distance represents a bonding interaction between the molecules. Another interesting feature of the 8-azaguanine structure was the absence of a hydrogen bond to N-8. The result of their structure analysis suggested that 8-azaguanine forms a charge-transfer self-complex in the crystals of the monohydrate.

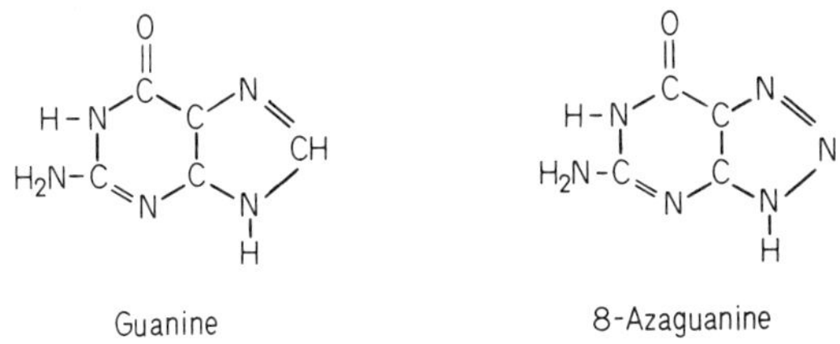

Fig. 1. Structure of guanine and 8-azaguanine

III. Synthesis and Metabolism

To study the substance effectively, MANDEL's group prepared 8-azaguanine labeled with [^{14}C] in the C-4 position (MANDEL et al., 1951). The reactions involved in this synthesis are shown in Fig. 2.

When radioactive 8-azaguanine was administered intraperitoneally to mice, it was found that twelve hours after the injection 3% of the original label remained in the animal (MANDEL, 1951) even though the peak action of the drug on tumor respiration was reported at 24 h after the drug had been administered (FINKELSTEIN et al., 1951).

MANDEL suggested, therefore, that azaguanine initiated some change in the animal which caused the maximum effect to appear after the drug was almost completely eliminated. The radioactive metabolite in urine was identified as 8-azaxanthine, both in mice and Macaca mulatta monkey (MANDEL et al., 1951). The deamination of 8-azaguanine to 8-azaxanthine is carried out by the enzyme guanine deaminase which also catalyzes the reaction of guanine to xanthine.

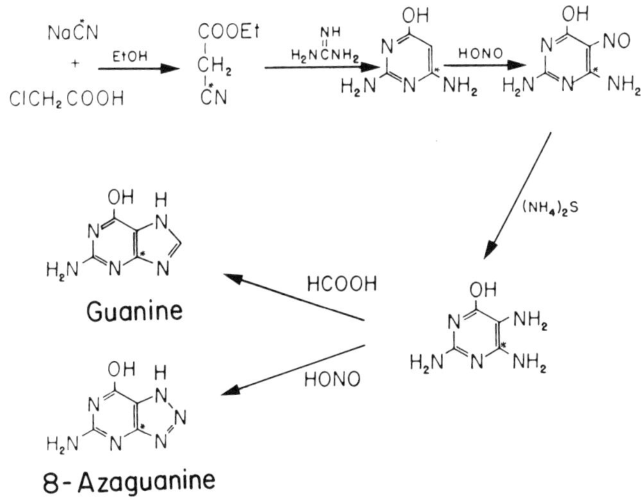

Fig. 2. Scheme of [^{14}C] 8-azaguanine synthesis

MANDEL (1961) showed that when both guanine and its analog were added to the cells, they incorporated the normal purine preferentially. Inhibition of growth was seen only when 8-azaguanine remained in the medium.

When *Pseudomonas aeruginosa* was allowed to grow in a minimal medium containing azaguanine (100 μg/ml), only 8-azaxanthine was detected in the medium 24 h later. The analog was deaminated by 8-azaguanine deaminase. The drug was more rapidly deaminated than guanine by both induced and non-induced cultures incubated anaerobically. Azaguanine was not found to act as an inducer for the deaminase, although it is a substrate of the enzyme (CLARKE and MEADOW, 1966).

Several groups of investigators have shown that azaguanine (azaG) is enzymatically converted to 8-azaGMP and 8-azaGTP (MITCHELL et al., 1950; MANDEL et al., 1954; SMITH and MATTHEWS, 1957; MANDEL and MARKHAM, 1958; WAY and PARKS, 1958; BROCKMAN et al., 1959; WAY et al., 1959). It was found that azaguanine did not block the incorporation of guanine into RNA, nor did it act by replacing guanine when RNA was formed, but rather it acted after its incorporation into nucleic acids (MANDEL and MARKHAM, 1958). LEVIN (1962) determined that polynucleotide phosphorylase catalyzed the formation of poly[azaG] from 8-azaGDP. The enzyme also catalyzed an exchange reaction between [^{32}P] orthophosphate and the terminal phosphate of 8-azaGDP. Takadiastase-T_1-ribonuclease and pancreatic ribonuclease degraded poly[azaG]-virtually completely, with primary products being 8-azaG-2′,3′-P(cyclic); 8-azaG-3′[2′]-P(noncyclic); and 8-azaGp8-azaG-2′,3′-P(cyclic).

IV. Mode of Action

BROCKMAN and his colleagues (1957, 1959) established that 8-azaguanine must be converted to its nucleotide derivative in order to exert its inhibitory effect. L-1210-leukemia and *Streptococci faecalis* cells were used in their experiments. The resistance to azaguanine was thought to be due to an inability of the cells to convert the analog to the nucleotide. The mechanism of action of the drug was postulated to be connected either with a general inhibition of protein synthesis, or with formation of a fraudulent RNA, or with the inhibition of a coenzyme function. The following section reviews the results of studies on the mode of azaguanine action.

A. Inhibition of Coenzyme Action

The possibility has been raised that some antimetabolites act by inhibiting the synthesis or functions of nucleotide coenzymes. ROY et al. (1961) found, however, that the ribonucleoside 5′-triphosphates of 8-azaguanosine did not inhibit the in vitro incorporation of amino acids into microsomal proteins. The 8-azaguanine 5′-triphosphate served as a partial substitute for GTP. They concluded that the possibility of 8-azaG acting by the formation of fraudulent triphosphate nucleosides competing with GTP was unlikely.

B. Incorporation into Nucleic Acids

Incorporation of the analog into the nucleic acids has been reported practically from the onset of azaguanine research (MITCHELL et al., 1950). The drug is incorporated into viral, bacterial, and mammalian RNA. LASNITZKY et al. (1954) found that azaguanine replaced up to 5% of the guanine residues when *Escherichia coli, Staphylococcus aureus,* and mice bearing subcutaneous and ascites tumors were investigated. Of the guanine residues 3% were replaced in tobacco virus (MATTHEWS, 1954) and 40% in *Bacillus cereus* (SMITH and MATTHEWS, 1957). LEVIN (1963) found an even higher percentage of replacement in *B. cereus.* KARON et al. (1965) demonstrated an 8% to 9% incorporation of the analog in place of the guanine residues in cultured human cells, claiming that the azaguanine incorporation into RNA in bacterial systems is about five times that of mammalian systems. An incorporation of the analog into DNA could not be demonstrated (HOLLINSHEAD, 1964). On the other hand, OTAKA (1960) observed that most RNA made in the presence of azaguanine was located in the supernatant after one hour of centrifugation of *B. cereus* extract at 100,000 rpm. Two hours after addition of the analog, however, very little RNA was found in the 30 and 50S ribosomal particles (CHANTRENNE, 1964). Similarly, OTAKA et al. (1962) and GRUNBERGER (1965) did not observe any azaguanine in the ribosomal particles. On the other hand, when GRUNBERGER and his colleagues (1964) compared pulse-labeled RNA made in the presence of azaguanine with that which had been made in the absence of the analog, a new broad peak was observed containing RNA rich in azaguanine. The properties of this RNA were those of rapidly labeled RNA. Several species of abnormal RNA were detected. Some behaved like mRNA, even though their half-life was longer than that of mRNA of growing bacteria. The other species were stable and were thought to be ribosomal precursors.

Since azaG inhibited protein synthesis very rapidly, it was reasoned by GRUNBERGER and MANDEL (1965) that azaguanine might act by incorporation into the only known species of RNA with a short lifetime, the mRNA. When *B. cereus* was incubated 30 min with 25 μg of azaguanine, pulse-labeled with uracil-2-[^{14}C], and the RNA was separated on a methylated albumin column, it was found that most of the radioactivity was located in fraction beyond 23S ribosomal RNA and the analog blocked the processing of ribosomal RNA precursors. Similar results were obtained by WEISS and PITOT (1974) in eukaryotic cells. They suggested that the inhibition of maturation of ribosomal RNA could be a common phenomenon to many purine and pyrimidine analogs. After 1 h of incubation of Novikoff hepatoma cells with 5×10^{-4}M azaguanine in the presence of [^{3}H]-uridine, the label was seen in the 38S RNA, but the labeling of 32S, 28S, and 18S RNA lagged behind that of control. At 2 h, even though the label appeared in the 28S and 18S RNA species, a marked inhibition of progression of the label was still found. Thus, it was demonstrated that the analog did not interfere with the 45S RNA synthesis, but rather slowed down the processing of the precursor to the mature 28S and 18S rRNA species.

LEVIN (1966) showed evidence for the existence of azaguanine-containing messenger RNA. As criteria for mRNA, he used the ability of this RNA to form a complex with DNA, to have a base composition complementary to DNA, migration of pulse-labeled RNA in the 6 to 14S region of sucrose density gradients, and high efficiency in stimulating polypeptide synthesis in *B. cereus* cell-free extracts.

A high level of azaG was also found in transfer RNA (LEVIN, 1963; WEINSTEIN and GRUNBERGER, 1965). Azaguanine residues in transfer RNA species were incorporated solely as a replacement for guanine, and no evidence for the formation of any unusual species of RNA was found (LEVIN, 1963). The secondary structure of the azaguanine-containing tRNA was less rigid than that of normal tRNA and was inversely related to the precentage of azaguanine incorporated (LEVIN, 1963). The early and rapid incorporation of azaguanine-[^{14}C] into RNA of the 4 to 6S region (KARON et al., 1965) confirmed the preferential incorporation of the drug into this species and into tRNA. When 19% of the guanine residues were replaced in *B. cereus* tRNA by the analog, the tRNA was able to retain the capacity to accept L-leucine, L-lysine, L-alanine, and L-valine in the presence of activating enzymes (LEVINE, 1965). Phenylalanine was also observed to be accepted by this tRNA and transferred to ribosomes. WEINSTEIN and GRUNBERGER (1965) confirmed the function of tRNA containing azaG in amino acid incorporation, and they observed no evidence of miscoding (anticodons containing azaguanine did not fit codons containing U instead of C).

The hypothesis that the azaguanine mode of action is due to its incorporation into RNA was further confirmed in a study using human epidermoid cells by NELSON et al. (1975). Inhibition of RNA synthesis by 6-azauridine and deoxycytidine afforded protection against azaguanine toxicity.

C. Inhibition of Protein Synthesis

Many investigators have shown that azaguanine is incorporated into several species of RNA where it replaced a certain fraction of guanine residues and then caused inhibition of protein synthesis. CHANTRENNE and DEVREUX (1958, 1960) demonstrated that two aspects of azaG action must be considered: the partial inhibition of the incorporation of amino acids into proteins, and the complete inhibition of the synthesis of some specific enzymes, such as catalase or constitutive penicillinase. When CHANTRENNE and LECLERCQ-CALINGAERT (1963) added guanosine to *B. cereus* cells within 15 min of azaguanine addition, a complete recovery of protein synthesis was noted. A less successful recovery was associated with a longer action of the analog. The short time required to inhibit protein synthesis by azaguanine led CHANTRENNE (1964) to propose messenger RNA as the primary site of 8-azaguanine action. LEVINTHAL et al. (1962) reported an average lifetime of two minutes for *Bacillus subtilis* mRNA. If azaguanine blocked the formation of mRNA, then the synthesis of proteins coded for by the short-lived messenger RNA would be inhibited once these molecules decayed. Since protein synthesis continued for many hours after the addition of the guanine analog, some amino acid incorporation was directed by messenger RNA formed in the presence of azaguanine (CHANTRENNE, 1964).

Formation of abnormal proteins, however, was not found when both enzymatic activities and serologic properties were tested. CHANTRENNE's group investigated the effect of azaguanine on the interaction between ribosomes and mRNA as another step in an effort to elucidate the mode of action of this analog. Polyribosomes from protoplasts of *Bacillus magaterium* were isolated and it was found that in the treated bacteria the polysome peaks (below 70S) were greatly diminished in comparison to the control. Azaguanine was seen to interfere with the formation of polysomes.

KARON et al. (1965) studied the effect of the analog on protein synthesis in human cells (KB). A 1×10^{-7}M solution of azaguanine did not inhibit the cellular growth while a 1×10^{-6}M concentration was lethal. Inhibition of protein synthesis at the latter concentration was evident within two hours. Protein synthesis at 1×10^{-7}M was also inhibited prior to that of the RNA.

When ZIMMERMAN and GREENBERG (1965) studied the effect of azaguanine on protein synthesis in the monolayer cultures of HeLa cells, they found that the analog inhibited the growth of cells at 4×10^{-5}M. The cells recovered from the drug effect within one to four days. Cells grown in suspension cultures in the presence of the analog at the same concentration did not recover, however. In a monolayer culture, azaguanine (6×10^{-5}M) inhibited protein synthesis by 75%; and cell growth was inhibited by only 42%. Thus, as in bacteria, azaguanine blocked in the HeLa cells preferentially protein synthesis. The same preference for inhibition of protein synthesis was observed in suspension cultures. The analog was also seen to decrease the amount of protein synthesized per unit of rRNA in the polysomes by 40% and, in addition, to decrease the number of polyribosomes when the cells were incubated for 24 h with 3×10^{-4}M of azaguanine. A four-hour exposure to azaguanine produced 27% and a 12 h exposure 53% inhibition of protein synthesis. In addition, they showed that azaguanine incorporation into RNA was essential for its action since there was no inhibition when a rabbit reticulocyte system (not synthesizing any RNA) was used.

GRUNBERGER (1965) investigated the function of normal ribosomes with attached abnormal mRNA in azaguanine-treated *B. cereus*. It appeared that after the incorporation of amino acids in the cell-free system about two-thirds of the synthesized proteins remained attached to the ribosomes and one-third was released into the supernatant. In the presence of ribosomes from azaG-treated cells only about one-fifth of the polypeptides formed were found in the supernatant. Amino acids probably formed incomplete proteins which remained attached to the ribosomes.

KLUBES and MANDEL (1966) found that GTP stimulated amino acid incorporation more strongly when added to the 30S fraction from normal cells than from azaguanine-treated *B. cereus*. The addition of ATP enhanced amino acid incorporation in the 30S fraction from normal but not from treated cells. They concluded that there were sufficient levels of GTP and ATP present endogenously in the 30S fraction of the treated cells to maintain a high level of amino acid incorporation. The insufficient intracellular level of ATP and/or GTP could then be eliminated as a cause of the inhibition of protein synthesis by azaguanine. To determine the level of this inhibition, ZIMMERMAN et al.

(1967) used poly[U] as an exogenous messenger. The azaguanine-treated cell-free extracts incorporated three to five times more [^{14}C]phenylalanine than control cells in the presence of poly[U]. The S-150 supernatant (tRNA and enzymes, but no ribosomes) was the site of the stimulation. Substitution of [^{14}C]phenylalanyl-tRNA for [^{14}C]phenylalanine as the substrate caused abolition of the stimulation of phenylalanine incorporation by azaguanine extracts, indicating that the stimulation was due to an enhanced synthesis of phenylalanyl-tRNA and not to an increased rate of polypeptide synthesis.

ZIMMERMAN (1968) showed further that there was no miscoding of the proteins present and that it was the incorporation of the analog into mRNA which caused the inhibition of protein synthesis in HeLa cells. When control aminoacyl-tRNA was added to the HeLa cell system, the inhibition of protein synthesis in azaguanine extracts was not reversed. It appeared unlikely that tRNA was the site of the azaguanine block, confirming previous results of LEVIN (1965), and WEINSTEIN and GRUNBERGER (1965) in bacterial systems. To pinpoint the site of azaguanine block, the ribosome fraction was further divided into polysomes and single ribosomes. Polysomes from the analog-treated cells were able to synthesize only 42% of the proteins as compared to control. To distinguish between the two possible sites of the block in protein synthesis, ribosomes or mRNA, exogenous messenger (poly[U]) was added to ribosomes and polyphenylalanine synthesis was followed. As in *B. cereus* (ZIMMERMAN et al., 1967), the HeLa extracts showed that single ribosomes from azaguanine-treated cells incorporated more phenylalanine than those from control extracts. The antimetabolite did not function by blocking either the initiation or releasing mechanisms (ZIMMERMAN, 1968). However, azaguanine caused a slight diminution in the relative size of proteins from molecular weights of over 200,000 to about 100,000.

MAHADEVAN and BHAGWAT (1969) studied the inhibition of protein synthesis in *Neurospora crassa*. They showed a continuing but depressed protein synthesis in the presence of the analog. The inhibition was about 35% to 50%. An accumulation of oligopeptides and small molecular weight proteins was seen in the cells, indicating synthesis of incomplete peptide chains due to the fraudulent RNA containing the modified base. This finding was in contrast to the observation of ZIMMERMAN (1968), who found no release of oligopeptides in the cell-free extracts of HeLa cells.

In rats, azaguanine resulted in the conversion of a portion of the polyribosomes in regenerating liver to functionally inactive monomers and dimers (KWAN and WEBB, 1967). The polyribosome degradation was generally increased under conditions which caused a greater extent of the incorporation of the antimetabolite into RNA. Some of these polyribosomes were found to be resistant to the azaguanine action. A portion of the short half-life mRNA was rendered defective und was unable to combine with ribosomes. LEVITAN and WEBB (1969, 1970) further demonstrated that the analog exhibited selectivity in the induction of tyrosine transaminase, but not that of tryptophan pyrrolase. Protein synthesis was inhibited by approximately 70% in 5 to 6 h after administration of 200 mg/kg of azaguanine in adrenalectomized rats (KWAN and WEBB, 1970). An additional 100 mg/kg of the drug did not increase the degree of inhibition indicating

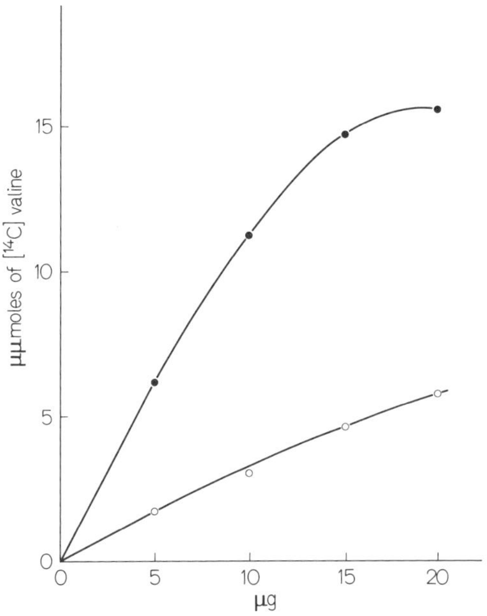

Fig. 3. The effect of poly[U_4,G] and poly[U_4,azaG] on [^{14}C]valine incorporation into proteins in S-30 *E. coli* extracts. ●—● poly [U_4,G], ○—○ poly[U_4,azaG]. Details described in GRUNBERGER et al. (1966b)

that about 30% of the synthesis was resistant to the analog. Membrane-free polyribosomes were converted preferentially to monomers and dimers by azaguanine. They were functionally inactive in vivo, but responded to poly[U] in vitro. KWAN and WEBB (1970) concluded that the antimetabolite selectively inhibited protein biosynthesis by incorporation into mRNA.

In an attempt to localize the site of action of the analog, GRUNBERGER et al. (1966a, 1966b, 1967, 1968) investigated the possibility of azaguanine action at the messenger RNA level and found that analog-containing synthetic polymers and triplet codons (e.g., poly[U_4,azaG], azaGpUpU, azaGpCpU) were less active in stimulating polypeptide synthesis in vitro and in tRNA binding to ribosomes than guanine-containing messengers (e.g., poly[U_4,G], GpUpU, GpCpU) (Figs. 3 and 4). The conclusion was drawn that azaguanine could replace guanine in some codons, but the template efficiency of the analog-containing codons was significantly lower.

LEVIN and LITT (1965) attempted to explain the weaker hydrogen bonding of the azaG-C base pairs. They assumed that the substitution of C-8 of the guanine ring by a N atom causes a reduction of the pK_a from 9.2 to 6.7 which could result in weaker hydrogen bonding with the cytidine residue. As a consequence of this decreased hydrogen bonding between azaguanine-containing codon and the anticodon there might be a block in one or more steps in the peptide bond formation. A more plausible explanation of the lower template activity of azaG containing mRNA could be derived from studies

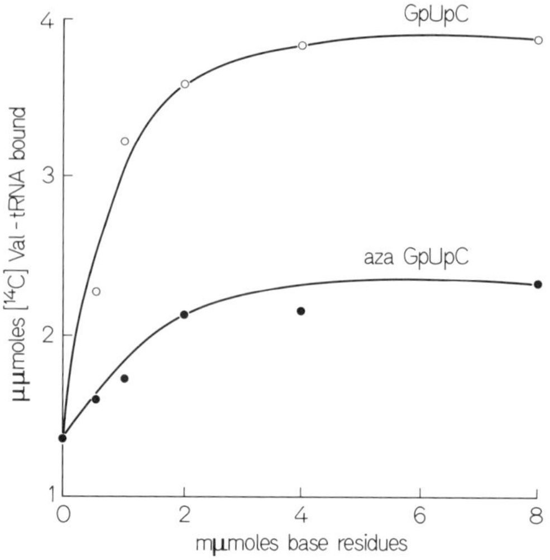

Fig. 4. The effect of GpUpC and azaGpUpC on the binding of [^{14}C]Val-tRNA to ribosomes. Experimental details described in GRUNBERGER et al. (1968)

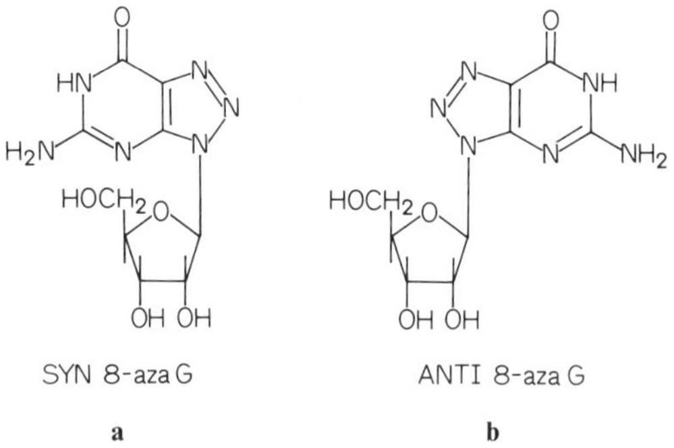

Fig. 5a and b. Structure of 8-azaguanine in **a** *syn* and **b** *anti* conformation

of WARD and REICH (1969). They suggested that incorporation of azaG into polynucleotides results in conformational changes of azaG residues at the glycosidic bonds. Although azaG possesses the normal C-N glycosyl bond, it is, in contrast to G, free of the steric conformational restraints produced by the C-8 H-sugar interactions. Therefore, the azaguanine base could rotate about the glycosidic bond from the more preferred *anti* towards *syn* conformation (Fig. 5). As a result of this conformational change, poly[azaG] is a substrate for pancreatic RNAse (LEVIN, 1962). Unlike normal pyrimidine substrates, this polymer is hydrolyzed mainly to 2′, 3′-cyclic azaGp. Similarly, the conformational changes produce a decrease in thermostability of the helical structure of RNA. The T_m of tRNA decreased progressively with increasing substitution of guanosine by azaG (LEVIN and LITT, 1965). Since the codon-anticodon recognition between mRNA and tRNA during translation is based on complementary base pairing which requires the *anti*-conformation, rotation of 8-azaguanine around the glycosidic bond towards *syn* would result in lower template activity of mRNA, containing azaG residues.

D. Interference with Control Mechanisms

The secondary effect of azaguanine in *B. cereus* on synthesis of penicillinase showed that restoration of synthesis did not occur for all proteins at the same time (CHANTRENNE and LECLERCQ-CALINGAERT, 1963). The synthesis of catalase and of the total protein material measured by the incorporation of [^{14}C]phenylalanine was found always to reappear earlier than that of constitutive penicillinase. The penicillinase-synthesizing system was inhibited regardless of its state of induction when under the azaguanine effect.

Azaguanine was found to inhibit sporulation of *B. cereus* strain T, but only when added to the cells prior to the transition from vegetative growth to presporulation (STAHLY et al., 1966). At the time of the transition, 80% to 85% of the analog was eliminated from RNA where it was solely incorporated. There were no degradative enzymes found and the phenomenon was thought to occur by increasing the ratio of natural purines to azaguanine in the intracellular pool and preferential incorporation of guanine. Addition of phosphate buffer resulted in a reversal of inhibition of sporulation and a 90% elimination of azaguanine from the cellular RNA.

The analog was shown to inhibit induction of xanthine oxidase and the uric acid oxidizing system only when it was added at equimolar concentration before the inducer (CLARKE and MEADOW, 1966). The antimetabolite also inhibited the formation of hemoglobin and incorporation of leucine into protein by blastodics of chicken embryo, explanted before the 6-somite stage (WAINWRIGHT and WAINWRIGHT, 1967). Total arrest of messenger RNA was observed. Delta-aminolevulinic acid reversed the inhibition of hemoglobin synthesis but not the inhibition of leucine incorporation. A charged bacterial transfer RNA reversed the inhibition of hemoglobin formation and partly the inhibition of leucine incorporation. These results were in accord with the hypotheses requiring synthesis of additional tRNA at the 3 to 5 somite stage for the regulation of the initiation of hemoglobin formation.

When rats starved for a short time, were re-fed by a high carbohydrate, low fat diet, an overshoot of glucose-6-phosphate dehydrogenase level occurred. Recovery of the levels of the enzyme was thought to be a process independent of de novo RNA synthesis, while a new synthesis was required for the overshoot (SZEPESI and FRIEDLAND, 1969). SZEPESI et al. (1971) observed that the overshoot of activities of glucose-6-phosphate dehydrogenase and malic enzyme was prevented by azaguanine.

V. Resistance

A partial or complete loss of hypoxanthine-guanine phosphoribosyl-transferase (HGPRT) activity was shown to be responsible for cellular resistance to azaguanine in established mouse lines, microorganisms, murine neoplasms, and mammalian cells in culture. The enzyme deficiency blocked the formation of GMP and its analog, as well as IMP in the salvage pathway. Three levels of resistance were studied by DAVIDSON et al. (1962); no detectable enzyme was encountered in any of them. LITTLEFIELD (1963) found that lines resistant to low (0.1 μg/ml) level of azaguanine possessed one-third of the enzyme activity of the wild type and a second line (resistant to 1 μg/ml) had no enzyme. He suggested that the low level might be expected of a heterozygote or hemizygote. MORROW (1970) reported the presence of two discrete levels of azaguanine resistance in an established mouse line. Intermediate HGPRT levels were found in lines isolated at less than 0.3 μg/ml of azaguanine and very low levels of the enzyme (about 1% of the wild-type) were demonstrated in lines isolated at 0.3 to 3.0 μg/ml of the analog. The resistant lines were found to be stable with a low frequency of reversion. In addition, resistance was not lost for at least one year of cultivation in the absence of azaguanine. No major chromosomal alterations were observed in the resistant lines, even though it was reported that increasing levels of azaguanine resistance in human cells might be due to the loss of a chromosome in the size-range of the human X. Azaguanine resistance behaved as a recessive character in a hybrid cell of a Chinese hamster cell line (CHU et al., 1969). Some azaguanine-resistant mutants of *Salmonella typhimurium* were shown to lack guanine and not hypoxanthine phosphoribosyltransferase activity (KALLE and GOTS, 1961). Azg-11, another azaguanine-resistant mutant of *S. typhimurium*, was found to be defective in a mechanism for incorporation and uptake of guanine, and possibly xanthine with no alteration in purine nucleotide pyrophosphorylases (THAKAR and KALLE, 1968).

References

Brockman, R.W., Sparks, M.C., Simpson, M.S.: A comparison of the metabolism of purines and purine analogs by susceptible and drug-resistant bacterial and neoplastic cells. Biochim. Biophys. Acta *26*, 671 (1957)

Brockman, R.W., Sparks, C., Hutchison, D.J., Slipper, H.E.: A mechanism of resistance to 8-azaguanine I. Microbiological studies on the metabolism of purines and 8-azaguanines. Cancer Res. *19*, 177 (1959)

Burchenal, J.H., Johnston, S.F., Burchenal, J.R., Kushida, M.N., Robinson, E., Stock, C.C.: Chemotherapy of leukemia. IV. Effect of folic acid derivatives on transplanted mouse leukemia. Proc. Soc. Exp. Biol. Med. *71*, 381 (1949)

Chantrenne, H.: Changes in patterns of nucleic acid and protein synthesis caused by a purine analogue. J. Cell Comp. Physiol. (Suppl.) *64*, 149 (1964)

Chantrenne, H., Devreux, S.: Dissociation of the synthesis of nucleic acids from that of protein by a purine analogue. Exp. Cell Res. (Suppl.) *6*, 152 (1958)

Chantrenne, H., Devreux, S.: Restoration de la synthese d'enzymes après inhibition per l'azaguanine. Biochim. Biophys. Acta *41*, 239 (1960)

Chantrenne, H., LeClercq-Calingaert, H.: Secondary effect of 8-azaguanine on the induced or constitutive synthesis of penicillinase in *B. cereus*. Biochim. Biophys. Acta *72*, 87 (1963)

Chu, E.H.Y., Brimer, P., Jacobson, K.B., Merrian, E.V.: Mammalian cell genetics. I. Selection and characterization of mutations auxotrophic for l-glutamine or resistant to 8-azaguanine in Chinese hamster cells *in vitro*. Genetics *62*, 359 (1969)

Clarke, P.H., Meadow, P.H.: The effect of 8-azaguanine on the inducible oxidation of guanine by *Pseudomonas aeruginosa*. J. Gen. Microbiol. *44*, 195 (1966)

Davidson, J.D., Bradley, T.R., Roosa, R.A., Law, L.W.: Purine nucleotide pyrophosphorylases in 8-azaguanine sensitive and resistant leukemias. J. Natl. Cancer Inst. *29*, 789 (1962)
Finkelstein, M., Winters, W.D., Thomas, P.A., Davison, C., Smith, P.K.: The effect of 8-azaguanine on tissue metabolism in mice bearing sarcoma 37. Cancer Res. *11*, 807 (1951)
Grunberger, D.: The character and function of ribosomes from 8-azaguanine-treated cells of *Bacillus cereus*. Coll. Czech. Chem. Commun. *30*, 128 (1965)
Grunberger, D., Mandel, H.G.: Enhanced messenger activity of RNA from 8-azaguanine-treated *Bacillus cereus*. Mol. Pharm. *1*, 157 (1965)
Grunberger, D., Maslova, R.N., Sorm, F.: Effect of 8-azaguanine on the synthesis of pulse-labelled ribonucleic acid in *Bacillus cereus*. Coll. Czech. Chem. Commun. *29*, 152 (1964)
Grunberger, D., Meissner, L., Holy, A., Sorm, F.: The effect of polymers and trinucleoside diphosphates containing 8-azaguanine upon the binding of [^{14}C]valine-sRNA to ribosomes. Biochim. Biophys. Acta *119*, 432 (1966a)
Grunberger, D., O'Neal, C., Nirenberg, M.: Stimulation of amino acid incorporation into protein by polyuridylic-8-azaguanylic acid. Biochim. Biophys. Acta *119*, 581 (1966b)
Grunberger, D., Meissner, L., Holy, A., Sorm, F.: The coding properties of polymers and trinucleoside diphosphates containing 8-azaguanosine. Coll. Czech. Chem. Commun. *32*, 2625 (1967)
Grunberger, D., Holy, A., Sorm, F.: Synthesis and coding properties of 8-azaguanosine-containing triribonucleoside diphosphates. Biochim. Biophys. Acta *161*, 147 (1968)
Hirschberg, E., Kream, J., Gellhorn, A.: Enzymatic deamination of 8-azaguanine in normal and neoplastic tissues. Cancer Res. *12*, 524 (1952)
Hollinshead, A.C.: Incorporation of 8-azaguanine and growth inhibition in mammalian spinner cultures. Exp. Cell. Res. *34*, 144 (1964)
Karon, M., Weissman, S., Meyer, C., Henry, P.: Studies of DNA, RNA and protein synthesis in cultured human cells exposed to 8-azaguanine. Cancer Res. *25*, 185 (1965)
Kelle, G.P., Gots, J.S.: Alterations in purine nucleotide pyrophosphorylases and resistance to purine analogs. Biochim. Biophys. Acta *53*, 166 (1961)
Kidder, G.W., Dewey, V.C.: The biological activity of substituted purines. J. Biol. Chem. *179*, 181 (1949)
Kidder, G.W., Dewey, V.C., Parks, R.E., Jr., Woodside, G.C.: Purine metabolism in Tetrahymena and its relation to malignant cells in mice. Science *109*, 511 (1949)
Kidder, G.W., Dewey, V.C., Parks, R.E., Jr., Woodside, G.C.: Further evidence on the mode of action of 8-azaguanine (guanazolo) in tumor inhibition. Cancer Res. *11*, 204 (1951)
Klubes, P., Mandel, H.G.: Effects of purine nucleoside triphosphates on amino acid incorporation in a cell-free system from 8-azaguanine-treated *Bacillus cereus*. Biochim. Biophys. Acta *129*, 594 (1966)
Kwan, S.W., Webb, T.E.: Study of the mechanism of polyribosome breakdown induced in the regenerating liver by 8-azaguanine. J. Biol. Chem. *242*, 5542 (1967)
Kwan, S.W., Webb, T.E.: Differential sensitivity of the protein synthesizing system of rat liver to 8-azaguanine. Life Sci. *9*, 975 (1970)
Lasnitzky, I., Matthews, R.E.F., Smith, J.D.: Incorporation of 8-azaguanine into nucleic acids. Nature (London) *173*, 346 (1954)
Law, L.W.: Studies of the effects of a guanine analog on acute lymphoid leukemia of mice. Cancer Res. *10*, 186 (1950)
Levin, D.H.: The polymerization of 8-azaguanosine 5′-diphosphate by polynucleotide phosphorylase. Biochim. Biophys. Acta *61*, 75 (1962)
Levin, D.H.: The incorporötion of 8-azaguanine into soluble ribonucleic acid of *Bacillus cereus*. J. Biol. Chem. *238*, 1098 (1963)
Levin, D.H.: Amino acid acceptor and transfer functions of sRNA containing 8-azaguanine. Biochem. Biophys. Res. Commun. *19*, 654 (1965)
Levin, D.H.: Evidence for an active messenger ribonucleic acid containing 8-azaguanine. Biochemistry *5*, 1618 (1966)
Levin, D.H., Litt, M.: Studies on the secondary structure of soluble ribonucleic acid containing 8-azaguanine. J. Mol. Biol. *14*, 506 (1965)
Levinthal, C., Keynan, A., Higa, A.: Messenger RNA turnover and protein synthesis in *B. subtilis* inhibited by actinomycin D. Proc. Natl. Acad. Sci. USA *48*, 1631 (1962)

Levitan, I.B., Webb, T.E.: Modification by 8-azaguanine of the effects of hydrocortisone on the induction and inactivation of tyrosine transaminase of rat liver. J. Biol. Chem. *244*, 341 (1969)
Levitan, I.B., Webb, T.E.: Posttranscriptional control in the steroid mediated induction of hepatic tyrosine transaminase. Science *167*, 283 (1970)
Littlefield, J.W.: The inosinic acid pyrophosphorylase activity of mouse fibroblasts partially resistant to 8-azaguanine. Proc. Natl. Acad. Sci. USA *50*, 568 (1963)
MacIntyre, W.M., Singh, P., Werkema, M.S.: The crystal and molecular structure of 8-azaguanine monohydrate. Biophys. J. *5*, 697 (1965)
Mahadevan, P.R., Bhagwat, A.J.: Inhibition of protein synthesis in *Neurospora crassa* by 8-azaguanine. Indian J. Biochem. *6*, 169 (1969)
Mandel, H.G.: Further studies on the modification of nucleic acid synthesis of *B. cereus* by 8-azaguanine. J. Pharm. Exp. Ther. *133*, 141 (1961)
Mandel, H.G., Markham, R.: The effects of 8-azaguanine on the biosynthesis of ribonucleic acid in *Bacillus cereus*. Biochem. J. *69*, 297 (1958)
Mandel, H.G., Alpen, E.L., Winters, W.D., Smith, P.K.: The urinary metabolites of 8-azaguanine in the mouse and the monkey. J. Biol. Chem. *193*, 63 (1951)
Mandel, H.G., Carlo, P.E., Smith, P.K.: The incorporation of 8-azaguanine into nucleic acids of tumor-bearing mice. J. Biol. Chem. *206*, 181 (1954)
Matthews, R.E.F.: Effect of purines on the multiplication of plant viruses. Nature (London) *169*, 500 (1952)
Matthews, R.E.F.: Effects of some purine analogues on tobacco mosaic virus. J. Gen. Microbiol. *10*, 521 (1954)
Mitchel, J.H., Jr., Skipper, H.E., Bennett, L.L., Jr.: Investigation of the nucleic acids of viscera and tumor tissue from animals injected with radioactive 8-azaguanine. Cancer Res. *10*, 647 (1950)
Morgan, H.R.: Factors related to the growth of *Psittacosis* virus (strain 6BC). II. Purines, pyrimidines, and other components related to nucleic acid. J. Exp. Med. *95*, 277 (1952)
Morrow, J.: Genetic analysis of azaguanine resistance in an established mouse cell line. Genetics *65*, 279 (1970)
Nelson, J.A., Carpenter, J.W., Rose, L.M., Adamson, D.J.: Mechanisms of action of 6-thioguanine, 6-mercaptopurine, and 8-azaguanine. Cancer Res. *35*, 2872 (1975)
Otaka, E.: Effect of 8-azaguanine on RNA and protein synthesis in *B. cereus*. Exp. Cell Res. *21*, 229 (1960)
Otaka, E., Osawa, S., Oota, Y., Ishikama, A., Mitsui, H.: Ribosomal RNA synthesis in growing bacterial cells. Biochim. Biophys. Acta *55*, 310 (1962)
Peterson, E.R., Murray, M.R.: 8-azaguanine metabolism of human glioblastoma *in vitro*. Proc. Am. Assoc. Cancer Res. *1*, 42 (1953)
Roblin, R.O., Jr., Lampen, J.O., English, J.P., Cole, Q.P., Vaughan, J.R., Jr.: Studies in chemotherapy. VIII Methionine and purine antagonists and their relation to the sulfonamides. J. Am. Chem. Soc. *67*, 290 (1945)
Roy, J.K., Kvam, D.C., Dahl, S.C., Parks, R.E., Jr.: Effect of triphosphate nucleosides of 8-azaguanine 6-thioguanine, and 6-mercaptopurine on amino acid incorporation in vitro into ribosomal protein. J. Biol. Chem. *236*, 1158 (1961)
Smith, J.D., Matthews, R.E.F.: The metabolism of 8-azapurines. Biochem. J. *66*, 323 (1957)
Stahly, D.P., Srinivasan, V.R., Halvorson, H.O.: Effect of 8-azaguanine on the transition from vegetative growth to presporulation in *Bacillus cereus*. J. Bacteriol. *91*, 1875 (1966)
Szepesi, B., Freedland, R.A.: Differential requirement for *de novo* RNA synthesis in the starved-refed rat; inhibition of the overshoot by 8-azaguanine after refeeding. J. Nutr. *99*, 449 (1969)
Szepesi, B., Berdainer, C.D., Diachenko, S.K., Moser, P.B.: Effect of length of starvation, refeeding, and 8-azaguanine on serum insulin and NADP-linked dehydrogenases of rat liver. J. Nutr. *101*, 1147 (1971)
Thaker, J.H., Kalle, G.P.: Defective guanine uptake in an 8-azaguanine-resistant mutant of *Salmonella typhimurium*. J. Bacteriol. *95*, 458 (1968)
Wainwright, S.D., Wainwright, L.K.: Regulation of the initiation of hemoglobin synthesis in the blood island cells of chick embryos. III. Qualitative studies of the effects of 8-azaguanine and preparations of transfer RNAs. Can. J. Biochem. *45*, 255 (1967)
Ward, D.C., Reich, E.: Relationship between nucleoside conformation and biological activity. Ann. Rep. Med. Chem. p. 272 (1969)

Way, J.L., Parks, R.E., Jr.: Enzymatic synthesis of 5′-phosphate nucleotides of purine analogues. J. Biol. Chem. *231*, 467 (1958)
Way, J.L., Dahl, J.L., Parks, R.E., Jr.: Polyphosphate nucleosides of purine analogues. J. Biol. Chem. *234*, 1241 (1959)
Webb, T.E.: Polyribosome breakdown in rat liver following administration of 8-azaguanine. Biochim. Biophys. Acta *138*, 307 (1967)
Weinstein, I.B., Grunberger, D.: Coding properties of sRNA containing 8-azaguanine. Biochem. Biophys. Res. Commun. *19*, 647 (1965)
Weiss, J.W., Pitot, H.C.: Inhibition of ribosomal ribonucleic acid by 5-azacytidine and 8-azaguanine in Novikoff hepatoma cells. Arch. Biochem. Biophys. *160*, 119 (1974)
Youngner, J.S., Ward, E.N., Salk, J.E.: Effect of 5-amino-7-hydroxy-H-V-triazolo(d)pyrimidine on growth and development of the chick embryo. Proc. Soc. Exp. Biol. Med. *75*, 157 (1950)
Zimmerman, E.F.: Azaguanine inhibition of protein synthesis, III. Site of action in HeLa cells. Biochim. Biophys. Acta *157*, 378 (1968)
Zimmerman, E.F., Greenberg, S.A.: Inhibition of protein synthesis by 8-azaguanine. I. Effects on polyribosomes in HeLa cells. Mol. Pharmacol. *1*, 113 (1965)
Zimmerman, E.F., Holler, B.W., Pearson, G.D.: Azaguanine inhibition of protein synthesis. II. Effects of poly[U] in *Bacillus cereus*. Biochim. Biophys. Acta *134*, 402 (1967)

Bleomycin

C.W. HAIDLE and R.S. LLOYD

I. Introduction

There have been many useful reviews published during the past few years concerning both the clinical and basic scientific aspects of research on the antineoplastic antibiotic, bleomycin. UMEZAWA, the discoverer of bleomycin (UMEZAWA et al., 1966) has written several reviews dealing primarily with the chemistry, structure, in vitro, and in vivo studies of bleomycin (UMEZAWA, 1975, 1976). Other articles dealing more specifically with the extracellular reaction between bleomycin and cellular macromolecules have appeared recently (MIYAKI and ONO, 1976; MÜLLER and ZAHN, 1976a, 1977; MÜLLER et al., 1976). Review articles have also been published concerning research on the effects of bleomycin on mammalian cell cultures and cell-cycle kinetics (BARRANCO and HUMPHREY, 1976; TERASIMA et al., 1976). An exhaustive review of the literature on both basic scientific studies and clinical studies has been prepared by CROOKE and BRADNER (1976). The reader is also referred to the Gann Monograph on Cancer Research (CARTER et al., 1976) which is devoted to articles on both fundamental and clinical studies.

The primary purpose of the present treatise is to present an updated review of the literature bearing on the question of the mechanism of action of bleomycin. Thus the emphasis is on those studies which detail the extracellular reaction and those cell culture studies which are germane to the mechanism of action. Since many of the details of the mode of action of this drug remain to be elucidated and since there are some apparent contradictions in the literature regarding this mechanism, we have attempted to point out and perhaps resolve some of these contradictory results and to indicate areas in need of more intensive investigation.

II. Chemistry and History

The bleomycins are a group of glycopeptide antibiotics produced by *Streptomyces verticillus* which were isolated as copper chelates by UMEZAWA et al. (1966) during a search for less toxic phleomycin-like antibiotics. The bleomycins were extracted from the fermentation broth by chromatography on Amberlite IRC-50 and further purified using alumina and Sephadex G-25 chromatography.

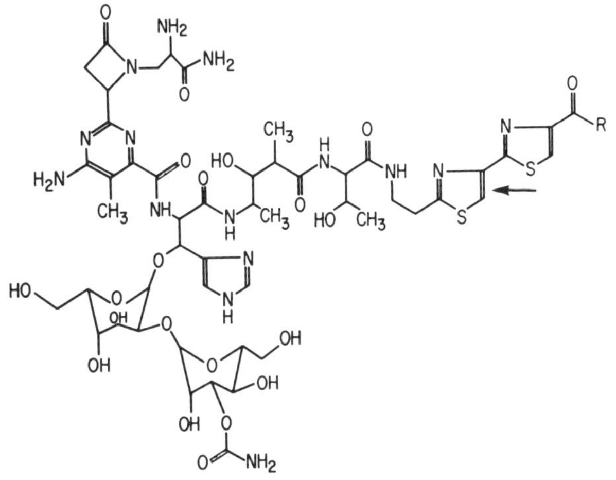

Bleomycinic acid	R:	-OH
A_2	R:	$-NH-(CH_2)_3-S^+(CH_3)_2\,X^-$
B_2	R:	$-NH-(CH_2)_4-NH-C(=NH)-NH_2$
A_2'-b	R:	$-NH-(CH_2)_3-NH_2$
A_5	R:	$-NH-(CH_2)_3-NH-(CH_2)_4-NH_2$
A_6	R:	$-NH-(CH_2)_3-NH-(CH_2)_4-NH-(CH_2)_3-NH_2$
B_1	R:	$-NH-CH(COOH)-(CH_2)_3-NH-C(=NH)-NH_2$

Fig. 1. Structure of bleomycin

Bleomycins could be separated into the A and B series by paper chromatography (UMEZAWA et al., 1966). Bleomycin A and B were further separated into the individual components (A_{1-6} and B_{1-5}) using CM-Sephadex C-25 chromatography (UMEZAWA et al., 1966).

The bleomycins differ from one another only in their terminal amine moieties. The main structural component, common to all bleomycins, is bleomycinic acid in which the amine moiety is replaced by an hydroxyl group (UMEZAWA, 1976). The basic structure of bleomycin together with a few of the more common amine moieties is shown in Fig. 1. Phleomycin differs from bleomycin in two respects; it has a saturated bond in one of the thiazole rings (arrow in Fig. 1), and it contains different amine (R) groups (TAKITA et al., 1972a, b).

It is possible to alter the normal production of bleomycin by adding specific amines to the fermentation broth so that the final bleomycin produced is enriched for bleomycin containing the added amine group (FUJII et al., 1974). Additionally, a semi-synthetic method has been devised to produce bleomycins with specific amine groups. This method involves the chemical cleavage of purified bleomycin A_2 followed by the addition of the desired amine group by aminolysis (TAKITA et al., 1973). For a complete discussion of the chemistry of the bleomycins the reader is referred to two reviews by UMEZAWA (UMEZAWA, 1975, 1976). The bleomycin (Blenoxane) currently in clinical use is a mixture of several of the individual bleomycins predominantly A_2 and B_2 (CROOKE and BRADNER, 1976).

III. Growth Inhibitory Properties and Toxicity

Bleomycin inhibits the growth of a wide variety of viruses, bacteria and mammalian cells. *Mycobacterium smegmatis, M. phlei* and *Bacillus subtilis* have been used as the test organisms for the determination of the activity of bleomycin in fermentation mixtures and in samples from treated animals. *B. subtilis* ATCC 6633 is considered to be the most sensitive bacterial test organism (UMEZAWA et al., 1966; ISHIZUKA et al., 1967; UMEZAWA et al., 1968; CROOKE and BRADNER, 1976). UMEZAWA et al. (1968) reported that both copper-free and copper-containing bleomycin were equally effective in their growth-inhibitory properties, but that the copper-containing form was more toxic in experimental animals. For a good description of the spectrum of antibacterial activity of bleomycin A and B, the reader is referred to the review article of CROOKE and BRADNER (1976).

UMEZAWA et al. (1966, 1967) were the first to observe the high therapeutic index of the bleomycins against Ehrlich carcinoma and sarcoma 180 in mice. These workers also noted a reversible toxicity in dogs after bleomycin administration. This toxicity was manifested by a hardening of the skin and foot pads and a reduction of liver function.

The first clinical trials of bleomycin were initiated in Japan (ICHIKAWA, 1976). The results of these trials demonstrated that bleomycin was very effective in the treatment of squamous cell carcinoma either alone or in combination with radiotherapy. These trials also showed that the most serious, life-threatening toxic effect of bleomycin therapy is pulmonary fibrosis. For a comprehensive review of the current status of bleomycin therapy against a variety of human malignancies the reader is referred to the Gann Monograph on Cancer Research No. 19 (CARTER et al., 1976).

IV. Cell-Free Reactions

One of the more interesting aspects of bleomycin research, from the biochemist's point of view, is the ability of this drug to cause extensive damage to isolated purified DNA. Since similar damage to intracellular DNA has also been observed, it may be possible to learn many of the details about the intracellular mode of action by studying the effect of the drug on isolated DNA. This section deals primarily with studies on the extracellular reaction which relate to the mechanism of action.

A. General Reaction Conditions

NAGAI et al. (1969) were the first to describe an effect of bleomycin on isolated DNA. They noted a decrease in the melting temperature (T_m) of bacterial DNA's in the presence of copper-free bleomycin and 2-mercaptoethanol or dithiothreitol. It was suggested that 2-mercaptoethanol reacts with the DNA, since DNA treated with 2-mercaptoethanol followed by dialysis and subsequent reaction with bleomycin alone exhibited the same decrease in T_m. NAGAI et al. (1969) also reported that H_2O_2 could substitute for 2-mercaptoethanol in the reduction of the T_m by bleomycin of salmon sperm and bacterial DNA's. In addition, these investigators reported that bleomycin plus H_2O_2 could induce single-strand breaks in DNA after a short incubation; however, no decrease in the molecular size of the DNA was observed in the absence of H_2O_2 even after 12 h incubation. In other reports, NAGAI et al. (1969) and SUZUKI et al. (1969) have shown that both reduction of the T_m and strand scission of bacterial DNA are mediated by bleomycin in the presence of 2-mercaptoethanol. HAIDLE (1971), using alkaline sucrose gradients, showed that bleomycin caused single-strand scissions in bacterial DNA in the absence of any reducing or oxidizing agents when incubated at 5 °C for 16 h. SHIRAKAWA et al. (1971) also demonstrated that reducing or oxidizing agents were not required for bleomycin-induced damage to ϕx174 bacteriophage DNA. It was concluded that oxidizing or reducing agents are not required for bleomycin activity, but that such agents greatly stimulate the DNA fragmentation reaction (HAIDLE, 1971; FUJIWARA and KONDO, 1973). However, UMEZAWA et al. (1973), using covalently closed-circular DNA from SV40 observed rather extensive single-strand scissions using 4.0 μg/ml of bleomycin B_2 during short incubations in the absence of any reducing agents; this reaction was stimulated 20-fold by the addition of 1 mM 2-mercaptoethanol. BEARDEN et al. (1977), using another covalently closed-circular DNA derived from the bacteriophage PM2, showed a much greater dependence on 2-mercaptoethanol to produce breakage comparable to that reported by UMEZAWA et al. (1973). ONISHI et al. (1975) reported that the reducing agents, 2-mercaptoethanol, dithiothreitol, L-ascorbic acid, or sodium borohydride, and the oxidizing agents, H_2O_2 or dehydroascorbic acid all stimulated the fragmentation reaction. We have found (unpublished results) that many thiol-containing chemicals (6-thioguanine, 6-mercaptopurine, 5-mercaptomethyl uracil, dithiouracil and thiouracil) stimulate the extracellular fragmentation of DNA. LOWN and SIM (1977) reported that either 10 mM 2-mercaptoethanol or 1 mM dithiothreitol alone caused extensive nicking of covalently closed circular PM2 DNA in 1 h at 37 °C. Other reports cited using these reagents report no such nicking albeit using different DNA's. BODE (1967) reported a nicking of superhelical DNA by dithiothreitol and ascorbate, but observed no appreciable nicking of the DNA by 2-mercaptoethanol after 14.5 h incubation. He concluded that the effect of such reducing agents might be dramatically influenced by metal ions or buffers. Our data (unpublished results) indicate that superhelical PM2 DNA is not nicked after 1 h at 37° C in the presence of 25 mM 2-mercaptoethanol. Certain intercalating agents also appear to stimulate the reaction on native double-stranded DNA but not denatured

DNA; these include proflavine, ethidium bromide and actinomycin D (BEARDEN and HAIDLE, 1975). MÜLLER et al. (1976), using the inhibition of DNA-dependent DNA polymerase I as a measure of bleomycin activity, showed a synergistic effect when bleomycin was used in the presence of steffimycin B (a possible intercalating agent) and Hoechst 33258 (an A·T specific non-intercalating DNA ligand). Using SV40 DNA, ASAKURA et al. (1975) found that actinomycin D stimulated the strand-scission reaction, but ethidium bromide inhibited it.

MÜLLER and ZAHN (1976a) using poly (dA·dT) as substrate, reported that after reaction with the poly (dA·dT) most of the bleomycin could be recovered in an active form thus suggesting a catalytic rather than a stoichiometric mechanism. However, ONISHI et al. (1975) reported that addition of fresh bleomycin to a bleomycin-DNA reaction which had come to completion caused increased degradation of the DNA. Other work (BEARDEN et al., 1977), using the percent of form I DNA (superhelical covalently closed-circular DNA) remaining after reaction with increasing drug concentrations reveals that the extent of reaction is proportional to the drug concentration. These results are best interpreted as reflecting a stoichiometric rather than a catalytic mechanism. This point needs further clarification.

B. Substrates

Viral, bacterial, and mammalian DNA's from a wide variety of sources are subject to breakage by bleomycin. Single-stranded, double-stranded and covalently closed-circular DNA's as well as many synthetic deoxyribo-polymers all serve as substrates for this breakage reaction (NAGAI et al., 1969; SUZUKI et al., 1970; HAIDLE, 1971; SHIRAKAWA et al., 1971; MÜLLER et al., 1972; UMEZAWA et al., 1973; BEARDEN et al., 1977). Using Sephadex gel filtration chromatography, MÜLLER et al. (1972) observed no small molecular weight fragments released from poly (dG·[^{3}H]dC), poly (dC·[^{3}H]dG), poly (dT·[^{3}H]dA), poly (dT) and poly (dI-dT).

RNA or synthetic ribopolymers do not serve as substrates for the reaction (SUZUKI et al., 1970; HAIDLE et al., 1972; MÜLLER et al., 1972; HAIDLE and BEARDEN, 1975; KUO et al., 1977). One of the unique features of the cell-free bleomycin reaction is its evident specificity for DNA. This lack of reactivity toward RNA has been demonstrated using natural RNA and the synthetic ribopolymers poly rA and poly rU (HAIDLE et al., 1972). Specificity for DNA could be the result of one or more of the following possibilities: (1) base composition difference between DNA and RNA i.e. thymine versus uracil, (2) differences in secondary structure, and (3) difference in the sugar moiety, i.e. deoxyribose versus ribose. The first possibility was ruled out since DNA from bacteriophage PBS-1, which contains uracil in place of thymine, was degraded by the drug with the release of free uracil. If one mixes poly rA and poly rU under appropriate conditions, a duplex molecule is formed with a structural configuration closely approximating DNA; the drug was found to be inactive in causing the degradation of such a duplex (HAIDLE et al., 1972). Additionally, HAIDLE and BEARDEN (1975), using an RNA–DNA hybrid molecule formed by the action of reverse transcriptase, reported the bleomycin-induced degradation of the DNA strand while leaving the RNA strand intact. Thus the specificity for DNA is not the result of secondary structural differences. One must assume that the deoxyribose plays a role in conferring specificity for bleomycin attack. Further evidence for the lack of damage to RNA was supplied by KUO et al. (1977) using globin mRNA in a wheat germ embryo translation system. When the globin mRNA was pretreated with high concentrations of bleomycin followed by removal of the drug and subsequent use of the mRNA in the translation system, there was no decrease in the biochemical activity of this mRNA to function as a template for the in vitro synthesis of globin.

MÜLLER and ZAHN (1976b) measured the release of thymine from chromatin isolated from proliferating and nonproliferating quail oviduct. They found that 1.6-fold more thymine was released from chromatin derived from the proliferating than from the nonproliferating cells. After treatment of the nonproliferating chromatin with KCl, the amount of thymine liberated by bleomycin was almost as great as that from untreated proliferating chromatin. It was concluded that the F1 histone protects DNA from the action of the drug.

It was also found (Dr. M. Tien KUO, personal communication), using chromatin from Chinese hamster cells, that unlike nucleases bleomycin attacked the "linker" DNA between the nucleosomes or nu bodies and did not affect the DNA associated with the nucleosomes. It was suggested that perhaps there are sequence differences between the linker DNA and nucleosomal DNA, or that the DNA in the nucleosome is in some sort of protected configuration.

C. Binding

SUZUKI et al. (1970) were the first to report a physical binding of bleomycin to purified DNA. This binding was assayed by passage of a mixture of tritiated bleomycin and DNA through a Sephadex G-100 column. It was found that a small proportion of the total bleomycin radioactivity was associated with the DNA after chromatography; a binding ratio of one bleomycin molecule/350 nucleotides was calculated. The amount of drug bound to single-stranded DNA was about 2-fold higher than for double-stranded DNA. The binding was observed in the presence or absence of 2-mercaptoethanol, but was inhibited by the presence of Cu^{2+}, Zn^{2+}, EDTA, or phleomycin. KRUEGER et al. (1973), using ultraviolet absorption and circular dichroism measurements, reported that bleomycin does bind to DNA and that this binding occurs without causing any extensive changes in the secondary structure of the DNA except for a possible increase in the regularity of the DNA helix. MÜLLER et al. (1972) noted a spectral shift after mixing bleomycin with DNA. MIYAKI et al. (1975) measured the binding of [^{14}C]-labeled bleomycin with DNA using equilibrium density gradient centrifugation. They reported a binding ratio of 1 mol bleomycin/ 1.1×10^8 daltons DNA using 15 µg/ml of bleomycin, and 1 mol/4.5×10^7 daltons using 30 µg/ml of bleomycin. The most definitive binding study to date was that of CHIEN et al. (1977) using fluorescence, proton magnetic resonance and viscosity measurements. It was found that approximately 1 molecule of bleomycin A_2 or tripeptide S (containing the bithiazole rings) binds to every 4–5 base pairs in DNA. It was suggested that the bithiazole rings and the dimethylsulfonium group (the R group of bleomycin A_2) are bound more tightly to DNA than other portions of the molecule. It was also noted that Mg^{2+} competitively inhibits the binding of bleomycin to DNA suggesting that charge interactions contribute to the binding.

D. DNA Strand-Scission

Although the earlier work cited in Sect. IV.A describes bleomycin-induced single-strand breaks determined by alkaline sucrose sedimentation velocity analyses and double-strand breaks determined under neutral conditions (HAIDLE, 1971), these methods are not sufficiently sensitive for quantitative determinations of the types of strand-scissions induced by this drug. Thus a system was developed which has the capacity to distinguish between single- and double-strand breaks and alkaline-labile damage (BEARDEN et al., 1977). This system employs a double-stranded superhelical, covalently closed-circular DNA extracted from the bacteriophage PM2 (ESPEJO and CANELO, 1968). After bleomycin treatment, the DNA was electrophoresed through agarose gels, thus achieving a total separation of form I (superhelical covalently-closed circles), form II (relaxed circles, formed by a single-strand break) and form III (linear molecules formed by a double-strand break). When testing to determine if alkaline labile sites were introduced into the DNA by the drug, the reactions were stopped using EDTA, and the pH of the DNA-containing solution was either allowed to remain at neutral pH or raised to a non-denaturing alkaline pH. At this nondenaturing pH, alkaline labile sites were hydrolyzed such that a form I molecule which contains an alkaline labile site would remain in the form I configuration at neutral pH but would be converted into a form II molecule under nondenaturing alkaline conditions. Also, an alkaline labile site on one strand opposite a single-strand break would be converted into a double-strand break. Data collected using these methods indicated that for every single-strand break introduced, one measurable alkaline labile site was also formed (LLOYD et al., 1977). Further characterization of these alkaline labile sites is presently underway in our laboratory.

We have also determined that double-strand breaks are introduced directly into PM2 DNA by bleomycin and their formation is not the result of an accumulation of random single-strand breaks (unpublished results). For every double-strand break measured under neutral assay conditions, an additional double-strand break can be measured under nondenaturing alkaline conditions (unpublished results).

E. Temperature and pH Dependence

The influence of temperature on the bleomycin-induced fragmentation of DNA has not been clearly defined. UMEZAWA et al. (1973), using bleomycin

B_2 on SV40 DNA, reported that the reaction had a temperature optimum of 20° C; however, the reaction proceeded more rapidly at 0° than at 10° C with almost no reaction at 37° C. On the other hand, TAKESHITA et al. (1976), using bleomycin A_2 in the ATP-stimulated degradation of vaccinia virus DNA, reported very little reaction at 0° C with an optimum at 37° C. HAIDLE (1971), using the clinically available mixture of bleomycin on *B. subtilis* DNA in the absence of 2-mercaptoethanol, showed a more complete reaction at 80° than at 40° or 20° C. Care must be exercised in the interpretation of these results especially at the higher temperatures since the DNA substrate undergoes helical transitions as the temperature is increased, which may be further complicated by the fact that the drug is known to decrease the T_m of DNA (NAGAI et al., 1969a, b).

There is general agreement that the optimum pH of the extracellular reaction is approximately 9.0 with little or no activity being observed at pH values less than 6 or above 13 (UMEZAWA et al., 1973; ASAKURA et al., 1975). UMEZAWA et al. (1973) reported three distinct pH maxima at approximately 8.6, 9.1 and 10 with most activity being observed at pH 9.1. ONISHI et al. (1975) reported that the optimum pH for the reaction varied depending on the oxidizing or reducing agent employed; these pH optima ranged from 6.4–7.0 using dehydroascorbic acid to 9.5 using 2-mercaptoethanol or dithiothreitol.

F. Metals

NAGAI et al. (1969) and SHIRAKAWA et al. (1971) noted that the copper-containing bleomycin was ineffective in cell-free reactions with DNA. It was also noted that addition of Cu^{2+}, Zn^{2+} and Co^{2+} to the reaction mixtures inhibited the reduction of the T_m and strand-scission of DNA using purified bleomycin A_2 (NAGAI et al., 1969; SUZUKI et al., 1970). UMEZAWA et al. (1973) reported that Cu^{2+} also inhibited the fragmentation of covalently closed-circular DNA by bleomycin B_2. NUNN (1976) noted that there were considerable differences between the metal complexes of bleomycin with indium, cobalt, or copper. He also noted differences in the rates of formation of these complexes. Several groups of investigators have reported a dramatic increase in the ability of bleomycin to degrade DNA in the presence of Fe^{2+} (ISHIDA and TAKAHASHI, 1975; SAUSVILLE et al., 1976; LOWN and SIM, 1977). ISHIDA and TAKAHASHI (1975) also noted a stimulation of the reaction in the presence of Fe^{3+}. We have also noted this Fe^{2+} effect (unpublished results); however, in view of the fact that Fe^{2+} alone causes extensive damage to DNA, we feel that it is impossible at present to conclude that Fe^{2+} plays a direct role in the bleomycin-induced DNA fragmentation reaction. TAKESHITA et al. (1976) reported that ATP, certain ATP analogs and other nucleotides stimulate the bleomycin-induced degradation of vaccinia virus DNA; this stimulation of DNA degradation was dependent on the presence of $MgCl_2$. We have shown (unpublished results) that both Mg^{2+} and Ca^{2+} (approximately 0.25 mM) stimulate the degradation by bleomycin of *B. subtilis* DNA. We also found that Zn^{2+}, Mn^{2+}, Cu^{2+}, Cu^{+}, Co^{2+} and Ni^{2+} inhibited the reaction, whereas Na^{+} and K^{+} at comparable concentrations showed no effect. ONISHI et al. (1975) reported an inhibition of the fragmentation reaction in the presence of 5 mM Mg^{2+}, 5 mM Ca^{2+} and 0.025 mM Mn^{2+}.

G. Chelating Agents

Conflicting reports have appeared in the literature concerning the role of EDTA in the extracellular reaction. Several groups of workers have reported that EDTA inhibits the binding of bleomycin to DNA, the bleomycin-mediated decrease in the T_m of DNA as well as the strand-scission of DNA (NAGAI et al., 1969; SUZUKI et al., 1970; SHIRAKAWA et al., 1971; FUJIWARA and KONDO, 1973; TAKESHITA et al., 1976). MÜLLER et al. (1972) reported no inhibition of the degradation of *E. coli* DNA in the presence of 10 mM EDTA. UMEZAWA et al. (1973) also reported that 10 mM EDTA did not inhibit the bleomycin-induced degradation of covalently closed circular DNA.

Using a variety of chelating agents, we have found (unpublished results) three chelators which inactivate bleomycin; these are in decreasing order of effectiveness, 1,2-diaminocyclohexane-N,N′tetraacetic (CDTA), ethylenediamine tetraacetic acid (EDTA) and [ethyleneglycolbis] (p-aminoethylether)-N,N′tetraacetic acid (EGTA). This inactivation reaction was time and temperature dependent. After reaction with any of these chelating agents, bleomycin was inactive in both the extracellular DNA fragmentation reaction and also in the inhibition of the growth of a bacterial test system.

H. Oxygen and Free-Radicals

Several groups have reported that the fragmentation of DNA by bleomycin proceeded more rapidly in the presence of O_2 compared with anaerobiosis (ISHIDA and TAKAHASHI, 1975; ONISHI et al., 1975; SAUSVILLE et al., 1976; LOWN and SIM, 1977).

NAGAI et al. (1969) demonstrated that catalase had no effect on the bleomycin-2-mercaptoethanol reaction on DNA. ISHIDA and TAKAHASHI (1975) reported that DNA fragmentation was enhanced in the presence of hypoxanthine and xanthine oxidase. This stimulatory effect disappeared when superoxide dismutase was added, but not when catalase was added. However, superoxide dismutase did not inhibit bleomycin-induced chain-breakage in the presence of 2-mercaptoethanol, dithiothreitol, ascorbic acid or H_2O_2. These authors concluded that the stimulation of fragmentation using the xanthine oxidase system proceeded by a different mechanism from that using 2-mercaptoethanol, dithiothreitol, ascorbic acid or H_2O_2. LOWN and SIM (1977), using a system containing Fe^{2+} alone or Fe^{2+} complexed with bleomycin, reported that the breakage of superhelical PM2 DNA was inhibited by superoxide dismutase, catalase, and more efficiently inhibited by a combination of the two enzymes. Free-radical scavengers also inhibited this bleomycin-Fe^{2+} fragmentation reaction. Another report also indicated that free-radical scavengers inhibited the bleomycin-induced fragmentation reaction (ONISHI et al., 1975); however, MÜLLER et al. (1972) reported that free-radical scavengers were without effect on the reaction.

I. End-Products

HAIDLE (1971) and HAIDLE et al. (1972), using paper chromatographic analyses, reported the release of all four bases from *B. subtilis* DNA after treatment with high concentrations of bleomycin. However, MÜLLER et al. (1972, 1976), using Sephadex chromatography and high pressure liquid chromatography, reported the release of only thymine, using much lower drug concentrations. These workers concluded that thymine was required for bleomycin action. However, as previously, discussed, HAIDLE et al. (1972) demonstrated the release of uracil from PBS-1 DNA, which contains uracil in place of thymine. ISHIDA and TAKAHASHI (1975), using Sephadex chromatography, confirmed that only thymine was released using low drug concentrations. It seems likely that thymine is preferentially released at lower drug concentrations. In addition, KUO and HAIDLE (1973) reported that bleomycin caused the rupture of phosphodiester bonds resulting in the production of 30% hydroxyl and 70% phosphoryl groups on the 5′-termini of the DNA with very few of the 3′ termini phosphorylated which indicated that the preponderance of the breaks were on the 3′-side of the sugar. They also noted the production of an aldehyde-like compound which presumably arose from the breakage of the deoxyribose moiety. MÜLLER et al. (1972) had also observed the production of aldehyde groups after bleomycin action; however, in the absence of thiol compounds during the bleomycin-DNA reaction, MÜLLER and ZAHN (1976a) could find no aldehyde groups. This question remains unresolved. KUO et al. (1973) reported that high concentrations of bleomycin resulted in the solubilization of approximately 80% of the DNA. The remaining 20% was resistant to further action of the drug and consisted of single-stranded oligonucleotides with a molecular weight of about 4000 daltons. The base composition of this resistant DNA was similar to the parental DNA from which it was derived.

J. Enzyme Inhibition

The reports on the effects of bleomycin on DNA polymerases in isolated enzyme systems have been contradictory. YAMAKI et al. (1971) reported that incubation of bleomycin A_2 in an *E. coli* B DNA polymerase system initially produced a stimulatory effect on the incorporation of [^{14}C]-dGMP into the acid-insoluble fraction, but a short time later, incorporation of dGMP was greatly reduced. These authors suggested that this inhibition was probably the result of bleomycin-induced strand scissions in DNA. However, MÜLLER et al. (1972) reported that concentrations of bleomycin up to 50 μg/ml did not inhibit DNA-dependent DNA polymerase isolated from mouse liver or *E. coli.* They also reported that low concentrations of bleomycin did inhibit DNA-dependent DNA polymerase from Rausher murine leukemia virus and that higher concentrations were needed to inhibit the RNA-dependent DNA polymerase from the same source. It should be noted that the Rauscher murine leukemia virus contains only an RNA-dependent DNA polymerase and that this same polymerase has the capacity to use DNA as a template. MÜLLER et al. (1975) have subsequently reported that bleomycin at 4–5 μg/ml concentrations causes a 50% inhibition of DNA-dependent DNA polymerases from mouse lymphoma cells and *E. coli*. DICIOCCIO and SRIVASTAVA (1976) demonstrated a bleomycin-induced inhibition of α and β DNA polymerases from Molt-4 cells while γ DNA polymerase was not affected. They also reported that addition of extra substrate would reverse the inhibition while extra enzyme would not. They concluded that this bleomycin inhibition was probably the result of the degradation of the DNA template.

TANAKA (1970) reported an inhibitory effect of bleomycin of the DNA dependent RNA polymerase derived from T4 bacteriophage and suggested that inhibition resulted from the binding of bleomycin to DNA thus preventing the elongation steps. MÜLLER et al. (1972) reported no inhibition of DNA-dependent RNA polymerase from mouse lymphoma cells in the presence of up to 50 μg/ml bleomycin. However, MÜLLER et al. (1975) later demonstrated significant inhibition of DNA-dependent RNA polymerase from mouse lymphoma cells and *E. coli* by 5 μg/ml of bleomycin. SHISHIDO (1973) also demonstrated an inhibition by bleomycin of RNA polymerase from T7 bacteriophage and *E. coli*. It was concluded that the drug did not interfere with initiation, and the mechanism of bleomycin action was postulated to be the result of the destruction of or binding to the template DNA. MIYAKI et al. (1971) and YAMAKI et al. (1971) reported that bleomycin inhibits the ligase reaction. This effect was probably also the result of bleomycin binding to the DNA, and not a direct effect on the ligase.

Conflicting results have appeared in the literature concerning the effect of the drug on the action of DNase I. YAMAKI et al. (1971) first demonstrated that bleomycin stimulates DNase action in an isolated system while MÜLLER et al. (1973) reported that bleomycin inhibited DNase I action. MÜLLER et al. (1973) also reported that bleomycin had minimal effects on DNase II and no effect on several RNA nucleases.

V. Cell-Culture Studies

Although much can be learned about the mechanism of action of bleomycin from the results of the cell-free studies, this knowledge has little meaning unless it can be related directly to intracellular damage and cell lethality and ultimately to the anticancer effects in animals and man. At present, there is little direct evidence linking the extracellular effects on DNA with the intracellular mechanism of action. This section describes the results of investigations which are germane to the generally held concept that the extracellular observed damage to DNA is related to the observed toxic effects on cells.

A. Cell-Cycle Specificity

Research on the effects of bleomycin on cell progression through the cell cycle has been actively pursued by numerous investigators. Even though no two studies have yielded identical results, and at times directly contradictory work has been reported, certain general features of bleomycin action on the cell cycle have emerged. The most prominent feature is the bleomycin-induced blockage of cells in the G_2 phase (KUNIMOTO et al., 1967; SUZUKI et al., 1968; BARRANCO and HUMPHREY, 1971; NAGATSU et al., 1972; TOBEY, 1972a, b; DREWINKO et al., 1973; HITTELMAN and RAO, 1974; WATANABE et al., 1974; WHEATLEY et al., 1974; BARLOGIE et al., 1976; REDDY et al., 1977). There is also general agreement that cells in the G_2 phase are more sensitive to the lethal effects of bleomycin (BARRANCO and HUMPHREY, 1971; NAGATSU et al., 1972; DREWINKO et al., 1973; CLARKSON and HUMPHREY, 1976; FERNÁNDEZ-GÓMEZ and DE LA TORRE, 1976). Many investigators have also demonstrated no significant bleomycin-induced time lag in the progression of cells from G_1 to S or from S to G_2 (KUNIMOTO et al., 1967; BARRANCO and HUMPHREY, 1971; TOBEY, 1972a, b; WATANABE et al., 1974; BARLOGIE et al., 1976).

The blockage of cells in G_2 by the action of bleomycin deserves further comment. Two groups have reported that maximum blockage at G_2 occurs if the cells were subjected to bleomycin in early S phase (KUNIMOTO et al., 1967; BARLOGIE et al., 1976). Further studies have demonstrated that this cell accumulation is confined to the first part of G_2 (WATANABE et al., 1974; WHEATLEY et al., 1974). In support of this finding, HITTELMAN and RAO (1974) reported that approximately one-half of the cells accumulated in G_2 did not enter mitosis. BARLOGIE et al. (1976), using a synchronous G_2 population treated with bleomycin, also showed that approximately one-half of the cells escape the G_2 block and enter mitosis. HITTELMAN and RAO (1974) have demonstrated that bleomycin, administered after release from a colcemid-block, does not inhibit the progression of cells through mitosis. WHEATLEY et al. (1974) have also reported similar results. FERNÁNDEZ-GÓMEZ and DE LA TORRE (1976) have reported results which suggest that some G_2 phase cells may be stimulated to enter early prophase by bleomycin.

Several hypotheses have been suggested to explain the accumulation of cells in G_2. BARRANCO and HUMPHREY (1971) proposed that the G_2 block could possibly be the result of the inhibition of essential proteins necessary to initiate chromosome condensation and division. WATANABE et al. (1974) suggested that the G_2 block could be caused by an interference with the mitotic apparatus, e.g., damage to the centrioles, spindles or nuclear membranes. HITTELMAN and RAO (1974) have presented evidence indicating that the G_2 block results from the accumulation of a critical amount of chromosomal damage, and that if a threshold level of chromosome damage was exceeded, the cells could not enter mitosis until the lesions were sufficiently repaired.

In contrast to the studies discussed above, TERASIMA and UMEZAWA (1970) reported that late G_1 and early S phase cells were more sensitive to the action of bleomycin than cells in other phases of the cell cycle. BARLOGIE et al. (1976) also showed that, in addition to the most effective cell killing at the G_2 phase, significant cell death was also observed in the G_1 phase. Using a whole animal test system, FUJIMOTO et al. (1976) reported that bleomycin was relatively non-cycle specific in killing mouse ascites tumor cells.

B. Survival and Repair

In many cell survival studies, treatment of exponentially growing and plateau cells with bleomycin results in the production of a biphasic survival curve (TERASIMA et al., 1972; BARRANCO et al., 1973; ONISHI et al., 1973; TWENTYMAN and BLEEHEN, 1973; BARRANCO et al., 1975; TWENTYMAN and BLEEHEN, 1975a; IQBAL et al., 1976; TWENTYMAN, 1976a). This biphasic survival curve is obtained if the surviving fraction of cells versus either bleomycin concentration or time of exposure to the drug is plotted. The initial part of the curve drops off sharply, followed by a leveling off as either the bleomycin concentration or the exposure time increases as shown in Fig. 2. Several investigators have offered explanations to account for this type of curve. One hypothesis states that cells are exponentially killed by the drug, followed by a build-up of resistance to bleomycin (TERASIMA et al., 1972; MAURO et al., 1974). This resistance is not a permanent one because when bleomycin is removed the resistance is subsequently lost. The cells return to their original sensitivity as a function of the time elapsed between bleomycin treatments. One possible explanation to account for such a gain and loss of resistance is that exposure to bleomycin causes the cells to produce an enzyme which can inactivate the drug, and as the drug is inactivated or removed, the intracellular concentration of this inactivating protein is diminished and cells again become sensitive to bleomycin; MÜLLER and ZAHN (1976c) have described such a bleomycin-inactivating enzyme.

Another explanation to account for the biphasic nature of the survival curve is that within any asynchronous cell population there exist some cells which are much more sensitive to bleomycin than others (DREWINKO et al., 1973). This sensitivity is most likely the result of the differences in sensitivity among cells in differing phases of the cell cycle. Also a biphasic curve representing DNA breakage in cells as measured by an alkaline elution assay has been described (IQBAL et al., 1976). These investigators postulated that the biphasic DNA elution curve indicates a selective sensitivity in the cell cycle, or possible selective breakage sites on the DNA.

The ability of bleomycin to kill exponentially growing cells in contrast to plateau phase cells has been examined by several groups. The results have been contradictory. BARRANCO et al. (1973) and RAY et al. (1973) have reported that bleomycin kills noncycling, plateau phase cells much more effectively than exponentially growing cells. However, TWENTYMAN and BLEEHEN (1973) using EMT6 mouse tumor cells, and MAURO et al. (1974) using Chinese hamster cells, reported that exponentially growing cells were more sensitive to the effects of bleomycin than plateau cells. TWENTYMAN and BLEEHEN (1975a) later concluded that plateau cells were, in fact, more sensitive than exponentially growing cells.

Bleomycin-treated mammalian cells have the capacity to repair at least part of the damage resulting from the action of the drug. Two basic types of damage relating to cell survival have been characterized from radiation studies: potentially lethal damage and sublethal damage (ELKIND and SUTTON, 1960; BACCHETTI et al., 1966; PHILLIPS and TOLMACH, 1966). Recovery from potentially lethal damage is measured by the increase in colony-forming ability as a function

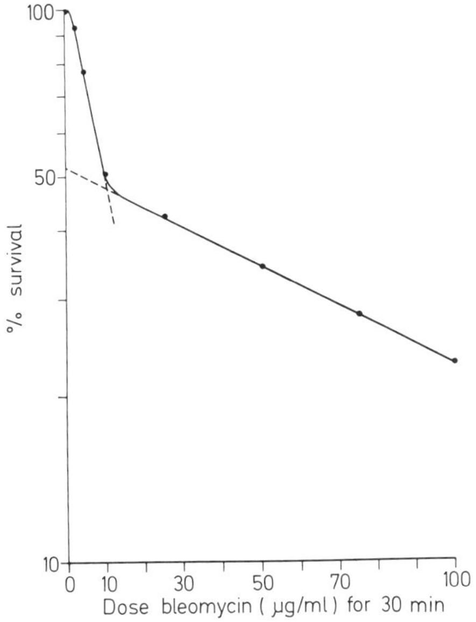

Fig. 2. Effect of bleomycin on survival in asynchronously growing CHO cells (BARRANCO and HUMPHREY, 1971)

of increasing time before subculturing after a single drug or radiation treatment. Recovery from sublethal damage is measured as an increase in cell survival as the time between successive drug or radiation treatments is increased.

Damage caused by bleomycin has been characterized as being more similar to X-ray than to UV damage (ONISHI et al., 1973; HAHN, 1976). These workers demonstrated that cells, which were treated with bleomycin and were allowed to recover from potentially lethal damage following drug removal, demonstrated recovery very similar to X-ray recovery (Fig. 3). Using exponentially growing cells exposed to varying concentrations of bleomycin for 1 h, BARRANCO et al. (1975) determined that cells plated immediately after drug removal versus subculturing 2 or 4 h later showed that the surviving fraction increased two-fold after 2 h and threefold after 4 h. Similar experiments using plateau phase cells demonstrated that a delay in subculturing of 2 and 6 h increased survival 4- and 7-fold respectively. These workers also reported that bleomycin-treated cells did not recover from sublethal damage.

TWENTYMAN and BLEEHEN (1975b) reported on factors which might influence cell recovery from potentially lethal damage following bleomycin treatment. Under the conditions used, an insignificant effect on cell survival was shown by altering the medium used, the number of cells plated, the temperature at which cells were exposed to the drug or the method for removing cells from the flasks.

As previously mentioned, bleomycin damage has been compared with X-ray damage to DNA. ONISHI et al. (1973), using *E. coli* strains that were very sensitive to ionizing radiation, reported that these cells were also very sensitive to bleomy-

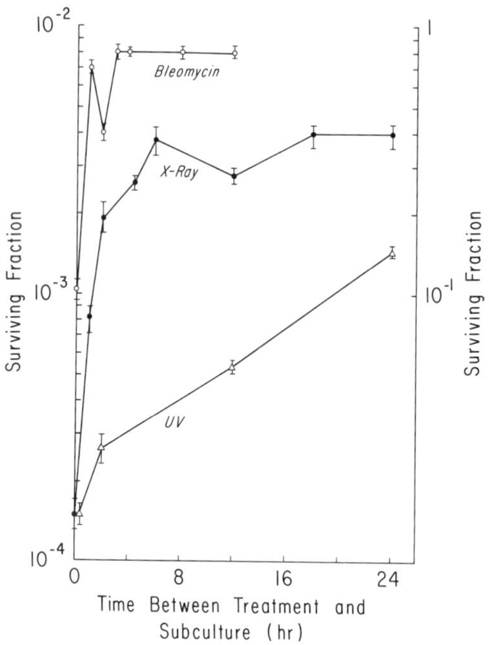

Fig. 3. Recovery of plateau-phase cells after exposure to 1500 rads of X-irradiation; 100 ergs/mm² of UV irradiation; or 20 µg/ml of bleomycin. X-irradiation and UV irradiation (*left ordinate*) and bleomycin (*right ordinate*). (Redrawn from HAHN, 1976)

cin treatment. This ionizing radiation sensitivity probably implied a lack of repair pathways or functional enzymes for the repair of this type of damage. In the same study, UV-sensitive mutants were able effectively to repair bleomycin damage, also implying that the mechanism for repair of UV damage was not significant in the repair of bleomycin damage. In support of this finding, IQBAL et al. (1976) reported that ultraviolet light-sensitive *Xeroderma pigmentosum* cells were able to repair bleomycin-induced damage as effectively as normal cells; this also suggests that the part of the ultraviolet repair pathway which is deficient in Xeroderma cells is not required for effective repair of bleomycin-induced damage.

Further evidence for bleomycin-induced repair synthesis was reported by FUJIWARA and KONDO (1973). These investigators determined that a 30 min exposure of either 25 or 100 µg/ml of bleomycin to cells which were not in the S phase, caused a low amount of unscheduled DNA synthesis; this was measured by [^{3}H]TdR incorporation and autoradiography. A DNA repair response to bleomycin treatment has also been described in isolated rat liver nuclei and rat hepatoma nuclei (SARTIANO et al., 1973, 1975, 1977; SPANGLER et al., 1976; COETZEE et al., 1977).

ROSS and MOSES (1976) have attempted to determine which enzymes and repair pathways might be necessary for bleomycin-induced DNA repair using a toluene-treated *E. coli* system. Toluene-treated cells require an exogenous source of ATP for semi-conservative DNA replication. These workers reported that when toluene-treated cells are exposed to bleomycin in the presence of ATP, DNA synthesis remains constant. Thus bleomycin does not inhibit semi-conservative DNA replication in this system. Analysis of the incorporation of bromodeoxyuridine 5′-triphosphate into DNA by density profile shifts revealed that parental and progeny DNA from ATP-stimulated synthesis in the presence of bleomycin were identical, again indicating that semi-conservative replication is not affected by bleomycin. Bleomycin-treated cells did not, however, require exogenous ATP to stimulate DNA synthesis. This DNA synthesis, in the absence of added ATP, was probably repair-type synthesis. In addition, if a temperature sensitive mutant for normal DNA replication were grown at nonpermissive temperatures in the presence of the drug, new DNA was synthesized. These workers have also shown that 5′ to 3′ exonuclease activity and DNA polymerase II are not required for repair of bleomycin-induced damage. However, a DNA polymerase I deficient mutant was not able to synthesize new DNA after bleomycin treatment indicating that DNA polymerase I is necessary for repair of bleomycin-induced damage.

C. Morphological Changes and Chromosome Damage

Cytological studies on the action of bleomycin on cultured mammalian cells have yielded interesting morphological findings as well as a complete description of chromosomal damage. Bleomycin alters the gross morphology of HeLa and mouse fibroblast cells, causing elongation and general cellular enlargement (SUZUKI et al., 1968; NAGATSU et al., 1972; KRISHAN, 1973; DESAI et al., 1974). Cells from various sources have also been shown to be multinucleate, indicating possible endoreduplication (NAGATSU et al., 1972; KRISHAN, 1973; DESAI et al., 1974). The DNA and protein content of these cells was also shown to be significantly higher than in normal cells (DESAI et al., 1974). Other distinctive morphological changes which have been noted were disrupted chromatin, decreased numbers of ribosomes, changes in nucleoli (OGAWA and ONOE, 1969) and hypertrophy of the Golgi apparatus and mitochondria (KRISHAN, 1973).

In addition to morphological alterations, bleomycin has been shown to induce chromosomal damage in cells from many sources (OHAMA and KADOTANI, 1970; BORNSTEIN et al., 1971; KUO, 1973; PAIKA and KRISHAN, 1973; TAMURA et al., 1974; HITTELMAN and RAO, 1974; PROMCHAINANT, 1975; BENEDICT et al., 1977). The most common chromosomal lesions found were breaks, achromatic gaps, deletions and fragments; these lesions were generally dependent on the concentration of bleomycin. Other chromosome abnormalities such as dicentric figures, ring chromosomes, and multi-radial translocations have also been reported (OHAMA and KADOTANI, 1970; PAIKA and KRISHAN, 1973). Utilizing the premature chromosome condensation technique, HITTELMAN and RAO (1974) reported that cells with extensive chromosome damage were blocked in G_2 and cells with extremely severe chromosome damage were prevented from entering mitosis. In a cytological study to analyze known environmental and chemical mutagens for sister chromatid exchange and chromosome breakage, bleomycin showed an extremely high frequency of chromosome breaks with a very low frequency of sister chromatid exchange (PERRY and EVANS, 1975). In addition, BENEDICT et al. (1977) demonstrated that bleomycin caused the transformation of 0.5% of mouse cells after 24 h exposure to 2.5 μg/ml of bleomycin.

D. Macromolecular Syntheses

It is very difficult to draw firm conclusions on the effects of bleomycin on macromolecular syntheses because of the diverse and often contradictory results reported in the literature. These contradictory results may be expected to arise from the different cells used having differing permeabilities and differing amounts of inactivating enzymes. One might also expect differences among cells in their ability to repair bleomycin-induced damage. One of the most serious objections to many of the experiments relating to macromolecular syntheses is the general failure to distinguish between semi-conservative replication and DNA repair synthesis. Another difficulty in interpreting experiments on the inhibition of DNA, RNA and protein syntheses results from the fact that most investigators report the gross incorporation of radioactive-labeled precursors into acid-precipitable material without considering the number of viable cells remaining after exposure to the drug.

SUZUKI et al. (1968) reported that DNA synthesis in growing HeLa cells was inhibited by approximately 80, 75, and 50% in the presence of 40 μg/ml of bleomycin A_2 incubated for 4, 8 and 24 h respectively. RNA and protein synthesis remained near control levels under the same experimental conditions. These workers also reported some inhibition of protein synthesis using Ehrlich carcinoma cells and some protein synthesis inhibition in *E. coli* grown in a low phosphate medium.

WHEATLEY et al. (1974), using synchronized HeLa S-3 cells in the presence of 5 μg/ml of bleomycin for 1, 4 and 8 h reported DNA synthesis to be 77, 57 and 43% of control values respectively while the incorporation of [^{14}C]-leucine remained near control values. Lower bleomycin concentrations, 1 μg/ml, showed no significant effect on DNA synthesis until 8 h after exposure to the drug, at which time DNA synthesis was 65% of the control value; minimal effects on protein and RNA synthesis were shown after 8 h.

WATANABE et al. (1973), using 20 μg/ml bleomycin for 1 h on mouse L5 cells showed that DNA synthesis was lowered to 40% of the control values while RNA and protein synthesis were only slightly affected, approximately 85% and 75% of control values respectively. Subsequently, MÜLLER et al. (1975) reported results using mouse lymphoma cells which were in good agreement with those described by WATANABE et al. (1973). Cells incubated for 1 h in the presence of 13 μg/ml of bleomycin showed approximately 50% inhibition of the incorporation of [^{3}H]-thymidine, while the incorporation of [^{3}H]-uridine and [^{3}H]-tryptophan were affected only slightly or not at all. Other groups have reported similar findings (KUNIMOTO et al., 1967; TOTSUKA et al., 1975).

In contrast to these studies, TOBEY (1972a) reported extensive cell killing and cell-cycle perturbance with little effect on macromolecular syntheses. Using

Chinese hamster ovary cells in the presence of 100 μg/ml of bleomycin for up to 6 h, he showed thymidine, uridine and leucine incorporation to be 80, and 90% of control values respectively. In support of these findings COHEN and I (1976) demonstrated only a slight inhibition of DNA synthesis and no RNA or protein synthesis inhibition at the time at which greater than 90% of the *E. coli* 15 TAU cells had been killed. DNA and RNA synthesis in vaccinia virus have been reported to be significantly inhibited by the action of bleomycin (TAKESHITA et al., 1974). SAUNDERS et al. (1972) also reported a significant inhibition of RNA and DNA synthesis in *B. subtilis*.

E. Intracellular DNA Damage

In the early stages of bleomycin research, it was determined by a number of groups, that bleomycin caused intracellular single-strand DNA scission (SUZUKI et al., 1969; YAMAKI et al., 1971; FUJIWARA and KONDO, 1973; MIYAKI et al., 1973; SAITO and ANDOH, 1973). Limited mitochondrial DNA scission by bleomycin was shown by OSIEKA et al. (1976). MIYAKI et al. (1973) reported the existence of intracellular alkaline labile sites produced as a result of bleomycin treatment. SAITO and ANDOH (1973) also demonstrated formation of DNA double-strand breaks in intact cells. The alkaline labile sites probably correspond to sites where bases have been excised, as reported in the in vitro work (HAIDLE et al., 1972; MÜLLER et al., 1972).

Various parameters affecting intracellular DNA breakage and cell toxicity have been reported. KOHN and EWIG (1976) reported that the extent of DNA scission and cytotoxicity increased as the pH of the bleomycin-incubation medium was increased from 6.6 to 7.6. The toxicity of various bleomycin derivatives was tested using various strains of *E. coli* (COHEN and I, 1976). Bleomycin A_5 was found to be the most lethal, followed by $A_{2\text{-b}}$, B_2, A_2 and bleomycinic acid. The lethality of bleomycin A_5 has been shown to be specifically and significantly blocked by hirudonine (1,8-diamidinospermidine; LAPI and COHEN, 1977). However, the toxicity of bleomycin A_5 or B_2 was not affected by hirudonine.

Using a double-layer agar assay as an antiphage screening test for various chemical agents, AOKI and SAKAI (1967) reported bacteriophage induction in *E. coli* W 3110 cells by 0.1 μg/ml bleomycin. HAIDLE et al. (1972) have also reported bleomycin-mediated induction of λ bacteriophage in *E. coli* K-12 (λ) and the defective bacteriophage PBSH in *B. subtilis* 168.

Several groups have suggested that bleomycin does not enter the cell or enters very poorly and consequently the DNA strand breakage in cell culture studies is an artifact arising from the extracellular fragmentation of DNA after cell lysis (FUJIWARA and KONDO, 1973; COX et al., 1974). FUJIWARA and KONDO (1973) observed that if cells were lysed in the presence of EDTA, a known inhibitor of the in vitro bleomycin-induced breakage reaction, only low amounts of DNA fragmentation were observed, while cell lysis without EDTA showed significant DNA breakage. In support of these findings, FUJIMOTO (1974) and FUJIMOTO et al. (1976), using autoradiography reported high concentrations of [^{14}C]-labeled bleomycin at the cell membrane of mouse tumor cells after 2 h of drug treatment and a subsequent high concentration of drug at the nuclear membrane after 4 h. Beyond 4 h, there was a sharp increase in necrotic cells. Cells in mitosis showed no concentration of grains in the nucleoplasm. However, the entry of these cells into mitosis could be caused by the failure of bleomycin to enter the cells and to induce a G_2 block as previously discussed. MIYAKI et al. (1974) demonstrated that bleomycin-induced breakage of a DNA-membrane complex occurred as a result of membrane disruption and DNA strand scission near the membrane-DNA attachment site.

F. Bleomycin in Combination with Other Agents

Several studies have described the action of bleomycin in combination with X-rays on mammalian cells and bacterial strains. MATSUZAWA et al. (1972) demonstrated that pretreatment with bleomycin enhances the cell killing effects of X-rays on mouse mammary carcinoma cells. Simple additive effects were demonstrated by BLEEHEN et al. (1974) in three bacterial strains and two mammalian cell lines. Whether bleomycin was present before radiation or present during radiation did not significantly affect the results. However, using the *E. coli* B/r strain, synergistic effects were shown if bleomycin treatment followed radiation. Using mouse L cells, BISTROVIC et al. (1976) reported a moderate synergistic effect if bleomycin and radiation were applied simultaneously. These investigators also reported that cellular recovery from X-ray damage was not affected by bleomycin. Identical recovery findings were reported by BYFIELD et al. (1976) using HeLa cells. Recently ALALAWI and CHAPMAN (1977) using asynchronous Ehrlich ascites cells in suspension culture demonstrated a synergistic effect if bleomycin were given in a split dose, before and after radiation; but only additive effects or less if the entire drug dose were given before, during, or after the X-rays.

Hyperthermia as an adjunct to radiation therapy and chemotherapy has been described only recently. BRAUN and HAHN (1975) studied the combination effects of bleomycin and 43° C hyperthermia on Chinese hamster cells. They reported a significant synergism when applied simultaneously. If cells were heated at 43° C immediately prior to bleomycin exposure at 37° C, a substantial sensitization to bleomycin was also produced. The authors speculated that the heat treatment must produce cellular effects rather than simply increasing the drug action at the higher temperature.

The effect of bleomycin in combination with pentamycin was reported by TWENTYMAN (1976b) to be synergistic when the drugs were administered consecutively rather than simultaneously.

VI. Proposed Mechanisms of Action

Several models for bleomycin interaction with isolated DNA have been proposed. Theories on the binding and interaction of different functional components of the drug will be discussed in conjunction with mechanistic models.

The bithiazole moiety of the tripeptide S portion of the bleomycin molecule has been suggested to undergo a partial intercalation reaction with DNA (MURAKAMI et al., 1973; MURAKAMI et al., 1976). These investigators have suggested that only one of the thiazole rings participates in this partial intercalation. Evidence supporting this hypothesis is an observed increase in the viscosity of the DNA after reaction with bleomycin resulting in an overall lengthening of the DNA (MURAKAMI et al., 1973; CHIEN et al., 1977). There was also thought to be a disturbance in base stacking forces and a general increase in helix instability as evidenced by a reduction in the melting temperature (MURAKAMI et al., 1973). However, KRUEGER et al. (1973) reported a possible increase in the regularity of the DNA helix. The exact site(s) on the DNA at which this intercalation occurs has not been unambiguously established. MURAKAMI et al. (1973) proposed that there could be preferential interaction between the thiazole ring and guanine bases. Theoretical evidence was presented which predicted an electrostatic stabilization and strong electronic affinity interactions. It was also postulated that electron transfer should occur between the strong electron donor, guanine, and the vacant $3d\pi$ atomic orbital of the sulfur atom in the thiazole ring. However, following the report by MÜLLER et al. (1972) that thymine was preferentially released from double-stranded DNA, MURAKAMI et al. (1976) examined the possible interaction of the bithiazole moiety and thymine of poly d(A·T). Even though the electrostatic forces between the bithiazole moiety and thymine are not as great as with guanine, a covalent-type of bond could be postulated between the N3 of thymine and the sulfur in the thiazole ring. This bond would be the result of transfer of the lone pair of electrons in the $2p\pi$ orbital of the N3 of thymine and the vacant $3d\pi$ of the sulfur. This electron transfer was postulated to be the initial step in the release of thymine as a free base. The subsequent steps involved in the conversion of the N1 of thymine from a trigonal planar state (sp^2) to a tetrahedral state (sp^3) followed by hydrogen transfer to the N1 atom would result in the liberation of thymine. Various thiol compounds could contribute significantly to this hydrogen transfer reaction. Proposed spatial relationships between the bleomycin molecule and one strand of the DNA helix are depicted in Fig. 4.

Another part of the bleomycin molecule which has been implicated in the release of thymine is the terminal β-amino-L-alanine moiety (MÜLLER and ZAHN, 1977). The amino group of this moiety was shown to have a pK of 7.3 (TAKITA et al., 1972), and the bleomycin breakage reaction was very slow below pH 7 (UMEZAWA et al., 1973). This evidence suggests that this amino group which exists in an unprotonated state is necessary for either DNA strand breakage, DNA binding or base release. UMEZAWA et al. (1973) have also determined that bleomycin loses activity if the carboxylamide group is hydrolyzed. On the basis of these findings, MÜLLER and ZAHN (1977) proposed a mechanism for thymine release. The first step involves a hydrogen bonding between the amide group of the carboxylamide moiety and the 2-keto group of thymine. Following hydrogen transfer to the thymine, the carboxylamide group becomes a negatively charged carboxylimide group. The carboxylimide group then binds a hydrogen from a water molecule, with the resulting free hydroxyl group

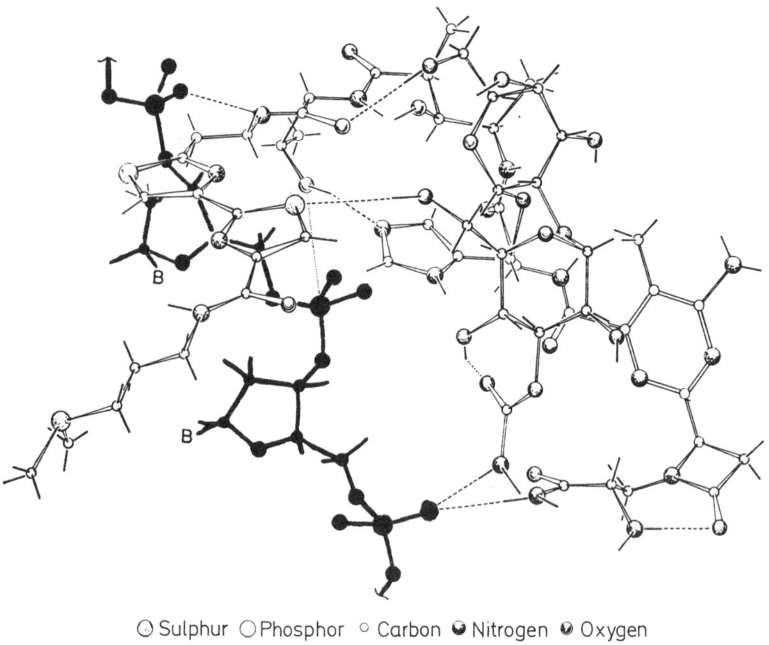

Fig. 4. Proposed configuration of one bleomycin molecule with one strand of a DNA phosphodiester backbone (*heavily darkened portion*). Three intermolecular hydrogen bonds between the "open" configuration of bleomycin and the DNA are proposed. (Redrawn from MURAKAMI et al., 1976)

transfered to the C1 of the deoxyribose moiety with the loss of thymine by glycosidic bond breakage.

This β-amino-L-alanine group has also been implicated as a part of a metal binding site (UMEZAWA et al., 1973; MURAKAMI et al., 1976; UMEZAWA, 1976; LOWN and SIM, 1977). The chelation of Cu^{2+} in this part of the molecule has been linked with the lack of activity of bleomycin-Cu^{2+} in the in vitro DNA breakage reaction (UMEZAWA et al., 1973; MURAKAMI et al., 1976; UMEZAWA, 1976). MURAKAMI et al. (1976) presented a model describing a possible Cu^{2+} chelation site formed by the free amino group of the α-carbon and the terminal amide of the β-amino-L-alanine moiety and nitrogen and oxygen atoms in the carbamoyloxy group located at the tip of the sugar moiety. Chelation of Fe^{2+} with the subsequent generation of free-radicals by this Fe^{2+} in the bleomycin molecule has been suggested by LOWN and SIM (1977) as a possible mechanism leading to DNA strand breakage.

Another portion of the bleomycin molecule which could theoretically bind metals was proposed by MURAKAMI et al. (1973). A tetrahedral metal chelation site was suggested to be formed by the threonine hydroxyl group, the imidazole nitrogen, the sulfur of the thiazole ring nearest the R-group, and the nitrogen of the other thiazole group.

Even though the location and/or orientation of the metal has not been completely established, supportive evidence exists which indicates metal involvement with drug. The various metals which cause breakage enhancement could possibly be required for proper stabilization and conformation of the bleomycin molecule to cause the observed DNA damage. Conversely, those metals which inhibit the reaction could fix the molecular structure in a configuration lacking the ability to break the DNA. DNA-metal interactions may also affect the activity of the drug. More evidence implicating metal ions with the action of bleomycin is that certain chelating agents (CDTA, EDTA, and EGTA) are capable of quickly stopping the bleomycin breakage reaction (unpublished results). These chelating agents could either bind to the metal-containing sites, and thus prevent drug binding to DNA, or they could sequester metals out of the putative bleomycin-metal complex which are necessary to maintain proper configuration to react with the DNA.

Several studies on the role of the different R-groups, which differentiate the various bleomycins, have been made. MÜLLER et al. (1972) reported that bleomycin B_2 was largely inactivated if urea was split from the guanidino group of the agmatine chain. ASAKURA et al. (1975), using SV40 DNA, reported that bleomycinic acid (R=OH) exhibited only 5% of the DNA strand breakage capacity as compared with bleomycin B_2. The bleomycin A_2 derivative (R=3-aminopropyl-dimethyl sulfonium) has probably been the most widely studied of all of the isolated bleomycin derivatives. MÜLLER et al. (1972) postulated that this side chain may act by a transmethylation reaction. MURAKAMI et al. (1973) and MURAKAMI et al. (1976) postulated that the dimethyl sulfonium ion being positively charged could interact with a phosphate of the DNA strand opposite the bithiazole intercalation site. CHIEN et al. (1977) also postulated strong bindings of not only the bithiazole moiety but also the dimethysulfonium group. Experimental evidence which supports the theory (MURAKAMI et al., 1973; MURAKAMI et al., 1976) that the drug may bind to both strands has been recently obtained. Bleomycin has been found directly to induce double-strand breaks in isolated PM2 DNA. These double-strand breaks are not the result of the accumulation of random single-strand breaks which suggests that the drug is binding to and breaking both strands of the DNA (unpublished results).

VII. Concluding Remarks

Although a great deal of research has been done on both the intra-and extracellular effects of bleomycin, the details of the mechanism of action remain unclear. A good theoretical working model for the physical interaction between the drug and DNA has been presented (MURAKAMI et al., 1973; MURAKAMI et al., 1976). Some aspects of this model have been verified experimentally (CHIEN et al., 1977). More work is needed to establish the details of the mechanism and the sequence of steps involved in the release of bases and rupture of the phosphodiester bonds. The role of reducing and oxidizing agents remains to be elucidated as well as the involvement of metal ions in the reaction. Several workers have concluded that the reaction proceeds via a free-radical mechanism with the involvement of Fe^{2+} (Sausville et al., 1976; Lown and Sim, 1977). However, since Fe^{2+} alone breaks DNA probably by a free-radical mechanism, care must be taken in interpreting such results. Since the bleomycin-induced DNA damage is very similar to that caused by X-rays and since the effect on the cell-cycle is also X-ray-like, one is tempted to postulate a similar mechanism i.e., free-radical involvement.

Müller and Zahn (1977) concluded that the drug remains active after the bleomycin-DNA reaction and refer to the reaction as a "quasi-enzyme reaction". It is felt that this conclusion, regarding the catalytic nature of the reaction is premature in light of the available evidence and must await further experimentation. One would also like to see further investigation into the temperature dependence of the extracellular reaction.

The studies on the inhibitory effects of bleomycin on macromolecular syntheses are also inconclusive at present. Further studies are required taking into account the various parameters discussed in the section on macromolecular synthesis.

From the results of all the studies on both the intra- and extracellular reaction, one gains the impression that DNA is likely the primary target of bleomycin-induced lethality. However it can be argued that the intracellular effects may be quite different from those observed extracellularly. It has even been suggested (Cox et al., 1974) that the observed intracellular damage is in fact an experimental artifact resulting from extracellular damage produced after cell lysis. Although the bulk of the evidence does not favor this theory, there is no direct experimental proof to refute it. Thus more work is needed to establish the exact relationships between the extracellular damage to DNA and the intracellular events leading to cell death.

Acknowledgments. The authors wish to express their appreciation to Ms. Janie Finch and Ms. Carol Martin for typing the manuscript and to Mr. Kenneth Kroll for his help in proofreading and organizing the manuscript.

The author's research was supported in part by Grant No. CA13246 awarded by the National Cancer Institute, DHEW, and Grant No. G-441 awarded by the Robert A. Welch Foundation.

Addendum

Several important observations pertinent to the mechanism of action of bleomycin have appeared in the literature since the initial writing of this article.

The first of these observations has been the unequivocal demonstration that bleomycin is capable of introducing direct double-strand breaks into DNA in the cell-free reaction (Povirk et al., 1977; Lloyd et al., 1978a, b) as had been previously suggested by Haidle (1971) and Lloyd et al. (1977). It has now been firmly established that the appearance of these double-strand breaks cannot be accounted for by the accumulation of many random single-strand breaks. In addition, Povirk et al. (1977) and Lloyd et al. (1978c) have confirmed the initial observation of Lloyd et al. (1977) that bleomycin introduces alkaline-labile sites in DNA; approximately one alkaline-labile site is introduced for each direct single-strand break. ROSS and MOSES (1978) also reported the appearance of alkaline-labile damage in the presence of bleomycin, but reported no single-strand breaks under neutral conditions.

LLOYD et al. (1978a) have made the unexpected observation that, using low concentrations of bleomycin (2.5 μg/ml bleomycin, 50 μg/ml DNA), there was a definite site specificity for bleomycin-mediated double-strand breaks in bacteriophage PM2 DNA. LLOYD et al. (1978b) were able to map physically 11 such specific sites of breakage on the PM2 genome using combined digestions with restriction endonucleases and bleomycin.

More recently, D'ANDREA and HASELTINE (1978), using the MAXAM and GILBERT (1977) DNA sequencing technique, showed a sequence-specific cleavage of regions of the lactose operon of *Escherichia coli* containing known nucleotide sequences. Using high drug concentrations (250 μg/ml bleomycin, 5 μg/ml DNA) in the presence of 2-mercaptoethanol, they observed a preferential cleavage at GC and GT sequences and a less preferential cleavage at TA sequences. When Fe^{2+} was substituted for 2-mercaptoethanol, bleomycin showed a different preference of cleavage; in this case the cleavage occurred at TT, AT, TA, GC, and GT sequences. TAKESHITA et al. (1978) observed a bleomycin-promoted cleavage at GT and GC sequences in the presence of Fe^{2+}.

Although it is difficult to compare the studies of LLOYD et al. (1978a, b) with those of D'ANDREA and HASELTINE (1978), because of the large differences in drug concentrations used and the fact that LLOYD et al. (1978a, b) were studying double-strand breakage while D'ANDREA and HASELTINE were studying single-strand breaks, some tentative conclusions can be drawn. It is quite possible that varying degrees of preference for strand breakage exist. For example, at low drug concentrations, bleomycin may bind preferentially to a certain specified sequence, while at higher drug concentrations these highly preferred sequences would be saturated and the drug might then bind to another less preferred sequence. It is therefore likely that, at physiological concentrations of the drug, the DNA would be broken at the most highly preferred sequences.

Two additional reports dealing with the involvement of Fe^{2+} in the cell-free reaction have also appeared (SAUSVILLE et al., 1978a, b), which constitute a further elaboration of the reaction in the presence of Fe^{2+} as previously reported (SAUSVILLE et al., 1976). These reports describe the stimulation by Fe^{2+} of the acid-solubilization of DNA by high concentrations of bleomycin. It is reported that the reaction requires molecular oxygen, is not inhibited by superoxide dismutase or catalase at high drug concentrations; at low drug concentrations superoxide dismutase does inhibit the reaction. Additionally, these workers reported the release of all four of the DNA bases, the production of nuclease-resistant small molecular weight oligonucleotides, and the production of a malondialdehyde-like compound indicating damage to the deoxyribose moiety. All of the foregoing observations are also characteristic of the bleomycin-2-mercaptoethanol-mediated breakage of DNA. They also reported that low concentrations of chelating agents inhibit the reaction, with deferoxamine mesylate being a more effective inhibitor than EDTA. Although it appears that Fe^{2+} does indeed stimulate the fragmentation of DNA under the reaction conditions used, the question arises as to the in vivo significance of using more or less equimolar amounts of bleomycin, Fe^{2+}, and DNA. It will be necessary to demonstrate the Fe^{2+} stimulation of the reaction using very low drug concentrations especially in light of the extensive damage to DNA by Fe^{2+} alone.

Further, LLOYD et al. (1978d, 1979) have observed the formation of intermolecular DNA–DNA cross-links by electron microscopy using purified supercoiled bacteriophage PM2 DNA in the presence of low concentrations of bleomycin and 2-mercaptoethanol. Approximately 16% of the DNA was observed in these cross-linked structures which consisted of dimers and higher oligomers of PM2 DNA. All three forms of DNA were observed in the cross-linked structures, but their initial formation was absolutely dependent upon the presence of supercoiled DNA. The cross-link bonds are thought to be noncovalent and may result from the association between bleomycin molecules bound to adjacent DNA molecules.

Finally, TAKITA et al. (1978) have presented evidence that the substituent at the 2-position of the pyrimidine ring of the original structure of bleomycin (Fig. 1) is in fact not a β-lactam ring. The revised structure of this portion of the bleomycin molecule exists as the "open" configuration of the β-lactam ring with an additional nitrogen which is present as an amide of the χ-aminocarboxylic acid moiety (TAKITA et al., 1972).

References to Addendum

D'Andrea, A.D., Haseltine, W.A.: Sequence specific cleavage of DNA by the antitumor antibiotics neocarzinostatin and bleomycin. Proc. Natl. Acad. Sci. USA *75*, 3608–3612 (1978)

Haidle, C.W.: Fragmentation of deoxyribonucleic acid by bleomycin. Mol. Pharmacol. *7*, 645–652 (1971)

Lloyd, R.S., Hewitt, R.R., Haidle, C.W.: Bleomycin-induced alkaline-labile damage and direct strand breakage in covalent-circular DNA. Fed. Proc. *36*, 694 (1977)

Lloyd, R.S., Haidle, C.W., Robberson, D.L.: Bleomycin-specific fragmentation of double-stranded DNA. Biochemistry *17*, 1890–1896 (1978a)

Lloyd, R.S., Haidle, C.W., Robberson, D.L., Dodson, M.L. Jr.: A physical map of bleomycin-specific fragmentation sites on PM2 bacteriophage DNA. Current Microbiol. *1*, 45–50 (1978b)

Lloyd, R.S., Haidle, C.W., Hewitt, R.R.: Bleomycin-induced alkaline-labile damage and direct strand breakage of PM2 DNA. Cancer Res. *38*, 3191–3196 (1978c)

Lloyd, R.S., Haidle, C.W., Robberson, D.L.: Bleomycin-mediated interstrand cross-links in PM2 DNA. Fed. Proc. *37*, 1670 (1978d)

Lloyd, R.S., Haidle, C.W., Robberson, D.L.: Non-covalent intermolecular cross-links are produced by bleomycin reaction with duplex DNA. Proc. Natl. Acad. Sci. USA, in press (1979)

Maxam, A.M., Gilbert, W.: A new method for sequencing DNA. Proc. Natl. Acad. Sci. USA *74*, 560–564 (1977)

Povirk, L.F., Wübker, W., Köhnlein, W., Hutchinson, F.: DNA double-strand breaks and alkali-labile bonds produced by bleomycin. Nucleic Acids Res. *4*, 3573–3580 (1977)

Ross, S.L., Moses, R.E.: Two actions of bleomycin on superhelical DNA. Biochemistry *17*, 581–586 (1978)

Sausville, E.A., Peisach, J., Horwitz, S.B.: A role for ferrous ion and oxygen in the degradation of DNA by bleomycin. Biochem. Biophys. Res. Commun. *73*, 814–822 (1976)

Sausville, E.A., Peisach, J., Horwitz, S.B.: Effect of chelating agents and metal ions on the degradation of DNA by bleomycin. Biochemistry *17*, 2740–2746 (1978a)

Sausville, E.A., Stein, R.W., Peisach, J., Horwitz, S.B.: Properties and products of the degradation of DNA by bleomycin and iron (II). Biochemistry *17*, 2746–2754 (1978b)

Takeshita, M., Grollman, A.P., Ohtsubo, E., Ohtsubo, H.: Interaction of bleomycin with DNA. Proc. Natl. Acad. Sci. USA *75*, 5983–5987 (1978)

Takita, T., Muraoka, Y., Yoshioka, T., Fujii, A., Maeda, K., Umezawa, H.: The chemistry of bleomycin. IX. The structures of bleomycin and phleomycin. J. Antibiot. *25*, 755–758 (1972)

Takita, T., Muraoka, Y., Nakatani, T., Fujii, A., Umezawa, Y., Naganawa, H., Umezawa, H.: Chemistry of bleomycin. XIX. Revised structures of bleomycin and phleomycin. J. Antibiot. *31*, 801–804 (1978)

References

Alalawi, F.A., Chapman, I.V.: Combined effects of bleomycin and X-rays on DNA synthesis in asynchronous Ehrlich ascites cells in suspension. Br. J. Cancer *36*, 78–83 (1977)

Aoki, H., Sakai, H.: Antiphage property as a screening test for antitumor agents. J. Antibiot. Ser. A *20*, 87–92 (1967)

Asakura, H., Hori, M., Umezawa, H.: Characterization of bleomycin action on DNA. J. Antibiot. *28*, 537–542 (1975)

Bacchetti, S., Cassandro, M., Elli, R., Falchetti, R., Mauro, F.: Relationship between recovery from sublethal damage by dose fractionation and the restoration of viability after delayed plating in diploid *Saccharomyces cerevisiae*. Radiat. Res. *29*, 295–315 (1966)

Barlogie, B., Drewinko, B., Schumann, J., Freireich, E.J.: Pulse cytophotometric analysis of cell cycle perturbation with bleomycin *in vitro*. Cancer Res. *36*, 1182–1187 (1976)

Barranco, S.C., Humphrey, R.M.: The effects of bleomycin on survival and cell progression in Chinese hamster cells *in vitro*. Cancer Res. *31*, 1218–1223 (1971)

Barranco, S.C., Humphrey, R.M.: The relevance of *in vitro* survival and cell cycle kinetics data to the clinical use of bleomycin. In: Gann monograph on cancer research No. 19. Fundamental and clinical studies of bleomycin. Carter, S.K., Ichikawa, T., Mathé, G., Umezawa, H. (eds.), pp. 83–95. Baltimore, London, New York: University Park 1976

Barranco, S.C., Novak, J.K., Humphrey, R.M.: Response of mammalian cells following treatment with bleomycin and 1,3-bis(2-chloroethyl)-1-nitrosourea during plateau phase. Cancer Res. *33*, 691–694 (1973)

Barranco, S.C., Novak, J.K., Humphrey, R.M.: Studies on recovery from chemically induced damage in mammalian cells. Cancer Res. *35*, 1194–1204 (1975)

Bearden, J.C., Jr., Haidle, C.W.: Stimulation of bleomycin-induced fragmentation of DNA by intercalating agents. Biochem. Biophys. Res. Commun. *65*, 371–377 (1975)

Bearden, J.C., Jr., Lloyd, R.S., Haidle, C.W.: Bleomycin-induced breakage of closed-circular DNA. Biochem. Biophys. Res. Commun. *75*, 442–447 (1977)

Benedict, W.F., Banerjee, A., Gardner, A., Jones, P.A.: Induction of morphological transformation in mouse C3H/10T$^1/_2$ clone 8 cells and chromosomal damage in hamster A(T_1)C1-3 cells by cancer chemotherapeutic agents. Cancer Res. *37*, 2202–2208 (1977)

Bistrovic, M., Maricic, Z., Kolaric, K.: Interaction of bleomycin and radiation in combined treatment on mouse L cells. Int. J. Cancer *18*, 540–542 (1976)

Bleehen, N.M., Gillies, N.E., Twentyman, P.R.: The effect of bleomycin and radiation in combination on bacteria and mammalian cells in culture. Br. J. Radiol. *47*, 346–351 (1974)

Bode, V.C.: Single-strand scissions induced in circular and linear λ DNA by the presence of dithiothreitol and other reducing agents. J. Mol. Biol. *26*, 125–129 (1967)

Bornstein, R.S., Hungerford, D.A., Haller, G., Engstrom, P.F., Yarbro, J.W.: Cytogenetic effects of bleomycin therapy in man. Cancer Res. *31*, 2004–2007 (1971)

Braun, J., Hahn, G.M.: Enhanced cell killing by bleomycin and 43° hyperthermia and the inhibition of recovery from potentially lethal damage. Cancer Res. *35*, 2921–2927 (1975)

Byfield, J.E., Lee, Y.C., Tu, L., Kulhanian, F.: Molecular interactions of the combined effects of bleomycin and X-rays on mammalian cell survival. Cancer Res. *36*, 1138–1143 (1976)

Carter, S.K., Ichikawa, T., Mathé, G., Umezawa, H. (eds.): Gann monograph on cancer research No. 19. Fundamental and clinical studies of bleomycin, p. 320. Baltimore, London, New York: University Park: 1976

Chien, M., Grollman, A.P., Horwitz, S.B.: Bleomycin-DNA interactions: Fluorescence and proton magnetic resonance studies. Biochemistry *16*, 3641–3647 (1977)

Clarkson, J.M., Humphrey, R.M.: The significance of damage in the cell cycle sensitivity of Chinese hamster ovary cells to bleomycin. Cancer Res. *36*, 2345–2349 (1976)

Coetzee, M.L., Sartiano, G.P., Klein, K., Ove, P.: Inhibition of bleomycin-induced [^{3}H]thymidine 5′-triphosphate incorporation into liver and hepatoma nuclei by N-ethyl maleimide and daunomycin. J. Antibiot. *30*, 163–171 (1977)

Cohen, S.S., I, J.: Synthesis and the lethality of bleomycin in bacteria. Cancer Res. *36*, 2768–2774 (1976)

Cox, R., Daoud, A.H., Irving, C.C.: Damage of rat liver deoxyribonucleic acid by bleomycin. Biochem. Pharmacol. *23*, 3147–3151 (1974)

Crooke, S.T., Bradner, W.T.: Bleomycin, a review. J. Med. *7*, 333–428 (1976)

Desai, L.S., Krishan, A., Foley, G.E.: Effects of bleomycin on cells in culture: A quantitative cytochemical study. Cancer *34*, 1873–1977 (1974)

DiCioccio, R., Srivastava, B.I.S.: Effect of bleomycin on deoxynucleotide-polymerizing enzymes from human cells. Cancer Res. *36*, 1664–1668 (1976)

Drewinko, B., Brown, B.W., Gottlieb, J.A.: The response of synchronized human lymphoma cells to bleomycin and 1,3-bis(2-chloroethyl)-1-nitrosourea. Cancer Res. *33*, 2732–2336 (1973)

Elkind, M.M., Sutton, H.: Radiation response of mammalian cells grown in culture. Radiat. Res. *13*, 556–593 (1960)

Espejo, R.T., Canelo, E.S.: Properties of bacteriophage PM2: A lipid containing bacterial virus. Virology *34*, 738–747 (1968)

Fernández-Gómez, M.E., De La Torre, C.: Action of bleomycin on proliferating plant cells. J. Antibiot. *29*, 1096–1101 (1976)

Fujii, A., Takita, T., Shimada, M., Umezawa, H.: Biosyntheses of new bleomycins. J. Antibiot. *27*, 73–77 (1974)

Fujimoto, J.: Radioautographic studies on the intracellular distribution of bleomycin-^{14}C in mouse tumor cells. Cancer Res. *34*, 2969–2974 (1974)

Fujimoto, J., Higashi, H., Kosaki, G.: Intracellular distribution of [^{14}C]bleomycin and the cytokinetic effects of bleomycin in the mouse tumor. Cancer Res. *36*, 2248–2253 (1976)

Fujiwara, Y., Kondo, T.: Strand-scission of HeLa cell deoxyribonucleic acid by bleomycin *in vitro* and *in vivo*. Biochem. Pharmacol. *22*, 323–333 (1973)

Hahn, G.M.: Recovery of cells from induced, potentially lethal damge. Cancer Treat. Rep. *60*, 1791–1798 (1976)

Haidle, C.W.: Fragmentation of deoxyribonucleic acid by bleomycin. Mol. Pharmacol. *7*, 645–652 (1971)

Haidle, C.W., Bearden, J., Jr.: Effect of bleomycin on an RNA-DNA hybrid. Biochem. Biophys. Res. Commun. *65*, 815–821 (1975)

Haidle, C.W., Kuo, M.T., Weiss, K.K.: Nucleic acid-specificity of bleomycin. Biochem. Pharmacol. *21*, 3308–3312 (1972a)

Haidle, C.W., Weiss, K.K., Kuo, M.T.: Release of free bases from deoxyribonucleic acid after reaction with bleomycin. Mol. Pharmacol. *8*, 531–537 (1972b)

Haidle, C.W., Weiss, K.K., Mace, M.L., Jr.: Induction of bacteriophage by bleomycin. Biochem. Biophys. Res. Commun. *48*, 1179–1184 (1972c)

Hittelman, W.M., Rao, P.N.: Bleomycin-induced damage in prematurely condensed chromosomes and its relationship to cell cycle progression in CHO cells. Cancer Res. *34*, 3433–3439 (1974)

Ichikawa, T.: Studies of bleomycin: Discovery of its clinical effect, combination treatment with bleomycin and radiotherapy, side effects, and long term survival. In: Gann monograph on cancer research No. 19. Fundamental and clinical studies of bleomycin. Carter, S.K., Ichikawa, T., Mathé, G., Umezawa, H. (eds.), pp. 99–115. Baltimore, London, New York: University Park: 1976

Iqbal, Z.M., Kohn, K.W., Ewig, R.A.G., Fornace, A.J., Jr.: Single-strand scission and repair of DNA in mammalian cells by bleomycin. Cancer Res. *36*, 3834–3838 (1976)

Ishida, R., Takahashi, T.: Increased DNA chain breakage by combined action of bleomycin and superoxide radical. Biochem. Biophys. Res. Commun. *66*, 1432–1438 (1975)

Ishizuka, M., Takayama, H., Takeuchi, T., Umezawa, H.: Activity and toxicity of bleomycin. J. Antibiot. Ser. A *20*, 15–24 (1967)

Kohn, K.W., Ewig, R.A.G.: Effect of pH on the bleomycin-induced DNA single-strand scission in L1210 cells and the relation to cell survival. Cancer Res. *36*, 3839–3841 (1976)

Krishan, A.: Bleomycin-induced fine structural alterations in cultured mouse fibroblasts and human lymphocytes of neoplastic origin. Cancer Res. *33*, 777–785 (1973)

Krueger, W.C., Pschigoda, L.M., Reusser, F.: Interaction of DNA with zorbamycin, phleomycin and bleomycin, Ultraviolet absorption and circular dichroism measurements. J. Antibiot. *26*, 424–428 (1973)

Kunimoto, T., Hori, M., Umezawa, H.: Modes of action of phleomycin, bleomycin, and formycin on HeLa S3 cells in synchronized culture. J. Antibiot. Ser. A *20*, 277–281 (1967)

Kuo, M.T.: Effects of bleomycin on DNA and mammalian chromosomes. Doctoral Dissertation. The University of Texas Health Science Center at Houston, Graduate School of Biomedical Sciences, 1973

Kuo, M.T., Haidle, C.W.: Characterization of chain breakage in DNA induced by bleomycin. Biochim. Biophys. Acta *385*, 109–114 (1973)

Kuo, M.T., Haidle, C.W., Inners, L.D.: Characterization of bleomycin-resistant DNA. Biophys. J. *13*, 1296–1306 (1973)

Kuo, M.T., Auger, L.T., Saunders, G.F., Haidle, C.W.: Effect of bleomycin on the synthesis and function of RNA. Cancer Res. *37*, 1345–1348 (1977)

Lapi, L., Cohen, S.S.: Inhibition of the lethality of bleomycin A_5 in L-cells by hirudonine. Cancer Res. *37*, 1384–1388 (1977)

Lloyd, R.S., Hewitt, R.R., Haidle, C.W.: Bleomycin-induced alkaline-labile damage and direct strand breakage in covalent-circular DNA. Fed. Proc. *36*, 694 (1977)

Lown, J.W., Sim, S.-K.: The mechanism of the bleomycin-induced cleavage of DNA. Biochem. Biophys. Res. Commun. *77*, 1150–1157 (1977)

Matsuzawa, T., Onozawa, M., Morita, K., Kakehi, M.: Radiosensitization of bleomycin on lethal effect of mouse cancer cell *in vitro*. Strahlentherapie *144*, 614–617 (1972)

Mauro, F., Falpo, B., Briganti, G., Elli, R., Zupi, G.: Effects of antineoplastic drugs on plateau-phase cultures of mammalian cells. II. Effects of bleomycin and hydroxyurea. J. Natl. Cancer Inst. *52*, 715–722 (1974)

Miyaki, M., Ono, T.: Mechanism of action of bleomycin. In: Gann monograph on cancer research No. 19. Fundamental and clinical studies of bleomycin. Carter, S.K., Ichikawa, T., Mathé, G., Umezawa, H. (eds.), pp. 37–50. Baltimore, London, New York: University Park 1976

Miyaki, M., Ono, T., Umezawa, H.: Inhibition of ligase reaction by bleomycin. J. Antibiot. *24*, 587–592 (1971)

Miyaki, M., Morohasi, S., Ono, T.: Single strand scission and repair of DNA in bleomycin-sensitive and resistant rat ascites hepatoma cells. J. Antibiot. *26*, 369–373 (1973)

Miyaki, M., Kitayama, T., Ono, T.: Breakage of DNA-membrane complex by bleomycin. J. Antibiot. *27*, 647–655 (1974)

Miyaki, M., Ono, R., Hori, S., Umezawa, H.: Binding of bleomycin to DNA in bleomycin-sensitive and -resistant rat ascites hepatoma cells. Cancer Res. *35*, 2015–2019 (1975)

Müller, W.E.G., Zahn, R.K.: Bleomycin: Mode of action on DNA. In: Gann monograph on cancer research No. 19. Fundamental and clinical studies of bleomycin. Carter, S.K., Ichikawa, T., Mathé, G., Umezawa, H. (eds.), pp. 51–62. Baltimore, London, New York: University Park 1976a

Müller, W.E.G., Zahn, R.K.: Effect of bleomycin on DNA, RNA, protein, chromatin and on cell transformation by oncogenic RNA viruses. Prog. Biochem. Pharmacol. *11*, 28–47 (1976b)

Müller, W.E.G., Zahn, R.K.: Determination of the bleomycin-inactivation enzyme in biopsies. Gann *67*, 425–430 (1976c)

Müller, W.E.G., Zahn, R.K.: Bleomycin, an antibiotic that removes thymine from double-stranded DNA. Prog. Nucl. Acid. Res. Mol. Biol. *40*, 21–57 (1977)

Müller, W.E.G., Yamazaki, Z., Breter, H.-J., Zahn, R.K.: Action of bleomycin on DNA and RNA. Eur. J. Biochem. *31*, 518–525 (1972a)

Müller, W.E.G., Yamazaki, Z., Zahn, R.K.: Bleomycin, a selective inhibitor of DNA dependent DNA polymerase from oncogenic RNA viruses Biochem. Biophys. Res. Commun. *46*, 1667–1673 (1972b)

Müller, W.E.G., Yamazaki, Z., Zöllner, J.E., Zahn, R.K.: Action of bleomycin on programmed synthesis influence on DNA and RNA nucleases. FEBS Lett. *31*, 217–221 (1973)

Müller, W.E.G., Totsuka, A., Nusser, I., Zahn, R.K., Umezawa, H.: Bleomycin inhibition of

DNA synthesis in isolated enzyme systems and in intact cell systems. Biochem. Pharmacol. *24*, 911–915 (1975)
Müller, W.E.G., Rohde, H.J., Steffen, R., Maidhof, A., Zahn, R.K.: Potentiation of the effectiveness of bleomycin by A·T-specific DNA ligands *in vitro* as well as *in vivo*. Cancer Lett. *1*, 127–132 (1976a)
Müller, W.E.G., Rohde, H.J., Zahn, R.K.: Effect of bleomycin on DNA, RNA, enzymes, chromatin and on local sarcoma. J. Mol. Med. *1*, 173–186 (1976b)
Murakami, H., Mori, H., Taira, S.: Active centre model on the structure and function of the bleomycin molecule as the prototype of esteratic enzymes. J. Theor. Biol. *42*, 443–460 (1973)
Murakami, H., Mori, H., Taira, S.: On the molecular embrace of bleomycin with helical DNA. J. Theor. Biol. *59*, 1–23 (1976)
Nagai, K., Suzuki, H., Tanaka, N., Umezawa, H.: Decrease of melting temperature and single-strand scission of DNA by bleomycin in the presence of 2-mercaptoethanol. J. Antibiot. *22*, 569–573 (1969a)
Nagai, K., Yamaki, H., Suzuki, H., Tanaka, N., Umezawa, H.: The combined effects of bleomycin and sulfhydryl compounds on the thermal denaturation of DNA. Biochim. Biophys. Acta *179*, 165–171 (1969b)
Nagatsu, M., Richert, R.M., Lambert, A.: Effects of bleomycin on the cell cycle of Ehrlich ascites carcinoma. Cancer Res. *32*, 1966–1970 (1972)
Nunn, A.D.: Interactions between bleomycins and metals. J. Antibiot. *29*, 1102–1108 (1976)
Ogawa, K., Onoé, T.: Nuclear changes produced by bleomycin in the 3-methyl-cholanthrene-induced mouse epidermal carcinoma cells. Gann *60*, 503–507 (1969)
Ohama, K., Kadotani, T.: Cytologic effects of bleomycin on cultured human leucocytes. Jpn. J. Human Genet. *14*, 293–297 (1970)
Onishi, T., Shimada, K., Takagi, Y.: Effects of bleomycin on *Escherichia coli* strains with various sensitivities to radiations. Biochim. Biophys. Acta *312*, 248–258 (1973)
Onishi, T., Iwata, H., Takagi, Y.: Effects of reducing and oxidizing agents on the action of bleomycin. J. Biochem. *77*, 745–752 (1975)
Osieka, R., Madreiter, H., Schmidt, C.G.: The effect of bleomycin on mitochondrial DNA. Z. Krebsforsch. *88*, 11–15 (1976)
Paika, K.D., Krishan, A.: Bleomycin-induced chromosomal aberrations in cultured mammalian cells. Cancer Res. *33*, 961–965 (1973)
Perry, P., Evans, H.J.: Cytological detection of mutagen-carcinogen exposure by sister chromatid exchange. Nature (London) *258*, 121–125 (1975)
Phillips, R.A., Tolmach, L.J.: Repair of potentially lethal damage in X-irradiated HeLa cells. Radiat. Res. *29*, 413–432 (1966)
Promchainant, C.: Cytogenetic effect of bleomycin on human leukocytes *in vitro*. Mutat. Res. *28*, 107–112 (1975)
Ray, G.R., Hahn, G.M., Bagshaw, M.A., Kurkjian, S.: Cell survival and repair of plateau-phase cultures after chemotherapy – relevance to tumor therapy and to the in vitro screening of new agents. Cancer Chemother. Rep. Part 1 *57*, 473–475 (1973)
Reddy, S.B., Linden, W.A., Zywietz, F., Baish, H., Struck, U.: Effects of acronycine, bleomycin and cytosine arabinoside on the cell cycle. Arzneimittelforschung/Drug Res. *27*, 1549–1553 (1977)
Ross, S.L., Moses, R.E.: Effect of bleomycin on deoxyribonucleic acid synthesis in toluene-treated *Escherichia coli* cells. Antimicrob. Agents Chemother. *9*, 239–246 (1976)
Saito, M., Andoh, T.: Breakage of a DNA-protein complex induced by bleomycin and their repair in cultured mouse fibroblasts. Cancer Res. *33*, 1696–1700 (1973)
Sartiano, G.P., Winklestein, A., Lynch, W.E., Boggs, S.S.: Effects of bleomycin on PHA-stimulated lymphocytes and isolated hepatic nuclei. J. Antibiot. *26*, 437–443 (1973)
Sartiano, G.P., Lynch, W., Boggs, S.S., Neil, G.L.: The demonstration of separate DNA polymerase activities in intact isolated rat liver nuclei by means of response to bleomycin and arabinosyl cytosine 5′-triphosphate. Proc. Soc. Exp. Biol. Med. *150*, 718–722 (1975)
Sartiano, G.P., Coetzee, M.L., Klein, K., Ove, P.: Effect of camptothecin and adriamycin on bleomycin-induced tritiated thymidine triphosphate incorporation in a rat nuclear system. J. Natl. Cancer Inst. *58*, 1357–1364 (1977)

Saunders, P.P., Schultz, G.A.: Mechanism of action of bleomycin-I Bacterial growth studies. Biochem. Pharmacol. *21*, 1657–1666 (1972)
Sausville, E.A., Peisach, J., Horwitz, S.B.: A role for ferrous ion and oxygen in the degradation of DNA by bleomycin. Biochem. Biophys. Res. Commun. *73*, 814–822 (1976)
Shirakawa, I., Azegami, M., Ishii, S.-I., Umezawa, H.: Reaction of bleomycin with DNA strand scission of DNA in the absence of sulfhydryl or peroxide compounds. J. Antibiot. *24*, 761–766 (1971)
Shishido, K.: Differential inhibition of transcriptions catalyzed by T7-specific and *Escherichia coli* RNA polymerases by bleomycin. J. Antibiot. *26*, 501–505 (1973)
Spangler, M., Sartiano, G.P., Coetzee, M.L., Ove, P.: Effect of bleomycin on [^{3}H]thymidine 5′-triphosphate incorporation into host liver and hepatoma nuclei. Cancer Res. *36*, 1339–1346 (1976)
Suzuki, H., Nagai, K., Yamaki, H., Tanaka, N., Umezawa, H.: Mechanism of action of bleomycin. Studies with the growing culture of bacterial and tumor cells. J. Antibiot. *21*, 379–386 (1968)
Suzuki, H., Nagai, K., Yamaki, H., Tanaka, N., Umezawa, H.: On the mechanism of action of bleomycin: Scission of DNA strands *in vitro* and *in vivo*. J. Antibiot. *22*, 446–448 (1969)
Suzuki, H., Nagai, K., Akutsu, E., Yamaki, H., Tanaka, N., Umezawa, H.: On the mechanism of action of bleomycin strand scission of DNA caused by bleomycin and its binding to DNA *in vitro*. J. Antibiot. *23*, 473–480 (1970)
Takeshita, M., Horwitz, S.B., Grollman, A.P.: Bleomycin, an inhibitor of vaccinia virus replication. Virology *60*, 455–465 (1974)
Takeshita, M., Grollman, A.P., Horwitz, S.B.: Effect of ATP and other nucleotides on the bleomycin-induced degradation of vaccinia virus DNA. Virology *69*, 453–463 (1976)
Takita, T., Muraoka, Y., Fujii, A., Itoh, H., Maeda, K., Umezawa, H.: The structure of the sulfur-containing chromophore of phleomycin, and the chemical transformation of phleomycin to bleomycin. J. Antibiot. *25*, 197–199 (1972a)
Takita, T., Muraoka, Y., Yoshioka, T., Fujii, A., Maeda, K., Umezawa, H.: The chemistry of bleomycin. IX. The structures of bleomycin and phleomycin. J. Antibiot. *25*, 755–758 (1972b)
Takita, T., Fujii, A., Fukuoka, T., Umezawa, H.: Chemical cleavage of bleomycin to bleomycinic acid and synthesis of new bleomycins. J. Antibiot. *26*, 252–254 (1973)
Tamura, H., Sugiyama, Y., Sugahara, T.: Effect of bleomycin on the chromosomes of human lymphocytes at various cell phases. Gann *65*, 103–107 (1974)
Tanaka, N.: Inhibition of transcription by pluramycin and bleomycin. J. Antibiot. *23*, 523–530 (1970)
Terasima, T., Umezawa, H.: Lethal effect of bleomycin on cultured mammalian cells. J. Antibiot. *23*, 300–304 (1970)
Terasima, T., Takabe, Y., Katsumata, T., Watanabe, M., Umezawa, H.: Effect of bleomycin on mammalian cell survival. J. Natl. Cancer Inst. *49*, 1093–1100 (1972)
Terasima, T., Watanabe, M., Takabe, Y., Miyamoto, T.: Action of bleomycin on proliferative capacity of mammalian cells. In: Gann monograph on cancer research No. 19. Fundamental and clinical studies of bleomycin. Carter, S.K., Ichikawa, T., Mathé, G., Umezawa, H. (eds.), pp. 63–81. Baltimore, London, New York: University Park 1976
Tobey, R.A.: Arrest of Chinese hamster cells in G_2 following treatments with the anti-tumor drug bleomycin. J. Cell. Physiol. *79*, 259–266 (1972a)
Tobey, R.A.: A simple, rapid technique for determination of the effects of chemotherapeutic agents on mammalian cell-cycle traverse. Cancer Res. *32*, 309–316 (1972b)
Totsuka, A., Müller, W.E.G., Zahn, R.K.: Bleomycin: Action on growth of oncogenic RNA viruses and on cell transformation. Arch. Virol. *48*, 169–179 (1975)
Twentyman, P.R.: Comparative chemosensitivity of exponential- versus pleateu-phase cells in both *in vitro* and *in vivo* model systems. Cancer Treat. Rep. *60*, 1719–1722 (1976a)
Twentyman, P.R.: The effect of bleomycin and pentamycin in combination on the survival of EMT6 mouse tumor cells *in vitro* and *in vivo*. Br. J. Cancer *33*, 459–464 (1976b)
Twentyman, P.R., Bleehen, N.M.: The sensitivity of cells in exponential and stationary phases of growth to bleomycin and to 1,3-bis(2-chloroethyl)-1-nitrosurea. Br. J. Cancer *28*, 500–507 (1973)
Twentyman, P.R., Bleehen, N.M.: Changes in sensitivity to radiation and to bleomycin occurring during the life history of monolayer cultures of a mouse tumor cell line. Br. J. Cancer *31*, 68–74 (1975a)

Twentyman, P.R., Bleehen, N.H.: Studies of "potentially lethal damage" in EMT6 mouse tumor cells treated with bleomycin either *in vitro* or *in vivo*. Br. J. Cancer *32*, 491–501 (1975b)

Umezawa, H.: Bleomycin. In: Antibiotics. Mechanism of action of antimicrobial and antitumor agents. Corcoran, J.W., Hahn, F.E. (eds.), Vol. III, pp. 21–33. Berlin, Heidelberg, New York: Springer 1975

Umezawa, H.: Bleomycin: Discovery, chemistry, and action. In: Gann monograph on cancer research No. 19. Fundamental and clinical studies of bleomycin. Carter, S.K., Ichikawa, T., Mathé, G., Umezawa, H. (eds.), pp. 3–36. Baltimore, London, New York: University Park 1976

Umezawa, H., Maeda, K., Takeuchi, T., Okami, Y.: New antibiotics, bleomycin A and B. J. Antibiot. Ser. A *19*, 200–209 (1966a)

Umezawa, H., Suhara, Y., Takita, T., Maeda, K.: Purification of bleomycins. J. Antibiot. Ser. A *19*, 210–215 (1966b)

Umezawa, H., Ishizuka, M., Maeda, K., Takeuchi, T.: Studies on bleomycin. Cancer *20*, 891–895 (1967)

Umezawa, H., Ishizuka, M., Hori, S., Chimura, H., Takeuchi, T.: The distribution of ^{3}H-bleomycin in mouse tissue. J. Antibiot. *21*, 638–642 (1968a)

Umezawa, H., Ishizuka, M., Kimura, K., Iwanaga, J., Takeuchi, T.: Biological studies on individual bleomycin. J. Antibiot. *21*, 592–602 (1968b)

Umezawa, H., Asakura, H., Oda, K., Hori, S., Hori, M.: The effect of bleomycin on SV40 DNA: Characteristics of bleomycin action which produces a single scission in a superhelical form of SV40 DNA. J. Antibiot. *26*, 521–527 (1973)

Watanabe, M., Takabe, Y., Katsumata, T., Terasima, T., Umezawa, H.: Response in macromolecular syntheses of mouse L cells to bleomycin, with special reference to cell-antibiotic interaction. J. Antibiot. *26*, 417–423 (1973)

Watanabe, M., Takabe, Y., Katsumata, T., Terasima, T.: Effects of bleomycin on progression through the cell cycle of mouse L-cells. Cancer Res. *34*, 878–881 (1974)

Wheatley, D.N., Muller, G.C., Kajiwara, K.: Anti-mitotic activity of bleomycin: Time of action in the mammalian cell cycle. Br. J. Cancer *29*, 117–131 (1974)

Yamaki, H., Suzuki, H., Nagai, K., Tanaka, N., Umezawa, H.: Effects of bleomycin A_2 on deoxyribonuclease, DNA polymerase and ligase reactions. J. Antibiot. *24*, 178–184 (1971)

Diphtheria Toxin and Exotoxin A from *Pseudomonas aeruginosa*

R.J. COLLIER

I. Introduction

A marked resurgence of interest in bacterial protein toxins has occurred in recent years, after a long period of relative neglect. Many of the classical toxins have been studied in greater depth, and new toxins have been discovered as well. As a result of the expanded interest and efforts there now exists a substantial and rapidly growing body of knowledge about the structures and activities of bacterial toxins from which one can begin to make meaningful generalizations.

One of the most intriguing generalizations to have emerged from the recent studies is the existence of unexpected biochemical unity in the modes of action of certain toxins. Until recently the available evidence (largely in the form of data on immunologic cross-reactivity and gross chemical and physical properties) left one with the impression that toxic proteins produced by unrelated or distantly related bacteria would prove to have independent origins. However, this view has been altered by studies on the actions of diphtheria toxin, exotoxin A from *Pseudomonas aeruginosa,* and cholera toxin. All three of these toxins have been shown to act by nicotinamide adenine dinucleotide (NAD) dependent reactions. Furthermore, diphtheria toxin and exotoxin A inactivate the same intracellular target protein by precisely the same NAD-dependent mechanism. Cholera toxin modifies the activity of a different intracellular target, but the biochemical mechanism of the modification is almost certainly similar to that of the diphtheria and *Pseudomonas* exotoxins. The evidence at hand suggests that these toxins, or at least certain domains or subunits thereof, have been derived from a common ancestral protein of unknown identity. Although it is unlikely that all of the major bacterial protein toxins will prove to share this biochemical activity, other toxins may well be found to have similar NAD-dependent mechanisms.

Below is reviewed the current knowledge of diphtheria toxin and exotoxin A from *Pseudomonas aeruginosa.* Several reviews on diphtheria toxin have been published in recent years, and readers are urged to consult these for more detailed discussions (GILL et al., 1973; PAPPENHEIMER and GILL, 1973; DIRKX, 1974; COLLIER, 1975, 1976; BIZZINI and TURPIN, 1976; MURPHY, 1976; PAPPENHEIMER, 1977). Other publications are cited as a guide to those who wish to obtain further information on the structure and activity of cholera toxin (FINKELSTEIN, 1973, 1976; GILL, 1977; MOSS and VAUGHAN, 1977).

II. Diphtheria Toxin

A. Diphtheria and Diphtheria Toxin

Diphtheria is one of the relatively few bacterial diseases in which the major symptoms are attributable to the action of a single, secreted toxin. In most cases of clinical diphtheria the causative organism, *Corynebacterium diphtheriae,* remains confined to the upper respiratory tract, where it proliferates on epithelial surfaces, and forms a leathery "pseudomembrane," composed of bacteria, necrotic cells, and fibrous exudate. In severe or lethal cases of the disease, however, one finds evidence of extensive tissue damage in diverse organs throughout the body. That such damage is produced by the action of a toxic substance secreted by the diphtheria bacillus in culture was demonstrated in the late 1800's. Subsequently it was found that immunization against the toxin protected against the disease, and widespread application of immunization against formalin-treated toxin (toxoid) has relegated clinical diphtheria to the status of a virtually unknown disease in many countries.

B. Structure of the Toxin

Diphtheria toxin is an acidic, globular protein (molecular weight 60,000–63,000; isoelectric point 4.1) which is excreted in the form of a single polypeptide chain (COLLIER, 1975). Under suitable conditions the toxin may be isolated in high yield from the culture fluids of toxinogenic *Corynebacterium diphtheriae* grown either in shake or still culture. The protein has been purified and crystallized in several laboratories, and the amino acid composition has been reported for several preparations. No unusual amino acids or nonprotein moieties have been found.

An interesting feature of the toxin, which is related to its toxic and enzymic activities, is its mode of scission by proteases specific for basic amino acids (DRAZIN et al., 1971; GILL and DINIUS, 1971). Low concentrations of trypsin, for example, cleave the intact 60,000 dalton toxin preferentially within a narrow region of the molecule, creating an amino terminal peptide representing about one third of the molecule (fragment A; molecular weight 21,145) and a carboxyl terminal peptide (fragment B; molecular weight about 39,000–40,000) representing about two thirds (Fig. 1). As detailed below, fragment A contains the enzymically active region of the molecule, whereas the B fragment seems to function in attachment and entry of the toxin into cells. If the tryptic cleavage is carried out in the absence of thiols or other reducing agents, the A and B fragments remain linked by a single disulfide bridge; this form has been termed "nicked toxin." A second disulfide bridge is contained within the carboxyl-terminal 17,0000 daltons of the B fragment. Neither fragment contains free sulfhydryl groups in the whole, unreduced toxin molecule.

Nicking of a small percentage of toxin almost always occurs during isolation or purification, through the action of bacterial proteases. Thus most preparations

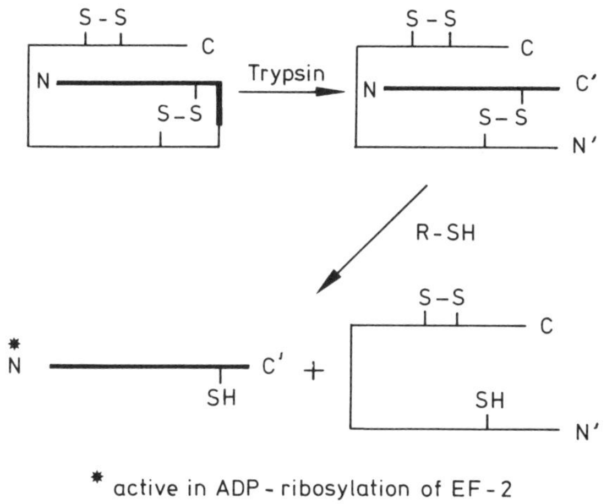

Fig. 1. Limited tryptic cleavage and reduction of diphtheria toxin

contain both nicked and intact forms of the toxin. Even after several steps of purification of the toxin, traces of proteases are present which cause increased nicking over long periods of storage. This may be minimized by addition of inhibitors of serine proteases and by storage at very low temperatures. Resolution of the nicked and intact forms of toxin has not been possible except after reduction and dissociation of the A and B fragments of the nicked form. Refolding of the reduced, intact toxin, which has been denatured with sodium dodecyl sulfate (SDS), into a toxic form has been observed recently after removal of the denaturant (EVERSE et al., 1977).

Treatment of nicked toxin with reducing agents, such as dithiothreitol, causes a relatively rapid reduction of the disulfide bridge linking the A and B fragments (COLLIER and KANDEL, 1971) and a slower reduction of the disulfide bridge which is internal within B. Dissociation of the A and B fragments can occur following reduction of the disulfide bridge linking them, but often the dissociation is incomplete, with a substantial fraction of the fragments remaining associated by noncovalent forces. Toxicity is lost upon dissociation of the A and B fragments, but the undissociated, reduced form retains high and perhaps full toxicity.

The A and B fragments released on dissociation of the reduced toxin differ markedly from one another in several properties. One notable difference is in stability. The A fragment remains in solution and retains almost full enzymic activity even after exposure to a pH of 2 or 12 at room temperature, or to 100° C at neutral pH. The fragment denatured with sodium dodecyl sulfate also folds back into an active form after removal of the detergent. In contrast, the B fragment rapidly precipitates from solution in most buffers even at 4° C. Recently it has been reported that the B fragment may be stabilized in solution with borate buffer (ZANEN et al., 1976) and that S-carboxymethylated fragment B remains soluble in tris(hydroxymethyl)amino methane buffer (BURGOYNE et al.,

```
                         10                                         20
H2N-Gly-Ala-Asp-Asp-Val-Val-Asp-Ser-Ser-Lys-Ser-Phe-Val-Met-Glu-Asn-Phe-Ser-Ser-Tyr-His-Gly-Thr-Lys-Pro-

                 30                                         40                                         50
Gly-Tyr-Val-Asp-Ser-Ile-Gln-Lys-Gly-Ile-Gln-Lys-Pro-Lys-Ser-Gly-Thr-Gln-Gly-Asn-Tyr-Asp-Asp-Asp-Trp-

                                    60                                         70
Lys-Gly-Phe-Tyr-Ser-Thr-Asp-Asn-Lys-Tyr-Asp-Ala-Ala-Gly-Tyr-Ser-Val-Asp-Asn-Glu-Asn-Pro-Leu-Ser-Gly-

                 80                                         90                                         100
Lys-Ala-Gly-Gly-Val-Val-Lys-Val-Thr-Tyr-Pro-Gly-Leu-Thr-Lys-Val-Leu-Ala-Leu-Lys-Val-Asp-Asn-Ala-Glu-

                                    110                                        120
Thr-Ile-Lys-Lys-Glu-Leu-Gly-Leu-Ser-Leu-Thr-Glu-Pro-Leu-Met-Glu-Gln-Val-Gly-Thr-Glu-Glu-Phe-Ile-Lys-

                 130                                        140                                        150
Arg-Phe-Gly-Asp-Gly-Ala-Ser-Arg-Val-Val-Leu-Ser-Leu-Pro-Phe-Ala-Glu-Gly-Ser-Ser-Val-Glu-Ser-Tyr-Ile-

                                    160                                        170
Asn-Asn-Trp-Glu-Gln-Ala-Lys-Ala-Leu-Ser-Val-Glu-Leu-Glu-Ile-Asn-Phe-Glu-Thr-Arg-Gly-Lys-Arg-Gly-Gln-

                 180                                        190       193
Asp-Ala-Met-Tyr-Glu-Tyr-Met-Ala-Gln-Ala-Cys-Ala-Gly-Asn-Arg-Val-Arg-Arg-COOH
```

Fig. 2. Amino acid sequence of fragment A from diphtheria toxin

1976). These findings open up new avenues of approach to the study of the activity of the B fragment.

Because of its inherent stability and its enzymic activity the A fragment has been studied in greater detail than fragment B. The complete primary structure of the A fragment (DeLange et al., 1976) is shown in Fig. 2. The sequence at the amino terminus is identical to that of whole diphtheria toxin. It was determined that heterogeneity existed at the carboxyl terminus. Three major forms of the fragment were found (190, 191, and 193 residues), which were apparently generated by attack of trypsin at any of the three basic residues within the sequence Arg-Val-Arg-Arg. The single half cystine residue of fragment A is located at position 186, only 7 residues from the terminal arginine of the longest form of the fragment. The half cystine in fragment B, which participates in the disulfide bridge to A, is known to be near the amino terminus of B, and it has been reported recently that the A-B disulfide bridge subtends a loop of only 14 residues (Pappenheimer, 1977). The trypsin-sensitive region therefore consists of a series of arginine residues contained within a short disulfide loop presumably exposed at the surface of whole toxin. Such a cluster of trypsin-sensitive residues suggests that this region may have evolved as a cleavage site.

The three major forms of fragment A may be resolved either by electrophoresis on polyacrylamide gels under nondenaturing conditions or by isoelectric focusing (Kandel et al., 1974). All three are enzymically active. Their isoelectric points are 4.56, 4.72, and 4.85.

Other interesting features of fragment A are that it contains only a single histidine residue (position 21) and two tryptophans (positions 50 and 153). Evidence has been reported suggesting that tryptophan 153 is necessary for enzymic activity and is possibly involved in NAD binding (KANDEL et al., 1974; MICHEL and DIRKX, 1977). Modification of a single tyrosine residue by treatment with tetranitromethane is also known to inactivate fragment A (BEUGNIER and ZANEN, 1977). It is noteworthy that all seven arginine residues in fragment A are present in the region from residues 126 to 193 and that only one aromatic residue is contained in the region between residues 66 and 122, despite an average of 13% of aromatic residues in the remainder of the molecule.

The structure of fragment B is less well characterized, but is being actively studied in the laboratory of DIRKX and co-workers in Belgium. Evidence for the presence of a hydrophobic domain near the amino terminus of B will be discussed below.

GOOR (1968) originally reported the existence of a dimer of whole diphtheria toxin present in some preparations of toxin. This molecule, which has a sedimentation coefficient of about 6.8, as contrasted with 4.2 for monomeric toxin, seems to be formed upon precipitation of toxin with ammonium sulfate (RELYVELD, 1970). There is also evidence for higher order aggregates of toxin in some preparations (ROBB, 1966; BERNARD and COLLIER, unpublished data), but the conditions under which these are formed have not been defined.

C. Toxic and Enzymic Properties

The toxin is lethal for a wide variety of animals, including guinea pigs, rabbits, monkeys, and man, at doses of about 100 ng per kg body weight (administered subcutaneously). With such doses death occurs only after 3–4 days. Although the period before death is shortened with higher doses, there is always a lag of about 10 h even with massive doses of toxin. Rats and mice are notably resistant to the toxin, requiring doses several orders of magnitude greater, per unit body weight, for a comparable effect.

The toxin shows little tissue specificity either in vivo or in vitro. Lesions comparable to those seen in clinical diphtheria are observed in a variety of internal organs in animals injected with the toxin, and cultured cells from a variety of organs are found to be sensitive to the toxin. Cultured cells from rats or mice exhibit insensitivity to toxin comparable to that of the parental animals (GABLIKS and SOLOTOROVSKY, 1962).

STRAUSS and HENDEE reported in 1959 a striking effect of diphtheria toxin on protein synthesis in HeLa cells. Using ^{35}S-methionine to measure incorporation of amino acids into protein, they observed that protein synthesis ceased in toxin-treated cells after a lag of at least 1 h, during which time synthesis proceeded normally. The duration of the lag was greater with lower concentrations of toxin.

Experiments by STRAUSS and HENDEE (1959) and other workers supported the hypothesis that the toxin might be affecting protein synthesis directly. For example, glycolysis, respiration, and the concentrations of ATP and GTP were found to be unaffected until long after protein synthesis had ceased in toxin-treated cells (STRAUSS and HENDEE 1959; COLLIER and PAPPENHEIMER, 1964a). Also, there appeared to be no early effect on plasma membrane permeability, as measured by transport of potassium ions (Kato and Pappenheimer, 1960), leakage of phosphorus containing compounds (Strauss, 1960) or amino acid transport (Moehring et al., 1967).

Subsequent studies in cell-free systems confirmed that the toxin did indeed act directly on protein synthesis, and furthermore that there was a requirement of a low molecular weight cellular component for the effect (Collier and Pappenheimer, 1965b). Early experiments revealed that amino acid incorporation was strongly inhibited by the toxin in cell-free systems in which the low molecular weight cellular components remained, but their removal by dialysis or gel filtration rendered the system completely insensitive to toxin. It was then found that dialyzed systems became sensitive to toxin if nicotinamide adenine dinucleotide (NAD) was added and that treatment of an undialyzed system with NADase rendered it insensitive. Later work showed that the oxidized form of NAD was specifically required for the inhibition of protein synthesis (Goor and Pappenheimer, 1967).

The intracellular target of the toxin in the presence of NAD was determined by fractionation of cell-free extracts from rabbit reticulocytes (Collier, 1967). Elongation factor II (EF II) was the only component of the system found to be inactivated by the toxin. EF II is a protein of molecular weight about 100,000, which is required for the translocation step of polypeptide chain elongation on ribosomes. Elongation factor I, which promotes binding of substrate aminoacyl-tRNA to ribosomes is not affected by the toxin. Also, EF-G, the functionally analogous protein in prokaryotic cells is not inactivated by the toxin (Johnson et al., 1968; Richter and Lipmann, 1970).

The mechanism of inactivation of EF II was elucidated largely by the work of Honjo et al. (1968, 1971). They incubated toxin with partially purified EF II in the presence of various preparations of radioactive NAD labeled in different parts of the molecule. Label from the adenosine, phosphate, or ribose moieties of NAD was incorporated into acid-insoluble material, whereas label from the nicotinamide moiety was released free into solution. The protein-bound label was localized to EF II and was found to be stable to brief exposure to 0.1 N HCl or 0.1 N NaOH. These results strongly suggested that the toxin promoted transfer of the adenosine diphosphate ribose moiety (ADP-ribose) of NAD into covalent linkage with EF II, with the release of nicotinamide and a proton (Fig. 3).

This reaction has now been thoroughly characterized, and there is no longer doubt that it is responsible for the inactivation of EF II. The equilibrium of the reaction is far to the right under physiologic conditions, but the reaction may be reversed by lowering the pH to about 5 and adding a high concentration of nicotinamide (0.1 M). Under these conditions EF II, active in protein synthesis, is regenerated, and the attached ADP-ribose moiety may be recovered as free NAD.

The nature of the side chain on EF II to which the ADP-ribose is attached remains uncertain. Robinson et al. (1974) have isolated a 15 residue tryptic peptide containing the attachment site and have determined the sequence to be Phe-Asp-Val-His-Asp-Val-Thr-Leu-His-Ala-Asp-Ala-Ile-X-Arg. The ADP-ribose group is attached to the residue designated X. This residue, present in

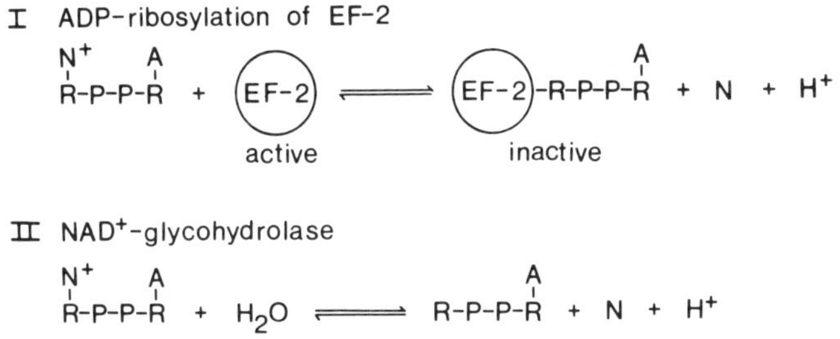

Fig. 3. Enzymic reactions associated with diphtheria toxin

a single copy per EF II molecule (even in EF II which has not yet been exposed to toxin), is weakly basic and does not correspond to any amino acid commonly occurring in proteins. Presumably, it results from post-translational modification of EF II.

EF II from all eukaryotic organisms tested, including rats and mice, yeast, and plants, acts as substrate of the ADP-ribosylation reaction, but EF-G from *E. coli* does not. No other protein substrate for the reaction has been found. Although small amounts of ADP-ribose can become attached to various proteins, including serum albumin (or even the toxin itself) upon prolonged incubation with the toxin (GILL and STEINHAUS, 1974), it seems probable, as suggested by PAPPENHEIMER (1977), that this is due to Schiff base formation of the protein with ADP-ribose liberated from NAD by the NAD glycohydrolase activity of the toxin described below.

Specificity with respect to the pyridine nucleotide substrate is also high. Reduced NAD and oxidized or reduced NADP are inactive as substrates. The NAD analogs thionicotinamide-AD, acetylpyridine-AD, and deamino-NAD show significant activity as substrates, although the latter two have K_M values about ten times higher than that for NAD.

The pH optimum of ADP-ribose transfer is 8.2 to 8.5. No requirements for specific ions have been well documented. The reaction is inhibited by high ionic strength, with inhibition of 25% to 40% reported for 30 mM NaCl. A stimulation of the reaction by thiols is observed under certain conditions, and this has been traced to a requirement for reduction of a disulfide bridge within the toxin for manifestation of ADP-ribosylation activity (COLLIER and KANDEL, 1971).

Adenine is a potent inhibitor of the reaction, but its K_i of about 30–40 μM is well above the K_M for NAD (5–10 μM) (KANDEL et al., 1974). Adenosine is tenfold less effective as an inhibitor, and AMP, ADP, ATP, and ADP-ribose are at least 100-fold less effective than adenine. Nicotinamide is a weak inhibitor of the reaction with K_i about 200 μM.

D. Fragment A and Enzymic Activity

The discovery of free fragment A in crude preparations of toxin prompted studies which led to the conclusion that whole toxin is in fact a proenzyme with respect to the ADP-ribosylation of EF II. Whole toxin, in either the intact or nicked form, appears to be inactive in this reaction, although both forms are toxic for animals or cultured cells. ADP-ribosylation activity is expressed only after reduction of the nicked form of the toxin, which releases fragment A, the active moiety in this reaction (DRAZIN et al., 1971; GILL and PAPPENHEIMER, 1971).

The properties of fragment A as an enzyme have been studied in some detail (KANDEL et al., 1974; CHUNG and COLLIER, 1977b). Work on the interaction of the fragment with NAD has been particularly fruitful. Early studies revealed that in the absence of EF II, fragment A catalyzed hydrolysis of NAD at a very low rate (Fig. 3), yielding ADP-ribose, nicotinamide, and a proton as products (KANDEL et al., 1974). Demonstration that all three electrophoretic forms of fragment A have this NAD glycohydrolase activity (EC 3.2.2.5) ruled out the possibility that the activity was due to contaminating traces of an unrelated NAD glycohydrolase. This reaction, because of its low rate, almost certainly does not contribute to toxicity. However, its existence implies a direct binding of NAD to fragment A and hence supports models of the reaction involving such a direct interaction.

Studies of NAD binding to fragment A by optical and dialysis methods have extended our knowledge of this interaction (KANDEL et al., 1974). The fragment has been found to contain a single, highly specific site for NAD, with a K_D of 8.3 μM. The bound NAD quenches tryptophan fluorescence dramatically (75%) and induces a weak broad band of absorbance with λ_{max} about 360 nm. Both optical effects may possibly be explained by the formation of a charge transfer complex involving the charged nicotinamide ring of NAD. This is supported by the finding that nicotinamide mononucleotide or N-methyl nicotinamide can induce similar optical changes in fragment A. Studies with various competitive inhibitors of NAD binding indicate that both the adenine and nicotinamide moieties of the dinucleotide contribute to binding, and that there is little contribution from the ribose or phosphate moieties.

Attempts to demonstrate interaction of fragment A with EF II in the absence of NAD have been unsuccessful (CHUNG and COLLIER, 1977b). EF II was unretarded when chromatographed on a fragment A-Sepharose affinity column, and no binding of the free fragment and EF II could be detected by equilibrium gel permeation.

On the basis of these results and studies on the kinetics of the ADP-ribosylation reaction CHUNG and COLLIER (1977b) recently proposed an ordered, sequential mechanism for the reaction, in which the sequence of binding of substrates is NAD, followed by EF II. This model assumes the existence of a ternary, noncovalent intermediate containing fragment A, EF II, and NAD. The existence of such an intermediate is further supported by the fact that attempts to detect an ADP-ribosyl-fragment A covalent intermediate have yielded uniformly negative results (KANDEL et al., 1974).

E. Fragment B and the Mechanism of Attachment and Entry

Free fragment A is essentially devoid of both toxicity for animals and capacity to inhibit protein synthesis in cultured cells, thus implying an essential role of the B fragment of the toxin in toxicity. Other experiments with nontoxic forms of the toxin obtained either by mutation of the tox gene or by chemical modification of whole toxin, have implied a role for the B moiety in attachment and entry into susceptible cells (PAPPENHEIMER and GILL, 1973; UCHIDA et al., 1972).

The structural gene for diphtheria toxin resides on the genome of corynephage β and certain other temperate corynephages, and nontoxic cross-reactive forms of the toxin have been obtained by mutagenizing such phage. One such form, CRM 197, has been particularly useful in studying the role of fragment B. CRM 197, which contains an enzymically inactive A moiety, but a fully functional B, has the interesting property of competitively inhibiting the activity of diphtheria toxin on whole cells (UCHIDA et al., 1972). Inasmuch as this protein does not inhibit the ADP-ribosylation of EF II catalyzed by fragment A in cell extracts, it has been proposed that CRM 197 acts on whole cells by blocking specific attachment of toxin to sites on the cell surface. Although the putative attachment sites have not yet been isolated or identified, the existence of specific receptors for the toxin still seems to be the most plausible explanation of the results obtained with CRM 197. The resistence of mouse and rat cells to diphtheria toxin may well be explained by the absence of specific receptors.

ZANEN et al. (1976), and BEUGNIER and ZANEN (1977) have reported that treatment of toxin with tetranitromethane produces concomitant loss of both enzymic activity and toxicity. This results from the nitration of a tyrosine residue of the fragment A moiety and produces modified toxin which, when completely detoxified (by reaction of at least 5 tyrosines per molecule) is a good antagonist for the action of toxin on HeLa cells.

Finally, it has also been reported that fragment B maintained in solution with borate buffer, can block the action of toxin in HeLa cells (ZANEN et al., 1976). The dissociation constant calculated in these experiments was approximately the same as reported for CRM 197, that is, about 1×10^{-8} M.

Assuming that the fragment B moiety of toxin binds whole toxin to specific cell surface receptors, one is next confronted with the question of the mechanism by which the protein penetrates into cells. (This aspect of the action of diphtheria toxin has been reviewed recently by PAPPENHEIMER, 1977.) Direct measurement of the attachment and entry of labeled toxin into cells has been plagued by difficulties arising from a high background of nonspecific binding to cells. BOQUET and PAPPENHEIMER (1976) have attempted to eliminate nonspecifically bound toxin by extensive washing with medium containing antitoxin, while BONVENTRE et al. (1975) employed trypsin treatment for the same purpose. After such treatments it is possible to measure the kinetics of appearance of cell-protected toxin; this represents, presumably, the sum of toxin taken up by pinocytosis of the fluid phase plus that protected by other means, such as perhaps binding to surface receptors. By making appropriate corrections for uptake of toxin in the fluid phase of pinocytotic vesicles, BOQUET and PAPPENHEIMER (1976) were able to estimate that about 4200 molecules of "specifically bound" iodinated toxin became protected from washing with antitoxin during a 1 h incubation at 37° C. Mouse L-cells showed no such specific binding, although they apparently took up as much toxin by pinocytosis of the bulk phase as did sensitive cells. The latter finding supports the idea that toxin taken up with the fluid phase of pinocytotic vesicles does not reach the cytosol in enzymically active form. Presumably, degradation occurs after fusion of the pinocytotic vesicles with liposomes.

There are at least two plausible models of toxin entry which are consistent with the available data. Both assume an initial attachment to specific cell-surface receptors. In the first it is assumed that the toxin is brought within the cell by endocytosis in membrane-bound form, and that subsequent rupture or dissolution of the vesicles permits the fragment A moiety to be released into the cytosol. NICOLSON (1974) has published evidence for entry of ricin, a toxic plant lectin, by this mechanism. Although present dogma holds that macromolecules entering cells within endocytotic vesicles are degraded and do not reach the cytoplasm in active form, there are instances in which fusion of endocytotic vesicles with lysosomes does not occur (for example, during pinocytosis of maternal proteins by oocytes). It has been suggested that this phenomenon is restricted to certain specialized systems, but it may be that certain specific ligands, such as some toxins, induce formation of endocytotic vesicles which fail to fuse with lysosomes.

A second plausible mode of toxin entry is by direct penetration of the plasma membrane. It is now clear that proteins destined for export from cells generally contain a "signal sequence" rich in hydrophobic residues at the amino terminus, and it has been proposed that this sequence facilitates or promotes transport across lipid bilayer barriers. Although fragment A, which corresponds to the amino terminus of diphtheria toxin, does not contain such a sequence, there is evidence for a highly hydrophobic region within the B portion which might serve a similar function in transport of toxin across the plasma membrane. BOQUET et al. (1976) have reported that diphtheria toxin and fragment B are capable of binding the nonionic detergent Triton X-100, if they are first denatured in 0.1% sodium dodecyl sulfate. CRM 45, a 45,000 dalton fragment of the toxin containing fragment A also binds Triton X-100 (even without denaturation by dodecyl sulfate), but fragment A does not. This evidence implies the presence of a Triton X-100 binding domain within approximately the central one third of the molecule. Such domains have been found within membrane-associated proteins, and may represent a region of the toxin which serves some function in transmembrane transport of the toxin.

Studies of inhibition of toxin action on whole cells by various chemicals have contributed relatively little to our understanding of the mechanism of entry. Perhaps the most intriguing of such inhibitors is ammonium ion. KIM and GROMAN (1965) identified an inhibitory effect of ammonium chloride on toxin action, and showed that adsorption of toxin was not blocked, but that absorbed toxin was maintained in an antitoxin-sensitive state at the cell surface for long periods. These observations have been confirmed in other laboratories. BOQUET (1977) has recently reported that CRM 45, at very high concentrations, can kill mouse L-cells in culture and that ammonium chloride blocks the action of CRM 45. This seems consistent with the results of KIM and GROMAN (1965) which imply that ammonium ion blocks some step in the entry process subsequent to adsorption. Other known inhibitors of toxin action on whole cells are sodium fluoride, arsenite, and ruthenium red (DUNCAN and GROMAN, 1969; IVINS et al., 1975; MIDDLEBROOK and DORLAND, 1977). No consistent theory to explain the actions of all these inhibitors on diphtheria toxin uptake has yet been proposed.

III. Exotoxin A from *Pseudomonas aeruginosa*

A. Pseudomonas Infections

There are strong contrasts between *P. aeruginosa* and *C. diphtheriae* both in cellular characteristics and patterns of infection (CLARKE and RICHMOND, 1975). For example, *P. aeruginosa* is gram-negative and capable of growing saprophytically in water, containing very low levels of nutrients, whereas *C. diphtheriae* is gram-positive and has much more complex growth requirements. *P. aeruginosa* is an opportunistic pathogen which only rarely causes infections in healthy individuals, except for infants. Most commonly, infections occur in individuals with impaired or overtaxed host defense mechanisms, such as those with genetic immunodeficiencies; those being treated with immunosuppressive drugs; or patients with extensive burns. As a result of its opportunistic nature and its capacity to grow in environments containing very low levels of nutrients, *P. aeruginosa* has become a major source of infections acquired in hospitals.

P. aeruginosa is capable of causing localized infections at various sites in the body, including the respiratory, urinary, and intestinal tracts, the ear, and the eye. Localized infections may progress to septicemia and generalized infections in patients with impaired host defense mechanisms. The fact that the organisms are insensitive to most antibiotics makes therapy difficult and contributes to the high mortality rate from generalized infections (approaching 100%).

Studies of the mechanisms of pathogenicity of *P. aeruginosa* have revealed a number of toxic factors including lecithinase, proteases, hemolysins, and various pigments. In addition, a protein toxin, which has been termed exotoxin A, has been isolated by LIU (1966). A high percentage of clinical isolates of *P. aeruginosa* are capable of producing this toxin in culture (BJORN et al., 1977; POLLACK et al., 1977). The toxin has been purified and shown to produce symptoms similar to those seen in animals infected with *P. aeruginosa*. LIU and HSIEH (1973) have shown that antiserum against the toxin prevents the lethal effects of infections of mice with the organism. Although it is still uncertain whether or not the toxin is a significant factor in human infections, neutralizing antitoxin in high titer was found in all of a group of 14 patients who recovered from serious pseudomonas infections (POLLACK et al., 1976).

B. Structure and Enzymology of Exotoxin A

Exotoxin A has been purified and studied in several laboratories. It has a mean lethal dose for a 20 g mouse of about 0.1 μg (LEPPLA, 1976). The toxin is composed of a single chain of molecular weight about 66,000, as estimated by electrophoresis on polyacrylamide gels in the presence of SDS (LEPPLA, 1976; CHUNG and COLLIER, 1977b). Its isoelectric point has been reported to be 5.0–5.1 (LEPPLA, 1976). The toxin has been shown to contain amino terminal arginine and has four disulfide bridges and no free sulfhydryls. The amino acid composition has been reported, with the most notable features being a high ratio of arginine to lysine (LEPPLA, 1976). Less than one residue of hexose per molecule was found using the anthrone test, and carbohydrate analysis by gas chromatography was negative.

Like diphtheria toxin, exotoxin A is cytocidal for a number of cell lines in culture and inhibits protein synthesis in such cells. The kinetics of inhibition of protein synthesis are similar to those observed with diphtheria toxin.

Studies in cell-free systems have shown that exotoxin A inhibits protein synthesis by the same mechanism as diphtheria toxin (IGLEWSKI and KABAT, 1975; IGLEWSKI et al., 1976). The inhibition of protein synthesis in cell-free systems is NAD-dependent, and one can show that label is incorporated from radioactive NAD (labeled in the ADPR moiety) specifically into EF II. Radioactivity is not incorporated from nicotinamide-labeled NAD. Evidence has been presented that label incorporated into EF II is attached to the same tryptic peptide which is labeled by diphtheria toxin. In addition, fragment A from diphtheria toxin catalyzes reversal of the reaction catalyzed by exotoxin A, as determined by release of labeled ADP-ribose (in the form of NAD) in the presence of high concentrations of nicotinamide. Thus there can be essentially no doubt that both toxins catalyze attachment of the ADP-ribose moiety of NAD to the same site on EF II, and with identical stereospecificity.

The identity of the reaction catalyzed by exotoxin A and diphtheria toxin raises questions concerning the similarities of structure–activity relationships between the two toxins. There is now clear evidence that exotoxin A, like diphtheria toxin, is synthesized in the form of a proenzyme, which has little if any capacity to catalyze the ADP-ribosylation of EF II (LEPPLA, 1976; CHUNG and COLLIER, 1977a; VASIL et al., 1977). This enzymic activity can be elicited by at least two methods (Fig. 4). The first involves cleavage of the toxin by an unidentified protease, present as a trace contaminant in purified toxin preparations. Such cleavage, which occurs upon prolonged storage of the purified exotoxin in the frozen state, yields as a major product a nontoxic 26,000 dalton peptide with high specific activity in catalyzing ADP-ribosylation of EF II. Reduction is not a required step in the activation by this pathway.

The second method of activation (Fig. 4) involves treatment of the toxin with reducing agents in the presence of a chaotropic agent such as urea. Under these conditions a 29 to 50-fold increase in specific activity in ADP-ribosylation has been observed (LEPPLA, 1976), and the activity may be shown to be associated with a molecule of about 66,000 daltons. Thus fragmentation of the toxin does not appear to occur during this treatment. Rather, unfolding of the molecule after reduction of certain of the disulfide bridges apparently exposes the enzymically active domain.

There is little evidence to suggest which of these mechanisms may be operative in the expression of enzymic activity in cells exposed to the toxin. One can

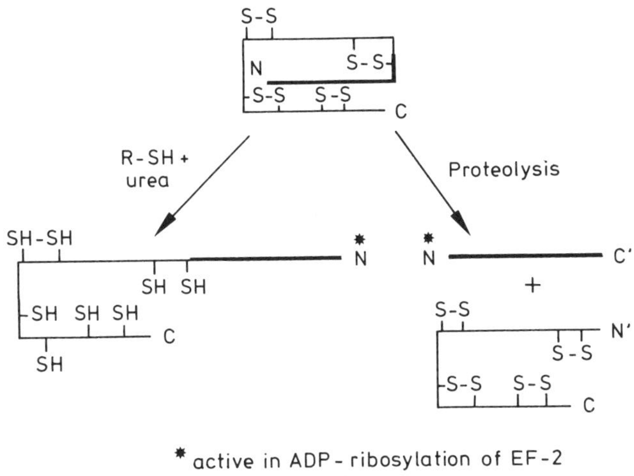

Fig. 4. Mechanism of conversion of exotoxin A from proenzyme to enzyme form

conceive that either or both may occur. Proteolytic attack within the cell or at the inner surface of the cell membrane might well release into the cytosol an active peptide similar or identical to the 26,000–27,000 dalton peptide described above. Alternatively, reduction of the whole toxin after penetration through the inner surface of the membrane could elicit such activity. Distortions of the toxin through interactions with the membrane or with cytoplasmic components might facilitate the reduction process and serve a function similar to that of urea in vitro.

The existence of structural domains within the toxin analogous (and possibly homologous) to the A and B fragments of diphtheria toxin is suggested by the available evidence. The enzymically active 26,000 dalton peptide of exotoxin A clearly documents the existence of a fragment A-like domain. In addition, the lack of toxicity of this peptide and of the reduced whole toxin implies that the integrity of the remainder of the molecule is necessary for toxicity. It may be surmised that the remainder of the molecule serves a role in binding to, or penetration of, cell surfaces, analagous to that of the B fragment of diphtheria toxin; but no data relevant to this question are available at present. A peptide of molecular weight 45,000, which may be compared to the B fragment of exotoxin A, has been observed in certain preparations of toxin, but attempts to isolate the fragment have been unsuccessful.

Studies of the detailed enzymic properties of exotoxin A are now in progress (S. Lory and R.J. Collier, unpublished data). It has been found that reduction of approximately two of the four disulfide bridges in the toxin is sufficient to elicit maximal ADP-ribosylation activity. NAD glycohydrolase activity is demonstrable in the partially or fully reduced molecule, but is negligibly low in the unreduced toxin. The kinetic constants and patterns of inhibition observed with various NAD analogs are similar to those measured with fragment A from diphtheria toxin.

More detailed studies have been performed with a 26,000 dalton, nontoxic, enzymically active peptide isolated from culture fluids of *P. aeruginosa* strain 103 (CHUNG and COLLIER, 1977a). This peptide probably corresponds to that produced during storage of purified whole toxin. The peptide catalyzes both ADP-ribosylation of EF II and hydrolysis of NAD (NAD-glycohydrolase), and shows strong similarities to fragment A from diphtheria toxin in specific activity, kinetic constants, pH optimum, and sensitivity to ionic strength. These results provide evidence for a high degree of homology in the active sites of the two fragments. The *Pseudomonas* peptide is clearly not identical to fragment A, however. It has a higher molecular weight, greater thermal and pH labilities, and an amino acid composition which is markedly different from that of fragment A in certain respects (notably, its proline content is high, and no half-cystine residues are present). In addition, there is no detectable reaction with, or neutralization by, antibody to diphtheria toxin fragment A. The intrinsic fluorescence of tryptophan in the peptide was maximally quenched by only about 20% upon binding of NAD; this contrasts with fragment A from diphtheria toxin, in which about 75% quenching is observed.

The mechanism of entry of exotoxin A into cells remains as obscure as that of diphtheria toxin. The fact that exotoxin A shows a different spectrum of cell sensitivity from that of diphtheria toxin (MIDDLEBROOK and DORLAND, 1977) suggests that the two toxins attach to different cell-surface receptors. MIDDLEBROOK and DORLAND (1977) have compared the effects of various potential inhibitors on the actions of diphtheria and pseudomonas exotoxins and found strong contrasts. For example, the action of exotoxin A was not inhibited by ammonium chloride, and sodium fluoride was found to potentiate the cytotoxicity of exotoxin A. This provides further evidence that there are major differences in the attachment and entry mechanisms of the two toxins, but little can be concluded about the nature of the entry of exotoxin A.

IV. Discussion

The data at hand strongly suggest that diphtheria toxin and exotoxin A, or at least those polypeptide domains forming the ADP-ribosyl transferase-active centers of the two toxins, may have had common evolutionary origins. Not only is the enzymic reaction catalyzed by the two toxins identical, but there are strong similarities in the detailed enzymic properties (e.g., kinetic constants, sensitivities to inhibitors, etc.). It can be argued to the contrary that these similarities may have resulted from convergent evolution of two unrelated proteins. However, it seems highly unlikely, given the potentially large number of ways a protein might evolve to catalyze a cytocidal reaction, that two such proteins would independently evolve active centers specific for transfer of the ADP-ribose moiety of NAD^+ to the same site on a single protein of the cell.

Assuming a common origin, it is apparent that considerable divergence has occurred even between the enzymically active peptides of the two toxins.

Thus, no immunologic cross reactivity has been found, and there are marked differences in amino acid composition between the two peptides. There is, as yet, no evidence for similarity in the B portions of the toxins, although the level of knowledge of the structure of these regions is insufficient to make truly meaningful judgments.

Studies of toxin antagonists on whole cells suggest that there may be major differences in the mechanisms of attachment and entry of the diphtheria and pseudomonas exotoxins into cells. It may well be, as implied above, that the ADP-ribosyl transferase-active center has been conserved as a domain and has become associated by genetic recombination with various other domains capable of serving attachment and transport functions. Cholera toxin may well be a third, markedly divergent example of this process, in which the product is a multi-subunit protein with ADP-ribosyl transferase activity directed toward a different protein acceptor (adenylate cyclase). The B subunits of cholera toxin are associated with the enzymically active A subunits of the toxin only by noncovalent forces, and appear, at least superficially, to be quite unrelated to the B domain of diphtheria toxin.

Although the evolutionary origins of the ADP-ribosyl transferase-active center are uncertain, there are some possible clues. ADP-ribosyl transferases are known to be formed during replication of at least two bacteriophages which infect *Escherichia coli* (SKORKO et al., 1977). Two such transferases are formed during infection by phage T4, both of which catalyze attachment of ADP-ribose to the α subunit of host RNA polymerase. One of these ("alteration" enzyme, MW 20,000), which is present in virions and apparently enters cells during infection, has relatively low target specificity; it promotes transfer to other proteins as well as the α subunit. The other enzyme ("modification" enzyme, MW 26,000) is not present in virions, but is formed as a "middle enzyme," with peak concentrations reached about four minutes after infection. The modification enzyme has much higher specificity for the α subunit of *E. coli* RNA polymerase. Both enzymes attach ADP-ribose to the same arginine residue of the α subunit.

Virions of coli phage N4 have also been shown to contain an ADP-ribosyl transferase (PESCE et al., 1976). This enzyme does not modify host RNA polymerase, but promotes transfer of ADP-ribose to a variety of host proteins in vivo, and certain proteins in vitro.

Finally, a brief report has appeared recently indicating that two enzymes (MW 60,000 and 20,000) apparently capable of transfering ADP-ribose from NAD^+ to a number of proteins including egg white lysozyme, are present in extracts from transport *E. coli* (SKORKO et al., 1977). Detailed properties of these enzymes have not been reported.

Although insufficient information is available at present to decide whether or not any of these enzymes may be related to the known ADP-ribosylation toxins, it is clear that NAD: protein ADP-ribosyl transferase activity is not unique to toxic proteins. From the present vantage point it seems probable that the ADP-ribosylating toxins may have evolved from a precursor enzyme containing an NAD binding site adapted to transfer of ADP-ribose, with mutations and recombinations giving rise to the singular protein substrate specificities and mechanisms of attachment and entry. With the expanding interest in bacterial toxins now evident, significant data pertinent to these general questions will undoubtedly be forthcoming within the next few years.

Acknowledgments. Research in the author's laboratory on diphtheria toxin and exotoxin A has been supported by USPHS grant AI-07877 and NSF grant GB-32406. Mrs. Patricia Bernard was responsible for preparation of the illustrations in this chapter.

References

Beugnier, N., Zanen, J.: Diphtheria toxin: The effect of nitration and reductive methylation on enzymatic activity and toxicity. Biochim. Biophys. Acta *490*, 225–234 (1977)
Bizzini, B., Turpin, A.: Les toxines bacteriennes. Recherche *7*, 444–451 (1976)
Bjorn, M.J., Vasil, M.L., Sadoff, J.C., Iglewski, B.H.: Incidence of exotoxin production by *Pseudomonas* species. Infect. Immun. *16*, 362–366 (1977)
Bonventre, P.F., Saelinger, C.B., Ivins, B., Woscinski, C., Amorini, M.: Interaction of cultured mammalian cells with (^{125}I) diphtheria toxin. Infect. Immun. *11*, 675–684 (1975)
Boquet, P.: Transport of diphtheria toxin fragment A across mammalian cell membranes. Biochem. Biophys. Res. Commun. *75*, 696–702 (1977)
Boquet, P., Pappenheimer, A.M., Jr.: Interaction of diphtheria toxin with mammalian cell membranes. J. Biol. Chem. *251*, 5770–5778 (1976)
Boquet, P., Silverman, M.S., Pappenheimer, A.M., Jr., Vernon, W.B.: Binding of Triton X-100 to diphtheria toxin, cross-reacting material 45, and their fragments. Proc. Natl. Acad. Sci. USA *73*, 4449–4453 (1976)
Burgoyne, R.D., Wolstenholme, J., Stephen, J.: The preparation of stable, biologically active B fragment of diphtheria toxin. Biochem. Biophys. Res. Commun. *71*, 920–925 (1976)
Chung, D.W., Collier, R.J.: Enzymatically active peptide from the adenosine diphosphate ribosylating toxin of *Pseudomonas aeruginosa*. Infect. Immun. *16*, 832–841 (1977a)
Chung, D.W., Collier, R.J.: The mechanism of ADP-ribosylation of elongation factor 2 catalyzed by fragment A from diphtheria toxin. Biochim. Biophys. Acta *483*, 248–257 (1977b)
Clarke, P.H., Richmond, M.H.: Genetics and biochemistry of *Pseudomonas*. London, New York, Sydney, Toronto: Wiley 1975
Collier, R.J.: Effect of diphtheria toxin on protein synthesis: Inactivation of one of the transfer factors. J. Mol. Biol. *25*, 83–98 (1967)
Collier, R.J.: Diphtheria toxin: mode of action and structure. Bacteriol. Rev. *39*, 54–85 (1975)
Collier, R.J.: Inhibition of protein synthesis by exotoxins from *Corynebacterium diphtheriae* and *Pseudomonas aeruginosa*. In: The specificity and action of animal, bacterial, and plant toxins, Series B. Cuatrecases, P. (ed.), Vol. 1, pp. 67–98. London: Chapman and Hall 1976
Collier, R.J., Kandel, J.: Structure and activity of diphtheria toxin. I. Thiol-dependent dissociation of a fraction of toxin into enzymically active and inactive fragments. J. Biol. Chem. *246*, 1496–1503 (1971)
Collier, R.J., Pappenheimer, A.M., Jr.: Studies on the mode of action of diphtheria toxin. I. Phosphorylated intermediates in normal and intoxicated HeLa cells. J. Exp. Med. *120*, 1007–1018 (1964a)
Collier, R.J., Pappenheimer, A.M., Jr.: Studies on the mode of action of diphtheria toxin. II. Effect of toxin on amino acid incorporation in cell-free systems. J. Exp. Med. *120*, 1019–1039 (1964b)
DeLange, R.J., Drazin, R.E., Collier, R.J.: Amino-acid sequence of fragment A, an enzymically active fragment from diphtheria toxin. Proc. Natl. Acad. Sci. USA *73*, 69–72 (1976)
Dirkx, J.: La toxine diphterique: biologie moleculaire d'une infection. Arch. Int. Physiol. Biochim. *82*, 157–170 (1974)
Drazin, R., Kandel, J., Collier, R.J.: Structure and activity of diphtheria toxin. II. Attack by trypsin at a specific site within the intact toxin molecule. J. Biol. Chem. *246*, 1504–1510 (1971)

Duncan, J.L., Groman, N.B.: Activity of diphtheria toxin. II. Early events in the intoxication of HeLa cells. J. Bacteriol. *98*, 973–969 (1969)
Everse, J., Lappi, D.A., Beglau, J.M., Lee, C.L., Kaplan, N.O.: Investigations into the relationship between structure and function of diphtheria toxin. Proc. Natl. Acad. Sci. USA *74*, 472–476 (1977)
Finkelstein, R.A.: Cholera. CRC Crit. Rev. Microbiol. *2*, 553–623 (1973)
Finkelstein, R.A.: Progress in the study of cholera and related enterotoxin. In: Mechanisms in bacterial toxinology. Bernheimer, A.W. (ed.), pp. 53–84. New York, London, Sidney, Toronto: Wiley 1976
Gabliks, J., Solotorovsky, M.: Cell culture reactivity to diphtheria, staphylococcus, tetanus, and *Escherichia coli* toxins. J. Immunol. *88*, 505–512 (1962)
Gill, D.M.: Mechanism of action of cholera toxin. Adv. Cyclic. Nucleotide Res. *8*, 85–118 (1977)
Gill, D.M., Dinius, L.L.: Observations on the structure of diphtheria toxin. J. Biol. Chem. *246*, 1485–1491 (1971)
Gill, D.M., Pappenheimer, A.M., Jr.: Structure-activity relationships in diphtheria toxin. J. Biol. Chem. *246*, 1492–1495 (1971)
Gill, D.M., Steinhaus, D.M.: Modification of diphtheria toxin by NAD^+. J. Hyg. Epidemiol. Microbiol. Immunol. *18*, 316–323 (1974)
Gill, D.M., Pappenheimer, A.M., Jr., Uchida, T.: Diphtheria toxin, protein synthesis, and the cell. Fed. Proc. *32*, 1508–1515 (1973)
Goor, R.S.: New form of diphtheria toxin. Nature (London) *217*, 1051–1053 (1968)
Goor, R.S., Pappenheimer, A.M., Jr.: Studies on the mode of action of diphtheria toxin. IV. Specificity of the cofactor (NAD) requirement for toxin action in cell-free systems. J. Exp. Med. *126*, 913–921 (1967)
Honjo, T., Nishizuka, Y., Hayaishi, O., Kato, I.: Diphtheria toxin-dependent adenosine diphosphate ribosylation of amino-acyl transferase II and inhibition of protein synthesis. J. Biol. Chem. *243*, 3553–3555 (1968)
Honjo, T., Nishizuka, Y., Kato, I., Hayaishi, O.: Adenosine diphosphate ribosylation of amino-acyl transferase II and inhibition of protein synthesis by diphtheria toxin. J. Biol. Chem. *246*, 4251–4260 (1971)
Iglewski, B.H., Kabat, D.: NAD-dependent inhibition of protein synthesis by *Pseudomonas aeruginosa* toxin. Proc. Natl. Acad. Sci. USA *72*, 2284–2288 (1975)
Iglewski, B., Elwell, L.P., Liu, P.V., Kabat, D.: ADP-ribosylation of elongation factor 2 by *Pseudomonas aeruginosa* exotoxin A and by diphtheria toxin. In: Proc. 4th Int. Symp. Interconversion of Enzymes. Shalfiel, S. (ed.), pp. 150–155. Berlin, Heidelberg, New York: Springer 1976
Ivins, B., Saelinger, C.B., Bonventre, P.F., Woscinski, C.: Chemical modulation of diphtheria toxin action on cultured mammalian cells. Infect. Immun. 665–674 (1975)
Johnson, W., Kuchler, R.J., Solotorovsky, M.: Site in cell-free protein synthesis sensitive to diphtheria toxin. J. Bacteriol. *96*, 1089–1098 (1968)
Kandel, J., Collier, R.J., Chung, D.W.: Interaction of fragment A from diphtheria toxin with nicotinamide adenine dinucleotide. J. Biol. Chem. *249*, 2088–2097 (1974)
Kim, K., Groman, N.B.: Mode of inhibition of diphtheria toxin by ammonium chloride. J. Bacteriol. *90*, 1557–1562 (1965)
Leppla, S.H.: Large scale purification and characterization of the exotoxin of *Pseudomonas aeruginosa*. Infect. Immun. *14*, 1077–1086 (1976)
Liu, P.V.: The roles of various fractions of *Pseudomonas aeruginosa* in its pathogenesis. III. Identity of the lethal toxin produced *in vitro* and *in vivo*. J. Infect. Dis. *116*, 481–489 (1966)
Liu, P.V., Hsieh, H.: Exotoxins of *Pseudomonas aeruginosa*. III. Characteristics of antitoxin A. J. Infect. Dis. *128*, 520–526 (1973)
Michel, A., Dirkx, J.: Occurrence of tryptophan in the enzymically active site of diphtheria toxin fragment A. Biochim. Biophys. Acta *491*, 286–295 (1977)
Middlebrook, J.L., Dorland, R.B.: Differential chemical protection of mammalian cells from the exotoxins of *Corynebacterium diphtheriae* and *Pseudomonas aeruginosa*. Infect. Immun. *16*, 232–239 (1977)
Moehring, T.J., Moehring, J.M., Kuchler, R.J., Solotorovsky, M.: The response of cultured mammalian cells to diphtheria toxin. I. Amino acid transport, accumulation, and incorporation in normal and intoxicated sensitive cells. J. Exp. Med. *126*, 407–422 (1967)

Moss, J., Vaughan, M.: Mechanism of action of choleragen. J. Biol. Chem. *252*, 2455–2457 (1977)

Murphy, J.R.: Structure activity relationships in diphtheria toxin. In: Mechanisms in bacterial toxinology. Bernheimer, A.W. (ed.), pp. 31–52. New York, London, Sidney, Toronto: Wiley 1976

Nicolson, G.L.: Ultrastructural analysis of toxin binding and entry into mammalian cells. Nature (London) *251*, 628–630 (1974)

Pappenheimer, A.M., Jr.: Diphtheria toxin. Annu. Rev. Biochem. *46*, 69–94 (1977)

Pappenheimer, A.M., Jr., Gill, D.M.: Diphtheria. Science *182*, 353–358 (1973)

Pesce, A., Casoli, C., Schito, G.C.: Rifampicin-resistant RNA polymerase and NAD transferase activities in coliphage N4 virions. Nature (London) *262*, 412–414 (1976)

Pollack, M., Callahan, L.T., III, Taylor, N.S.: Neutralizing antibody to *Pseudomonas aeruginosa* exotoxin in human sera: Evidence for in vivo toxin production during infections. Infect. Immun. *14*, 942–947 (1976)

Pollack, M., Taylor, N.S., Callahan, L.T., III.: Exotoxin production by clinical isolates of *Pseudomonas aeruginosa*. Infect. Immun. *15*, 776–780 (1977)

Reylveld, E.H.: Formation de la toxine diphterique lourde. C.R. Acad. Sci. Paris *270*(D), 410–413 (1970)

Richter, D., Lipmann, F.: Separation of mitochondrial and cytoplasmic peptide chain elongation factors from yeast. Biochemistry *9*, 5065–5070 (1970)

Robb, L.A.: Separation of diphtheria toxin proteins. Can. J. Microbiol. *12*, 573–579 (1966)

Robinson, E.A., Henriksen, O., Maxwell, E.S.: Elongation factor 2. Amino acid sequence at the site of adenosine diphosphate ribosylation. J. Biol. Chem. *249*, 5088–5093 (1974)

Skorko, R., Zillig, W., Rohrer, H., Fujiki, H., Mailhammer, R.: Purification and properties of the NAD^+: Protein ADP-ribosyltransferase responsible for the T4-phage-induced modification of the subunit of DNA-dependent RNA polymerase of *Escherichia coli*. Eur. J. Biochem. *79*, 55–66 (1977)

Strauss, N.: The effect of diphtheria toxin on the metabolism of HeLa cells. II. Effect on nucleic acid metabolism. J. Exp. Med. *112*, 351–359 (1960)

Strauss, N., Hendee, E.D.: The effect of diphtheria toxin on the metabolism of HeLa cells. J. Exp. Med. *109*, 144–163 (1959)

Uchida, T., Pappenheimer, A.M., Jr., Harper, A.A.: Reconstitution of diphtheria toxin from two nontoxic cross-reacting mutant toxins. Science *175*, 901–903 (1972)

Uchida, T., Pappenheimer, A.M., Jr., Gregory, R.: Diphtheria toxin and related proteins. I. Isolation and properties of mutant proteins serologically related to diphtheria toxin. J. Biol. Chem. *248*, 3838–3844 (1973)

Vasil, M.L., Kabat, D., Iglewski, B.H.: Structure-activity relationships of an exotoxin of *Pseudomonas aeruginosa*. Infect. Immun. *16*, 353–361 (1977)

Zanen, J., Muyldermans, G., Beugnier, N.: Competitive antagonists of the action of diphtheria toxin in HeLa cells. FEBS Lett. *66*, 261–263 (1976)

Echinomycin, Triostin, and Related Antibiotics

M.J. WARING

Introduction

Quinoxaline antibiotics are of widespread occurrence in nature. They are heterodetic cyclic depsipeptides characterized by the possession of quinoxaline-2-carboxylic acid moieties, and the whole group may conveniently be subdivided into two families, the quinomycins and triostins (SHOJI and KATAGIRI, 1961; YOSHIDA et al., 1961; OTSUKA and SHOJI, 1965).

The best-known mumber of the series is echinomycin (KELLER-SCHIERLEIN et al., 1959) which is identical to quinomycin A. In general, quinoxalines are powerful antimicrobial agents, cytotoxic to mammalian cells in culture, and display significant inhibitory activity towards a variety of tumors in experimental animals. All these aspects, together with the basic chemistry, biochemistry and microbiology of the antibiotics have been expertly reviewed by KATAGIRI et al. (1975). Consequently, the present review will be concentrated largely on new developments which have occurred since the article of KATAGIRI et al. (1975) was prepared, particularly in respect of new chemical findings and the detailed insights which have been gained into the mode of action of these antibiotics at the molecular level (WARING, 1977).

Chemical Structure

An important development has been the revision of the structure of quinomycin antibiotics, reported independently in April 1975 by two groups of workers in Britain and the USA (DELL et al., 1975; MARTIN et al., 1975). The impetus for these investigations was provided, in both instances, by preliminary nuclear magnetic resonance (NMR) measurements which revealed significant discrepancies from expectations based on the published formulae (KELLER-SCHIERLEIN et al., 1959; Fig. 1). In the author's laboratory the 100 MHz proton NMR spectrum of echinomycin was found to lack the magnetic equivalence expected for pairs of symmetry-related protons in the structure of Fig. 1a and to contain resonances corresponding to the presence of some four more protons than could be accounted for by that structure (J. FEENEY, G.C.K. ROBERTS and M.J. WARING, unpublished observations). The American group noted the apparent presence of an S–CH_3 group, inconsistent with the published structure

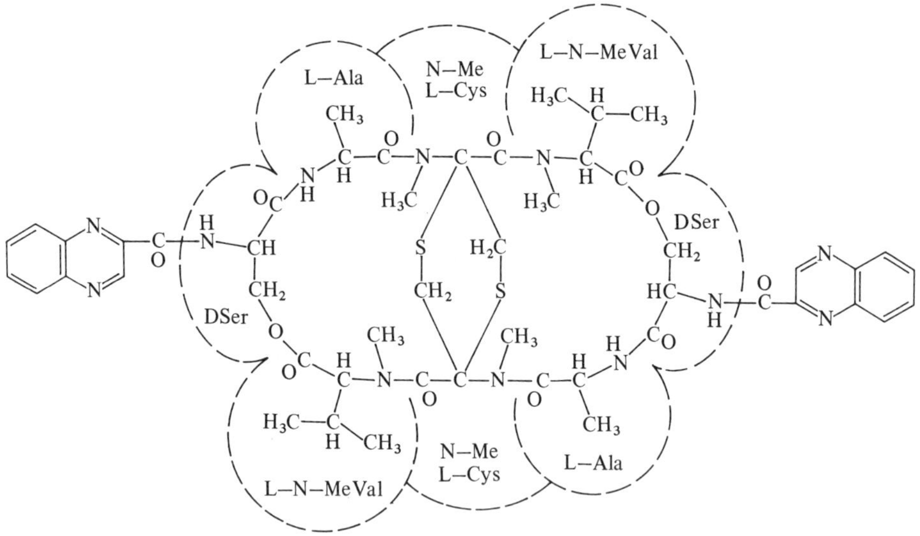

a

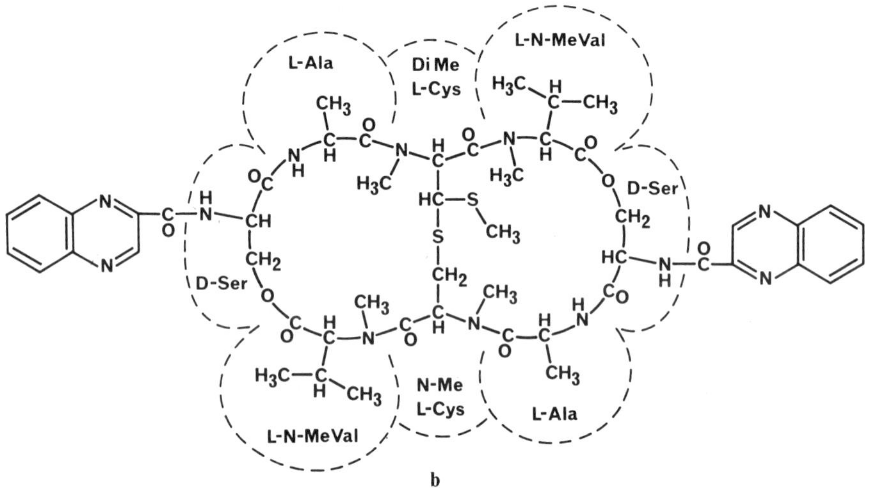

b

Fig. 1. a Structure of echinomycin as originally proposed by Keller-Schierlein et al. (1959). **b** Revised structure of echinomycin (quinomycin A) reported by Dell et al. (1975) and Martin et al. (1975). Other members of the quinomycin family have amino acid replacements at the N-methyl valine sites; in quinomycin C both residues are dimethyl-allo-isoleucine. **c** Structure of triostin A as confirmed by Otsuka et al. (1976). Other triostins have different amino acids in place of N-methyl valine (two moieties of dimethyl-allo-isoleucine in the case of triostin C). TANDEM (des-N-tetramethyl triostin A) lacks the methyl substituents on the Ala-Cys and Cys-Val peptide bonds

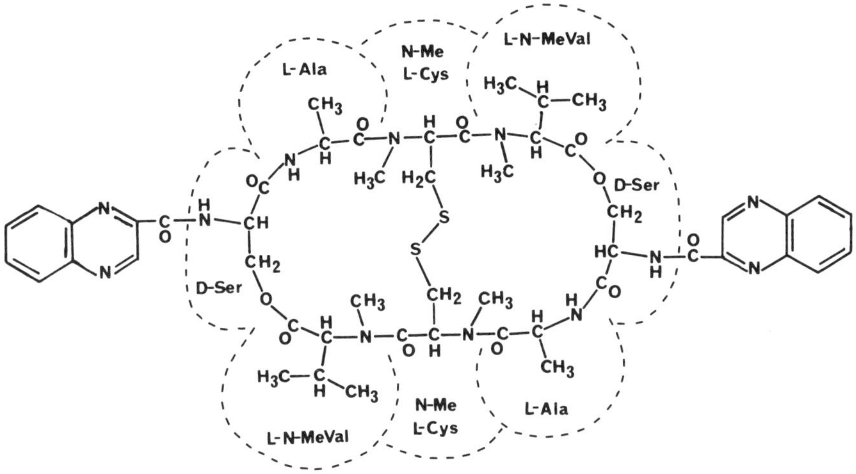

Fig. 1c

(MARTIN et al., 1975). Both groups undertook high-resolution ^{1}H and ^{13}C NMR studies as well as field desorption mass spectrometry to establish the correct structure of echinomycin (quinomycin A). The most significant of their combined findings are summarized below:

1. The NMR spectra reveal the presence of 64 protons (four exchangeable) and 51 carbons (including 10 carbonyls) corresponding to a molecular formula of $C_{51}H_{64}O_{12}N_{12}S_2$ which is greater by CH_4 than that originally proposed.
2. Resonances corresponding to the N–CH_3 groups on the Ala-Cys and Cys-Val peptide bonds can be identified, as also can an S–CH_3 signal, but the expected isolated bridge methylene protons are absent; instead the two units –CHH′–CH–Y and W–CH–CH–Z can be detected.
3. The molecule contains a total of three (not four) methylene carbons, and none of the aliphatic carbons are quaternary.
4. The magnetic nonequivalence of the two halves of the molecule is evident, a particularly striking feature being the appearance of two nonequivalent single protons at low field due to the 3H's of the quinoxaline rings.
5. The molecular formula calculated in (1) requires a molecular weight of 1100.421. The molecular ion detected by mass spectrometry has, indeed, m/e 1100. In addition, the complete mass spectrum of echinomycin reveals a pattern of fragmentation which confirms the sequence of amino acids in the antibiotic as well as the nature of the sulfur-containing cross-link.

On the basis of these, as well as other observations, DELL et al. (1975) and MARTIN et al. (1975) proposed the amended formula represented in Fig. 1b in which the dithian cross-link bridging across the two equivalent halves of the peptide rings is replaced by an asymmetric thioacetal. Since the structures of quinomycins B_0, C, D, B and E are based on analogy with echinomycin (KATAGIRI et al., 1975) it is presumed that the nature of the cross-link in these antibiotics should be modified in the same way. MARTIN et al. (1975) went on to confirm this for an antibiotic apparently identical to quinomycin C by comparison of NMR spectra and by showing that field desorption mass spectrometry afforded a molecular ion at m/e 1156 as required by the revised molecular formula $C_{55}H_{72}N_{12}O_{12}S_2$.

An interesting consequence of the asymmetry between the two halves of the molecule imparted by the thioacetal cross-bridge is that one must expect the occurrence of positional isomers for a quinomycin antibiotic such as E which has different amino acids at the variable positions (cf. Fig. 1b). In quinomycin E these sites are occupied by one residue each of N-methyl-allo-isoleucine and dimethyl-allo-isoleucine. SHOJI et al. (1976) showed that careful examination of ^{13}C-NMR spectra of quinomycin E in $CDCl_3$ solution revealed pairs of signals for the α–CH and γ–CH_3 of these residues, attributable to positional nonequivalence as predicted, but the two isomers were not present in equal proportions. On the contrary, they appeared in approximately 4:1 ratio as judged by the ratio of peak intensities. However, despite determined efforts the isomers were not separable by high performance liquid chromatography (SHOJI et al., 1976), perhaps because they are relatively large molecules whose structure is not far from symmetrical. The isomerism only results from the disposition of the S–CH_3 group, the effect of which may be quite small in relation to the large molecular size.

Prompted by the outcome of the NMR studies on quinomycins, OTSUKA et al. (1976) undertook similar investigations on triostin A. They were able to detect the signals of the Cα and Cβ protons of the N-methyl cysteine residues and to confirm the presence of the disulfide cross-link in this molecule; moreover, their assignments of the majority of resonances in the ^{1}H and ^{13}C spectra provided confirmation of the validity of the previously proposed structure (Fig. 1c). However, they made the surprising observation that despite the exact symmetry implicit in the structural formula in Fig. 1c the spectrum of triostin A in $CDCl_3$ solution contained well-resolved pairs of signals for chemically equivalent protons and carbon atoms in the two halves of the molecule. In deuterated dimethylsulfoxide (DMSO), however, the pairs coalesced to single signals as expected for a totally symmetrical molecule. OTSUKA et al. (1976) interpreted their results to indicate that although the triostin A molecule is constructed from two chemically equivalent halves each half does not adopt an equivalent conformation in $CDCl_3$, hence the observed magnetic nonequivalence. However, BLAKE et al. (1977) subsequently showed that the two resonances for each pair of symmetry-related protons were unequal in intensity, being approximately in the ratio 3:2, and that the observed ratio could be altered at will by varying the polarity of the solvent. They concluded that triostin A can adopt two symmetrical conformations which interconvert slowly on the NMR time-scale, but that the presence of an asymmetrical conformation is excluded (BLAKE et al., 1977). They reinforced this conclusion by showing that the two conformers could be physically resolved by thin-layer chromatography on silica gel plates at low temperature, that they equilibrated readily when the temperature was raised, and that the energy barrier between the conformers was about 22 kcal/mol. One, designated the "polar" conformer, is favored by such solvents as pyridine and DMSO in which it represents the sole species present; the "nonpolar" conformer is preferred in solvents containing a high proportion of benzene, chloroform or CCl_4 (BLAKE et al., 1977).

Synthesis of Quinoxalines

Significant progress towards the total synthesis of a naturally occurring quinoxaline antibiotic has been reported by OLSEN's group (CHEN et al., 1975; CIARDELLI and OLSEN, 1977). They have achieved the total synthesis of des-*N*-tetramethyl triostin A (acronym: TANDEM) which only differs from triostin A in lacking the N-methylation of four peptide bonds. TANDEM was synthesized by classical solution techniques involving the stepwise addition of protected amino acids to benzyloxycarbonyl-D-serine, yielding two tetradepsipeptide fragments which were then coupled and cyclized to produce the basic octapeptide lactone ring. After the appropriate removal of protecting groups the disulfide cross-bridge was closed and finally the quinoxaline-2-carbonyl chromophores were attached (CIARDELLI and OLSEN, 1977). Although TANDEM has less than 1/20th the antibacterial activity of echinomycin or triostin A against *Staphylococcus aureus* in a disc-agar diffusion assay (D. GAUVREAU and M.J. WARING, unpublished observations) it interacts strongly with DNA and the characteristics of its binding are of some considerable interest (see below).

References to the biosynthesis of quinoxalines were collated by KATAGIRI et al. (1975). Now that the structure of the quinomycin series has been revised it is feasible to postulate a route for their biogenesis; granted that both echinomycin and triostin can be produced by strains related to *Streptomyces aureus*, it can be postulated that triostins are immediate precursors of quinomycins, the conversion involving monomethylation of the disulfide cross-bridge followed by a facile rearrangement (DELL et al., 1975).

Inhibition of Nucleic Acid Synthesis

The characterization of echinomycin as a powerful, selective inhibitor of nucleic acid synthesis in vivo (WARD et al., 1965; SATO et al., 1967; KATAGIRI et al., 1975) has been confirmed and extended in a study of its effects on *Bacillus megaterium* (WARING and MAKOFF, 1974). By measuring the decay of pulse-labeled RNA in this organism as a function of antibiotic concentration it is possible to study quite sensitively the specificity, rapidity of action, and relative potency of inhibitors of RNA synthesis (FOK and WARING, 1972). Echinomycin totally suppresses the incorporation of ^{3}H-uridine into RNA by *B. megaterium* within 5–10 s or less after its addition to an exponentially growing culture. Incorporation of ^{3}H-thymidine into DNA persists for much longer, of the order of 60–100 s, and only after several minutes is there extensive breakdown of polysomes, reflecting secondary impairment of protein synthesis (WAR-

ING and MAKOFF, 1974). In respect of these phenomena echinomycin is at least as selective an inhibitor of RNA synthesis as actinomycin D, and on a molar basis it appears 4–5 times more potent. Even at concentrations 50–100-fold higher than the minimum necessary to block RNA synthesis completely there is no evidence for abnormal breakdown of pulse-labeled RNA, suggesting that the action of the antibiotic as an inhibitor of RNA synthesis is, to all intents and purposes, "clean". The more limited data reported for triostins A and C indicate that their action is essentially similar to that of echinomycin (WARING and MAKOFF, 1974), and the same appears true of analogs of echinomycin in which one or both of the quinoxaline chromophores are replaced by quinoline-2-carbonyl moieties (D. GAUVREAU and M.J. WARING, unpublished observations).

Binding to DNA

Although the ability of echinomycin to form a complex with DNA and to inhibit its capacity to serve as a template for DNA-directed RNA synthesis has been known for several years (WARD et al., 1965; SATO et al., 1967), precise data on its interaction with nucleic acids have only recently become available. The chief problem is that echinomycin, in common with all the other quinoxaline antibiotics, is relatively insoluble in aqueous solution (Table 1) which presents formidable difficulties for the determination of accurate binding parameters. In particular, despite the occurrence of a small but definite hypochromic-bathochromic spectral shift when echinomycin binds to DNA (WARD et al., 1965; SATO et al., 1967; WARING et al., 1975), the sheer insolubility of the antibiotic precludes the usual spectrophotometric method as a means of assaying the binding reaction. The breakthrough came with the development of a novel solvent-partition method for measuring the binding of drugs to DNA (WARING et al., 1975). The antibiotic, dissolved in a water-immiscible organic solvent, is brought into equilibrium with a nucleic acid in aqueous buffer solution by vigorous shaking. If the partition coefficient of the antibiotic between the organic and aqueous phases is known this enables direct determination of c, the free ligand concentration in the aqueous phase, from a measurement of its concentration in the organic phase (e.g., by spectrophotometry). The extent of antibiotic binding to the nucleic acid can be estimated from a measurement of the total ligand concentration in the aqueous phase (e.g., by spectrophotometry after dissociation of the complex by addition of DMSO to 50%) less c; it is usually expressed in terms of r, the number of antibiotic molecules bound per nucleotide of the polymer. This method is generally applicable to the study of interactions between ligands and nucleic acids, but it is particularly well suited to rather hydrophobic, sparingly water-soluble substances like the quinoxalines. Its only potentially serious disadvantage lies in the finite solubility of most organic solvents in the aqueous phase. Practical details and rules for optimizing the choice of solvent, together with specific examples of application to the study of quinoxaline antibiotics, are given by WARING et al. (1975).

Table 1. Physical properties of quinoxaline antibiotics

mpound	Mol. wt.	Approximate aqueous solubility (μM)	Partition coefficient	Solvent system	Molar extinction coefficient	
					Organic phase	Aqueous phase
inomycin	1,100	5	111±4 (20° C) 106±7 (30° C) 159±9 (40° C)	IPA / 0.01 SHE	11,500 (315 nm)	11,500 (325 nm) 48,200 (245 nm)
			136±6 (20° C) 125±3 (30° C) 121±6 (40° C)	IPA / 0.1 SHE		
			138±5	IPA / 0.5 SHE		
			113±5	IPA / 0.05 *M* tris-HCl pH 7.9		
inomycin C	1,156	1.7	928±35	70/30 IPA/heptane / 0.01 SHE	12,870 (315 nm)	11,800 (325 nm) 50,800 (243 nm)
ostin A	1,086	1.7	943±23	IPA / 0.01 SHE	12,100 (317 nm)	10,900 (325 nm) 53,100 (243 nm)
ostin C	1,142	0.8	–	–	–	–
NDEM	1,030	6.0	67.6±1	70/30 IPA/heptane / 0.01 SHE	12,410 (316 nm)	12,130 (323 nm) 57,850 (245 nm)

NDEM is an acronym (LEE and WARING, 1978b) for the synthetic analogue of a naturally-occurring quinoxaline, -*N*-tetramethyltriostin A (CIARDELLI and OLSEN, 1977). The values cited for aqueous solubility refer to 0.01 E buffer (2 m*M* HEPES, 10 μ*M* EDTA, 9.4 m*M* NaCl, pH 7.0 at 20° C, total ionic strength 0.01 mol/l). er SHE buffers referred to in the column "solvent system" contain added NaCl to provide the indicated c strength. IPA is iso-amyl (iso-pentyl) acetate; 70/30 IPA/heptane is a 70%–30% (v/v) mixture of iso-pentylace- and n-heptane. Partition coefficients are given as the equilibrium ratio of concentration in the organic se divided by that in the aqueous phase. (From WARING et al., 1975; WAKELIN and WARING, 1976; LEE and WARING, 1978a, b).

The most important consideration affecting the choice of solvent is the partition coefficient of the antibiotic, for it is this parameter which effectively determines the amplification factor by which small values of c, the free antibiotic concentration in equilibrium with the complex, can be determined. For quinoxaline antibiotics a partition coefficient lying in the range 100–1000 was found most suitable, and this could generally be achieved using iso-amyl (pentyl) acetate as the organic phase. This could be supplemented if need be with 30% (v/v) *n*-heptane to reduce the solubility of the antibiotic and lower the partition coefficient. Table 1 includes data on partition and extinction coefficients for the five quinoxaline compounds whose interaction with nucleic acids has been investigated to date. In general they were found to partition according to a simple linear relationship at all accessible concentrations up to saturation of the aqueous phase; the example of triostin A is illustrated in Fig. 2.

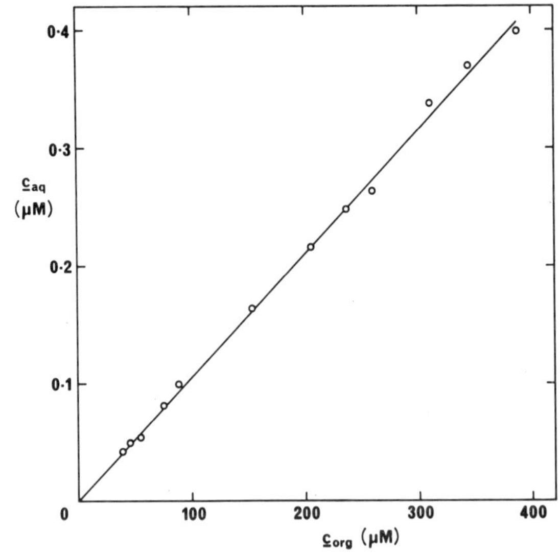

Fig. 2. Partition of triostin A between iso-amyl acetate and 0.01 SHE buffer at 20° C. The slope of the computer-fitted least-squares line, which was constrained to pass through the origin, gives the partition coefficient as 943 ± 23. (From WARING et al., 1975)

Characterization of Quinoxaline Antibiotic-DNA Complexes

The first studies performed using the new solvent-partition method confirmed the findings of previous workers (WARD et al., 1965; SATO et al., 1967) that echinomycin binds specifically to DNA, not RNA, and that it requires the presence of a helical structure in the DNA (WARING and WAKELIN, 1974). However, the most important advances stemmed from measurements of the effects of echinomycin binding to circular DNA and short rod-like fragments of sonicated DNA, which clearly identified it as a bifunctional DNA-intercalating agent – the first such substance ever described (WARING and WAKELIN, 1974). The two techniques concerned are established methods for investigating unwinding and extension of the DNA helix as demanded by the intercalation model (COHEN and EISENBERG, 1966, 1969; WARING, 1970) and their application to characterize ligand-DNA complexes has been fully described elsewhere (WARING, 1972, 1975, 1977; REINERT, 1973). In the present context the argument runs that a bifunctional intercalating agent may be expected to unwind and extend the DNA helix about twice as much per bound ligand molecule as does a simple monofunctional intercalating drug. The only difficulty lies in deciding what to adopt as the standard, ideal monofunctional intercalator; at least for the present the best choice seems to be ethidium (see reviews previously cited). The validity of the argument about bifunctional intercalation has recently received strong support from studies of homologous series of synthetic diacridines (LE PECQ et al., 1975; WAKELIN et al., 1976, 1978). As the length

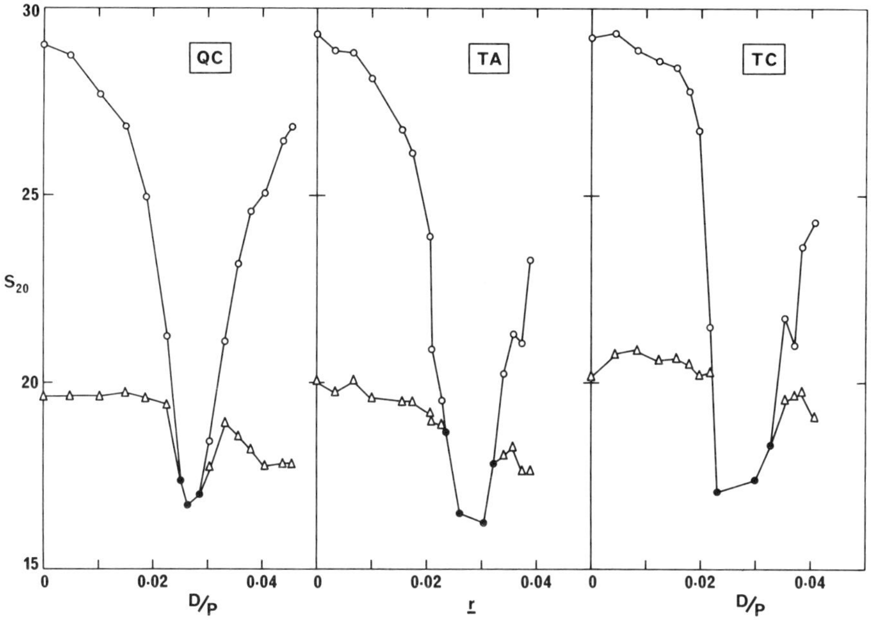

Fig. 3. Effects of quinomycin C (*left*), triostin A (*center*) and triostin C (*right*) on the sedimentation coefficient (S_{20}) of PM2 DNA in 0.01 SHE buffer, ionic strength 0.01, pH 7.0. The DNA preparations contained 80%–90% closed circular duplex molecules whose S_{20} is represented by O. The S_{20} of the nicked circles is shown by △, and when the two DNA components co-sedimented as a single unresolved boundary the symbol ● is plotted. For triostin A the abscissa shows the average number of antibiotic molecules bound per nucleotide (r) determined by the solvent-partition method. For quinomycin C and triostin C the abscissa shows the drug to nucleotide molar ratio (D/P). (After LEE and WARING, 1978a)

Table 2. Apparent intercalation events per DNA-bound molecule of quinoxaline antibiotic

Compound	Ionic strength (mol/l)	ϕ_{rel} from S_{20} plot	ϕ_{rel} from cross-over	$m/2$ from L/L_0 plot
Echinomycin	0.01	1.82 ± 0.30	1.89	1.87 ± 0.05
	0.036	1.74 ± 0.30	–	–
	0.10	1.54 ± 0.25	–	1.50 ± 0.05
	0.50	1.18 ± 0.19	–	1.16 ± 0.03
Quinomycin C	0.01	$\geqq 1.92 \pm 0.20$	–	–
Triostin A	0.01	1.82 ± 0.40	1.85	1.79 ± 0.10
Triostin C	0.01	$\geqq 1.81 \pm 0.40$	–	$\geqq 1.95 \pm 0.10$
TANDEM	0.01	1.75 ± 0.23	–	–

ϕ_{rel} is the helix-unwinding angle of the antibiotic relative to that of ethidium, calculated from the equivalence binding ratio required to effect complete relaxation of the supercoiling of closed circular duplex DNA, determined by sedimentation experiments of the type illustrated in Fig. 3 or by measurement of the cross-over point of binding isotherms to nicked and closed circular species of PM2 DNA (cf. Fig. 4). $m/2$ represents half the gradient of a plot of L/L_0 versus r or D/P for sonicated rod-like fragments of calf thymus DNA (cf. Fig. 5). For an ideal monofunctional intercalation process both ϕ_{rel} and $m/2$ may be expected to be approximately unity; for a purely bifunctional reaction they may be expected to approximate to 2. (From WAKELIN and WARING, 1976, LEE and WARING, 1978a, b).

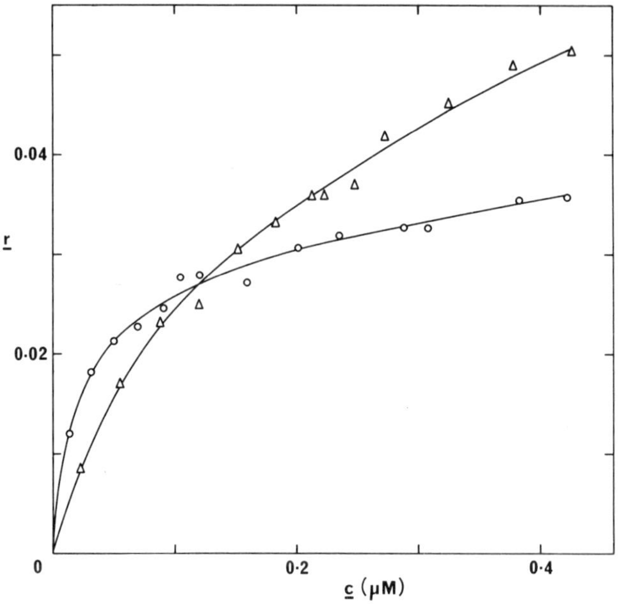

Fig. 4. Binding of triostin A to closed (○) and nicked (△) circular PM2 DNA in 0.01 SHE buffer. The binding ratio r (antibiotic molecules bound per nucleotide) is plotted as a function of the free triostin concentration in the aqueous phase, c. (After LEE and WARING, 1978a)

of flexible aliphatic chain connecting two potentially intercalative acridine chromophores is increased, there is an abrupt change in the helix-unwinding angle and helix extension to values about double those seen with shorter homologs when the transition from monofunctional to a bifunctional mode of binding occurs.

In Fig. 3 the effects of three quinoxaline antibiotics on the sedimentation behavior of closed circular duplex DNA are illustrated. All cause the decisive removal and reversal of supercoiling typical of intercalating agents.

The equivalence binding ratios, derived from the minimum in the curve for the closed circular molecules, are all in the region of 0.027 antibiotic molecules bound per nucleotide – almost half the value seen with ethidium under the same conditions (0.051) – leading to estimates of helix-unwinding angles relative to that of ethidium (ϕ_{rel}) as shown in Table 2. Similar results were obtained at ionic strength 0.01 for echinomycin (WARING and WAKELIN, 1974) and TANDEM (LEE and WARING, 1978b). Equivalence binding ratios can also be determined from inspection of binding isotherms to closed circular and nicked circular DNA molecules (Fig. 4). Whereas the isotherm for nicked circles is fairly normal in appearance, that for closed circles is substantially distorted because of the effect of the varying superhelix free energy on the binding reaction. For quinoxaline antibiotics, because of their uniquely high helix-unwinding angles, the effect is quite pronounced and leads to a good estimate of ϕ_{rel} from the cross-over point (WARING and WAKELIN, 1974; LEE and WARING, 1978a; Table 2).

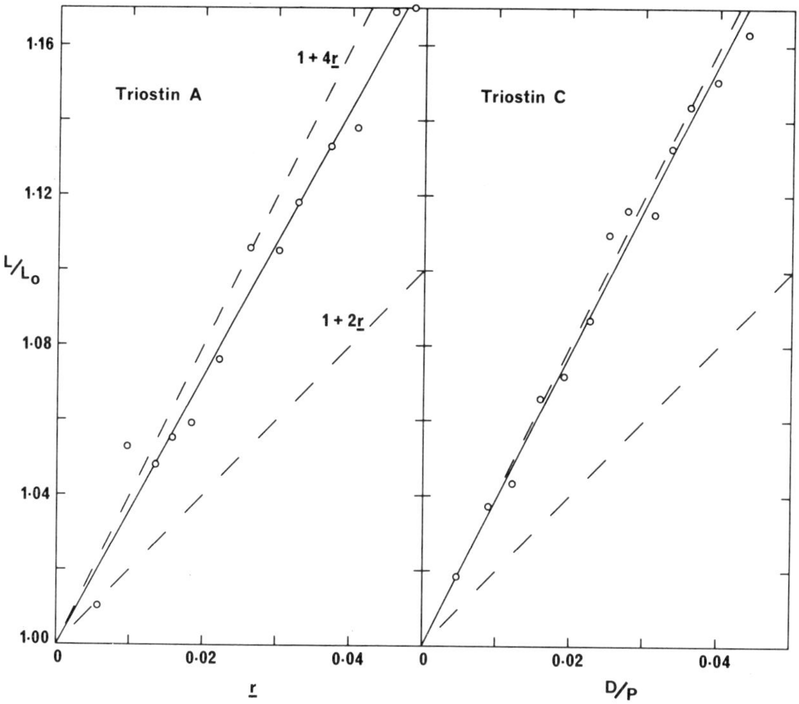

Fig. 5. Effects of triostin A (*left*) and triostin C (*right*) on the relative contour length L/L_0 of sonicated calf thymus DNA fragments, M_r 5×10^5. L/L_0 was calculated from viscosity measurements as described by COHEN and EISENBERG (1966, 1969). The abscissa represents the binding ratio r for triostin A and the drug to nucleotide ratio D/P for triostin C. Also shown are theoretical lines corresponding to the lengthening expected for ideal monofunctional intercalation $(1+2r)$ and for ideal bifunctional intercalation $(1+4r)$. The lines passing through the experimental points were fitted by the method of least squares and constrained to pass through the origin (0,1). Their slopes correspond to $1+(3.57\pm0.2)r$ (triostin A) and $1+(3.89\pm0.2)D/P$ (triostin C). (After LEE and WARING, 1978a)

The third line of evidence for bifunctional intercalation is illustrated for the triostin antibiotics in Fig. 5. With a simple monofunctional intercalation process the relative contour length of the DNA fragments is expected to increase according to the relation $L/L_0=1+2\,r$ assuming that the intercalated molecule is sandwiched parallel to the base-pairs each side of it and that it occupies the same space (3.4 Å) along the helix axis as an additional base-pair. By an analogous argument the relation expected for ideal bifunctional intercalation should be $L/L_0=1+4\,r$. Thus if m is the observed gradient of a plot of L/L_0 versus r (which can be approximated to D/P if the binding is known to be tight) the value of m/2, like that of ϕ_{rel}, should approach a value of 2 for a bifunctional reaction.

Table 2 reveals excellent agreement between ϕ_{rel} and m/2 for all quinoxalines at low ionic strength, and on this basis their interaction with DNA is identified as bifunctional intercalation. At least for echinomycin, however, there is a change if the ionic strength is raised: both parameters indicate a steady transition towards more nearly monofunctional reaction at high salt concentration. The origins and significance of this effect remain uncertain (WARING and WAKELIN, 1974; WAKELIN and WARING, 1976).

Sequence-Specificity in the Binding of Quinoxaline Antibiotics to DNA

It has been argued elsewhere (WARING and WAKELIN, 1974; WAKELIN and WARING, 1976; WARING, 1977) that true specificity for recognizing different DNA nucleotide sequences can only be achieved by polyfunctional ligands having multiple centers of specificity combined within one molecule. Thus a bifunctional drug molecule might be expected to display substantially higher selectivity for different types of nucleotide sequence than simple monofunctional agents. With this in mind, considerable efforts have been made to compare the binding of different quinoxaline antibiotics to different DNAs, primarily to investigate whether nucleotide sequence-selectivity can be detected and, if so, to relate it to the molecular structure of the antibiotic(s). The experiments were conducted at low ionic strength in order to preserve the bifunctional intercalative character of the interaction as evidenced by the parameters recorded in Table 2.

A set of data for the interaction between echinomycin and 8 naturally occurring DNA's is presented in Fig. 6. It is evident that the binding differs significantly depending upon the source of the DNA, but it does not correlate in any simple way with the gross base composition. Parameters of interaction derived from these plots are collected in Table 3. There seems to be a tendency for DNA's richer in G+C to bind the antibiotic more tightly – the highest binding constant was found for *Micrococcus lysodeikticus* DNA, the lowest for *Clostridium perfringens* DNA – but between these limits the association constant is not monotonically related to the mole fraction of G+C. In particular, a significant difference can be seen when the binding curves for *Escherichia coli* and *Salmonella typhimurium* DNA's are compared (Fig. 6), yet these species share the same overall base composition. On the other hand, the parameters determined for calf thymus and nicked PM2 DNA's (both 42% G+C) are practically the same, notwithstanding the extreme difference in their origins and genetic complexity. When the apparent frequencies of binding sites reflected in the site-size parameter n are compared, there is no relation at all to the base composition. For double-helical natural DNA's n lies within the range 9.5 ± 2.4 nucleotides per binding site. It is of interest that the DNA of the echinomycin-producing organism, *Streptomyces echinatus,* is not immune from attack by the antibiotic and indeed yields the second highest binding constant observed with any nucleic acid (Fig. 7; Table 3). Evidently the producing organism is not protected from possible toxic effects of its own metabolite by any peculiarity of its DNA, which appears normal in all respects including its GC-rich base composition which is typical of the genus *Streptomyces* (HILL, 1966).

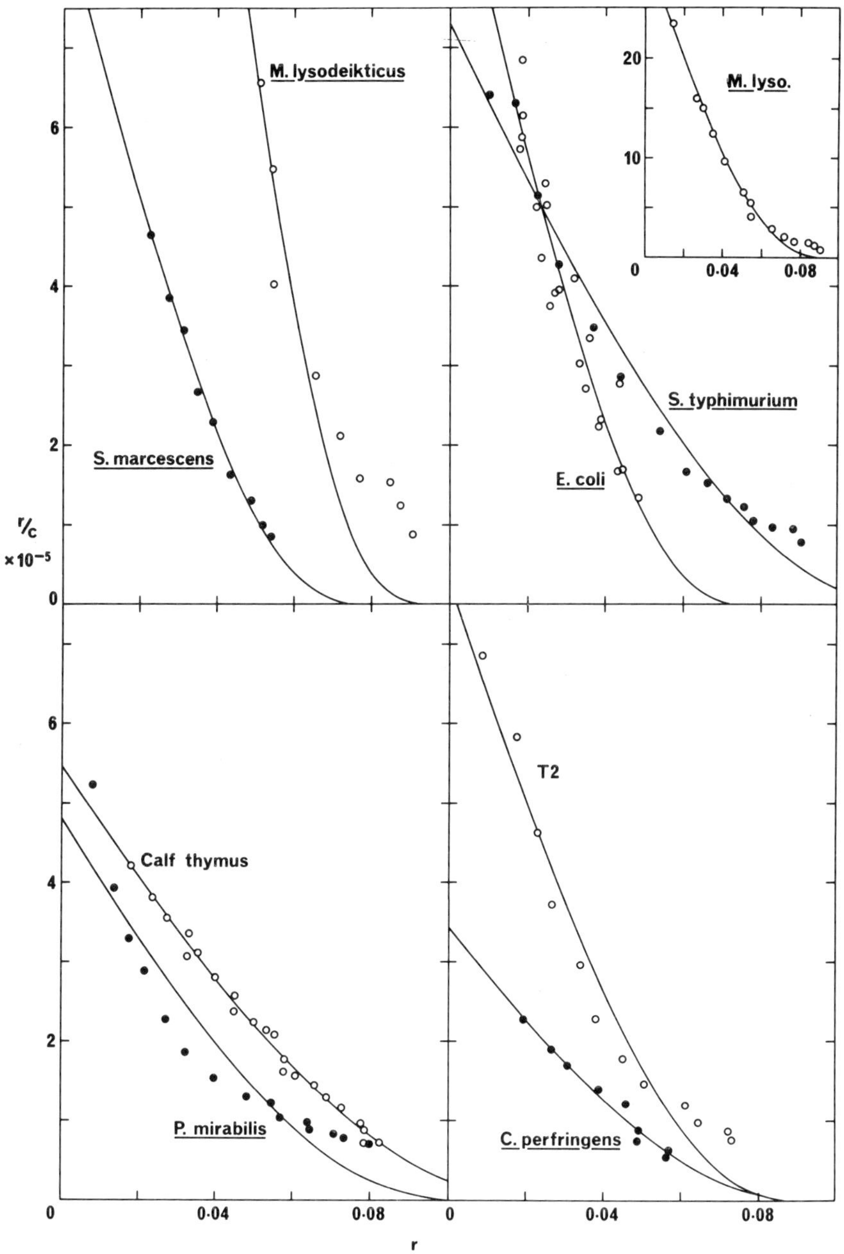

Fig. 6. Effects of base composition on the binding of echinomycin to DNA. The data are presented in the form of the Scatchard plot, where r is the binding ratio (echinomycin molecules bound/DNA nucleotide) and c is the free antibiotic concentration. The ionic strength was 0.01, pH 7.0. For ease of comparison the same scale is used throughout, except for the inset (*top right*), where the data for *M. lysodeikticus* DNA are replotted with a contracted ordinate scale in order to include points at low values of r. The curves are theoretical, computed to fit Eq. (10) of McGhee and von Hippel (1974) using the values of K(0) and n listed in Table 3. (After Wakelin and Waring, 1976)

Table 3. Parameters of interaction between echinomycin and nucleic acids

DNA	G+C (%)	Ionic strength (mol/l)	Temperature (° C)	$10^{-5} \times K(0)$ (M^{-1})	n
Calf thymus	42	0.01	20	5.48	7.17
Calf thymus	42	0.01	30	4.62	6.60
Calf thymus	42	0.01	40	3.96	6.68
Calf thymus	42	0.10	20	1.47	4.77
Calf thymus	42	0.10	30	1.14	5.56
Calf thymus	42	0.10	40	1.01	2.76
Calf thymus	42	0.50	20	1.04	6.57
Calf thymus (heat-denatured)	42	0.01	20	1.40	19.49
Bacteriophage fd	42	0.01	20	1.21	11.37
Micrococcus lysodeikticus	72	0.01	20	31.0	9.85
Streptomyces echinatus	71	0.01	20	26.0	9.73
Serratia marcescens	58	0.01	20	8.71	11.61
Escherichia coli	50	0.01	20	9.80	11.88
Salmonella typhimurium	50	0.01	20	7.38	7.58
Bacteriophage PM2 (nicked)	42	0.01	20	5.07	7.75
Proteus mirabilis	40	0.01	20	4.79	8.69
Bacteriophage T2	34	0.01	20	7.78	9.97
Clostridium perfringens	30	0.01	20	3.44	9.46
Poly(dG)·poly(dC)	100	0.01	20	15.1	9.09
Poly(dG–dC)	100	0.01	20	5.53	5.48
Poly(dA–dT)	0	0.01	20	3.12	5.65

Measurements of r, the number of antibiotic molecules bound per nucleotide, and c, the free ligand concentration, were made by solvent-partition analysis using saline-HEPES-EDTA buffers of pH 7.0 at 20° C and the indicated ionic strength (WAKELIN and WARING, 1976). The binding parameters were computed by an iterative procedure designed to satisfy Eq. (10) of MCGHEE and VON HIPPEL (1974):

$$\frac{r}{c} = K(0)(1-nr)\left[\frac{1-nr}{1-(n-1)r}\right]^{n-1}$$

given the experimentally determined values of r and c and an initial guess of n, the number of nucleotides occluded by a bound antibiotic molecule. The program (devised by J.D. MCGHEE and operated by G. UGHETTO) was made to recycle until K(0) and n changed by less than 1%, and then to print out the final values of K(0) and n together with a calculated binding isotherm at 5%-saturation increments. The calculated isotherm was then checked for "goodness of fit" to the original data; examples are shown in Figs. 6, 7, 8 and 9. It should be noted that the binding (association) constant K(0) calculated by this procedure is the intrinsic binding constant to an isolated site, given by the intercept of the calculated curve on the axis of r/c (MCGHEE and VON HIPPEL, 1974). In the corresponding treatment of SCATCHARD (1949) this intercept would be interpreted as K/n. In addition, n as defined here is the reciprocal of the binding-site parameter which results from SCATCHARD (1949) analysis.

In an effort to clarify the issue of specificity by studying simpler models the interaction between echinomycin and seven synthetic double-helical polynucleotides was investigated (WAKELIN and WARING, 1976). Four were found to interact barely at all, or only very weakly, with the antibiotic: poly dI·poly dC, poly (dI-dC), poly dA·poly dT and poly rA·poly rU. The other three bound the antibiotic well (Table 3). The tightest binding was observed with poly dG·poly dC, whose binding constant was exceeded only by that of *M. lyso-*

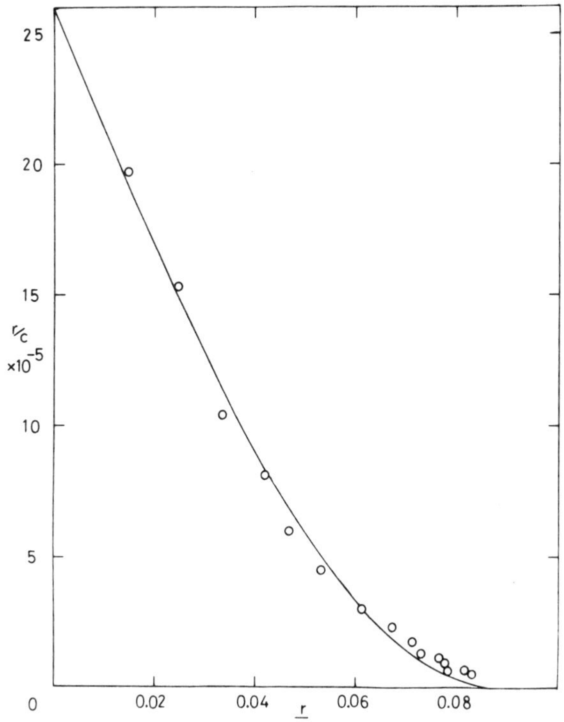

Fig. 7. Scatchard plot for the interaction between echinomycin and DNA from *Streptomyces echinatus*. Details as described in the legend to Fig. 6. The DNA was extracted from a mycelial cake derived from a culture which was producing antibiotic at typical levels, i.e., 15–30 mg/l. (Unpublished experiment of J.S. LEE, D. GAUVREAU and M.J. WARING)

deikticus and *S. echinatus* DNAs. Poly (dG-dC) yielded a binding constant of the same order as seen with several natural DNA's, while that of poly (dA-dT) fell below the range found with native double-helical DNA's. Substantially higher levels of binding were attained with the two alternating polydeoxynucleotides than with other DNA's, reflected in the computed values of n (Table 3), suggesting that a potential binding site in these polymers might be formed by as little as 5–6 nucleotides (2.5–3 base-pairs).

Thus there is undoubtedly selectivity in the interaction between echinomycin and different DNA nucleotide sequences. Particularly striking is the failure of poly dA · poly dT to bind the antibiotic while its sequence isomer poly (dA-dT) binds it well (WARING and WAKELIN, 1974). Since the association constant for *M. lysodeikticus* DNA is twice as high as that for the best of the synthetic polynucleotides, poly dG · poly dC, it may be that the base sequence (or sequences) generating the optimum conditions for binding of echinomycin contains all four nucleotides. There are evidently considerable subtleties in the preference of echinomycin for available DNA binding sites and those preferences are clearly different from those of actinomycin, its nearest equivalent among previously studied DNA-binding peptide antibiotics (WELLS and LARSON, 1970).

Table 4. DNA-binding parameters for Quinomycin C and Triostin A

DNA	G+C (%)	Quinomycin C		Triostin A	
		$10^{-6}\times K(0)$ (M^{-1})	n	$10^{-6}\times K(0)$ (M^{-1})	n
M. lysodeikticus	72	8.26	8.34	1.13	7.73
Calf thymus	42	2.60	8.30	0.70	7.29
Nicked PM2 DNA	42	–	–	0.42	9.42
Cl. perfringens	30	0.91	9.56	0.49	8.52
poly(dG-dC)	100	3.36	6.12	0.43	7.41
poly(dA-dT)	0	0.57	7.02	0.97	4.76

K(0), the intrinsic association constant, and n, the number of nucleotides occluded by the binding of one molecule, were evaluated from measurements of binding in 0.01 SHE buffer (pH 7.0, ionic strength 0.01) using equation (10) of McGHEE and VON HIPPEL (1974) as described in the legend to Table 3. (From LEE and WARING, 1978a).

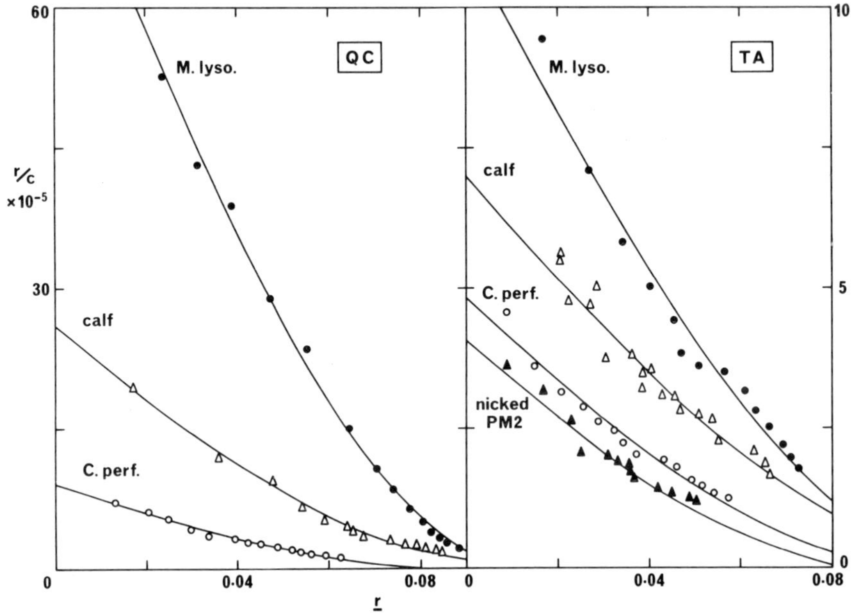

Fig. 8. Effects of base composition on the binding of quinomycin C (*left*) and triostin A (*right*) to DNA. Details as described in the legend to Fig. 6. The resulting values of binding parameters are given in Table 4. (From LEE and WARING, 1978a)

Most intriguing is the discovery that the pattern of sequence-selectivity differs among closely related quinoxaline antibiotics. There is no great change in proceeding from echinomycin to quinomycin C (i.e., in replacing both N-methylvaline residues with dimethyl-allo-isoleucine) – the binding constants all rise, perhaps related to the diminished hydrophilicity of quinomycin C, but among the different DNA's they fall in the same ranking order as was found for

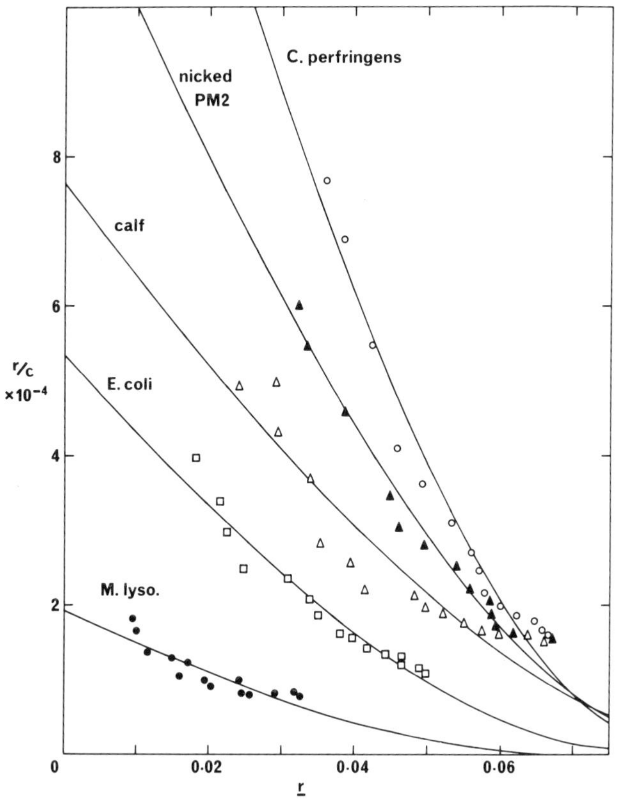

Fig. 9. Binding of TANDEM to DNAs of different base composition (see legend to Fig. 6 for details). Values of K (0) and n corresponding to the curves drawn are collated in Table 5. (From LEE and WARING, 1978b)

echinomycin (Fig. 8 and Table 4; cf. also Table 3). Not so for triostin A, which differs from echinomycin only in the replacement of the thioacetal cross-bridge by a disulfide link (Fig. 8). Binding constants for triostin A (Table 4) vary much less than they do for the quinomycins, covering only a threefold range compared to a range of 10–20 for echinomycin and quinomycin C, and there are clear differences in the ranking order of K(O) values for different DNA's. Echinomycin binds almost equally tightly to nicked PM2 and calf thymus DNA's, whereas triostin clearly prefers the latter, and their relative binding constants for nicked PM2 and *Cl. perfringens* DNA's are reversed. A bigger difference is apparent when the binding constants for the two synthetic alternating polydeoxynucleotides are compared; whereas the quinomycins bind much better to poly (dG-dC) than to poly (dA-dT) the reverse is true for triostin. It is curious that triostin A should show an almost twofold preference for the synthetic AT-polymer, while preferring the most GC-rich among the natural DNA's.

The synthetic quinoxaline depsipeptide TANDEM shows even more striking changes in sequence-selectivity (Fig. 9). With this compound the preference is

Table 5. Parameters of binding of TANDEM to nucleic acids

Nucleic acid	G+C (%)	$10^{-4} \times K(0)$ (M^{-1})	n
M. lysodeikticus DNA	72	1.94	12.13
E. coli DNA	50	5.35	10.55
Calf thymus DNA	42	7.64	8.89
Nicked PM2 DNA	42	12.10	9.50
Cl. perfringens DNA	30	18.46	10.02
poly (dG-dC)	100	<0.2	–
poly (dI-dC)	–	0.63	8.41
poly dA·poly dT	0	<0.3	–
poly rA·poly rU	0	0.52	8.01
poly (dA-dT)	0	[1500]	7.40

K(0), the intrinsic association constant, and n, the number of nucleotides occluded by the binding of one molecule, were evaluated from an analysis of binding data in 0.01 SHE buffer (pH 7.0, ionic strength 0.01) using equation (10) of McGHEE and VON HIPPEL (1974) except for poly (dA-dT) where the cooperative equation (15) was employed with ω, the parameter of cooperativity, set equal to 15. For poly (dG-dC) and poly dA·poly dT the very low levels of binding observed did not permit any theoretical analysis; the values of K(0) quoted for these polymers are upper limit estimates based on the maximum value attained by r/c. (From LEE and WARING, 1978b).

clearly for the more AT-rich among the natural DNA's, and the ratio of binding constants for the two extreme examples (*M. lysodeikticus* and *Cl. perfringens* DNA's) approaches 10 (Table 5). At the same time the discrimination between the synthetic alternating polydeoxynucleotides becomes extreme; interaction with poly (dG-dC) is barely detectable at all, while the binding to poly (dA-dT) becomes so tight that it is difficult to detect dissociation of the complex with the existing solvent-partition conditions (LEE and WARING, 1978b). In fact, there is clear evidence of cooperativity in the Scatchard plot for binding of TANDEM to poly (dA-dT), a phenomenon which may also be present though less noticeable in the corresponding data for the natural quinoxaline antibiotics (WAKELIN and WARING, 1976; LEE and WARING, 1978a, b). Theoretical considerations suggest that the "best" DNA-binding site for TANDEM may contain as many as three successive AT nucleotide-pairs, whereas that for echinomycin and quinomycin C might have 2–3 successive GC pairs; the relatively weak preferences of triostin A detected in Fig. 8 would, on this basis, be explicable in terms of preferential affinity for sites containing a single GC pair (LEE and WARING, 1978a, b).

With regard to their chemical structures the differences between the quinoxalines referred to above are quite small. More drastic alterations, such as breakage of the lactone links in the peptide ring, cleavage of the cross-bridge, replacement of the chromophores with benzyloxycarbonyl substituents, or alteration of the stereoisomerism of the serine residues from D- to L-, are known to reduce the interaction with DNA drastically or abolish binding altogether (LEE and WARING, 1978b). Evidently the integrity and/or precise conformation of the octapeptide ring in these antibiotics is a crucial feature required for their biological activity and DNA-binding properties, to say nothing of its likely influence on their sequence-selectivity. Whatever the exact nature of that selectivity, which remains to be precisely defined, it must ultimately derive from a capacity to recognize distinct nucleotide sequences either by direct interaction between functional groupings on the antibiotic molecule and the base-pairs or indirectly via recognition of a local conformational peculiarity of the DNA associated with a particular type or types of sequence. The latter is a real possibility, at least in theory, though the large differences in antibiotic-binding properties of the synthetic polynucleotides cannot be simply related to what is known of their conformational characteristics in drawn fibers or in solution (WAKELIN and WARING, 1976; LEE and WARING, 1978a, b). Nevertheless, the possibility that polynucleotide polymorphism plays an important part in determining the suitability of DNA-binding sites for quinoxaline antibiotics must be borne in mind in any discussion of molecular models.

Conformational Studies

Much interest is attached to the problem of relating the unique features of the interaction between quinoxaline antibiotics and DNA to their three-dimensional conformation. So far, no crystal structure is available for any member of the group, though diffraction data have been collected for triostin A (G.M. SHELDRICK, L.P.G. WAKELIN and M.J. WARING, unpublished). However, detailed NMR measurements have been made (DELL et al., 1975; MARTIN et al., 1975; BLAKE et al., 1977; CHEUNG et al., 1978; KALMAN et al., 1979) and preliminary molecular model-building studies have been undertaken using conformational information derived from NMR coupling constants together with semi-empirical potential energy calculations. For echinomycin, the results of these studies (CHEUNG et al., 1978; UGHETTO and WARING, 1977) have served to establish that only a limited number of possible conformations are feasible on stereochemical as well as energetic grounds, primarily because of the severe constraints on conformational flexibility imposed by the cyclic nature of the octapeptide ring and its thioacetal cross-bridge. It is clear that the whole peptide ring behaves essentially as a rigid unit, with most of its constituent groupings lying approximately within a single plane (CHEUNG et al., 1978; UGHETTO and WARING, 1977). The overall shape of the molecule is thus like a rigid disk, with the quinoxaline chromophores at opposite ends extending away approximately perpendicular to the plane of the disk, and the S–CH_3 function of the cross-bridge projecting from the middle (Fig. 10). In all models there are substantial elements of twofold rotational symmetry between the two halves of the molecule, and the chromophores project from the same side of the peptide disk with their planes roughly parallel and approximately 10 Å apart. These features are almost ideally in accord with expectations based on the requirements of a bifunctional DNA-intercalation model (WARING and WAKELIN, 1974; CHEUNG et al., 1978; UGHETTO and WARING, 1977; WARING, 1977) and the space between the quinoxaline rings appears exactly right to accommodate two DNA base-pairs.

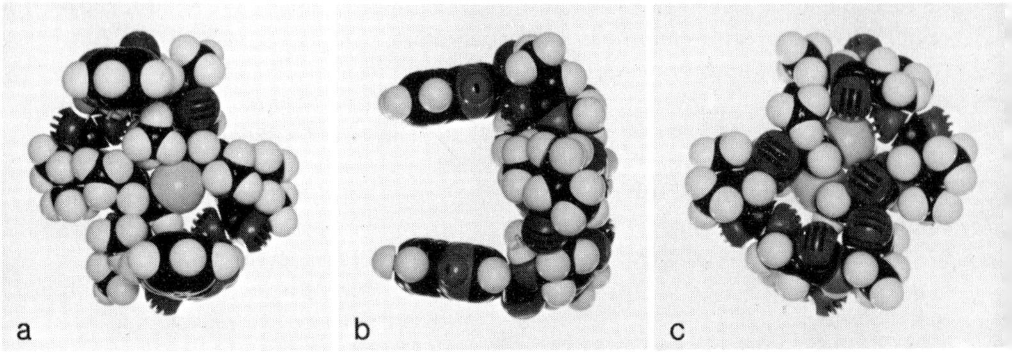

Fig. 10a–c. CPK model of a suggested conformation for echinomycin, viewed along its quasi-dyad axis (*outer panels*) or at right angles to it (**b**). **a** The quinoxaline chromophores project forward towards the viewer; **c** they project away from the direction of view and are completely obscured by the N-methylvalyl-O-seryl-alanyl sequences of the peptide ring. (From UGHETTO and WARING, 1977)

While it would be imprudent to rely too heavily on existing molecular models to seek explanations for the characteristics of quinoxaline antibiotic binding to DNA, it is of interest to speculate how the different nucleotide sequence preferences of quinomycins, triostins, and TANDEM (whatever their precise nature) might arise. The NMR evidence indicates that the conformation of the peptide ring is much the same in echinomycin, triostin A ("polar" conformer) and TANDEM, (CHEUNG et al., 1978; KALMAN et al., 1979; J.R. KALMAN, personal communication) suggesting that it really is the nature and disposition of the sulfur-containing cross-bridge which critically determines the relative affinity of the ligand for different types of site in DNA. If, as seems likely, the S–CH_3 of the thioacetal cross-bridge in echinomycin projects from the peptide ring on the side opposite the chromophores this would effectively maximize the space between the intercalative quinoxaline rings, so as to accommodate a substituent in the DNA like the 2-amino group of guanine which might additionally form a hydrogen bond to an alanine carbonyl group (CHEUNG et al., 1978; LEE and WARING, 1978b). On the other hand, if the bulky sulfur atoms of the disulfide cross-bridge were to lie permanently (TANDEM) or transiently (triostin A) out of the peptide plane on the same side as the chromophores (KALMAN et al., 1979; J.R. Kalman, personal communication) that space would be more occluded, which might provoke a distinct shift towards preference for nucleotide sequences lacking such substituents (LEE and WARING, 1978b). In any event, the evidence that the peptide ring behaves as a substantially rigid unit tends to argue against the possibility that major conformational changes affecting the disposition of peptide bonds might accompany complex formation with DNA, though the steric relationships between the chromophores and the peptide ring might alter (COSTANTINO et al., 1978).

Acknowledgments. It is a pleasure to record the contributions of my collaborators in this work, particularly Drs. H. BICKEL, A. DELL, J. FEENEY, P.J. FOK, R. GOSLING, J.R. KALMAN, J.S. LEE, A. MAKOFF, J.D. MCGHEE, J. MÜLLER, J. NÜESCH, R.K. OLSEN, G.C.K. ROBERTS, K. SCHEIBLI, G.M. SHELDRICK, G. UGHETTO, L.P.G. WAKELIN, V.B. WHITMARSH and D.H. WILLIAMS, and Messrs T.J. BLAKE, A. FIELDES, K.R. FOX, D. GAUVREAU and D. MARTIN. These and other colleagues provided invaluable advice, assistance, criticism, and samples of experimental materials. Original work reported here was supported by grants from the Medical Research Council, the Science Research Council, the Cancer Research Campaign and CIBA-Geigy Ltd.

References

Blake, T.J., Kalman, J.R., Williams, D.H.: Two symmetrical conformations of the triostin antibiotics in solution. Tetrahedron Lett. *30*, 2621–2624 (1977)

Chen, W.Y., Hsu, M.L., Olsen, R.K.: Synthesis of a model depsipeptide lactone related to the quinoxaline antibiotics. J. Org. Chem. *40*, 3110–3112 (1975)

Cheung, H.T., Feeney, J., Roberts, G.C.K., Williams, D.H., Ughetto, G., Waring, M.J.: The conformation of echinomycin in solution. J. Am. Chem. Soc. *100*, 46–54 (1978)

Ciardelli, T.L., Olsen, R.K.: Synthesis of Des-N-methyltriostin A, a bicyclic octadepsipeptide related to the quinoxaline antibiotics. J. Am. Chem. Soc. *99*, 2806–2807 (1977)

Cohen, G., Eisenberg, H.: Conformation studies on the sodium and caesium salts of calf thymus DNA. Biopolymers *4*, 429–440 (1966)

Cohen, G., Eisenberg, H.: Viscosity and sedimentation study of sonicated DNA-proflavine complexes. Biopolymers *8*, 45–55 (1969)

Costantino, P., De Santis, P., Ughetto, G., Waring, M.J.: Circular dichroism studies on the echinomycin-DNA complex. FEBS Lett. **88**, 349–352 (1978)

Dell, A., Williams, D.H., Morris, H.R., Smith, G.A., Feeney, J., Roberts, G.C.K.: Structure revision of the antibiotic echinomycin. J. Am. Chem. Soc. *97*, 2497–2502 (1975)

Fok, J., Waring, M.J.: Breakdown of pulse-labelled RNA in *Bacillus megaterium* revealed by exposure to the antibiotics mithramycin, chromomycin and nogalamycin. Mol. Pharmacol. *8*, 65–74 (1972)

Hill, L.R.: An index to DNA base compositions of bacterial species. J. Gen. Microbiol. *44*, 419–437 (1966)

Kalman, J.R., Blake, T.J., Williams, D.H., Feeney, J., Roberts, G.C.K.: J. Chem. Soc. Perkin I, 1313–1321 (1979)

Katagiri, K., Yoshida, T., Sato, K.: Quinoxaline antibiotics. In: Antibiotics. Mechanism of action of antimicrobial and antitumour agents. Corcoran, J.W., Hahn, F.E. (eds.), Vol. III, pp. 234–251. Berlin, Heidelberg, New York: Springer 1975

Keller-Schierlein, W., Mihailovič, M.L., Prelog, V.: Stoffwechsel produkte von Actinomyceten. Über die Konstitution von Echinomycin. Helv. Chim. Acta *42*, 305–322 (1959)

Lee, J.S., Waring, M.J.: Bifunctional intercalation and sequence-specificity in the binding of quinomycin and triostin antibiotics to DNA. Biochem. J. **173**, 115–128 (1978a)

Lee, J.S., Waring, M.J.: Interaction between synthetic analogues of quinoxaline antibiotics and nucleic acids: changes in mechanism and specificity related to structural alterations. Biochem. J. **173**, 129–144 (1978b)

Le Pecq, J.B., Le Bret, M., Barbet, J., Roques, B.: DNA polyintercalating drugs: DNA binding of diacridine derivatives. Proc. Natl. Acad. Sci. USA *72*, 2915–2919 (1975)

Martin, D.G., Mizsak, S.A., Biles, C., Stewart, J.C., Baczynskyj, L., Meulman, P.A.: Structure of quinomycin antibiotics. J. Antibiot. *28*, 332–336 (1975)

McGhee, J.D., von Hippel, P.H.: Theoretical aspects of DNA-protein interactions: cooperative and non-cooperative binding of large ligands to a one-dimensional homogeneous lattice. J. Mol. Biol. *86*, 469–489 (1974)

Otsuka, H., Shoji, J.: The structure of triostin C. Tetrahedron *21*, 2931–2938 (1965)

Otsuka, H., Shoji, J., Kawano, K., Kyogoku, Y.: Structure confirmation of triostin A by ^{1}H and ^{13}C magnetic resonance. J. Antibiot. *29*, 107–110 (1976)

Reinert, K.E.: DNA stiffening and elongation caused by the binding of ethidium bromide. Biochim. Biophys. Acta *319*, 135–139 (1973)

Sato, K., Shiratori, O., Katagiri, K.: The mode of action of quinoxaline antibiotics. Interaction of quinomycin A with DNA. J. Antibiot. Ser. A *20*, 270–276 (1967)

Scatchard, G.: The attractions of proteins for small molecules and ions. Ann. N.Y. Acad. Sci. *51*, 660–672 (1949)

Shoji, J., Katagiri, K.: Studies on quinoxaline antibiotics. III. New antibiotics, triostin A, B and C. J. Antibiot. Ser. A *14*, 335–339 (1961)

Shoji, J., Konaka, R., Kawano, K., Higuchi, N., Kyogoku, Y.: Presence of isomers in quinomycin E. J. Antibiot. *29*, 1246–1248 (1976)

Ughetto, G., Waring, M.J.: Conformation of the DNA-binding peptide antibiotic echinomycin based on energy calculations. Mol. Pharmacol. *13*, 579–584 (1977)

Wakelin, L.P.G., Waring, M.J.: The binding of echinomycin to DNA. Biochem. J. *157*, 721–740 (1976)

Wakelin, L.P.G., Romanos, M., Canellakis, E.S., Waring, M.J.: Diacridines as bifunctional DNA-intercalating agents. Stud. Biophys. *60*, 111–118 (1976)

Wakelin, L.P.G., Romanos, M., Glaubiger, D., Canellakis, E.S., Waring, M.J.: Structural limitations on the bifunctional intercalation of diacridines into DNA. Biochemistry **17**, 5057–5063 (1978)

Ward, D., Reich, E., Goldberg, I.H.: Base specificity in the interaction of polynucleotides with antibiotic drugs. Science *149*, 1259–1263 (1965)

Waring, M.J.: Variation of the supercoils in closed circular DNA by binding of antibiotics and drugs: evidence for molecular models involving intercalation. J. Mol. Biol. *54*, 247–279 (1970)

Waring, M.J.: Inhibitors of nucleic acid synthesis. In: The molecular basis of antibiotic action. Gale, E.F., Cundliffe, E., Reynolds, P.E., Richmond, M.H., Waring, M.J. (eds.), pp. 173–277. London: Wiley 1972

Waring, M.J.: Structural constraints in the binding of drugs to DNA. In: Topics in infectious diseases. Drug-receptor interactions in antimicrobial chemotherapy. Drews, J., Hahn, F.E. (eds.), Vol. I, pp. 77–90. Wien, New York: Springer 1975

Waring, M.J.: Structural and conformational studies on quinoxaline antibiotics in relation to the molecular basis of their interaction with DNA. In: Drug action at the molecular level. Roberts, G.C.K. (ed.), pp. 167–189. London: Macmillan 1977

Waring, M.J., Makoff, A.: Breakdown of pulse-labelled RNA and polysomes in *Bacillus megaterium:* Actions of streptolydigin, echinomycin and triostins. Mol. Pharmacol. *10*, 214–224 (1974)

Waring, M.J., Wakelin, L.P.G.: Echinomycin: a bifunctional intercalating antibiotic. Nature (London) *252*, 653–657 (1974)

Waring, M.J., Wakelin, L.P.G., Lee, J.S.: A solvent-partition method for measuring the binding of drugs to DNA. Application to the quinoxaline antibiotics echinomycin and triostin A. Biochim. Biophys. Acta *407*, 200–212 (1975)

Wells, R.D., Larson, J.E.: Studies on the binding of actinomycin D to DNA and DNA model polymers. J. Mol. Biol. *49*, 319–342 (1970)

Yoshida, T., Katagiri, K., Yokozawa, S.: Studies on quinoxaline antibiotics. II. Isolation and properties of quinomycins A, B and C. J. Antibiot. Ser. A *14*, 330–334 (1961)

Ellipticine

K.W. KOHN, W.E. ROSS, and D. GLAUBIGER

Introduction

In an examination of Australian plants for substances with antitumor activity, extracts of two botanically related species, *Ochrosia moorei* and *Excavatia coccinea*, were tested by the National Cancer Institute, U.S.A. They were found active against several transplantable tumors in mice; the activity was mostly accounted for by two alkaloids, ellipticine and 9-methoxy-ellipticine (DALTON et al., 1967). These alkaloids are widely distributed in the related genera *Aspidosperma* and *Ochrosia*. Ellipticine was first identified in extracts of leaves of *O. elliptica* Labill. (family Apocynaceae), a small tropical evergreen tree (GOODWIN et al., 1959); the genus *Ochrosia* is a member of the tribe Plumiereae along with the alkaloid-producing genus *Rauwolfia*. Ellipticine and reserpine alkaloids, which are both based on indole, often occur together in the same plant material. KILMINSTER et al. (1972), in a search for a good botanical source of the alkaloids, extracted ellipticines from various parts of the plant *Bleekeria vitiensis,* a small tree indigenous to the island of Fiji. Ellipticine itself was not present in the leafy material but occurred in other organs of the plant; 9-methoxyellipticine was the major alkaloid and occurred in all parts of the plant examined, the bark and wood being an especially rich source. Several chemical syntheses of ellipticines have been devised (see GUTHRIE et al., 1974 for references).

Ellipticine and its derivatives are of interest both in regard to the mechanisms of their interactions with macromolecules and because of their promise as anti-cancer agents active in man (MATHE et al., 1970; ANSARI et al., 1975; JURET et al., 1977).

Chemistry

Ellipticine is a 4-ring planar aromatic molecule containing two heterocyclic nitrogen atoms and bearing two methyl groups (Fig. 1).

The bond distances, bond angles and deviations from planarity have been determined by X-ray diffraction (COURSEILLE et al., 1974). The molecule tends

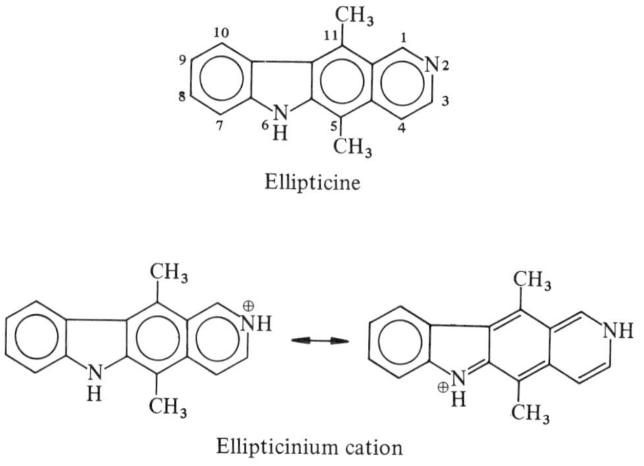

Fig. 1. Structure of ellipticine

to become protonated at the N_2 position ($pK_a = 6.8$[1]; LE PECQ et al., 1974); the resultant positive charge is delocalized over the ring system between the two nitrogen atoms, thereby generating a quadrupole moment (Fig. 1).

The size and shape of the molecule closely resembles that of a purine–pyrimidine complementary base pair (Fig. 2), providing a favorable condition for intercalation in double-stranded nucleic acids. The evidence for intercalative binding will be summarized later. LE PECQ et al. (1974b) suggested that the orientation of the quadrupole moment may influence the helix unwinding angle resulting from intercalation of various ellipticine derivatives.

The ellipticine structure is notable in that, unlike some intercalating antibiotics, the polycyclic ring system bears no side chains and the molecule is not sensitive to oxidation-reduction. At physiologic pH ellipticine exists both in the unprotonated and protonated form. The unprotonated form has a very low solubility in water, and tends to deposit on glass surfaces thus complicating some physical and biological studies. In the protonated form, however, ellipticine is water-soluble and stable. Like many other intercalating drugs, ellipticines tend to self-associate in aqueous solution (DELBARRE et al., 1976), the flat aromatic surfaces of the molecules apposing to form multi-unit stacks. The molecules may be stacked in an anti-parallel fashion, so as to minimize electrostatic repulsion (DELBARRE et al., 1976). These inferences were based on shifts in the proton magnetic resonance peaks as a function of drug concentration. Self-association constants for several ellipticines at pH 4.7 were estimated to be approximately 700 M^{-1}. The dependence of the self-association constant of

1 The anomalously high values of $pK_a > 9$ originally reported for ellipticine, 9-aminoellipticine and 9-hydroxyellipticine (LE PECQ et al. 1974a, b) have been redetermined at very low drug concentrations and were found to be 6.8, 4.9 and 6.6, respectively (J.B. LE PECQ, personal communication). The pK_a values of ellipticine derivatives differing in regard to methylation at positions 5, 6 and 11 or in regard to substitution at position 9 of OH, OCH_3 or $OOCH_3$ all were found to be between 6.1 and 6.9 (J.B. LE PECQ, personal communication).

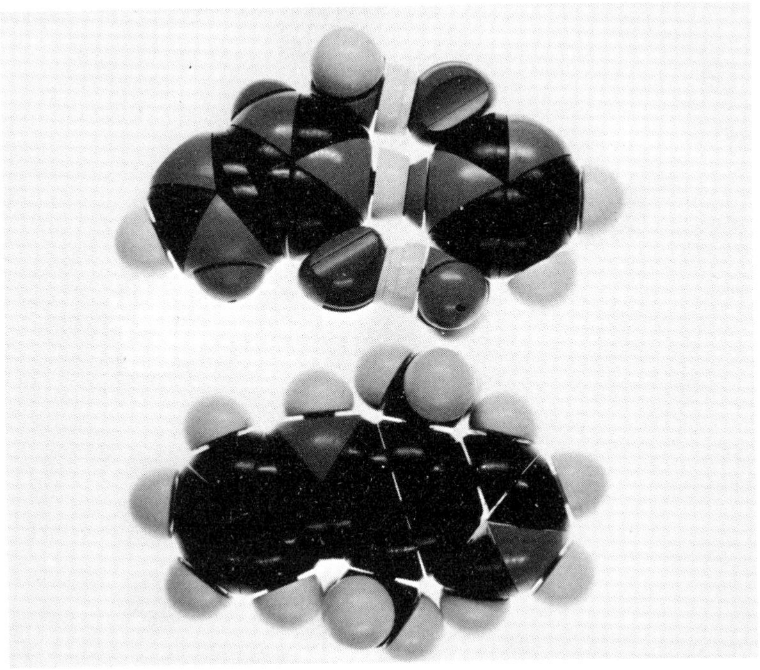

Fig. 2. Molecular models of GC base-pair (*top*) and ellipticine (*bottom*)

9-OH-ellipticine on temperature suggested the thermodynamic values $\Delta H° = 15.6$ kcal/M^{-1}, $\Delta S° = 39$. Self-association is favored by an increased salt concentration which tends to neutralize the repulsion between the positively charged molecules. With the loss of charge at neutral pH, the molecules should have a greater tendency to self-associate.

Binding to Nucleic Acids

The best explanations for some of the major biological effects of ellipticines currently stem from the intercalative binding to double-helical regions of nucleic acids, both DNA and RNA. The binding of ellipticine to DNA is accompanied by the changes in absorption spectrum shown in Figs. 3 and 4. Free ellipticine at pH 7.0 has a multi-component spectrum which becomes markedly altered when DNA is added (Fig. 3). The absorption peak is shifted to longer wavelengths (bathochromism), the amplitude of the peak is reduced (hypochromism), and the multi-component structure is lost. The results with native and denatured DNA were similar, except that larger amounts of denatured DNA were needed to produce comparable effects, and the spectral curves in the case of denatured DNA did not intersect in an isobestic point as well as they did in the case of native DNA. Since the pK_a of ellipticine is 6.8 (J.B. Le Pecq, personal

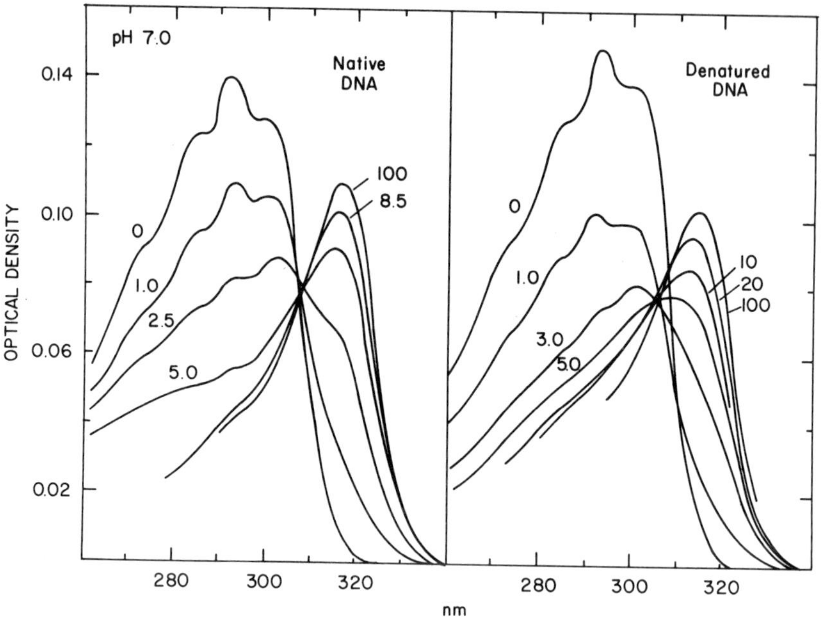

Fig. 3. Spectral changes of ellipticine due to interaction with native and denatured calf thymus DNA at pH 7.0 (0.06 M sodium phosphate). Ellipticine concentration 3.8 μM; 5-cm light path. Mol ratios of DNA nucleotides to ellipticine are indicated (KOHN et al., 1975)

communication), free ellipticine at pH 7.0 should exist both in the protonated and unprotonated form, and this is reflected in the multi-component spectrum. At pH 4.7 (Fig. 4), well below the pK_a, the ellipticine spectrum is dominated by a single peak at 301 nm, which must correspond to the protonated species. In contrast to the large spectral differences between pH 7.0 and 4.7 for free ellipticine, the spectrum of DNA-bound ellipticine was the same at the two pH values. This indicates that the acid-base dissociation of DNA-bound ellipticine is suppressed; bound ellipticine is almost certainly in the protonated form. The binding to native DNA both at pH 7.0 and 4.7 showed a distinct isobestic point, indicating that there is only one mode of binding, or, if several modes exist, they all produce the same spectral change. In the case of denatured DNA, the spectra did not all go through the same point, suggesting some heterogeneity of binding modes.

Ellipticine binding increases the melting temperature (T_m) of DNA, depending on base composition; T_m elevation was seen with poly[d(A–T)] but not with poly[d(G–C)] (BHUYAN et al., 1972). However, association constants measured for ellipticine and a variety of naturally occurring DNA of varying base composition indicate relatively little specificity of the binding for A–T or G–C base pairs (MÜLLER and CROTHERS, 1975).

The strength of binding to DNA is difficult to evaluate because the Scatchard plots are curved (KOHN et al., 1975) indicating heterogeneity of binding constants. The binding constant appears to decrease as the extent of binding in-

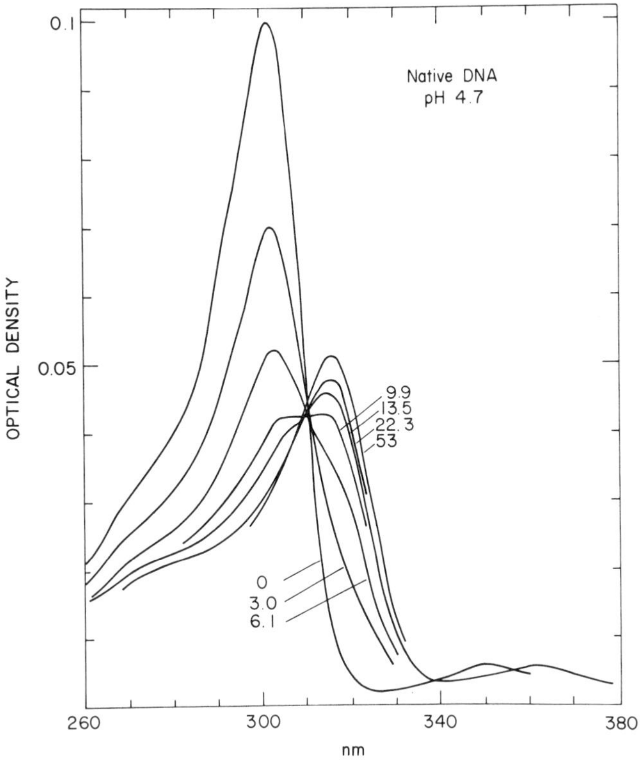

Fig. 4. Spectral changes of ellipticine due to interaction with native calf thymus DNA at pH 4.7 (0.05 M acetic acid-0.05 M sodium acetate-0.05 M NaCl). Ellipticine concentration, 3.0 μM; 10-cm light path. Mol ratios of DNA nucleotides to ellipticine are indicated (KOHN et al., 1975)

creases, suggesting that a bound ellipticine molecule tends to block the binding of other ellipticine molecules nearby. It is clear however that the binding to native DNA is stronger than to denatured DNA. The apparent association constants of ellipticine with calf thymus DNA at a binding ratio of 1 ellipticine/20 nucleotides at pH 7.0, 0.1 M Na^+, 25° C were estimated to be 1.0×10^7 l/mol for native DNA and 0.4×10^7 for denatured DNA. These estimates were based on the slopes of the Scatchard plots at the indicated binding ratio, which was the lowest extent of binding at which the slopes could be reliably estimated. At lower extents of binding the apparent association constants are higher, and at higher extents of binding they are lower.

Thus the association constant of ellipticine with native DNA is remarkably high, being at least as great as that of actinomycin (MÜLLER and CROTHERS, 1968). Actinomycin exhibits slow components in the DNA association and dissociation kinetics, which have been attributed to conformational changes of the side chains in the process of their fitting into the DNA minor groove (MÜLLER and CROTHERS, 1968). Ellipticine is a simple molecule lacking side chains, so that one would not expect slow components in the kinetics (although

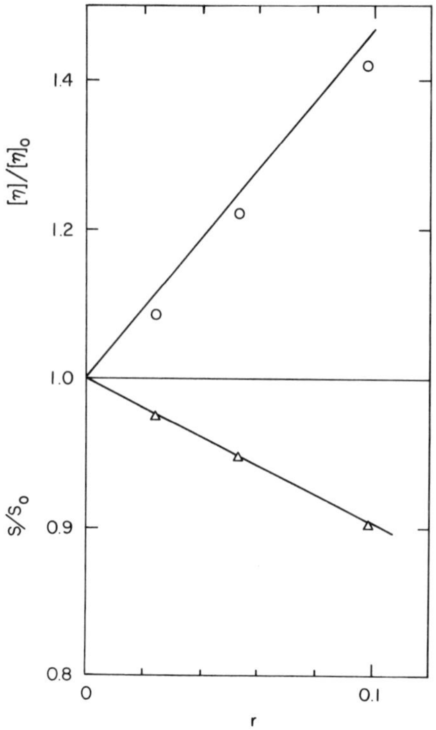

Fig. 5. Dependence of viscosity and sedimentation constant on mol ratio of ellipticine to DNA nucleotides (r). (For details see KOHN et al., 1975)

this expectation remains to be verified). The interesting point is that ellipticine and actinomycin have comparable DNA binding affinities but may have different binding kinetics which may explain differences between the actions of these two antibiotics (MÜLLER and CROTHERS, 1968; KANN and KOHN, 1972).

Lower estimates for the association constant of ellipticines with DNA were derived from measurements of competition with ethidium for DNA binding sites (LE PECQ et al., 1974b). This discrepancy might be due to a reduction in binding constants at DNA sites close to existing sites of intercalation. In any case, the binding of ellipticines was found to be stronger than the binding of ethidium.

There is good evidence that ellipticine and some of its derivatives bind to DNA by intercalation between base-pairs. The ellipticine ring system has dimensions very close to the size and shape of a DNA base pair (Fig. 2). The flat aromatic character of the ellipticine molecule also meets the requirements for intercalation, and the positive charge of the protonated form of ellipticine would further stabilize the intercalated complex. The classic hydrodynamic criteria for intercalation, which consist of an increase in intrinsic viscosity accompanied by a drecrease in sedimentation constant (LERMAN, 1961) were met for the binding of ellipticine to calf thymus DNA (KOHN et. al., 1975).

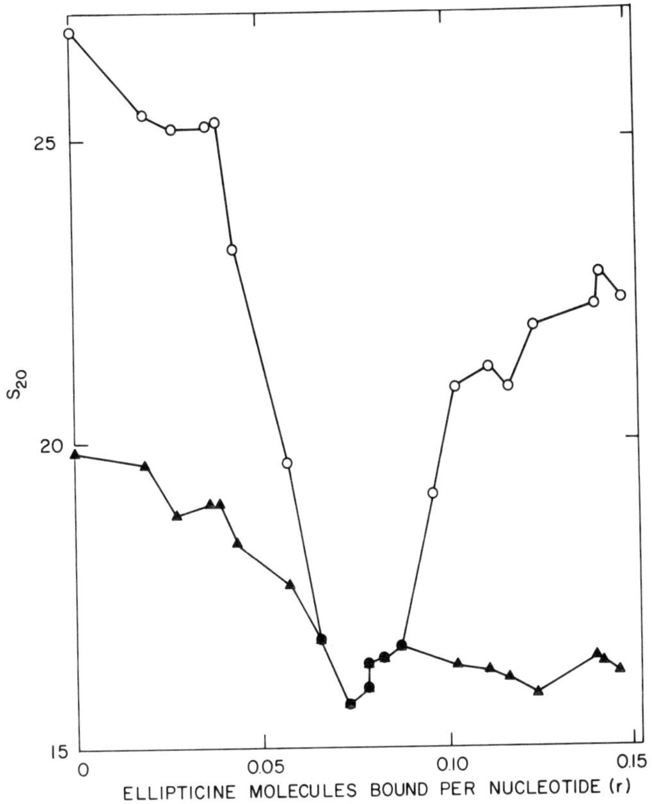

Fig. 6. Effect of ellipticine on sedimentation constant of closed circular DNA helix of phage PM2. (For details see KOHN et al., 1975)

When sonicated DNA is used, these hydrodynamic changes reflect an increase in the length of the rod-like DNA molecules. The increase in length per intercalation should be nearly independent of the identity of the intercalating agents. In accord with this expectation, the effect of 9-methoxyellipticine on the intrinsic viscosity of sonicated calf thymus DNA was quantitatively similar to the effect of ethidium (FESTY et al., 1971). The effects of ellipticine on intrinsic viscosity and sedimentation were similar to those of proflavin (KOHN, et al., 1975) (Fig. 5).

A second line of evidence is the elimination and redevelopment of supercoils in closed circular DNA as the extent of intercalator binding is increased (WARING, 1970). The expected behavior was observed for ellipticine using sedimentation constant as the measure of supercoiling (KOHN et al., 1975) (Fig. 6), and for 9-methoxyellipticine using intrinsic viscosity as the measure of supercoiling (FESTY et al., 1971). In principle, both of these measures of supercoiling permit estimation of the angle of unwinding of the DNA helix per intercalation (WARING, 1970). Although the absolute values of unwinding angles are still uncertain (WANG, 1974), the values for 9-methoxyellipticine (FESTY et al., 1971) and ellipticine (KOHN et al., 1975) both appear to be less than the unwinding angle for ethidium. LE PECQ et al. (1974a, b) estimated unwinding angles for several intercalating ellipticine derivatives to range from 4° to 12° C, relative to an assumed angle of 12° for ethidium. There may be a relationship between unwinding angle and the orientation of the quadrupole axis in the ellipticine ring system (LE PECQ et al., 1974b).

A third type of evidence for intercalation of ellipticine stems from measurements of electric dichroism, which demonstrates that the ellipticine ring system is oriented parallel to the DNA bases (KOHN et al., 1975).

Biochemical Effects

Most of the known biochemical effects of ellipticines seem to be attributable to their binding to double-helical nucleic acids. LI and COWIE (1974) found that ellipticine inhibited DNA polymerase activity in a crude enzyme preparation from L1210 cells, whether primed by salmon sperm DNA, poly[d(A–T)] or poly(dG)·poly(dC). DNA polymerase from *Micrococcus lysodeikticus* was also inhibited by ellipticine, especially when primed by poly(dG)·poly(dC). Ellipticine did not inhibit RNA polymerase activity in isolated mouse liver nuclei. The relative potencies for inhibition of specific eukaryotic polymerases have not been determined.

BENARD and RIOU (1977) studied the effect of 9-hydroxyellipticine on transcription of linear and circular DNA from Trypanosome kinetoplasts by *Escherichia coli* RNA polymerase. The drug was a more effective inhibitor than ethidium. The inhibition seems to be due to an action on DNA rather than on the enzyme, since inhibition could be overcome by adding excess DNA. Both initiation and elongation of RNA chains appeared to be inhibited. The drug was more potent in inhibiting kinetoplast DNA than nuclear DNA from Trypanosomes.

Ellipticine behaves similarly to other DNA intercalating agents (e.g., proflavin and ethidium) in its effects on RNA synthesis and metabolism in L1210 cells in vitro (KANN and KOHN, 1972). In the concentration range 3–20 μM, ellipticine caused a prompt concentration-dependent inhibition both of nuclear and nucleoplasmic RNA synthesis. As with the other intercalating agents, nucleolar RNA synthesis was inhibited to a greater degree than nucleoplasmic RNA synthesis. Thus the synthesis of ribosomal RNA precursors may be inhibited more strongly than the synthesis of messenger RNA precursors.

Ellipticine, like other intercalators, affects RNA metabolism by inhibiting the cleavage steps in the maturational processing of high molecular weight RNA precursors (SYNDER et al., 1971). This is most clearly demonstrable for the cleavage of the 45s rRNA precursors to the 32s stage. Evidence has also been obtained for the inhibition of the cleavage of high molecular weight heterogeneous nucleoplasmic RNA (KOHN et al., 1973). It was hypothesized that this type of action may be due to intercalation at sites in the RNA where there are helical "hairpin" loops which may be supposed to act as recognition sites for specific cleavage or excision in the course of RNA maturation. Thus ellipticine inhibits the formation in cells of functional rRNA and mRNA molecules both by inhibiting RNA synthesis and by inhibiting the maturational processing of large precursor molecules.

Ellipticine and other intercalators have been found to inhibit RNA methylase reactions in isolated nucleoli (LIAU et al., 1977). Nucleoli from Novikoff ascites hepatoma were more sensitive than rat liver nucleoli to the inhibition of rRNA methylation by ellipticine, ethidium and lucanthone. In a soluble methylase system from tumor nucleoli, ellipticine inhibited tRNA methylation mainly at adenine sites and, at a higher drug concentration at guanine sites. Ellipticine may bring about this inhibition by distorting the tRNA molecule by intercalation at specific helical sites in the tRNA molecule. Interestingly, methylation of histones in rat liver nuclei by S-adenosyl-methionine and lysine methyltransferase was stimulated by 9-OH ellipticine and 2-methyl-9-OH ellipticine (BYVOET and SAYRE, 1977). The distortion of helical structure in DNA due to intercalation of 9-hydroxyellipticine appears to interfere with the DNA binding of uterine estradiol-receptor complex (ANDRE et al., 1976). Ellipticine, like other intercalating agents, has recently been found to produce DNA single-strand breaks that appear to be associated with DNA-protein crosslinks (ROSS et al., 1978).

Effects on Cells

The previously discussed chemical characteristics of the ellipticine molecule would be expected to bear on its effects on cells, as well as on its pharmacologic behavior. The non-polar polycyclic aromatic character of the molecule confers a very low water solubility and a high lipid solubility at physiologic pH. The octanol/water partition ratio is of the order of 10^2 (CHADWICK et al., 1978) or 10^4 (HANSCH, 1972). The flat, highly aromatic ring system should promote adherence to surfaces having a low degree of polarity, such as membranes and appropriately conformed hydrophobic regions of proteins, as well as to nucleic acids. The ability of the ellipticine molecule to become protonated and positively charged with the pK_a not far below physiologic pH, would be expected to favor binding to hydrophobic surfaces associated with negative charge, as has been discussed for the binding of cationic ellipticine to DNA. Similar binding circumstances may apply to cell membranes and to certain protein molecules, so that cellular and pharmacologic effects could arise from interaction of the drug with several types of macromolecules.

The affinity of ellipticine for cell membranes is illustrated by its interaction with erythrocytes (HERMAN et al., 1971, 1974; LEE, 1975). LEE (1976) reported binding of ellipticine to erythrocytes in isotonic NaCl. The uptake of ellipticine by erythrocytes was rapid (occurring within 1 min) and independent of temperature, and the apparent concentration in the erythrocyte compartment was much greater than in the external medium. Most of the ellipticine remained in hemolysed ghosts, suggesting localization in the membrane. Upon isolation and separation of various lipid fractions of the erythrocyte membrane, most of the ellipticine was recovered in phospholipid fractions. Although the association of ellipticine with phospholipids after isolation procedures does not imply that this relationship exists in intact cells or membranes, phospholipids do meet the suggested requirements for strong ellipticine binding in having negative charges as well as hydrophobic character.

Ellipticine concentrations above a critical value of about 10^{-4} M produced rapid hemolysis (LEE, 1976); this correlated with the micellar concentration of the drug in that the same ellipticine concentration produced a sharp drop in surface tension. Hemolysis could result from accumulation of a critical ellipticine concentration in the erythrocyte membrane. Hemolysis did not occur with the slightly less hydrophobic 9-methoxy-and 11-demethyl ellipticines.

Another possible manifestation of an affinity for membrane or hydrophobic sites, is the effect of ellipticine on mitochondrial function (GOSALVEZ et al., 1974). Ellipticine appeared to uncouple oxidative phosphorylation and, under some conditions, to inhibit respiration. Ehrlich ascites tumor cells were more affected than pig leukocytes.

ALAZARD et al. (1976) studied the effects of 9-hydroxy-ellipticine on *E. coli*. Growth rate (measured turbidimetrically) decreased linearly with increasing drug concentration, but viability remained unimpaired up to 15 μM (2-h drug exposure), beyond which it declined rapidly. In the sublethal concentration range (< 15 μM), the growth inhibition could be immediately reversed by filtering and washing the bacteria and resuspending them in fresh warm medium. It was also possible to reverse the growth inhibition by raising the Mg^{2+} concentration in the medium from 0.1 mM to 10 mM. At a sublethal drug concentration of 12 μM, there was an immediate 40% reduction of precursor incorporation rates into protein and RNA, but little change in the rate of thymidine incorporation into DNA. At 20 μM, which killed 55% of the organisms in 2 h, all three of the macromolecular syntheses were completely inhibited.

Several studies in mammalian cells have characterized the effects of ellipticines on cell proliferation and survival, and have examined some effects on macromolecular syntheses. LI and COWIE (1974), studying mouse leukemia L1210 cells found that the cells continued to proliferate exponentially in the presence of 0.7 μM of ellipticine or 9-methoxyellipticine, although the doubling time was increased by approximately a factor of 2. Proliferation was almost completely inhibited at a concentration of 4 μM of either drug. The inhibited proliferation was not reversed by increasing the medium concentrations of various metabolites, such as purines, pyrimidines, vitamins or amino acids. The inhibition of proliferation by ellipticine could not be reversed after a contact period of 15–120 min, probably because of the tightness of binding of the drug to nucleic acids and possibly other sites, or the inadequacy of the wash procedure. Indeed, BHUYAN et al. (1972) found that survival of L1210 cells or DON cells was progressively reduced as a function of drug exposure times covering many hours; these survival experiments entailed large dilution factors of the cells for the cloning assays, thereby facilitating the removal of drug. In the cloning assays of BHUYAN et al. (1972), 50% loss of colony-forming ability resulted from 1 h treatments at ellipticine concentrations of 4 μM for L1210 cells and 16 μM for DON cells. These same treatments inhibited DNA, RNA, and protein synthesis to the extents of approximately 55%, 70% and 30%, respectively in L1210 cells; and 70%, 70% and

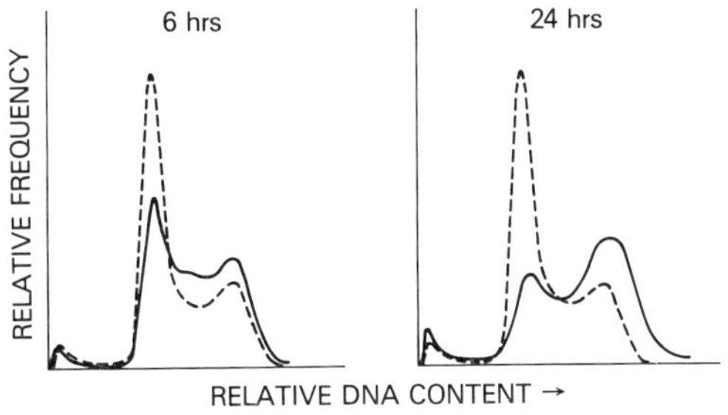

Fig. 7. Effect of ellipticine on DNA content distribution in an exponentially growing L1210 cell culture. Cells were grown in RPMI 1630 medium containing 20% fetal calf serum with (——) or without (– – –) 2.5 μM ellipticine. In the presence of drug, proliferation rate was reduced 50%. Cells were stained with propidium iodide in hypotonic medium and analysed by flow microfluorometry. (Data of R. DION and V. BONO, JR., unpublished data)

45% respectively in DON cells (1-h precursor incorporation periods coincident with drug exposure). These data suggest RNA synthesis inhibition as a possible correlate of proliferative survival in different cell types. An ellipticine:DNA complex has also been shown to exhibit cytotoxicity towards L1210 cells in culture (SORACE and SHEID, 1977).

Small differences in sensitivity to ellipticine have been observed as a function of time in the cell cycle (BHUYAN et al., 1972). Cell survival, measured in DON cells by cloning at various times after mitotic selection, was most sensitive to the drug near the end of S phase and became most insensitive near the time of mitosis. An initial high drug sensitivity of newly planted mitotic cells was observed, but this could have resulted in part from a surface effect of the drug rather than to an intrinsically high sensitivity of this phase of the cycle. There was no appreciable variation in ^{14}C-ellipticine uptake through the cell cycle, nor did there appear to be any correlation between cell cycle sensitivity and macromolecular synthesis inhibition, but this question demands further study.

TOBEY et al. (1972) studied drug effects on the cell cycle of CHO cells by means of an autoradiographic technique, and concluded that ellipticine blocks the onset of S phase but does not prevent continued DNA synthesis in cells already in S at the time of drug addition. They concluded also that the drug inhibits the completion of G2 phase. This latter type of effect appeared to be the dominant one in L1210 cells studied by flow microfluorimetry (R. DION and V.H. BONO, JR., unpublished data; Fig. 7). The DNA content distribution after 6 h of treatment with 2.5 μM ellipticine suggested a slowing of DNA synthesis and an interference with cell division after completion of DNA synthesis. After 24 h, most of the cells appeared to be blocked at or near G2 phase.

As is the rule with DNA-reactive compounds, ellipticine produces marked chromosomal abnormalities (BHUYAN et al., 1972). The abnormalities noted included achromatic gaps, chromatid breaks, chromatid interchanges and fragmented chromosomes. Ellipticine and many of its congeners are mutagenic by the Ames test and mutagenicity is enhanced if the test is performed in the presence of hepatic microsomes (J.B. LE PECQ, personal communication). Interestingly, the quaternized derivative 2-methyl-9-OH ellipticine is devoid of mutagenicity.

Pharmacology and Toxicology

The previously described properties of the ellipticine molecule, particularly its lipophilicity and acid-base properties, are key elements in the drug's pharmacologic behavior.

Intravenously administered ellipticine (CHADWICK et al., 1978) or 9-hydroxy-ellipticine (LE PECQ, personal communication) distribute very quickly to different tissues; the compounds disappear from the blood in a very rapid phase within a few minutes, followed by a slower phase. CHADWICK et al. (1978) administered ellipticine-1-^{14}C intravenously into several species of mammals and studied its physiologic disposition. Within 2 min after administration, over 90% of the drug had disappeared from the circulating blood compartment; the apparent volume of distribution was between 2.6 and 6.8 l/kg, depending on the species. This very rapid removal of drug from the circulation into an apparent distribution volume much greater than the total body water compartment may reflect binding to tissue surfaces or macromolecules and concentration in lipid phases. The drug remaining in the blood following the rapid phase of distribution is probably bound to blood cells and perhaps also to plasma proteins. The remaining ellipticine then disappears from the blood with half-times between 20 and 200 min, depending upon the species of animal. Most of this elimination rate is due to conversion of ellipticine to metabolic products. The elimination half-times for the metabolites were between 140 and 320 min.

The main elimination path for ellipticine is by metabolism in the liver and secretion of conjugated metabolites into the bile. The mono-oxygenase system of rat liver hydroxylates ellipticine mainly at position 9, and to a lesser degree at one or more other, as yet undetermined, positions (LESCA et al., 1976, 1978; CHADWICK et al., 1978). This activity is probably a function of cytochrome P-448, and can be induced by pretreatment of rats with 3-methylcholanthrene and less effectively with phenobarbital. Ellipticine itself is an effective inducer (LESCA et al., 1978). Ellipticine also tends to inhibit its own hydroxylation, as well as that of benzypyrene, probably by binding to the iron atoms of the cytochromes (LESCA et al., 1978).

The expected mechanism of hydroxylation would involve epoxidation across positions 9 and 10, followed by an "NIH shift" of the hydrogen (or deuterium) atom from position 9 to 10. Deuterium atoms at position 9 of ellipticine however failed to be retained in the molecule, contrary to NIH shift specifications, and an explanation of how the deuterium atom might be lost is suggested by REINHOLD and BRUNI (1976). The hydroxylated compounds are conjugated in the liver to the glucuronide and sulfate; the formation of these two conjugates of 9-hydroxy-ellipticine has been verified by mass spectrometry (BRANFMAN et al., 1978). Whether ellipticine may be metabolized in tissues other than liver is uncertain. Both conjugates are negatively charged and hence probably do not enter cells; they are probably inactive metabolites, although they have not been tested for anti-tumor activity. 9-Hydroxyellipticine however is fully active.

The conjugated and nonconjugated ellipticine derivates can be distinguished on the basis of extractability into ethyl acetate; the conjugated derivatives are charged and therefore unextractable, whereas the unconjugated forms are readily extracted. The conjugated metabolites are secreted into the bile. CHADWICK et al., 1978 found 60% of an intravenously injected dose of ellipticine-1-^{14}C secreted into the bile of rats in a 24 h period; almost all was in conjugated form.

Ellipticine or its unconjugated metabolites may be sequestered into the gastointestinal tract through the stomach wall (CHADWICK et al., 1978) by the mechanism of ion trapping. At the gastric pH, which is far below the ellipticine pK_a of approximately 6, the acid-base equilibrium heavily favors the ionized form of the drug which perhaps does not permeate the mucosal lining. This mechanism may account for the finding that the fraction of ellipticine in nonconjugated form is greater in feces than in bile (CHADWICK et al., 1978). LE PECQ (personal communication) however suggests that 9-hydroxyellipticine glucuronide is partly hydrolyzed in the small intestine back to 9-hydroxyellipticine.

PAOLETTI et al. (1977) report that a derivative that is not glucuronidated or otherwise metabolized is 2-methyl-9-hydroxyellipticinium. This cationic derivative, which retains anti-tumor activity, reportedly differs from most nonquaternary ellipticines in being nonmutagenic. The mutagenic activity of nonquarternary ellipticines is said to be increased by incubation with microsomal enzymes in the Ames system, while the quarternary compounds are unaffected by these enzymes (PAOLETTI et al., 1977; LE PECQ, personal communication). Orally administered ellipticine is fully effective in anti-tumor treatment of mice, although 2–4 times the intraperitoneal dose may be required (NCI Screening data). The acid medium of the stomach would tend to dissolve and dilute the drug; the acid form of the drug however would probably not be absorbed. Absorption could occur after passage to the alkaline regions of the small intestine.

Ellipticine or its metabolites are excreted primarily in feces and secondarily in urine (HARDESTY et al., 1972; CHADWICK et al., 1978). CHADWICK et al. recovered 70%–80% of an intravenous dose of ellipticine-1-^{14}C in the feces and 8%–15% in urine. In mouse, rat, and dog this excretion was complete within 24 h, whereas in monkeys it occurred gradually over a 5-day period. The slower fecal excretion by monkeys could be due to a possibly more effective reabsorption of the compounds from the gastrointestinal tract, thus producing a more extensive enterohepatic circuit.

Ellipticine is rapidly distributed into most, or all, animal tissues, including brain (HARDESTY et al., 1972; CHADWICK et al., 1978). Within 24 h, almost all of the drug was either eliminated or conjugated, and no detectable unconjugated drug remained in any tissue of dog, rat, monkey or mouse (CHADWICK et al., 1978). Small quantities, remaining tightly bound to specific sites, may of course go undetected. The tissues accumulating the greatest concentrations of unconjugated drug included liver, pancreas, adrenals, spleen, lymph nodes, and kidney, but this varied somewhat depending on animal species and the time after drug administration. The amounts detected in brain, heart, lung, and bone marrow tended to be smaller but still substantial.

The cationic charge of quaternary ellipticines would be expected to retard the passage through membrane barriers and therefore to affect tissue distribution. Thus methylation at the N_2 position was found to eliminate the ability of the drug to concentrate in lungs and pancreas and to increase accumulation in the intestinal walls and in the thyroid (LE PECQ, personal communication). The charge would be expected also to interfere with entry into the brain. Within the brain, ellipticine especially localizes in the Purkinje neurons and granular cells of the cerebellum. This was demonstrated by whole body radio-autography after administration of ^{14}C-ellipticine to mice. The Purkinje cells exhibited alterations of ultrastructure which affected polysomes and the endoplasmic reticulum of the Nissl substance, and perhaps relates to the neurologic toxicity of the drug.

9-hydroxyellipticine, like ellipticine, produces preferential lesions of cerebellar Purkinje cells which appear to be responsible for locomotor disturbances in mice (CROS et al., 1975).

In addition to the neurologic toxicity attributable to effects on the cerebellum, 9-hydroxyellipticine depressed granulocyte and lymphocyte counts and caused transient hypothermia in mice and dogs (CHANH et al., 1974; CROS et al., 1975). The mechanism of ellipticine-induced hemolysis has been previously discussed. This hemolysis was reported to be prevented by adding citrate or EDTA to the solvent (LEE, 1976). Hemolysis in vivo however occurred only during the injection period of a few minutes. Since ellipticine is quite stable (in slightly acidic medium in the dark), hemolysis and other immediate toxicities (HERMAN et al., 1971) should be avoidable by slow intravenous infusion or by oral administration.

Ellipticine and its congeners exert complex dose-dependent effects on the cardiovascular system. HERMAN et al. (1974) found that low doses of ellipticine (5–20 mg/kg) administered intravenously to monkeys produced transient decreases in arterial blood pressure and heart rate while carotid artery blood flow increased. These parameters returned to normal 5–10 min post-injection. Higher doses (27–40 mg/kg) resulted in irreversible cardiovascular and respiratory depression (HERMAN et al., 1971). Qualitatively similar results were obtained by HERMAN et al. (1974) for 9-methoxyellipticine, 7, 10-dimethylellipticine and 11-demethylellipticine. Interestingly CHANH et al. (1976) reported that intravenous 9-OH ellipticine, 1–10 mg/kg, produced only positive inotropic effects in the anesthetized dog. In an isolated perfused dog heart preparation, ellipticine caused a brief (5 min) reduction in rate and force of contraction which was followed by recovery to supranormal values. This recovery was blocked by the beta-adrenergic antagonist *dl*-propranolol and by reserpine which depletes intramyocardial catecholamine stores. Higher concentrations of ellipticine, produced prolonged depression in force and rate of contraction. In summary, ellipticine and its congeners cause cardiac depression which, at lower doses, is overcome by mechanisms which appear to involve release of endogenous catecholamines. At higher doses the depression is less easily reversed. No data are available concerning cumulative myocardial toxicity and further studies are needed.

Anti-Tumor Activity

The anti-tumor activity of ellipticine derivatives has in general correlated with their capacity for intercalative DNA binding. Thus, disturbing the aromatic planarity of the ring system, for example by hydrogenating the 3 and 4 positions, destroys anti-tumor activity (Screening data of the National Cancer Institute's Developmental Therapeutics Program). LE PECQ et al. (1974a) tested several ellipticine derivatives both for anti-tumor activity (mouse leukemia L1210 system) and for DNA intercalation. They found that substitution of $-OH$ or $-OCH_3$ at position 9 or substitution of $-CH_3$ at the N_6 position yielded compounds that were both active and strongly intercalating (high association constant). Substitution of an isopentyl group at N_6 abolished both activity and ability to intercalate. Removing the ellipticine methyl groups greatly reduced the DNA binding constant and eliminated activity. 9-Bromoellipticine was inactive although it bound strongly to DNA; however the binding was not by intercalation. 9-Aminoellipticine seemed to present a contradiction, since it bound strongly by intercalation, but was inactive; HAYAT et al. (1974) however found this compound to have activity. The correlation between anti-tumor activity and DNA intercalation therefore in this series of compounds remains untarnished.

HANSCH (1972) analyzed strategies for drug design using ellipticine as an example. Since substitution of even a few types of substituents at all possible positions of the ellipticine ring, and in all possible combinations, would lead to millions of derivatives to be synthesized and tested, some strategy is needed to guide the choice of structures. HANSCH discussed strategies based on the use of substituent constants and regression analysis. Although nearly 100 ellipticine derivatives have now been tested, the available information is still fragmentary, and a concerted effort to apply a guided approach such as that suggested by HANSCH remains to be attempted.

The structure-activity data summarized below was derived from the Developmental Therapeutics Program of the National Cancer Institute, unless otherwise indicated. All of the data are based on intraperitoneally inoculated mouse leukemia L1210. The results of substitutions at various positions of ellipticine lead to the following inferences.

Position 1. Methylation preserves activity, but substitution of a Br, butyl, or phenyl group leads to inactive derivatives.

Position 2. Methylation (which introduces a positive charge) preserves activity. N-oxide derivatives are inactive.

Position 3. Methylation inactivates.

Position 4. No data.

Position 5. Removal of both methyl groups from ellipticine inactivates.

Position 6. Substitution introduces a positive charge. Substitutions of methyl, allyl, hydroxethyl, or epoxyproyl preserved activity, but larger substitutions usually inactivate. PAOLETTI et al. (1977) however report active derivatives bearing at this position diethylaminoethyl or 1-piperidinyl-ethyl.

Position 7. 7, 10-dimethylellipticine is inactive.

Position 8. No data.

Position 9. LE PECQ et al. (1974a) reported that 9-hydroxellipticine is more active than ellipticine when tested using a single intraperitoneal injection. The NCI Developmental Therapeutics Program however used multiple-injection schedules and failed to find a significant difference between the drugs. The 9-methoxy derivative also is active. The Br derivative is inactive (LE PECQ et al., 1974), as are derivatives bearing at this position Cl, methyl or phenyl (NCI data).

Position 10. 7, 10-dimethylellipticine is inactive.

Position 11. Removal of the 11-methyl group was reported by LE PECQ et al. (1974a) and HAYAT et al. (1974) to destroy activity; extensive tests by the NCI, however, indicated retention of a high degree of activity. There is agreement that removal of both methyl groups inactivates.

Thus ellipticine can be modified by attaching groups at several positions without loss of activity. Opportunities for design of improved structures exist but have not been fully exploited.

In the treatment of L1210 leukemia, ellipticine was fully effective when given by the oral route, although two to four times the intraperitoneal dose was required for equal effectiveness (NCI screening data). SVOBODA et al. (1968) had shown the effectiveness of oral therapy of 9-methoxyellipticine against several rodent tumors.

LE PECQ et al. (1976) compared the intraperitoneal and intravenous routes of administration of 9-hydroxyellipticine. When tested against intraperitoneally inoculated L1210 tumor, the drug was much more effective administered intraperitoneally than intravenously. In the case of an intravenously inoculated tumor however, the two routes of drug injection gave identical results. The simplest explanation for these findings would appear to be that some of the intraperitoneally administered drug, perhaps because of its limited solubility or surface sticking tendencies, remains localized in the peritoneal cavity for a period of time, and that tumor cells localized in the peritoneal cavity are therefore exposed to a relatively high drug concentration.

NCI screening tests showed ellipticine to be active against mouse leukemias L1210, P388 and AKR, melanoma B16, colon tumors 26 and 28 of mice, and Walker 256 tumor of rats. No consistent activity was seen against Lewis lung carcinoma or mouse ependymoblastoma.

Since ellipticine penetrates into the central nervous system, one might hope for activity against intracranial tumors. Although the NCI screening program has obtained a few positive results, the results are insufficient for a firm conclusion. Le Pecq et al. (1976) bioassayed L1210 cells located in mouse brain after intraperitoneal inoculation and observed an action of 9-hydroxyellipticine against these cells.

Perspective

Ellipticine is of interest both as an experimental tool and for its anti-cancer potential. Its simple chemical structure and clearly defined properties make it suitable for studies of the details of interactions with macromolecules and for exploration of structure-activity relations. It may be considered to be the sine-qua-non of intercalating agents because of its close approximation to the geometry of a purine–pyrimidine base pair and lack of such complicating structural features as side chains or groups highly sensitive to oxidation–reduction or the formation of free radicals. Considering the simplicity of the molecule, it has an unusually high binding affinity for helical nucleic acids.

A particularly noteworthy feature of its chemistry, which distinguishes it from other simple intercalators, is the acid-base equilibrium which allows the molecule to assume either a cationic or an uncharged state under physiologic conditions. Thus the binding to nucleic acids is stabilized by the acquisition of a positive charge, while the uncharged species readily penetrates membrane barriers. These features confer to the drug both desirable and undesirable properties from the pharmacologic standpoint. Particularly notable are the ability of the drug to penetrate the central nervous system and its activity by the oral route. It is not surprising, in view of the structural simplicity upon which the drug's actions are founded, that there are multiple sites of action some of which may lead to undesirable effects. The molecule however is suitable for systematic exploration of structure modification in search of compounds with optimized features.

Acknowledgments. We are grateful to Dr. J.B. Le Pecq for copies of manuscript pre-prints and for the unpublished data quoted in the text as personal communications. We also thank Drs. J.A.R. Mead, D. Abraham, and V.H. Bono, Jr., Mssrs. G. Hazard and R. Dion, and Ms. R. Davis for unpublished information from the National Cancer Institute.

References

Alazard, R., Boquet, P.L., Paoletti, C.: Effects of 9-hydroxyellipticine on growth and macromolecular synthesis in *Escherichia coli*. FEBS Lett. *63*, 278–282 (1976)

Andreé, J., Pfeiffer, A., Rochefort, H.: Inhibition of estrogen-receptor-DNA interaction by intercalating drugs. Biochem. *15*, 2964–2969 (1976)

Ansari, B.M., Thompson, E.N.: Methoxy-9-ellipticine in refractory acute myeloid leukemia. Postgrad. Med. J. *51*, 103–105 (1975)

Bénard, J., Riou, G.: Effects of 9-hydroxy ellipticine on in vitro transcription of *Trypanosoma cruzi* DNAs. Biochem. Biophys. Res. Commun. *77*, 1189–1195 (1977)

Bhuyan, B.K., Fraser, T.J., Li, L.H.: Cell cycle phase specificity and biochemical effects of ellipticine on mammalian cells. Cancer Res. *32*, 2538–2544 (1972)

Branfman, A.R., Bruni, R.J., Reinhold, V.N., Silveira, D., Chadwick, M., Yesair, D.W.: Characterization of the metabolites of ellipticine in rat bile. Drug Metab. Dispos. *6*, 542–548 (1978)

Byvoet, P., Sayre, D.: Stimulation of histone methylation by intercalating anti-tumor drugs. Proc. Am. Assoc. Can. Res. *17*, 156 (1977)

Chadwick, M., Platz, B.B., Hayes, D., Silveria, D.: Comparative physiological disposition of ellipticine in several animal species after intravenous administration. Drug Metab. Dispos. (in press, 1978)

Chanh, P.H., Sorbara, R., Dat-Xuong, N., Le Pecq, J.B., Paoletti, C.: Action cardiovasculaire et toxicite de l'hydroxy-9-ellipticine chez le chien. C.R. Acad. Sci. D. *279*, 1039–1043 (1974)

Chanh, P.H., Dat-Xuong, N., Le Pecq, J.B., Paoletti, C.: Cardiovascular activity of 9-hydroxy-ellipticine. Pharmacology *14*, 490–498 (1976)

Courseille, P.C., Busetta, B., Hospital, M.: Structure cristalline et moleculaire du dimethyl-5,11 6H-pyrido[4,3-b] carbazole (ellipticine). Acta Cryst. *30*, 2628–2631 (1974)

Cros, S., Sorbara, R., Moisand, Ch., Dat-Xuong, N., Lecointe, P., Paoletti, C.: Toxicological and pharmacological studies on 9-hydroxy-ellipticine in mice. Toxicol. Appl. Pharmacol. *33*, 484–497 (1975)

Dalton, L.K., Demerac, S., Elmes, B.L., Loder, J.W., Swan, J.M., Teitei, T.: Synthesis of the tumor-inhibitory alkaloids, ellipticine, 9-methoxyellipticine, and related pyrido[4,3-b]carbazoles. Aust. J. Chem. *20*, 2715 (1967)

Delbarre, A., Roques, B.P., Le Pecq, J.B., Lallemand, J.Y., Dat-Xuong, N.: PMR studies of the self-association of DNA intercalating ellipticine derivatives in aqueous solution. Biophys. Chem. *4*, 275–279 (1976)

Festy, B., Poisson, J., Paoletti, C.: A new DNA intercalating drug: methoxy-9-ellipticine. FEBS Lett. *17*, 321–323 (1971)

Goodwin, S., Smith, A.F., Horning, E.C.: Alkaloids of ochrosia elliptica labill. J. Am. Chem. Soc. *81*, 1903 (1959)

Gosalvez, M., Blanco, M., Hunter, J., Miko, M., Chance, B.: Effects of anticancer agents on the respiration of isolated mitochondria and tumor cells. Eur. J. Cancer *10*, 567–574 (1974)

Guthrie, R.W., Brossi, A., Mennona, F.A., Mullin, J.G., Kierstead, R.W.: Ellipticine derivatives. J. Chem. *18*, 755–760 (1974)

Hansch, C.: Commentary: strategy in drug design. Cancer Chemother. Rep. *56*, 433–441 (1972)

Hardesty, C.T., Chaney, N.A., Mead, J.A.R.: The effect of route of administration on the distribution of ellipticine in mice. Cancer Res. *32*, 1884–1889 (1972)

Hayat, M., Mathe, G., Janot, M.M., Potier, P., Dat-Xuong, N., Cave, A., Sevenet, T., Kan-Fan, C., Poisson, J., Miet, J., Le Men, J., Le Goffic, F., Gouyette, A., Ahond, A., Dalton, L.K., Connors, T.A.: Experimental screening of 3 forms and 19 derivatives or analogs of ellipticine: oncostatic effect on L1210 leukemia and immunosuppressive effect of 4 of them. Biomedicine *21*, 101–106 (1974)

Herman, E., Vick, J., Burka, B.: The cardiovascular actions of ellipticine. Toxicol. Appl. Pharmacol. *18*, 743–751 (1971)

Herman, E.H., Chadwick, D.P., Mhatre, R.M.: Comparison of the acute hemolytic and cardiovascular actions of ellipticine (NSC-71795) and some ellipticine analogs. Cancer Chemother. Rep. *58*, 637–642 (1974)

Juret, P., Tanguy, A., Girard, A., Le Talaer, J.Y., Dat-Xuong, N., Le Pecq, J.B., Paoletti, C.: Preliminary trial of 9-hydroxy-2-methylellipticinium (NSC 264-137) in advanced human cancers. Eur. J. Can. (in press, 1977)

Kann, H.E., Jr., Kohn, K.W.: Effects of deoxyribonucleic acid-reactive drugs on ribonucleic acid synthesis in leukemia L1210 cells. Mol. Pharmacol. *8*, 551–560 (1972)

Kilminster, K.N., Sainsbury, M., Webb, B.: Alkaloids and terpenoids of bleekevia vitiensis. Phytochemistry *11*, 389 (1972)

Kohn, K.W., Snyder, A.L., Kann, H.E., Jr.: Size distributions of high molecular weight RNA synthesized by L1210 cells: effects of DNA-reactive drugs. Biochim. Biophys. Acta *324*, 93–109 (1973)

Kohn, K.W., Waring, M.J., Glaubiger, D., Friedman, C.A.: Intercalative binding of ellipticine to DNA. Cancer Res. *35*, 71–76 (1975)

Lee, I.P.: A possible mechanism of ellipticine-induced hemolysis. J. Pharmacol. Exp. Ther. *196*, 525–535 (1976)

Le Pecq, J.B., Dat-Xuong, N., Goose, C., Paoletti, C.: A new antitumoral agent: 9-hydroxyellipticine. Possibility of a rational design of anticancerous drugs in the series of DNA intercalating drugs. Proc. Natl. Acad. Sci. USA *71*, 5078–5082 (1974a)

Le Pecq, J.B., LeBret, M., Goose, Ch., Paoletti, C.: Interest of quantum mechanical calculations for the design of anticancerous drugs in the series of ellipticines. In: Molecular and quantum pharmacology. Bergmann, E., Pullman, B. (eds.), pp. 515–535. Dordecht-Holland: D. Reidel 1974b

Le Pecq, J.B., Goose, C., Dat-Xuong, N., Cros, S., Paoletti, C.: Antitumor activity of 9-hydroxyellipticine (NSC 210717) on L1210 mouse leukemia and the effect of route of injection. Cancer Res. *36*, 3067–3076 (1976)

Lerman, L.S.: Structural considerations in the interaction of DNA and acridines. J. Mol. Biol. *3*, 18 (1961)

Lesca, P., Lecointe, P., Paoletti, C., Mansuy, D.: Induction des mono-oxygenases hepatiques par l'ellipticine chez le rat: formation de cytochrome P_{488} activite hydroxylante. C.R. Acad. Sci. D *282*, 1457–1460 (1976)

Lesca, P., Lecointe, P., Paoletti, C.: The hydroxylation of the antitumor agent, ellipticine, by liver microsomes from differently pretreated rats. Biochem. Pharmacol. *27*, 1203–1209 (1978)

Li, L.H., Cowie, C.H.: Biochemical effects of ellipticine leukemia L1210 cells. Biochim. Biophys. Acta *353*, 375–384 (1974)

Liau, M.C., Lin, G.W., Knight, C.A., Hurlbert, R.B.: Inhibition of RNA methylation by intercalating agents. Cancer Res. *37*, 4202–4210 (1977)

Mathe, G., Hayat, M., De Vassal, F., Schwatzenberg, L., Schneider, J.R., Schlumberger, C., Jasmin, C., Rosenfeld, C.: Methoxy 9-ellipticine lactate III. Clinical screening: its action in acute myeloblastic leukemia. Rev. Eur. Etud. Clin. Biol. *15*, 541 (1970)

Müller, W., Crothers, D.M.: Studies of the binding of actinomycin and related compounds to DNA. Eur. J. Biochem. *35*, 251–290 (1968)

Müller, W., Crothers, D.M.: Interactions of heteroaromatic compounds with nucleic acids. 1. The influence of heteroatoms and polarizability on the base specificity of intercalating ligands. Eur. J. Biochem. *54*, 267–277 (1975)

Mullin, J.G., Kierstead, R.W., Grunberg, E.: Ellipticine derivatives. J. Med. Chem. *18*, 755–760 (1975)

Paoletti, C., Le Pecq, J.B., Dat-Xuong, N., Lesca, P., Lecointe, P.: New anticancer derivatives in the ellipticine series. Proc. 10th Int. Cancer Congr. (in press, 1977)

Reinhold, V.N., Bruni, R.J.: Aromatic hydroxylation of ellipticine in rats: lack of an NIH shift. Biomed. Mass Spectromet. *3*, 335–339 (1976)

Ross, W., Glaubiger, D., Kohn, K.W.: Protein-associated DNA breaks in cells treated with adriamycin or ellipticine. Biochim. Biophys. Acta *519*, 23–30 (1978)

Snyder, A.L., Kann, H.E., Jr., Kohn, K.W.: Inhibition of the processing of ribosomal precursor RNA by intercalating agents. J. Mol. Biol. *58*, 555–565 (1971)

Sorace, R.A., Sheid, B.: Anti-tumor effects of DNA-ellipticine and DNA-ellipticine: daunomycin on the L1210(A) leukemia. Fed. Proc. *36*, 335 (1977)

Svoboda, G., Poore, G.A., Montfort, M.L.: Isolation of the alkaloids and study of the antitumor properties of 9-methoxyellipticine. J. Pharm. Sci. *57*, 1720–1725 (1968)

Tobey, R.A.: A simple, rapid technique for determination of the effects of chemotherapeutic agents on mammalian cell-cycle traverse. Cancer Res. **32**, 309–316 (1972)

Wang, J.C.: The degree of unwinding of the DNA helix by ethidium. I. Titration of twisted PM2 DNA molecules in alkaline cesium chloride density gradients. J. Mol. Biol. *89*, 783 (1974)

Waring, M.: Variation of the supercoils in closed circular DNA by binding of antibiotics and drugs: evidence from molecular models involving intercalation. J. Mol. Biol. *54*, 247 (1970)

2-Hydroxy-3-Alkyl-1,4-Naphthoquinones

J.G. OLENICK

Introduction

At the outbreak of the Second World War, Japanese troops overran the Dutch East Indies, thereby cutting off the Allied Forces from their major source of the antimalarial drug quinine. Faced with entirely inadequate supplies of quinine coupled with the grim prospect of waging tropical warfare in some of the world's worst malaria-infested regions, the Allied Powers instituted a comprehensive program of research in the chemotherapy of malaria. This program, sponsored and supported by the Committee on Medical Research of the Office of Scientific Research and Development, involved active participation and joint cooperation by academic institutions, pharmaceutical firms, private individuals, and the United States Army, Navy, and Public Health Service.

As part of the program, compounds were screened for antimalarial potency against an avian malaria test system. Antimalarial activity was found in compounds derived from a variety of structural types. The finding of activity in samples of hydrolapachol (a naturally occurring pigment which is 2-hydroxy-3-isoamyl-1,4-naphthoquinone) and two related quinones, originally prepared in 1936 by HOOKER, led to the synthesis by FIESER and his colleagues of a number of other 3-alkyl derivatives of 2-hydroxy-1,4-naphthoquinone. Some members of the group were highly active against avian malaria but had little activity against human malaria, presumably owing to rapid metabolic inactivation in the human body. However, lapinone, which has a hydroxylated alkyl side chain (Table 1), was shown to be resistant to metabolic degradation and to be a potent antimalarial against *Plasmodium vivax*, but suffered from the disadvantage of having to be administered parenterally in high doses.

After the Second World War and with the discovery of the very effective 4-aminoquinoline antimalarials, the problems of malaria chemotherapy were adjudged to be solved. It was felt that, with technical implementation, the cure and eradication of malaria were inevitable. Accordingly, most research efforts aimed at developing new drugs were discontinued. Subsequently, however, the appearance of resistance to 4-aminoquinolines in certain strains of plasmodia shattered this overly optimistic assessment. After the first report of drug-resistant cases of falciparum malaria from South America in 1959, considerable evidence accumulated to indicate the occurrence of similar cases in Southeast Asia. The existence of this phenomenon and the prevalence of highly endemic falciparum malaria in Vietnam prompted the establishment of

Table 1. Molecular structures of various 2-hydroxy-3-alkyl-1,4-naphthoquinones

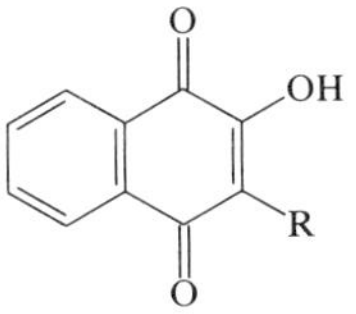

R	Compound
$-CH_2CH_2-C(H)(CH_3)-CH_3$	Hydrolapachol
$-(CH_2)_7-CH_2-C(OH)(CH_2-(CH_2)_3-CH_3)-CH_2-(CH_2)_3-CH_3$	Lapinone
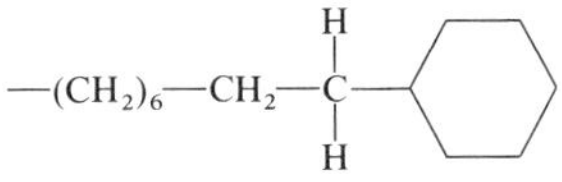	Menoctone
$-CH_2-C(H)(CH_3)-(CH_2)_5-CH_3$	2-hydroxy-3-(2-methyloctyl)-1,4-naphthoquinone
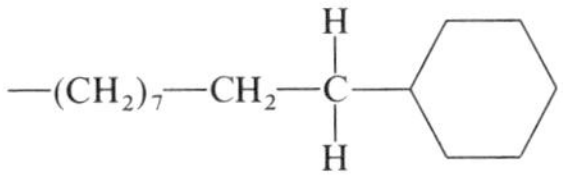	2-hydroxy-3-(9-cyclohexylnonyl)-1,4-naphthoquinone
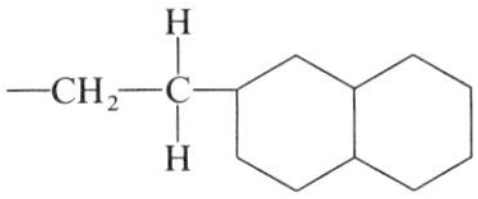	2-hydroxy-3-(decalylethyl)-1,4-naphthoquinone
$-CH_2CH_2-C(H)(CH_3)-(CH_2)_3-C(H)(CH_3)-CH_3$	2-hydroxy-3-(3,7-dimethyloctyl)-1,4-naphthoquinone
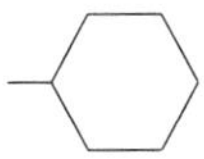	2-hydroxy-3-(cyclohexyl)-1,4-naphthoquinone
$-CH_2-C(H){=}C(CH_3)-CH_3$	Lapachol
$-CH_2-C(H){=}C(CH_3)-CH_2OH$	Lomatiol
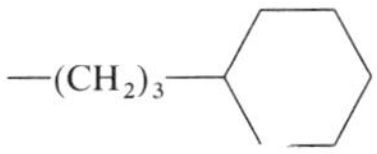	2-hydroxy-3-(cyclohexylpropyl)-1,4-naphthoquinone

Compounds are listed in the order in which they are discussed.

a massive research program initiated by the United States Army Medical Research and Development Command. Malaria became a top priority military medical problem and the 2-hydroxy-3-alkyl-1,4-naphthoquinones, which had received investigative scrutiny during the Second World War, were once again being explored. From this second look at naphthoquinone derivatives, the most active compound to emerge has been 2-hydroxy-3-(8-cyclohexyloctyl)-1,4-naphthoquinone (menoctone). Menoctone is effective in rodents infected with drug-resistant strains of *Plasmodium berghei*. The human antimalarial dose has not yet been determined.

Physical and Chemical Properties

The 2-hydroxy-3-alkyl-1,4-naphthoquinones are generally crystalline yellow solids melting at 70–150° C and having molecular weights of 200–400. These compounds are very slightly soluble in water but dissolve readily in benzene, ether, or acetic acid, with moderate solubility in alcohol or ligroin. A typical compound dissolves easily in a mixture of ethanol and aqueous alkali to give a deep red solution of the sodium salt but is only sparingly soluble in aqueous alkali. The sodium salt, however, dissolves freely in ether or in isoamyl alcohol and may be extracted from aqueous media by these solvents in the presence of excess sodium ion. Electrometric titrations in acetone-water, 50% (v/v), indicate a pK value of approximately 7 with the nonionized form predominating at pH 6. The oxidation-reduction potentials have been inferred to be approximately −200 millivolts.

Structure–Antimalarial Activity Relationships

As previously noted, the finding of antimalarial activity in samples of hydrolapachol led to the synthesis of additional naphthoquinone derivatives by FIESER et al. (1948). Increasing the length of the isoalkyl side chain of hydrolapachol by inserting more methylene groups increases the activity against *Plasmodium lophurae* in parasitized ducks. A maximum is reached with a C_9-side chain, beyond which activity decreases. Naphthoquinones of the normal alkyl series or with branched side-chains of various types show the same relationship and the same peak of activity. Identical structure–activity requirements of side-chain length were demonstrated by BERBERIAN and SLIGHTER (1968) for *Plasmodium berghei* infections in mice. Replacement of the quinonoid 2-hydroxyl group with OCH_3, H, CH_3, Cl, $NHCOCH_3$, or SH results in a loss of activity. Substitutions (CH_3, Br, OCH_3) in the benzenoid ring cause a complete or extensive loss of activity. A decrease in activity occurs with substitutions in the hydrocarbon side chain of halogen, nitrogen, or a double bond.

Antirespiratory Activity

WENDEL (1946), in studying the action of 2-hydroxy-3-alkyl-1,4-naphthoquinones, was first to observe that these compounds inhibited the in vitro oxygen uptake of duck erythrocytes parasitized with *P. lophurae*. With normal erythrocytes, 100 times as high a concentration of naphthoquinone was required to affect an equal reduction of oxygen consumption. The inhibitory effect on respiration was markedly dependent on pH. The ability of the drugs to depress the respiration of the malarial parasite paralleled their antimalarial efficacy in vivo.

The direct relationship between the antimalarial and antirespiratory activities was confirmed by BALL et al. (1974) and was extended to include the inhibitory action of alkyl-hydroxynaphthoquinones on succinate oxidation. Using as test materials a beef-heart succinoxidase preparation and monkey red blood cells parasitized with *Plasmodium knowlesi*, they found a striking similarity in the inhibitory action of these compounds on the succinate oxidase system and upon the respiration of the malarial parasite. The oxidation of succinate was completely inhibited by certain 2-hydroxy-3-alkyl-naphthoquinones at concentrations as low as 1×10^{-6} M. However, the pH of the assay mixture considerably influenced the degree of inhibition. As the pH was increased, less inhibition was produced; an effect similar to that reported by WENDEL (1946) for the malarial antirespiratory activity of these naphthoquinones. BALL et al. (1947) suggested, but considered unlikely, that alterations in the degree of dissociation of the 2-hydroxy group may account for variations of naphthoquinone action with changes in pH. HOWLAND (1963) considered this a plausible explanation, noting that ionization of the 2-hydroxy group at higher pH lowers the lipophilic properties of the drug, thus preventing it from reaching the lipid-rich regions of the mitochondrial membrane, where presumably the inhibition occurs. Indeed, TAPPEL (1960) found that inhibition of electron transport by a variety of naphthoquinone derivatives was increased with increases in the lipophilic character of the side chains. The possession of lipid solubility by alkyl-hydroxynaphthoquinones does not mean, however, that mitochondrial lipids must be directly involved as reactants in the elaboration of inhibitory events.

Protein has been implicated as the mitochondrial constituent taking part in the inhibitory action of naphthoquinones. HEYMANN and FIESER (1948) demonstrated that naphthoquinones were bound by human and animal plasma and that mitochondrial succinoxidase inhibition produced by naphthoquinones was reversed by addition of serum albumin. This reactivation by serum albumin was studied by REIF and POTTER (1953); they classified the alkyl-hydroxynaphthoquinones as pseudo-irreversible inhibitors. They further inferred that the cytochrome c component of the succinoxidase system was involved in the binding to naphthoquinones, since raising the level of cytochrome c in the enzyme system lowered the inhibitory action of naphthoquinones on succinate oxidation. Although the foregoing observations suggest that the inhibitory effect of antimalarial naphthoquinones on succinate oxidation may be a consequence of protein interaction, the effect of lipid solubility must not be discounted. As previously mentioned, the degree of inhibition exhibited by these compounds was related to the extent of their lipid solubility. Accordingly, in order to produce an inhibitory response, at least two events must take place: (1) permeation of a lipid barrier or a lipid-protein interface, and (2) binding by, and affinity for, specific proteins of the mitochondrion.

Attempts at pinpointing the specific site of naphthoquinone action in the respiratory chain of enzymes were made initially by BALL et al. (1947). They measured the catalytic activities of various portions of the naphthoquinone-inhibited succinoxidase system; 2-hydroxy-3-(2-methyloctyl)-1,4-naphthoquinone prevented the reoxidation of reduced cytochrome b, but succinic dehydrogenase and cytochrome oxidase were unaffected. These observations led them to conclude that the 2-hydroxy-3-alkyl-naphthoquinones act at a locus between cytochromes b and c. WIDMER et al. (1954) reported that cytochrome c_1, as well as cytochrome b, were reduced by succinate in the presence of 2-hydroxy-3-(2-methyloctyl)-1,4-naphthoquinone. They postulated, therefore, that the inhibitory block was between cytochromes c_1 and c. ESTABROOK (1958) obtained similar results, but, while measuring the reduction of cytochrome c_1, he noted that the initial rate was not influenced by the naphthoquinone and that, after a rapid phase of reduction the cytochrome was slowly reoxidized. Rather than postulating an inhibitory block per se, he suggested instead that naphthoquinones exert their inhibitory action only after some component between dehydrogenase and cytochrome c_1 was reduced.

BALL et al. (1947) also reported that reactions catalyzed by respiratory enzymes requiring pyridine nucleotides as coenzymes do not appear to be inhibited by the alkyl-hydroxynaphthoquinones. This is somewhat misleading, since, in spite of the fact that dehydrogenase activity for NADH is, indeed, not affected by naphthoquinones, the oxidase activity for this substrate is strongly inhibited. Moreover, HATEFI et al. (1961) demonstrated that NADH-cytochrome c reductase preparations, essentially free of succinic-cytochrome c reductase and cytochrome oxidase activities, were also completely inhibited by 2-hydroxy-3-(2-methyloctyl)-1,4-naphthoquinone. Thus, the main inhibitory effect of naphthoquinones on respiration appears to be limited to an action upon some component gearing the oxidation of metabolites by dehydrogenases to the reduction of cytochrome c.

As early as 1947, BALL et al. (1947) considered the possibility that the inhibitory action of alkyl-hydroxynaphthoquinones might be due to their competition with a naturally occurring naphthoquinone and they unsuccessfully attempted to release the respiratory inhibition by 2-hydroxy-3-(2-methyloctyl)-1,4-naphthoquinone with the addition of vitamin K. Ten years later, the isolation of a benzoquinone (coenzyme Q) from beef heart mitochondria (CRANE et al., 1957) and the demonstration of its coenzymic activity in the oxidation of succinate (CRANE et al., 1959) and of NADH (CRANE, 1960) prompted further investigations into the possibility that the alkyl-hydroxynaphthoquinones were competitively inhibiting at the coenzyme Q site. CRANE (1960), and HENDLIN and COOK (1960) demonstrated that the inhibitory effect of naphthoquinones on the succinoxidase system of beef heart electron transport particles can be released by coenzyme Q_{10} and a variety of its analogs, as well as by a number of other lipophilic substances, including alpha-tocopherol, squalene, and vitamin K_1. However, reversal occurred only at low levels of inhibitor and required large (100- to 200-fold) molar excesses of the lipophilic material. TAKEMORI and KING (1964) found that the inhibition produced by 2-hydroxy-3-(9-cyclohexylnonyl)-1,4-naphthoquinone against succinate-cytochrome c reductase was not reversed by coenzyme Q_2, except at low levels of naphthoquinone. This inhibition against an isolated segment of the respiratory chain required less excessive (20-fold) amounts of coenzyme Q_2 for complete reversal. TAPPEL (1960) succeeded in restoring the activity of a smaller portion of the respiratory chain of enzymes, succinate-coenzyme Q reductase, partially inhibited by 2-hydroxy-3-(decalyl-ethyl)-1,4-naphthoquinone, with equivalent quantities of coenzymes Q_{10}, Q_7, and Q_2, and also of vitamin K_1. At higher concentrations of naphthoquinone, only coenzyme Q_2 was able to release the inhibition of succinate-coenzyme Q reductase. The observed effects of high levels of lipophilic substances coupled with their lack of specificity and inability to displace higher inhibitory concentrations of naphthoquinone cast some doubt on the hypothesis that naphthoquinones act competitively at the coenzyme Q locus.

Uncoupling Activity

Adopting a suggestion by HÜLSMANN (1958) that certain electron transport inhibitors might react with the same component of the mitochondrial respiratory apparatus as do uncoupling agents, HOWLAND (1963a) succeeded in demonstrating the reversal of hydrolapachol inhibition of succinate oxidation in intact mitochondria by adding the uncoupler, 2,4-dinitrophenol. Such a finding indicates that, superimposed upon inhibition of electron transport, there may be additional effects of 2-hydroxy-3-alkyl-naphthoquinones due to inhibition of energy transfer pathways. HOWLAND (1963b) further studied the influence of naphthoquinones on oxidative phosphorylation, employing conditions where the antirespiratory inhibition site was bypassed, by using ascorbate (plus tetramethyl-paraphenylenediamine as carrier) to donate electrons to cytochrome c. One group of alkyl-hydroxynaphthoquinones, including 2-hydroxy-3-(3,7-dimethyloctyl)-1,4-naphthoquinone, 2-hydroxy-3-(cyclohexyl)-1,4-naphthoquinone, and 2-hydroxy-3-hydroxy-3-(3-methylbutyl)-1,4-naphthoquinone (hydrolapachol), were shown to have characteristics of inhibitors of oxidative phosphorylation – inhibiting ATP synthesis and preventing the stimulation of respiration by phosphate acceptor. On the other hand, 2-hydroxy-3-(3-methyl-2-butenyl)-1,4-naphthoquinone (lapachol) and 2-hydroxy-3-(4-hydroxy-3-methyl-2-butenyl)-1,4-naphthoquinone (lomatiol) appeared to act as uncouplers of oxidative phosphorylation – stimulating respiration in the absence of phosphate acceptor and eliminating ATP synthesis. Of the alkyl-hydroxynaphtoquinones studied by HOWLAND (1963b), those which were shown to uncouple possessed a 2′,3′-unsaturated side chain at the 3-position; those saturated at this bond act as phosphorylation inhibitors. Lapachol and hydrolapachol, which differ only at the 2′,3′-bond of the C-3-side chain, clearly exemplify this distinction. It is noteworthy that a 2′,3′-double bond is an absolute requirement for one of the proposed mechanisms of respiratory ATP synthesis, which involves a cyclization between the 2′,3′-unsaturated bond of the 3-position side chain of a benzoquinone (coenzyme Q) or of a naphthoquinone (vitamin K) and the 4-position oxygen (BRODIE et al., 1957; CHMIELEWSKA, 1960; VILKAS and LEDERER, 1962; GUTNICK and BRODIE, 1965).

Naphthoquinones of the vitamin K type, as well as benzoquinones, are widely distributed in microorganisms (LESTER and CRANE, 1959; JACOBSEN and DAM, 1960; BISHOP et al., 1962). Vitamin K is the respiratory quinone of most of the aerobic gram-positive bacteria; coenzyme Q is found in the gram-negative types. Certain bacteria contain both benzo- and naphthoquinones and are referred to as having mixed quinone systems. BRODIE (1961) found that respiration and phosphorylation in UV-irradiated extracts of *Mycobacterium phlei* can be restored by addition of vitamin K_1 or closely related homologs and that only naphthoquinones which can cyclize and form a chromanyl ring are capable of restoring oxidative phosphorylation. Saturation of the phytyl side chain of vitamin K_1 had a marked influence on phosphorylation resulting in the restoration of only oxidation. As a matter of fact, this compound, 2,3-dihydrophytyl vitamin K_1, acted as an uncoupling agent when added to nonirradiated preparations. Uncoupling agents, which are structurally similar to vitamin K_1 (notably lapachol), were found to be competitive inhibitors of phosphorylation with respect to vitamin K_1 (BRODIE and BALLANTINE, 1960). Lapachol is theoretically capable of cyclizing, although the 2-hydroxyl group contributes an orthoquinoid character to the system and should affect the formation and stability of the chromanyl ring. Evidence favoring this explanation for the inhibitory action of lapachol on phosphorylation has been obtained by BRODIE and BALLANTINE (1960), who showed that methyl lapachol, which differs from lapachol by the substitution of a methyl for a hydroxyl group in the C-2-position of the naphthoquinone ring, can reactivate both oxidation and phosphate esterification in extracts of *M. phlei* that had been inactivated by UV-irradiation. Lapachol reactivates only oxidation, favoring the suggestion that the 2-hydroxyl group may interfere with the formation of the chromanyl ring.

Antibacterial Activity

A number of substituted 1,4-naphthoquinones, primarily differing from the 2-hydroxy-3-alkyl-1,4-naphthoquinones by lacking a 2-hydroxyl substituent, were found by LEAHY et al. (1968) to be bacterial growth inhibitors. The action was bacteriostatic and was postulated to occur due to competitive inhibition with the endogenous naphthoquinone or benzoquinone, thus decreasing the effectiveness of the latter as oxidative phosphorylating agents.

A representative of the alkyl-hydroxynaphthoquinones, 2-hydroxy-3-(cyclohexylpropyl)-1,4-naphthoquinone (a lower homolog of menoctone), was shown by OLENICK et al. (1971) to inhibit the growth of the gram-positive bacterium, *Bacillus megaterium*, at concentrations of the order of 6×10^{-6} M to 10^{-5} M.

The antibacterial spectrum was limited to only a few other species of gram-positive bacteria. All growth inhibitory concentrations within this narrow range were bactericidal and even resting suspensions of cells were killed, indicating that growth and metabolism were not prerequisites for the elaboration of inhibitory events. Bactericidal concentrations instantly arrested the incorporation of ^{14}C-labeled uracil, thymidine, leucine, or ^{3}H-labeled diaminopimelic acid, demonstrating complete and simultaneous failure of biosyntheses of RNA, DNA, protein, and the cell-wall polymer. At a time when all major biosyntheses had failed, no change was produced in the rate of oxygen consumption by cells growing on glucose and no significant depletion was detected in the level of the intracellular ATP pool. Experiments by OLENICK and HAHN (1974) that measured the total uptake of ^{14}C-uracil and its incorporation into RNA revealed that 2-hydroxy-3-(cyclohexylpropyl)-1,4-naphthoquinone blocked the entry of uracil into cells of *B. megaterium*; the chasing of preloaded radioactive uracil from the cells by excess nonradioactive uracil was also prevented. Although the total uptake of only uracil was tested, it was assumed (in view of the identical inhibitory patterns) that the transport of the other radioactively labeled precursors was also blocked. Based on these results, coupled with the demonstration of preferential binding of 2-hydroxy-3-(cyclohexylpropyl)-1,4-naphthoquinone to the membrane fraction of *B. megaterium*, OLENICK and HAHN (1974) postulated that the mode of action on susceptible bacteria is to deny access of essential metabolites through the membrane into the interior of the cell.

References

Ball, E.G., Anfinsen, C.B., Cooper, O.: The inhibitory action of naphthoquinones on respiratory processes. J. Biol. Chem. *168*, 257–270 (1947)

Berberian, D.A., Slighter, R.G., Jr.: The schizonticidal activity of hydroxynaphthoquinones against *Plasmodium berghei* infections in mice. J. Parasitol. *54*, 999–1005 (1968)

Bishop, D.H.L., Pandya, K.P., King, H.K.: Ubiquinone and vitamin K in bacteria. Biochem. J. *83*, 606–614 (1962)

Brodie, A.F.: Vitamin K and other quinones as coenzymes in oxidative phosphorylation in bacterial systems. Fed. Proc. *20*, 995–1004 (1961)

Brodie, A.F., Ballantine, J.: Oxidative phosphorylation in fractionated bacterial systems. III. Specificity of vitamin K reactivation. J. Biol. Chem. *235*, 232–237 (1960)

Brodie, A.F., Weber, M.M., Gray, C.T.: The role of vitamin K_1 in coupled oxidative phosphorylation. Biochim. Biophys. Acta *25*, 448–449 (1957)

Chmielewska, I.: Oxidative and photosynthetic phosphorylation involving 2-methylquinones. Biochim. Biophys. Acta *39*, 170–171 (1960)

Crane, F.L.: Quinones in electron transport. I. Coenzymatic activity of plastoquinones, Coenzyme Q and related natural quinones. Arch. Biochem. Biophys. *87*, 198–202 (1960)

Crane, F.L., Hatefi, Y., Lester, R.L., Widmer, C.: Isolation of a quinone from beef heart mitochondria. Biochim. Biophys. Acta *25*, 220–221 (1957)

Crane, F.L., Widmer, C., Lester, R.L., Hatefi, Y.: Studies on the electron transport system. XV. Coenzyme Q (Q275) and the succinoxidase activity of the electron transport particle. Biochim. Biophys. Acta *31*, 476–489 (1959)

Estabrook, R.W.: The spectral and enzymatic characterization of cytochrome c_1 of liver mitochondria. J. Biol. Chem. *230*, 735–750 (1958)

Fieser, L.F., Berliner, E., Bondrus, F.J., Chang, F.C., Dauben, W.G., Ettlinger, M.G., Fawaz, G., Fields, M., Fieser, M., Heidelberger, C., Heymann, H., Seligman, A.M., Vaughan, W.R.,

Wilson, A.G., Wilson, E., Wu, M., Leffler, M.T., Hamlin, K.E., Hathaway, R.J., Matson, E.J., Moore, E.E., Moore, M.B., Rapala, R.T., Zaugg, H.E.: Naphthoquinone antimalarials. I. General survey. J. Am. Chem. Soc. *70*, 3151–3155 (1948)

Gutnick, D.L., Brodie, A.F.: Phosphate-dependent incorporation of tritium into a naphthoquinone during oxidative phosphorylation. J. Biol. Chem. *240*, PC 3698–3699 (1965)

Hatefi, Y., Haavik, A.G., Jurtshuk, P.: Studies on the electron transport system. XXX. DPNH-cytochrome c reductase I. Biochim. Biophys. Acta *52*, 106–118 (1961)

Hendlin, D., Cook, T.M.: The reversible inhibition of succinoxidase by naphthoquinones. Biochem. Biophys. Res. Commun. *2*, 71–75 (1960)

Heymann, H., Fieser, L.F.: Naphthoquinone antimalarials. J. Biol. Chem. *176*, 1359–1362 (1948)

Howland, J.L.: The reversibility of inhibition by 2-heptyl-4-hydroxyquinoline-N-oxide and 2-hydroxy-3-(3-methylbutyl)-1,4-naphthoquinone of succinate oxidation. Biochim. Biophys. Acta *73*, 665–667 (1963a)

Howland, J.L.: Uncoupling and inhibition of oxidative phosphorylation by 2-hydroxy-3-alkyl-1,4-naphthoquinones. Biochim. Biophys. Acta *77*, 659–662 (1963b)

Hülsmann, W.C.: Over het mechanisme van de ademhalingsketenphosphorylering. M.D. Thesis, Klein Offset Drukkerij, Amsterdam (1958)

Jacobsen, B.K., Dam, H.: Vitamin K in bacteria. Biochim. Biophys. Acta *40*, 211–216 (1960)

Leahy, G.J., Currie, D.J., Holmes, H.L., Maltman, J.R.: Growth-inhibitory activities of some 1,4-naphthoquinones and related compounds on *Staphylococcus aureus* and *Escherichia coli*. Can. J. Microbiol. *14*, 661–666 (1968)

Lester, R.L., Crane, F.L.: The natural occurrence of Coenzyme Q and related compounds. J. Biol. Chem. *234*, 2169–2175 (1959)

Olenick, J.G., Hahn, F.E.: Bactericidal action of a 2-hydroxy-3-alkyl-1,4-naphthoquinone: Blockade of metabolite permeation across the membrane. Ann. N.Y. Acad. Sci. *235*, 542–552 (1974)

Olenick, J.G., Cook, T.M., Hahn, F.E.: Bactericidal action of 2-hydroxy-3-(cyclohexylpropyl)-1,4-naphthoquinone on *Bacillus megaterium*. J. Bacteriol *107*, 528–534 (1971)

Reif, A.E., Potter, V.R.: Studies on succinoxidase inhibition I. Pseudoirreversible inhibition by a naphthoquinone and by antimycin A. J. Biol. Chem. *205*, 279–290 (1953)

Takemori, S., King, T.E.: Reconstitution of respiratory chain enzyme systems. XIII. Sequential fragmentation of succinate oxidase: preparation and properties of succinate-cytochrome c reductase and the cytochrome b-c_1 particle. J. Biol. Chem. *239*, 3546–3558 (1964)

Tappel, A.L.: Inhibition of electron transport by antimycin A, alkyl hydroxynaphthoquinones and metal coordination compounds. Biochem. Pharmacol. *3*, 289–296 (1960)

Vilkas, M., Lederer, E.: Sur un mecanisme possible de la phosphorylation oxydative. Experientia *18*, 546–549 (1962)

Wendel, W.B.: The influence of naphthoquinones upon the respiratory and carbohydrate metabolism of malarial parasites. Fed. Proc. *5*, 406–407 (1946)

Widmer, C., Clark, H.W., Neufeld, H.A., Stotz, E.: Cytochrome components of the soluble SC factor preparation. J. Biol. Chem. *210*, 861–867 (1954)

Hydroxystilbamidine

B. FESTY

I. Introduction

Hydroxystilbamidine (OH.SA.) is hydroxy-4-4′ diamidino stilbene used as diisethionate; as other diamidine compounds (pentamidine, propamidine, stilbamidine, berenil, etc.), it shows strong activity against bacteria, protozoa, and fungi. It is clinically used in systemic mycosis, mainly North American blastomycosis, visceral leishmaniasis, and secondarily in prophylaxis and treatment of African trypanosomiasis, and in cases of malignancy, e.g., multiple myeloma. Pharmacology of OH.SA. has not been studied in such detail as of stilbamidine (SA); its properties are roughly the same but OH.SA. is experimentally and clinically less toxic than SA. So far no resistances have been extensively described. Its mechanism of action is not known well but recent work has shown in vitro or/and in vivo affinity of OH.SA. for nucleic acids, mainly DNA, and biologic effects such as modifications of the kinetoplast-mitochondrial system of Trypanosoma with alteration of extranuclear circular DNA replication. Mitochondrial DNA affinity of OH.SA. can be shown by cytoplasmic mutations in yeast. OH.SA. is a good nonintercalative chemical instrument for nucleic acids conformation studies.

II. Development and Physico-Chemical Properties

OH.SA. is a member of the aromatic diamidine series of compounds which were synthesized in the research laboratories of May and Backer Ltd – Dagenham, Essex, England (ASHLEY et al., 1942; ASHLEY and HARRIS, 1946) in the course of investigations on trypanocidal properties of diguanidine derivatives (LOURIE and YORKE, 1939). It soon became evident that a series of diamidines in which the central alkyl chain was replaced by aryl groups led to molecules with a greater trypanocidal activity in vitro or in experimental animal infections than any drug hitherto known. The most important members of this series were stilbamidine (SA), pentamidine, propamidine, phenamidine, hydroxystilbamidine, dihydroxystilbamidine and dimethylstilbamidine, whose properties have now been widely studied (HAWKING, 1963). Berenil (Ber.), another aromatic diamidine, was synthesized in 1954 (NEWTON, 1975). These aromatic diamidines have polyvalent activity against bacteria, protozoa, fungi, and tumor cells

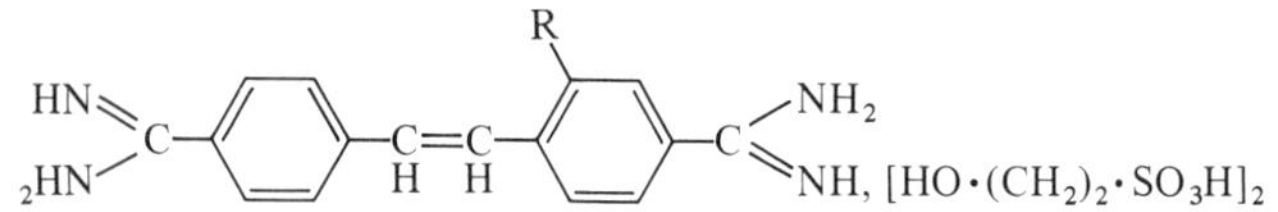

Fig. 1. Stilbamidine (SA) diisethionate (R = H). Hydroxystilbamidine (OHSA) diisethionate (R = OH) OHSA: mw = 532.5

(SCHOENBACH and GREENSPAN, 1948; SNAPPER et al., 1952b). Members of this series were extensively used in prophylaxis and treatment of African Trypanosomiasis and against antimony-resistant cases of Kala-Azar. Some of them were the first active chemotherapeutic agents applied to North American blastomycosis, extending their activity to other systemic mycosis, such as moniliasis and actinomycosis. Stilbamidine was at first extensively used, but as it was responsible for a neuropathic syndrome with distressing sequelae in many patients, OH.SA. was then preferred for clinical use.

OH.SA. diisethionate or di (*β* hydroxy ethane sulfonate) (Fig. 1), as free base, is a yellow crystalline solid, discolored by light and decomposed near 275°–300° C. It is freely soluble in water (1 g/100 ml in alkaline solution) but practically insoluble in ether. Aqueous solutions are weakly acid (1%→pH near 4.5) and weakly fluorescent under UV light. Although far more stable than SA. or Ber., OH.SA. solutions should be freshly prepared, especially for clinical use.

The commercial product is described as monohydrate without well-defined physical constants. It is not clear whether OH.SA. is the trans or cis form or a mixture of these two isomers. Crystallographic study (COURSEILLE et al., 1972) shows that OH.SA. may be obtained as dihydrate, and that the two aromatic rings of the molecule make a 12° angle in contrast to SA. in which they are coplanar.

An extensive study of physico-chemical properties of OH.SA. was undertaken (FESTY, 1971). The commercial product is heterogeneous, as shown by thin layer chromatography on silica gel and UV fluorescence. Chromatography on G-15 Sephadex gave three fractions: the major component is pure OH.SA. (about 95%); the other compounds as identified by their spectroscopic properties are SA and dihydroxystilbamidine. Absorption and fluorescence spectra of the pure dye are very characteristic; the absorption spectrum is pH-dependent because of the equilibrium between the protonated form (Am^+ OH Am^+) and the zwitterion (Am^+ O^- Am^+), the corresponding pK of OH group being close to 8 in the ground state. The fluorescence spectrum at pH 5 is, surprisingly, composed of two emission bands in the blue and the red areas of the spectrum. But they correspond to an identical excitation spectrum. This unusual feature, all contamination source being excluded, should be related to the ionization of the phenolic group in the excited state and to the large change in pK. Fluorescence properties in the pH range studied could be correlated with the existence of both molecular species (Am^+ OH Am^+ and Am^+ O^- Am^+) seen in variable relative amounts. A possible explanation relies on comparison between the lifetime of the excited state and the rate of proton transfer. When the latter is strongly reduced, only the blue form is detected, as observed at very low temperatures or in a medium of high viscosity such as glycerol. In other cases, the two emissions are present generally with a prominence of the red form. OH.SA. fluorescence is strongly enhanced by various organic solvents (as well as with some macromolecules in aqueous solutions or within animal cells). Its unusually high value of the fluorescence polarization coefficient (0.20–0.30) in aqueous solution might be correlated with a very short fluorescence life time.

Besides radioactive and biologic methods of limited value because of their difficult application, various chemical methods have been described for diamidines determination in aqueous solution or biologic samples (SNAPPER et al., 1951a; HAWKING, 1963). They are useful but generally not very sensitive or specific. Fluorescence techniques may be used directly for SA or after obtaining fluorescent glyoxalidone derivatives of aromatic amidines. Enhancement of fluorescence with DNA may also be used to determine OH.SA. concentrations in aqueous solution (FESTY, 1971): this property was made use of to study the stoichiometry of the DNA-OH.SA. association.

III. Pharmacologic Properties and Clinical Use[1]

The pharmacology of OH.SA. has not been studied in such detail as that of SA (SCHOENBACH and GREENSPAN, 1948; SNAPPER et al., 1952b; HAWKING, 1963); but the properties of the two drugs are generally similar in activity, absorption, distribution, and excretion. The major advantage of OH.SA. is its lower toxicity.

A. Experimental Studies

1. Absorption, Distribution, and Excretion

The diamidines compounds are not well absorbed by the oral route. After subcutaneous injection they are moderately absorbed according to the dose used, and local fixation is observed. After intravenous or intraperitoneal injection, blood concentration decreases rapidly but drugs are retained for long periods of time in the body (HAWKING, 1963).

The fate of OH.SA. in the body shows a similar pattern to that of SA. It seems that its absorption through the gastro-intestinal tract is very weak or incomplete: OH.SA. is ineffective when given orally to mice for pulmonary blastomycosis treatment but is effective when given subcutaneously (SOLOTOROVSKY et al., 1954). Distribution of the two amidines into animals and man have been studied (SNAPPER et al., 1951a), sometimes after long periods of administration. It was seen that SA and OH.SA. have long biologic lifetimes and that they are retained in various parenchymatous tissues and tumor cells;

1 Many older references may be found in May and Baker (1957).

measurable amounts of the drugs were found in liver and adrenals several months after administration. Urinary excretion of the two drugs has been compared in rats (HAMPTON, 1947); after repeated doses of each diamidine an initial delay was followed by a marked rise in excretion. But for equivalent doses of the two drugs this delay in the case of OH.SA. was about half of the one observed with SA. On the other hand, excretion of the two drugs was proportionately not so high for daily doses (10 mg/kg) as it was for weekly doses (1 mg/kg). OH.SA. is not so persistent as SA; this is of interest in explaining differences in clinical toxicity.

2. Toxicity

The acute toxicities for mice of diamidine compounds are related (HAWKING, 1963): propamidine and pentamidine seem to be the more toxic, berenil the least toxic, SA and phenamidine having an intermediate position (SA:LD_{50}S.C. = 180 mg/kg; Max. Tol. dose i.p. = 50 mg/kg). For SA in rabbits a single subcutaneous dose of 50 mg/kg causes death after one to ten days. In mice or rabbits subacute doses produce general depression of the central nervous system with stimulation and then depression of breathing, resulting in death. A transient fall of blood pressure occurs with smaller doses. Toxic action on the kidney is evident with impairment of renal function. SA liberates histamine from mast cells. Chronic effects were also described with SA in rats after repeated administration of one-fifth of the toxic dose: decrease of growth, vasodilatation of ear, nose, and feet, occasional tremors; lowered body temperature was also registered.

Experimental acute or subacute toxicities of SA and OH.SA. are of the same kind. The median lethal intravenous and subcutaneous doses in mice are respectively 0.25 and 0.15 mg per gram (MAY and BAKER, 1957). OH.SA. is less toxic than SA for the liver of experimental animals. A significant increase of toxicity (50% for 24 h) does occur after exposure of drug solutions to light; this phenomenon is not so pronounced as with SA, but it is important enough to be kept in mind for clinical administration.

3. Chemotherapeutic Activity

After SA, OH.SA. was studied for its activity against various microorganisms. Its action is relatively broad; it shows some activity against bacteria, especially gram-positive bacteria; but it is mainly active against fungi and protozoa. Moreover, it has also some effect against tumor cells (SCHOENBACH and GREENSPAN, 1948; SNAPPER et al., 1952b).

Fungi (TASCHDJIAN, 1954). Historically, propamidine is the first aromatic diamidine whose activity on *Blastomyces dermatitidis* was reported. Then it was shown that OH.SA. inhibits the growth of this fungus and of *Histoplasma capsulatum* in vitro at concentrations of a few micrograms per ml (SNAPPER et al., 1952b). This in vitro activity was confirmed against *Blastomyces dermatitidis* inhibited by concentrations of no more than 2.5 µg/ml (SOLOTOROVSKY et al., 1954); a moderate activity was also reported against other fungi, as *Cryptococcus neoformans, Candida albicans, Trichophyton mentagrophytes, Epidermophytes floccosum,* and *Microsporum canis*. Other authors found OH.SA. less active in vitro: 1 mg/ml against fungus species including *Candida, Nocardia, Cryptococcus, Histoplasma,* and *Aspergillus,* or 100 µg/ml for complete inhibition of *Coccidioides immitis*. But OH.SA. activity is found always against *Blastomyces dermatitidis* in vitro and a comparative study of various amidines including OH.SA. showed a more marked action of drugs against the yeast form than the mycelial form. By the subcutaneous route OH.SA. is also active against *Blastomyces dermatitidis* in experimental mouse infections (SOLOTOROVSKY et al., 1954). But OH.SA. is ineffective in mouse experimentally infected with *Candida* or *Coccidioides immitis* at subtoxic levels.

Protozoa. Diamidines and OH.SA. are active against various protozoa, especially *Leishmania, Trypanosoma,* and *Amoeba*.

As leishmanicides, aromatic diamidines and antimony derivatives are the most important drugs. But diamidines, unlike antimony drugs, are active against flagellates in vitro. OH.SA. was shown active in vitro at a concentration of 10^{-6} (COLLIER and LOURIE, 1946); under the same experimental conditions OH.SA. had only a 50% efficiency. Nevertheless, the activity of the two drugs was found equivalent in blood agar medium (SNAPPER et al., 1952b). In vivo, OH.SA. is as effective as SA when given intraperitoneally at repeated doses to hamsters infected with *L. donovani;* repeated doses of SA (and then OH.SA.) necessary to cure hamsters with light and heavy infections are respectively 2 and 2.5–5 mg/kg (BEVERIDGE, 1963); 10 doses of 20 mg/kg three times a week are curative. But OH.SA. was reported to be inactive therapeutically and prophylactically with a single intramuscular dose of 50 mg/kg in the same animal. On the other hand, 14 daily doses of 12.5 mg/kg were inactive against cutaneous *L. braziliensis* infection of mice (ERCOLI, 1961).

Aromatic diamidines are also well known as trypanocides (LOURIE and YORKE, 1939; FULTON, 1944). Experimental studies have been mainly with pentamidine, propamidine, and SA active against *T. gambiense*, or Ber. active on *T. congolense*. A detailed review of this subject described (HAWKING, 1963) their in vitro trypanocidal activity against *T. equiperdum* (0.04 µg/ml for 24 h at 37° C) and possible structure–activity relationships. In vivo diamidines are mainly efficient against *T. rhodesiense* and *T. congolense,* and possibly *T. vivax* (Ber) but have no action against *T. cruzi*. OH.SA. has not been studied so much as the other aromatic diamidines; nevertheless it was shown to have a curative action against experimental trypanosome infections of mice with *T. rhodesiense* or *T. gambiense*; but it is ineffective against *T. congolense* and *T. cruzi*. Its prophylactic action against *T. rhodesiense* is as good or better than that of SA (FULTON, 1944).

In vitro, amebicidal and amebistatic actions against strains of *Acanthamoeba*, isolated from eye infections, and *Naegleria gruberi* were tested for several compounds: some of them including OH.SA. and related drugs which influence the molecular biology of nucleic acids, such as acriflavine and proflavine, were found active (NAGINGTON and RICHARDS, 1976).

Some in vitro or in vivo experimental studies have shown activity of diamidines including SA and/or OH.SA. against *Babesia, Trichomonas, Plasmodium*, and *Pneumocystis carinii*.

4. Other Activities

OH.SA. produces immunosuppression (FOLDS et al., 1975): it is a potent suppressor of the plaque-forming cell response of mice injected with heterologous erythrocytes. OH.SA. suppresses both the primary and the secondary immune responses to bovine serum-albumin, which cannot be explained alone by a toxic effect on spleen cells. Stilbamidines also have cortisone-like effects on lysosomes and connective tissue (COTTY and HARRIS, 1967; HIRSCHHORN et al., 1969; WEISSMANN et al., 1970).

B. Clinical Studies

The use of OH.SA. in human diseases has met with mixed success.

1. Fungal Infections and Systemic Mycosis

OH.SA. has been used successfully in the treatment of a number of systemic fungal diseases, particularly blastomyces and candida infections. The introduction of SA and OH.SA. has revolutionized the therapy of blastomycosis.

North American Blastomycosis (Blastomyces dermatitidis). Following the successful use of SA, OH.SA. was tried because of its lower toxicity (SNAPPER, 1952a; SNAPPER et al., 1953); these references describe its use in four patients, three suffering from the systemic form and one from the cutaneous form of the infection. In the four cases, intravenous administration of several grams (4.5 to 19.6) of OH.SA. in the course of a few months (with complementary diet and treatment) was followed by cure with disappearance of clinical and biologic symptoms. Several months later there was no evidence of remaining lesions and extensive laboratory tests showed no abnormalities in any functions tested. This success was confirmed by several authors, but some of them drew attention to the necessity of other therapeutic interventions, such as resection of affected lung after control of active disease by OH.SA. therapy. Others reported successful results in cases of relapse. OH.SA. is recognized as the best chemotherapeutic agent for North American blastomycosis (SUTLIFF and MILLS, 1961; DOWNER et al., 1966; PICKAR and WALKER, 1968; LOCKWOOD et al., 1969; BUSEY, 1972).

South American Blastomycosis (Paracoccidioides braziliensis). OH.SA. has a greater activity on this fungus than SA, but does not seem able to lead to any improvement in cases of generalized South American blastomycosis. This negative result may be diagnostically useful to distinguish between the two blastomycosis (LISBOA et al., 1957).

Moniliasis (Candida albicans). OH.SA. has been used successfully in the treatment of candida infections. WOLFF et al. (1955) described their experience in three cases of newborn infants with thrush esophagitis. The disease did not respond to classical therapy but intravenous OH.SA. treatment (15 mg every 12 h) caused improvement after one or a few days with some side effects as venospasm and thrombophlebitis. Associated complications were stabilized by antibiotics. Many additional cases were subsequently described.

Miscellaneous Mycosis. OH.SA. has been used successfully in the treatment of some cases of actinomycosis after penicillin failure. The compound is highly active in vitro against *Cryptococcosis neoformans.* Cases of generalized torulosis (cryptococcosis) were cured by intravenous administration of a few grams of the drug over a few days. Its preventive effect of dissemination of infection has also been described. Histoplasmosis cases were treated with OH.SA. with partial success; the drug is of little value in the disseminated form of the disease. Coccidioidomycosis treatment with OH.SA. gave disappointing results. It seems that OH.SA. might influence the evolution of pulmonary aspergillosis due to *Aspergillus fumigatus.* Intravenous administration of OH.SA. is interesting in view of the saprophytic form of the disease; direct injection in mycetoma or inhalation of OH.SA. have been successfully used in some cases. Improvement has been described in treatment of the generalized form of sporotrichosis due to *Sporotrichum schencki.* Being active in vitro against *Microsporum audouini,* OH.SA. was injected intramusculary in cases of *Tinea capitis* (Dermatomycosis) with incomplete success.

2. Protozoan Infections

Diamidines are efficient as leishmanicides (Sen Gupta, 1950, 1953): (1) They are used for kala-azar treatment. Because of its delayed toxicity, SA was replaced by OH.SA. which shows the same activity but is less toxic. It was successfully used in 42 patients with visceral kala-azar, both fresh or relapsed cases resistant to classic chemotherapy. OH.SA. was given by the intravenous or the intramuscular routes in 10–26 injections of a few grams. In cases of resistance or hypersensitivity to antimony compounds, diamidines and OH.SA. seem to be particularly important drugs. (2) Pentamidine and OH.SA. have been also successfully used against cutaneous leishmaniasis (Snapper, 1952a; Ercoli, 1961).

Diamidines are well known as animal and/or human trypanocides (Hawking, 1963). Pentamidine is the more effective for prophylaxis and treatment of *T. gambiense*; it is less active against *T. rhodesiense.* Propamidine and SA are less effective than pentamidine in the treatment of human trypanosomiasis. Although OH.SA. has the same activity as S.A., it seems to have been used more often in experimental models of trypanosomiasis than in human or veterinary medicine.

3. Miscellaneous Uses

Once again, chiefly SA and later OH.SA. were applied for myelomatosis treatment. Bone pain can be relieved and in a few cases temporary arrest of the malignant process may occur (Snapper, 1948; Pointon, 1961; Mihich and Muhlhern, 1966; Schwarzenberg et al., 1966).

4. Side Effects and Contraindications

Clinical application shows that the drug is generally well tolerated when given by slow intravenous injection or drips (Sen Gupta, 1950; Oberman and Gilbert, 1958; Lockwood et al., 1969; Weissmann et al., 1970). If injections are too fast or too frequent, side effects may occur, such as giddiness, palpitations and fall in blood pressure, due perhaps to histamine release; preventive use of antihistaminics is proposed. Concentrated solutions may cause thrombophlebitis, particularly in small veins. A generalized pruritus has also been observed. No fifth nerve neuropathy has been reported. Clinical application has not shown any absolute contraindication, but it is not advised to use OH.SA. in gross kidney or liver damage.

5. Resistances

Drug resistance in vitro and/or in vivo is a well-known and alarming phenomenon. Diamidines are no exceptions: this is the case for Ber. and SA. Resistance to SA has been described for *Babesia, Trichomonas* (Schnitzer, 1963), and *Trypanosoma* (Hawking, 1963); there is scarce information about OH.SA. but resistances of fungi were reported (Schnitzer, 1963). The same problems may exist for OH.SA. (Taschdjian, 1954) and SA. In spite of these restrictions OH.SA., as other diamidines, may help to palliate resistance of various microorganisms to other drugs.

IV. Biologic Studies and Mechanism of Action of OH.SA.

Several theories have been proposed concerning the mechanism of action of aromatic diamidines on microorganisms, particularly trypanosomes (Schoenbach and Greenspan, 1948). One proposal has been that they interfere with the intrinsic aerobic glucose metabolism of the cell. It has also been suggested a long time ago that diamidines may interfere with nucleoproteins or nucleic acids. Further biologic studies were done at cellular and molecular levels.

A. Cellular Studies In Vitro or In Vivo

SA and OH.SA. are known to localize in myeloma cells and to combine with nucleic acids (Snapper et al., 1951 b), giving fluorescent complexes useful for histological and pharmacologic studies. SA (and presumably other diamidines) is rapidly absorbed by the trypanosomes in which local concentration may be as much as 1400 times that of the external environment (Hawking, 1963). Extensive studies were made with various diamidines and trypanosomes as cellular models (Ormerod and Shaw, 1963) to follow the drugs, and with morphological alterations in relationship to pharmacologic activity.

1. Trypanosomes

OH.SA. activity was studied on in vitro cultures of *T. cruzi* (DELAIN et al., 1970, 1971; RIOU et al., 1970; FESTY, 1971). Effect on growth was evident after five days at a concentration over 10 μg/ml. OH.SA. was selectively found in the kinetoplasts by specific fluorescence. A few days after culture with 10 μg/ml OH.SA. 30–40% of the trypanosomes were dyskinetoplastic as judged by Giemsa staining or loss of kinetoplastic fluorescence. These phenomena were studied in greater detail by electron microscopy in cells treated by 5 μg/ml OH.SA. within 7 days. Characteristic and selective alterations of kinetoplasts occur after 15 h: the double-layered pattern of kinetoplast DNA (K-DNA) is rearranged into elongated fibrillar bodies; then all regular fibrillar structure disappears and later stages are characterized by the progressive loss of K-DNA: dyskinetoplastic cells appear after 6–7 days, containing only a small amount of amorphous kinetoplastic material. Irregular division may occur. Similar global results have been described for *T. gambiense* (ONO and INOKI, 1975) and *T. rhodesiense* in mice (MACADAM and WILLIAMSON, 1972); Ber, OH.SA., and pentamidine have been found to produce similar and specific lesions in the structure of *Trypanosoma rhodesiense,* with no effect on the nucleus but disintegration of the K-DNA core into granules and fibrils. These modifications of kinetoplastic organization suggest effects on extranuclear DNA replication as with Berenil (BRACK et al., 1972; DELAIN et al., 1970; NEWTON, 1975). In a previous study (RIOU et al., 1970) analytic ultracentrifugation of DNA revealed no modification of nuclear DNA by OH.SA. (or Ber.), but modifications in relative proportions of the two chondriome satellite DNAs. No abnormal circular DNA molecules were induced as by ethidium.

2. Yeast

Experimental studies showed (FESTY, 1971) that OH.SA. concentrations of 10^{-6}–10^{-5} M were without effect on growth of *Saccharomyces cerevisiae* in culture over a 28 h period. Under these conditions, OH.SA. is a very efficient mutagen producing "petite" colonies, like the intercalative drugs acriflavine and ethidium (3×10^{-6} M OH.SA. produced 97% mutants within 28 h). This can be compared to other active diamidines such as berenil (FESTY and GRAZZINI, 1974).

3. Bacteria

OH.SA. shows some antibacterial activity; it is also able to cure bacteria from their resistance plasmids (BOUANCHAUD, 1969) as do some intercalative dyes.

B. Physico-Chemical Studies In Vitro at the Molecular Level

Interactions of diamidines with nucleic acids in vivo or in vitro have been studied in detail with SA (TRUHAUT et al., 1966), Ber. (NEWTON, 1975), and

OH.SA. (FESTY, 1968, 1971; FESTY and DAUNE, 1973; FESTY et al., 1975). DNA association with SA or OH.SA. was proved by several physico-chemical methods: spectroscopic modifications of the dye, sedimentation, chromatography, and thermal stabilization of DNA. OH.SA. is a nonintercalative drug and a fluorescent probe of nucleic acid conformation. This latter property is associated with the specific modifications of fluorescence of OH.SA., induced by nucleic acids: both blue and red emissions are enhanced when the dye is bound to DNA; but only the blue emission is present when OH.SA. is bound to RNA or synthetic polyribonucleotides. In the case of DNA the enhancement of blue fluorescence increases linearly with the square of the percentage of A+T. Isotherms describing the binding of OH.SA. to DNA show two different sets of binding sites, the first one characterized by a higher binding constant, and a topological specificity for A-T. pairs. OH.SA.-DNA association involves two ion pairs, an almost purely entropic free energy of binding, and a large enhancement of the blue fluorescence of OH.SA. when the site corresponds to three adjacent A-T. pairs. From the geometry of the dye and its selective binding to double stranded structures, OH.SA. in the first set of sites is probably situated in the small groove of DNA, the phenolic group playing probably a major role in the selective binding.

A T-jump relaxation study of this association (STURM et al., 1975) clearly indicates two groups of sites and the kinetic model is in good agreement with those from the previous stoichiometric studies. Fluorescence confirms OH.SA. as a probe of conformation and dynamic structure of polydeoxyribonucleotides. The fluorescence properties of OH.SA. have also been used to study in vitro DNA accessibility to histones.

OH.SA.-nucleic acid associations are also of enzymatic interest. OH.SA. is an in vitro inhibitor of DNases I and II and of DNA-polymerase; this could probably be explained by template toxicity. The stimulation of the RNA polymerase of *Escherichia coli* (FESTY, 1971) is surprising and can be related to that observed with some diamines or the basic peptide H Factor of RNA synthesis.

C. Relationship Between Pharmacologic, Cellular, and Molecular Data

The occurrence, specificity, and enzymatic consequences in vitro of the OH.SA.-DNA association must be compared to biologic effects induced by the drug in trypanosoma or yeast. It is tempting to relate characteristics of in vitro OH.SA.-DNA association to in vivo affinity of OH.SA. to "nude" and AT-rich extranuclear DNA, to inhibition of its replication, and to cytoplasmic mutation in yeast induced by the drug. These molecular or cellular data afford a first attempt at understanding the pharmacologic activity of OH.SA. particularly in trypanosomiasis. OH.SA. activity can be compared to effects induced by other aromatic diamidines such as berenil: the two drugs have similar biologic properties and are representative of the same chemical series. In certain respects they differ from intercalative drugs such as acridines or phenanthridines

(LE PECQ, 1971) whose pharmacologic and clinical importance approaches that of diamidines.

Acknowledgment. The author wishes to thank May and Baker Ltd for supplies of diamidines and useful documentation.

References

Ashley, J.N., Harris, J.O.: Attempts to find new chemotherapeutic amidines. Part III. Nuclear substituted derivatives of 4:4′- and 3:3′-diamidinostilbene. J. Chem. Soc., 567 (1946)

Ashley, J.N., Barber, H.J., Ewins, A.J., Newbery, G., Self, A.D.H.: A chemotherapeutic comparison of the trypanocidal action of some aromatic diamidines. J. Chem. Soc., 103–116 (1942)

Beveridge, E.: Chemotherapy of leishmaniasis. In: Experimental chemotherapy. Schnitzer, R.J., Hawking, F. (eds.), Vol. II, pp. 257–287. New York, London: Academic Press 1963

Bouanchaud, D.: Personal communication (1969)

Brack, Ch., Delain, E., Riou, G., Festy, B.: Molecular organization of the kinetoplast DNA of Trypanosoma cruzi treated with berenil, a DNA interacting drug. J. Ultrastruct. Res. *39*, 568–579 (1972)

Busey, J.F.: Blastomycosis-3 – a comparative study of 2-hydroxystilbamidine and amphotericine B therapy. Am. Rev. Respir. Dis. *105*, 812–818 (1972)

Collier, H.O., Lourie, E.M.: The action in vitro of diamidines and other compounds on Leishmania donovani. Ann. Trop. Med. Parasitol. *40*, 88 (1946)

Cotty, V.F., Harris, A.F.: Action of amidines on epiphyseal cartilage of the rachitic rat and on chondroitin sulfate. Bull. N.J. Acad. Sci. *12*, 7–11 (1967)

Courseille, C., Busetta, B., Hospital, M.: Etude cristallographique des composés se fixant sur les acides nucléiques. Structure cristalline du diiséthionate d'hydroxystilbamidine. C.R. Acad. Sci. *274*, 1921–1924 (1972)

Delain, E., Brack, Ch., Riou, G., Festy, B.: Ultrastructure of trypanosomes treated with trypanocides: Selective effects on cytoplasmic DNA. J. Parasitol. *56*, 416 (1970)

Delain, E., Brack, Ch., Riou, G., Festy, B.: Ultrastructural alterations of Trypanosoma cruzi kinetoplast induced by the interaction of a trypanocidal drug (hydroxystilbamidine) with the kinetoplast DNA. J. Ultrastruct. Res. *37*, 200–218 (1971)

Downer, J.G., Batson, B.E., Busey, J.F., Allison, F., Lockwood, W.R.: Indications for the use of hydroxystilbamidine for the treatment of North American blastomycosis. Clin. Res. *14*, 94 (1966)

Ercoli, N.: Chemotherapeutic studies on cutaneous leishmaniasis. Proc. Soc. Exp. Biol. Med. *106*, 787–790 (1961)

Festy, B.: Interaction de l'hydroxystilbamidine avec les acides nucléiques in vitro et ses incidences enzymatiques. C.R. Acad. Sci. *266*, 1433–1436 (1968)

Festy, B.: Interaction de l'hydroxystilbamidine avec les acides nucléiques. Etud. Physicochim. Biol. Thesis (1971)

Festy, B., Daune, M.: Hydroxystilbamidine. A non intercalating drug as a probe of nucleic acid conformation. Biochemistry *12*, 4827–4833 (1973)

Festy, B., Grazzini, A.: Personal communication (1974)

Festy, B., Sturm, J., Daune, M.: Interaction between hydroxystilbamidine and DNA. I. Binding isotherms and thermodynamics of the association. Biochim. Biophys. Acta *407*, 24–42 (1975)

Folds, J.D., Orlando, G., Spitznagel, J.K.: Immunosuppression by hydroxystilbamidine isethionate, a lysosome stabilizing, antiproteolitic, antifungal drug. Infect. Immun. *11*, 441–444 (1975)

Fulton, J.D.: The prophylactic action of various aromatic diamidines in trypanosomiasis in mice. Ann. Trop. Med. Parasitol. *38*, 78 (1944)

Hampton, J.W.F.: The excretion of stilbamidine and some related compounds in experimental animals. Ann. Trop. Med. Parasitol. *41*, 226 (1947)

Hawking, F.: Chemotherapy of trypanosomiasis. In: Experimental chemotherapy. Schnitzer, R.J., Hawking, F. (eds.), Vol. I, pp. 129–256. New York, London: Academic Press 1963

Hirschhorn, R., Davies, P., Krakauer, K., Weissmann, G.: Stilbamidines: cortisone-like effects on lysosomes and connective tissue. Clin. Res. *17*, 354 (1969)

Le Pecq, J.B.: Use of ethidium bromide for separation and determination of nucleic acids of various conformational forms and measurement of their associated enzymes. In: Methods of biochemical analysis. Glick, D. (ed.), Vol. 20, pp. 41–86. New York: John Wiley and Sons, Inc. 1971

Lisboa, M.J., Torrico, M.A., Netto, L.A.G.B.: The use of 2-hydroxystilbamidine in lutz mycosis (South American blastomycosis), Sect. VI. Excerpta Med. *11*, 1406 (1957)

Lockwood, W.R., Allison, F., Batson, B.E., Busey, J.F.: The treatment of North American blastomycosis. Ten years experience. Am. Rev. Resp. Dis. *100*, 908–910 (1969)

Lourie, E.M., Yorke, W.: Studies in chemotherapy. XXI. The trypanocidal action of certain aromatic diamidines. Ann. Trop. Med. Parasitol. *33*, 289 (1939)

Macadam, R.F., Williamson, J.: Drug effects on the fine structure of Trypanosoma rhodesiense. Trans. R. Soc. Trop. Med. Hyg. *66*, 897–904 (1972)

May, Baker: Hydroxystilbamidine. Amidine therapy. 1° ed. (1957)

Mihich, E., Mulhern, A.I.: Synergistic antileukemic action of certain bisguanylhydrazones in combination with hydroxystilbamidine. Proc. Am. Assoc. Cancer Res. *7*, 49 (1966)

Nagington, J., Richards, J.E.: Chemotherapeutic compounds and Acanthamoebae from eye infections. J. Clin. Pathol. *29*, 648–651 (1976)

Newton, B.A.: Berenil: a trypanocide with selective activity against extranuclear DNA. In: Antibiotics. Mechanism of action of Antimicrobial and Antitumor Agents. Corcoran, J.W., Hahn, F.E. (eds.), Vol. III, pp. 34–47. Berlin, Heidelberg, New York: Springer 1975

Oberman, J.W., Gilbert, E.F.: The toxicity of 2-hydroxystilbamidine: probable fatal toxic reaction during treatment of blastomycosis. Ann. Intern. Med. *48*, 1401–1414 (1958)

Ono, T., Inoki, S.: Effect of hydroxystilbamidine on the kinetoplast of Trypanosoma gambiense in mice. Biken J. *18*, 257–265 (1975)

Ormerod, W.E., Shaw, J.J.: A study of granules and other changes in phase-contrast appearance produced by chemotherapeutic agents in trypanosomes. Br. J. Pharmacol. Chemother. *21*, 259–272 (1963)

Pickar, D.N., Walker, R.: Therapy of blastomycosis: a twenty-year study. Am. Rev. Resp. Dis. *98*, 119–120 (1968)

Pointon, R.C.S.: Chemotherapy of multiple myelomatosis. Clin. Radiol. *12*, 17–19 (1961)

Riou, G., Brack, Ch., Festy, B., Delain, E.: Kinetoplast DNA: Action of trypanocidal drugs on its biosynthesis. J. Parasitol. *56*, 464 (1970)

Schnitzer, R.J.: Drug resistance in chemotherapy. In: Experimental chemotherapy. Schnitzer, R.J., Hawking, F. (eds.), Vol. I, pp. 81–114. New York, London: Academic Press 1963

Schoenbach, E.B., Greenspan, E.M.: The pharmacology, mode of action and therapeutic potentialities of stilbamidine, pentamidine, propamidine and other aromatic diamidines. A review. Medicine *27*, 327 (1948)

Schwarzenberg, L., Schneider, M., Cattan, A., Amiel, J.L., Schlumberger, J.R., Mathé, G.: Le traitement des leucémies aigues par la méthyl-glyoxal-bis(guanylhydrazone) et son association avec la 2-hydroxystilbamidine. Sem. Hop. *42*, 2955–2959 (1966)

Sen Gupta, P.C.: Hydroxystilbamidine in the treatment of indian Kala-Azar. Indian Med. Gaz. *85*, 547 (1950)

Sen Gupta, P.C.: Chemotherapy of leishmanial diseases. A resume of recent researches. Indian Med. Gaz. *88*, 20 (1953)

Snapper, I.: Influence of 2-hydroxystilbamidine on the course of multiple myeloma. J. Mount Sinai Hosp. *15*, 156 (1948)

Snapper, I.: American mucocutaneous leishmaniasis successfully treated with 2-hydroxystilbamidine. Am. J. Med. *13*, 655 (1952)

Snapper, I., Lieben, F., Greenspan, E.M., Schneid, B.: Determination of stilbamidine and 2-hydroxystilbamidine deposited in parenchymatous organs and tumours. Cancer *4*, 1246 (1951 a)

Snapper, I., Schneid, B., Lieben, F., Gerber, I., Greenspan, E.: Influence of nucleic acid upon the fluorescence of nucleic and cytoplasm after injection of aromatic diamidines. J. Lab. Clin. Med. *37*, 562 (1951 b)

Snapper, I., Schneid, B., McVay, L., Lieben, F.: Pharmacology and therapeutic value of diamidine derivatives, particularly of 2-hydroxystilbamidine. Trans. N.Y. Acad. Sci. *14*, 269 (1952)

Snapper, I., McVay, L., Schneid, B.: The treatment of North American blastomycosis with 2-hydroxystilbamidine. Am. J. Med. *15*, 603 (1953)
Solotorovsky, M., Ironson, E.J., Gregory, F.J., Winsten, S.: Activity of certain diamidines against blastomycosis and Candida infections in mice. Antibiot. Chemother. *4*, 165 (1954)
Sturm, J., Zana, R., Daune, M.: Interaction between hydroxystilbamidine and DNA. II. Temperature jump relaxation study: dynamics of nucleic acids and polynucleotides. Biochim. Biophys. Acta *407*, 43–60 (1975)
Sutliff, W.D., Mills, D.: Chemotherapy of North american blastomycosis cases observed from 2 to 10 years. Antimicrob. Agents Chemother., 364–370 (1961)
Taschdjian, C.L.: Resistance of Trichophyton rubrum and Microsporum audouini to 2-hydroxystilbamidine induced in vitro. J. Invest. Derm. *23*, 385 (1954)
Truhaut, R., Festy, B., Le Talaer, J.Y., Jeanteur, P.: Interaction de la stilbamidine avec les acides nucléiques et son incidence sur quelques systèmes enzymatiques. C.R. Acad. Sci. *262*, 1905–1908 (1966)
Weissmann, G., Davies, P., Krakauer, K., Hirschhorn, R.: Studies on lysosomes -13- Effects of stilbamidine and hydroxystilbamidine on in vitro and in vivo systems. Biochem. Pharmacol. *19*, 1251–1261 (1970)
Wolff, O.H., Petty, B.W., Astley, R., Smellie, J.M.: Thrush oesophagitis with pharyngeal incoordination treated with hydroxystilbamidine. Lancet *1955 I*, 991

5-Iodo-2′-Deoxyuridine

W.H. PRUSOFF, M.S. CHEN, P.H. FISCHER, T.S. LIN, and G.T. SHIAU

I. History of Development

Iodinated pyrimidines were first synthesized by JOHNSON and JOHNS (1905–1906), and a systematic study of the biologic activities of various purine and pyrimidine base analogs was initiated by HITCHINGS et al. (1945) and extended by THOMPSON et al. (1949). The clinical potential of base analogs, whether halogenated or not, has been well recognized in chemotherapy. Furthermore, such compounds have proven to be powerful tools for elucidation of many intricate biochemical events of importance to molecular biology. Halogenated pyrimidine bases (ClUra, BrUra, IUra) are readily incorporated into the DNA of various microorganisms, however they are poorly utilized for the biosynthesis of DNA in mammalian systems in contrast to the corresponding deoxyribonucleosides (CldUrd, BrdUrd, IdUrd).

5-Iodo-2′-deoxyuridine (IUdR, IdU, IdUrd; Fig. 1) was first synthesized (Prusoff, 1959) as part of an anticancer program (WELCH and PRUSOFF, 1960). The finding by HERRMANN (1961) that IdUrd inhibited the replication of several DNA containing viruses (vaccinia and herpes simplex) in cell culture, resulted subsequently in the demonstration by KAUFMAN et al. (1962a, b), and GORDON and KARNOFSKY (1963) that this compound was effective in the topical therapy of an established virus infection in man (herpetic keratitis). Since systemic administration of IdUrd is associated with toxicity, programs concerned with the development of antiviral agents with decreased toxicity when administered systemically were initiated in many laboratories. From such a program evolved the 5′-amino analog of IdUrd. This compound, 5-iodo-5′-amino-2′,5′-dideoxyuridine (AIU, AIdUrd, Fig. 1), was synthesized by LIN et al. (1976) and found to be less potent than IdUrd as an antiviral agent (CHENG et al., 1975) in vitro, but to have the unique property of being nontoxic to either cells in culture or to day-old or adult mice (ALBERT et al., in press). AIdUrd has been shown to be highly effective in the treatment of herpes simplex keratitis in rabbits, although at molar doses higher than that required for IdUrd (ALBERT et al., 1976; PULIAFITO et al., 1977).

The chemical, physical and biologic properties of IdUrd have been recently reviewed extensively by PRUSOFF and GOZ (1975), and by LANGEN (1975). Because of the very close relationship of BrdUrd to IdUrd, where appropriate, either or both analogs will be discussed.

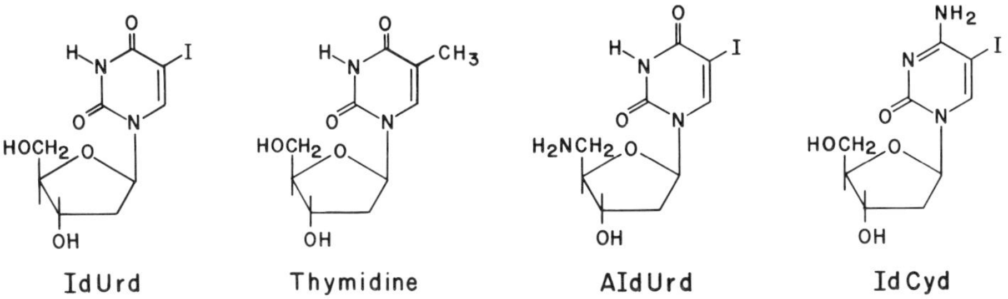

Fig. 1. Structure of 5-iodo-2′-deoxyuridine (IdUrd), 5-iodo-5′-amino-2′,5′-dideoxyuridine (AIdUrd), 5-iodo-2′-deoxycytidine (IdCyd), and thymidine (dThd)

II. Growth Inhibitory Properties of 5-Iodo-2′-Deoxyuridine

A. Bacteria

There are several reviews which describe in detail the effect of halogenated uracil analogs on microbial systems (HANDSCHUMACHER and WELCH, 1960; BROCKMAN and ANDERSON, 1963; HITCHINGS and ELION, 1963; LANGEN, 1975). HITCHINGS and co-workers (1945) first demontrated that 5-iodo-, 5-bromo, and 5-chlorouracil inhibited the replication of *Lactobacillus casei.*

5-Iodo-2′-deoxyuridine but not the corresponding ribonucleoside, 5-iodouridine, is almost as effective as iodouracil as an inhibitor of the growth of *Streptococcus faecalis* (ATCC 8043) when grown in media supplemented with thymine, thymidine or pteroylglutamic acid (PRUSOFF, 1959). Whereas IdUrd exerted complete inhibition of this microorganism, 5-iodouracil produced an inhibition of not more than 30% to 50% even at saturation levels (GUNTHER and PRUSOFF, 1963).

GUNTHER and PRUSOFF (1963) isolated a mutant strain of *Streptococcus faecalis* (ATCC 8043) that was 7,500-fold and 230-fold more resistant than the parent strain to the inhibition of growth produced by 6-azathymine and 6-azathymine-2′-deoxyribonucleoside, respectively. The growth of this mutant was stimulated fourfold by the addition of 5-iodouracil or of 5-iodo-2′-deoxyuridine to media supplemented with a suboptimal concentration of thymidine; however, in the absence of the latter no growth was observed. The parent and mutant strains possessed similar nucleoside phosphorylase activities. The mutant organism, in comparison to the parent strain, demonstrated a decreased efficiency in the utilization of thymidine for the biosynthesis of DNA-thymidine, because the mutant strain did not readily utilize the free thymine formed by the effect of nucleoside phosphorylase activity. Iododeoxyuridine was able to spare thymidine competitively from this catabolic reaction, and thereby enabled the cell to utilize more efficiently, for maximal growth and incorporation into DNA, an otherwise suboptimal amount of thymidine. The possibility that the mutant strain utilized IdUrd in lieu of thymidine for the synthesis of DNA was excluded experimentally, however there was some incorporation of labeled IdUrd into the bacterial DNA.

The observation that thymidine is more efficiently utilized by a pyrimidine-resistant strain of *S. faecalis* when in the presence of an analog is not a unique phenomenon. HITCHINGS et al. (1945), PRUSOFF (1954), and VISSER et al. (1960) previously found that analogs of pyrimidines stimulated microbial growth.

B. Mammalian Cells in Cell Culture

Replication of mammalian cells in cell culture is readily inhibited by IdUrd as well as the corresponding bromo-analog (5-bromo-2′-deoxyuridine, BUdR, BdU, BrdUrd). The kinetics of inhibition of L1210 cells by IdUrd in culture was studied by WILKOF et al. (1970) who found that kinetic parameters were independent of concentration and could be described by the Gompertz function. The inhibition exerted by IdUrd or BrdUrd can be increased by combination with antifolates. Thus BrdUrd in combination with methotrexate was found to exert an irreversible inhibition of HeLa cells (HAKALA, 1958, 1959). The inhibition of thymidylate synthetase by methotrexate prevents the de novo synthesis of dTMP, and hence affords the efficient utilization of BrdUrd or IdUrd for DNA biosynthesis after phosphorylation via the salvage pathway (thymidine kinase). Thus 50% replacement of DNA-thymidine by BrdUrd during a single cell cycle prevented further cellular replication. Other cell lines such as Sarcoma 180, L cells, and human uterine fibroblasts were able to undergo two to three replicative cycles before inhibition set in.

Mutant cell lines have been isolated by DJORDJEVIC and SZYBALSKI (1960), which showed no impairment of replication when grown continuously in the presence of 33 μM BrdUrd, a concentration that produced 14% substitution of DNA-thymidine. However, a fivefold increase in BrdUrd concentration increased DNA-thymine substitution to 39% with impairment of cell viability. SIMON (1963) has also described cells that are tolerant to the presence of BrdUrd in the media and can incorporate this analog into their DNA without apparent detriment. Mutant Syrian hamster melanoma cells which could replace 50% of DNA-thymidine with BrdUrd were characterized as being dependent on BrdUrd since in its absence these cells grew very poorly (DAVIDSON and BICK, 1973).

IdUrd is considerably more inhibitory than BrdUrd to human cell line D985, since growth in the presence of merely 14 μM IdUrd reduced viability markedly (DJORDJEVIC and SZYBALSKI, 1960). Similarly MATHIAS et al. (1959) and MATHIAS and FISCHER (1962) found that as little as 10 μM IdUrd allowed only one replication of murine leukemia L5178Y cells with concomitant loss of viability. The inhibitory effect of IdUrd was prevented by inclusion of thymidine in the medium. Analysis of the DNA derived from these murine leukemic lymphoblasts grown in the presence of 30 μM [^{131}I]-IdUrd indicated that two-thirds of DNA-thymidine in the progeny DNA had been replaced by this analog (MATHIAS et al., 1959). Replication of HEp cells in media supplemented with either BrdUrd or IdUrd allowed a single replication, and in the presence of 140 μM IdUrd about 25% of the DNA-thymidine had been substituted with IdUrd (EIDINOFF et al., 1959; CHEONG et al., 1960). MORRIS and CRAMER (1966, 1968) found IdUrd allowed only one replication of cell number and DNA when P8154 murine mast tumor cells were allowed to grow in the presence of 100 to 200 μM of this analog. These investigators (CRAMER and MORRIS, 1966) found that DNA synthesis took place in half of the population of cells inhibited by IdUrd. There have been many other studies of the inhibition by IdUrd and BrdUrd of replication of a variety of mammalian cells (ERIKSON and SZYBALSKI, 1961; MOHLER and ELKIND, 1963; SIMON, 1963; EY et al., 1964; KAJIWARA and MUELLER, 1964; GEERAETS et al., 1965; COGGIN et al., 1967; KIM et al., 1967; FUJWARA et al., 1970).

A lack of thymidine kinase is primarily responsible for cellular resistance to these halogenated nucleosides (KIT et al., 1963, 1966; LITTLEFIELD, 1965; DUBBS et al., 1967). Phosphorylation of IdUrd by this enzyme to the monophosphate derivative, IdUMP, is required for subsequent phosphorylation to the diphosphate, IdUDP, by thymidylate kinase, and then to the triphosphate, IdUTP, by nucleoside diphosphokinase. Since IdUTP and dTTP are alternate substrates for DNA polymerase, once IdUTP is formed it may then be incorporated into DNA with resultant inhibition of cellular replication (Fig. 2).

Marked cytologic damage to cells in culture is produced by these halogenated nucleosides which include lengthening of centromeric regions, secondary constrictions, and chromatid breaks (HSU and SOMERS, 1961, 1962; HSU et al., 1961; HUMPHREY and HSU, 1965; IZUTSU and BISELE, 1966).

Both 5-iodo-2′-deoxyuridine and 5-bromo-2′-deoxyuridine have been reported to have a variety of effects on enzyme activities in a number of different cell lines: induction, inhibition, alteration (STELLWAGEN and TOMKINS, 1971a, b; GOZ, 1974; BICK and SOFFER, 1976; BULMER et al., 1976; GURR et al., 1977).

C. Viruses

The potential of nucleoside analogs as antiviral agents, and of IdUrd and BrdUrd more specifically, has been extensively reviewed by PRUSOFF and GOZ (1975), and PRUSOFF and WARD (1976). THOMPSON and co-workers (1949) reported a modest inhibition by 5-bromouracil of the replication of vaccinia virus in cell culture, and VISSER et al. (1952) described the antiviral activity of 5-chlorouridine against Theiler's mouse encephalitis virus in mouse brain cultures. BrdUrd was found by SMITH et al. (1960) to inhibit the replication of polyoma virus in mouse embryonic cells, and HERRMANN (1961) found both BrdUrd and IdUrd to inhibit the replication of vaccinia and herpes simplex virus in cell culture. Although about 21 viruses were listed as being susceptible to the inhibitory effects of BrdUrd and IdUrd, only the inhibition of herpes simplex virus is of clinical utility (PRUSOFF and GOZ, 1975).

Studies by SMITH (1963), and SMITH and DUKES (1964) support the view that IdUrd does not prevent adsorption of herpes virus to cells. The virus particles formed in the presence of IdUrd, which are noninfectious, appear ragged and often empty, as shown for vaccinia virus (PRUSOFF et al., 1963), herpes zoster virus (RAPP and VANDERSLICE, 1964), herpes simplex virus (SMITH and DUKES, 1964), and SV40 virus (RAPP et al., 1965). SMITH and DUKES (1964) found IdUrd allowed only partial assembly of the herpes virion, rather than inhibiting the production of viral components. Similar findings with pseudorabies virus were made by KAPLAN et al. (1965).

ROIZMAN et al. (1963) found IdUrd exerted its inhibition of the replication of herpes simplex virus at 3 to 4 h after infection, and after 4 h the inhibition could not be reversed by thymidine. Thus inhibition was initiated during the process of viral DNA synthesis, and presumably once IdUrd is incorporated into the DNA, the biologic consequences can not be altered. Incorporation of halogenated nucleosides into viral DNA has been shown in vaccinia virus by PRUSOFF et al. (1963), and by EASTERBROOK and DAVERN (1963); in pseudorabies virus by KAPLAN et al. (1965); in herpes simplex virus by SCHIEK and SCHIEK (1969), CHEN et al. (1976); in SV-40 virus by BUETTNER and WERCHAU (1973), and CALOTHY et al. (1973); in polyoma virus by HIRT (1966); and in adenovirus by WIGAND and KLEIN (1974).

It has been postulated that incorporation of IdUrd into viral DNA is the critical event required to inhibit viral replication (PRUSOFF et al., 1965). FISCHER et al. (1977) found with herpes simplex virus type 1 a direct parallelism between the incorporation of IdUrd and 5-iodo-5′-amino-2′-dideoxyuridine into viral DNA and the degree of inhibition of herpes virus replication. BUETTNER and WERCHAU (1973) had previously isolated infectious DNA from SV40 virions and shown a relationship between loss of infectivity and the extent of substitution of SV40 DNA-thymidine by IdUrd.

Studies of the molecular event affected by incorporation of halogenated nucleosides into viral DNA found in general that the synthesis of specific viral antigens was not prevented, even though formation of infectious virus was (references cited in PRUSOFF and GOZ, 1975). However, MAASS and HAAS (1966) found a marked decrease in the formation of virus-specific SV40 antigens when the virus replicated in the presence of 280 μM IdUrd.

Studies with a bacterial virus (phage T_4) by GOZ and PRUSOFF (1968) indicated that infection with IdUrd-substituted phage T_4 resulted in the induction of markedly decreased levels of viral enzymes such as deoxycytidylate hydroxymethylase, dihydrofolate reductase, and lysozyme. This was apparently due to a reduced synthesis of enzyme molecules rather than to the formation of inactive protein (AAMODT and GOZ, 1970). Different gene products were affected to different extents (GOZ and PRUSOFF, 1970).

Analysis of the capsid proteins derived from adenovirus grown in the presence of IdUrd showed no difference in several physiologic and immunologic characteristics relative to control virions (WIGAND and KLEIN, 1974). KAN and PRUSOFF (1976) studied the effect of various levels of IdUrd on adenovirus-2 induction of polypeptides and found no effect on the rate of synthesis of early proteins. However, the synthesis of late proteins was uniformly depressed. It is conceivable that the analytic methods used may not have detected small but critical changes in amount of a specific protein, the appearance or disappearance of polypeptides present normally in small amounts or having mobilities identical to a protein present in large amounts, or small changes induced in molecular weight. PENNINGTON (1976) similarly had investigated the effect of BrdUrd on the formation of vaccinia virus-induced polypeptides. Under a viral inhibitory concentration of BrdUrd most polypeptides were nevertheless synthesized, but a few post-replicative polypeptides were markedly inhibited.

Following the observation that IdUrd and BrdUrd inhibit the replication of herpes simplex virus in vitro by HERRMANN (1961), the efficacy of IdUrd against herpes keratitis in rabbits and in humans was demonstrated by KAUFMAN (1962) and KAUFMAN et al. (1962a, b). The studies of experimental herpes keratitis in rabbits were confirmed by PERKINS et al. (1962), who also established the structural requirement of the pentose moiety of IdUrd since the corresponding *ribo*nucleoside of 5-iodouracil was biologically inactive. An unexplained finding by MAICHUK et al. (1973) is the inhibitory effect of 5-bromouridine on the replication of herpes simplex virus in cell culture which could be prevented by uridine, as well as the therapeutic effectiveness of 5-bromouridine in the therapy of herpes keratitis both in rabbits and clinically. The pyrimidine moiety of IdUrd, 5-iodouracil, neither prevented the replication of herpes simplex virus nor affected the synthesis of DNA (HANNA, 1966). Acetylation of the 3′- and 5′-hydroxyls of IdUrd produced a compound that was equally as efficacious as IdUrd in the therapy of experimental herpes keratitis in rabbits (PERKINS et al., 1962).

A comparison of the antiviral activity of IdUrd and 9-β-D-arabinofuranosyladenine (ara-A) against herpes simplex type 1 and 2 infections in vitro and in rabbit cornea in vivo by NORTH and PAVAN-LANGSTON (1976) showed araA to be more effective than IdUrd in vitro against both viruses; both were very effective, however, under in vivo conditions with no significant differences between the two drugs. RENIS (1977) compared the in vitro antiviral activity against herpes simplex virus type 2 of IdUrd, 1-β-D-arabinofuranosylcytosine (ara-C), 9-β-D-arabinofuranosyladenine (ara-A), and disodium phosphonoacetate (PAA) with the in vivo antiviral activity of these compounds in female hamsters with genital herpes simplex virus type 2 infection. He found not only *no* positive correlation existed, but rather, if anything, an inverse relationship. Thus IdUrd and ara-C were most inhibitory in vitro but were least active in vivo, whereas ara-A and PAA which were least active in vitro were most active in vivo. Thus great care should be exerted relative to the amount of enthusiasm generated from in vitro antiviral studies alone. There are obvious limitations in translation of findings not only from in vitro to animal studies, but also, as has been found with many other potential drugs, from animal studies to man.

Thus IdUrd represents the first antiviral agent which is effective clinically in an established virus infection. The efficacy of this drug in the therapy of herpes simplex infection of the corneal epithelium in man, a disease which is the major cause of blindness due to a corneal infection, has been unequivocally established in the United States and approved by the FDA for such use. JUEL-JENSEN (1973, 1974) has reviewed the clinical utility of IdUrd in man and, in addition to the therapy of herpes keratitis, beneficial results have been obtained in the therapy of herpetic whitlow, genital herpes, cutaneous herpes, herpes zoster, vaccinia lesions, and vaccinia whitlow (JUEL-JENSEN, 1973, 1974).

Successful treatment of herpes zoster topically with solutions of IdUrd in 100% dimethylsulfoxide (DMSO) as a solvent has been reported (JUEL-JENSEN et al., 1970; DAWBER, 1974). JUEL-JENSEN and MACCALLUM (1974) have treated over 1,000 patients with a 40% or a 35% IdUrd solution; DAWBER (1974) used 5% IdUrd in DMSO topically in a randomized double-blind control trial in 118 patients, and also significantly decreased the vesicular phase, healing time, and duration of pain. JUEL-JENSEN and MACCALLUM (1974) reiterate that 40% idoxuridine in DMSO continuously applied for 4 days was superior to 5% intermittently applied with a P value of <0.00001.

The early enthusiastic reports of the efficacy of IdUrd in the therapy of herpes encephalitis in man (BREEDEN et al., 1966; other references cited in GOZ and PRUSOFF, 1970) are in question because, in general, they were not randomized controlled experiments. Such a controlled study was initiated (Boston Interhospital Virus Study Group and cosponsor, 1975) but was terminated prematurely because myelosuppression was observed. Since this and other toxicities of IdUrd have been well documented in the literature (CALABRESI et al., 1961), such toxicity should not have been unexpected. Nevertheless, of the six patients with proven herpes simplex virus encephalitis treated, only one survived and that patient had received intraventricularly as well as intravenously administered IdUrd. That the mode of administration is very important is supported by the findings of LAUTER et al. (1975) who found that only one patient out of five treated with IdUrd against herpes encephalitis had a significant concentration of IdUrd in the cerebral spinal fluid, the others had none. Thus an intrathecal infusion is clearly indicated as being the appropriate manner of administration. Although the decision to terminate further study of the use of IdUrd in this condition may be correct, one wonders if careful attention to the proper pharmacologic use of this agent would have modified the clinical outcome. Furthermore, six cases may not be adequate to establish the efficacy or lack of efficacy of a drug in the therapy of herpes encephalitis because the condition of the patient being treated is critical. GURWITH et al. (1971) in reviewing mortality rates in this disease reported a 30% survival of patients who became comatose and an 85% survival of those who do not progress into coma.

Since IdUrd in appropriate concentration is toxic to normal cells, it is logical to ask what is the basis for its beneficial effect in those conditions such as herpes keratitis. References to studies concerned with this problem have been presented (PRUSOFF and GOZ, 1975). Fortunately for man, herpes simplex virus aids in its own demise by the induction of high levels of thymidine kinase in the infected cells. Thus IdUrd is trapped by phosphorylation in these cells for subsequent additional phosphorylation and incorporation into viral-DNA. The IdUrd not phosphorylated is subject to catabolism to inactive substances, primarily in the liver, as well as to urinary excretion. Those uninfected tissues, such as bone marrow, that are engaged in active DNA synthesis also have high thymidine kinase activity and may incorporate toxic amounts of IdUrd into their DNA. KAPLAN and BEN-PORAT (1967) found however a marked difference in the amount of IdUrd incorporated into the DNA of infected cells relative to noninfected cells, when incubated with low levels of drug (up to 1 μg/ml). Thus, judicious use of this agent may minimize toxicity.

Resistance to IdUrd develops rapidly following several passages in cell culture which contain the analog with vaccinia virus (LODDO and COLLA, 1973), and with herpes simplex virus (SMITH, 1963; BUTHALA, 1964). However, this does not appear to be a major problem clinically. Resistance as well as dependence of pox- and herpes-virus to IdUrd and BrdUrd have been reviewed by LODDO and COLLA (1973).

There have been a number of publications (cited in SUAREZ et al., 1976) that describe an enhancement of production of cytomegalovirus, adenovirus 7, Rubella virus, and SV40 virus in cells treated with IdUrd prior to infection. The mechanism is unknown, but incorporation into cellular DNA appears to be required.

D. Neoplasms

IdUrd was originally prepared as part of an anticancer program (PRUSOFF, 1959; WELCH and PRUSOFF, 1960), however its use today is primarily as an antiviral agent. JAFFEE and PRUSOFF (1960) found that IdUrd, when injected into mice in amounts of 100 or 150 mg/kg daily for 6 days, inhibited significantly the growth of Sarcoma 180, and lymphoma L1210 and L5178Y without evidence of toxicity. In no instance was a "cure" obtained, but marked inhibition of tumor growth was found. Even at concentrations which produced severe host toxicity and over 95% inhibition of tumor growth, the remaining neoplasia retained viability (JAFFEE and PRUSOFF, 1960).

Although JAFFEE and PRUSOFF (1960) found only additive inhibitory effects in the growth of murine lymphoma L1210 when combined with azaserine, 6-azathymine, 6-azauridine, FdUrd, or methotrexate, other investigators found IdUrd potentiated the activity of FdUrd in mice or rats bearing various neoplasms (BURCHENAL et al., 1960; HEIDELBERGER et al., 1960). GOLDIN et al. (1961) found IdUrd to be only 20% as effective as methotrexate in advanced murine leukemia L1210. BOOTH and SARTORELLI (1963) found that IdUrd in combination with uracil mustard resulted in a potentiation of the antitumor activity in Sarcoma 180 bearing mice.

Halogenated uracil derivatives, when incorporated into DNA, sensitize bacteria (GREER and ZAMENHOF, 1957; GREER, 1960) and mammalian cells in culture (DJORDJEVIC and SZYBALSKI, 1960) to the lethal effects of UV and X-ray radiations. These findings stimulated the experiments of BERRY and ANDREWS (1962a, b) who demonstrated a marked potentiating inhibitory effect on the growth of P-388 lymphocytic leukemia in mice by combination of IdUrd and X-ray radiations. Iodinated substrate analogs, when bound to the active site of an enzyme, may enhance the ultraviolet inactivation of specific enzymes (CYSYK and PRUSOFF, 1972; VOYTEK et al., 1972; KU and PRUSOFF, 1974; VOYTEK, 1975; CHEN et al., 1976; CHEN and PRUSOFF, 1977). The mechanism of radiation sensitization of these enzymes involves a dehalogenation with formation of a uracylil-free radical (RUPP and PRUSOFF, 1964; RUPP and PRUSOFF, 1965a, b) which subsequently interacts and inactivates the enzyme.

Studies in man by CALABRESI et al. (1961) provided evidence of modest tumor inhibition in 6 of 16 patients who had a variety of advanced neoplastic diseases with daily doses of IdUrd (17 to 124 mg/kg; i.v. within 1 to 3 h for 2 to 7 days). IdUrd therapy, when combined with radiation of a specific tumor area, was followed by prolonged arrest of growth at the irradiated site. PAPAC et al. (1962) also found treatment with IdUrd to be beneficial to patients with certain neoplastic diseases. The efficacy of IdUrd alone against neoplastic disease however does not appear to be promising. Whether combination therapy either with other drugs or radiation would offer any significant advantage, remains to be established.

BAGSHAW and DOGGETT (1969), KAPLAN (1970), and VERMUND (1971) have reviewed the potential of chemotherapeutic agents to enhance radiation therapy. Several studies have been performed but these were very limited in scope (WELCH and PRUSOFF, 1960; CALABRESI et al., 1961; GOLLIN et al., 1964; BAGSHAW et al., 1967; SANO et al., 1965, 1968; HOSHINO and SANO, 1969; LANDOLT, 1971).

IdUrd and BrdUrd are potent inducers of endogenous C-type viruses, and these viruses have been considered for a role in carcinogenesis. On the other hand the potent carcinogens are poor inducers of these viruses. Whereas LAZAR et al. (1975) found IdUrd-induced oncorna viruses ultimately led to carcinogenesis in vivo, JONES et al. (1976) found IdUrd did *not* produce transformation in a murine cell line even though oncornaviruses were induced by this nucleoside analog. The frequency of induction of C-type viruses by IdUrd is markedly augmented by polycyclic hydrocarbons (YOSHIKURA and ZAJDELA, 1976; YOSHIKURA et al., 1977), however there was *no* parallelism between such enhancement and in vivo carcinogenicity (Yoshikura et al., 1977).

III. Toxicity

That IdUrd is a cytotoxic agent was indicated by PRUSOFF (1959), JAFFEE and PRUSOFF (1960), and MATHIAS and FISCHER (1962) among others. The toxicity of IdUrd in mice, dogs, and man has been reviewed by WELCH and PRUSOFF (1960). The acute toxicity of intraperitoneally administered IdUrd in Swiss mice indicated an LD_{50} of 2.5 g/kg (PRUSOFF et al., 1960). The daily administration of 18 μmol (about 250 mg/kg) to mice produced 100% lethality, however the daily administration of half this amount was nontoxic. The lethality of IdUrd (18 μmol/day) could be prevented by the prior administration of thymidine (100 μmol). Thymidine may have saturated either the transport mechanism involved in the passage of IdUrd into cells or thymidine kinase within the cells for a sufficient period of time to allow catabolism and excretion of IdUrd thereby causing a reduction in the intracellular pools of IdUrd and its phosphorylated derivatives to a nontoxic level. Toxicity presumably is related to the amount of incorporation of IdUrd into the DNA of sensitive tissues.

Newborn rats were injected subcutaneously with IdUrd at the rate of 200 or 400 mg/kg per day for 5 days beginning at 1 day of age and killed at 20 days of age (PERCY et al., 1973). The growth rate was significantly reduced as well as growth of hair, and in addition developmental defects in the eye, cerebellum, and kidney were found. Rats and mice treated postnatally by PERCY and ALBERT (1974) with IdUrd showed defects in cerebellar, retinal and renal cortical development. PERCY (1975) treated pregnant mice and rats daily with IdUrd on 3 consecutive days, beginning on day 16 and 18 of pregnancy respectively. All offspring of mice treated with a massive concentration of 400 mg/kg were stillborn or died within 2 days. The teratogenic effects of IdUrd were minimal and were induced by dosages much higher than normally used in man. Thus damage produced in these animals by prenatal treatment with IdUrd were minimal compared with those treated postnatally.

The halogenated deoxyribonucleosides 5-chloro-2′-deoxyuridine, BrdUrd and IdUrd are teratogenic in mice, rats, and hamsters (CHAUBE and MURPHY, 1964; RUFFOLO and FERM, 1965; SKALKO et al., 1971; SKALKO and PACKARD, 1973). IdUrd at an equivalent dosage was found to be more embryotoxic than BrdUrd in mice (SKALKO and PACKARD, 1973). SKALKO et al. (1975) found pregnant female mice, administered a teratogenic dose of tritium labeled IdUrd on the 10th day of gestation, incorporated the analog into the DNA of mitotically active tissues of maternal organs, placentas, and embryos.

ITOI et al. (1975) administered 1 drop of 0.1% IdUrd solution into the eyes of rabbits six times on the sixth day of gestation and thereafter four times a day for 12 days. On the 28th day of gestation the animals were killed and the fetuses were removed. Teratogenic effects included exophthalmus-like deformities and clubbed forelegs. Although IdUrd has produced teratogenic effects in rabbits (ITOI et al., 1975), no teratogenic effect was found when this drug was given systemically to rats. Thus a striking species difference appears to exist, and the question raised is of what relevance are these findings to man?

The daily intraperitoneal administration of IdUrd (100 mg/kg) to dogs caused, within 10–20 days, loss of appetite, a gradual fall in the total leukocyte and thrombocyte counts, and the appearance of small amounts of blood in the feces. Histological examination revealed marked inhibition of cellular proliferation in the lymphoid elements and in the small intestine, the latter showed signs of epithelial desquamation (WELCH et al., 1960).

CALABRESI et al. (1961) found toxicity of systemically administered IdUrd in man to be concentration-dependent, the major toxic effects with doses of 100 to 120 mg/kg, when infused intravenously for periods of 2 to 3 h daily for 5 or 6 days, being stomatitis, leukopenia, and alopecia. The toxic manifestations of IdUrd in man such as alopecia and stomatitis were prevented by infusion of thymidine into the external carotid artery, while IdUrd was administered intravenously; however the effects of IdUrd on bone marrow were not abolished (CALABRESI, 1962; MARK and CALABRESI, 1962).

Topical therapy of herpes keratitis in man with IdUrd is not without hazards. These have been reviewed by MCGILL et al. (1974) and include contact dermatitis, punctate epithelial keratopathy, follicular conjunctivitis, narrowing and occulation of the puncta, lid changes, and lacrimation.

Of theoretical concern not only with IdUrd but also any drug that is incorporated to DNA or interacts with this polymer, are: (1) potential mutagenic effects, (2) carcinogenesis, (3) teratogenesis, and (4) activation of latent oncogenic viruses (AARONSON et al., 1971; LOWY et al., 1971; KLEMENT et al., 1971, and STEWART et al., 1972). Thus use of such compounds should be restricted to therapy of diseases of either high lethality or great morbidity, such as blindness.

IV. Synthesis

IdUrd can be isolated from enzymic-degraded DNA derived from microorganisms, such as *Escherichia coli* grown in media supplemented with 5-iodouracil (DUNN and SMITH, 1954, 1957; ZAMENHOF et al., 1956). IdUrd may also be prepared enzymically by incubation of 5-iodouracil, deoxyribose-l-phosphate, and the enzyme thymidine phosphorylase (FRIEDKIN and ROBERTS, 1954).

Synthetic IdUrd was prepared by PRUSOFF (1959), and CHEONG et al. (1960) by iodination of deoxyuridine in dilute nitric acid [dUrd (400 mg), iodine (400 mg), chloroform (2 ml), and HNO_3 (lN, 4 ml) are refluxed gently for 2 h during which time white needle crystals of IdUrd form]; in alkaline solution (PRUSOFF, 1959); with iodic acid (CHANG and WELCH, 1963); and with iodine monochloride (BROWNSTONE, 1963; BUI et al., 1965).

Radioactive IdUrd labeled with ^{125}I, ^{131}I or ^{132}I is readily prepared by any of these procedures (BROWNSTONE, 1963; SILVESTER and WHITE, 1963; BUI et al., 1965). A precaution in the measurement of ^{125}I isotope was reported by BAKHLE et al. (1964) who observed that some solvents or electrolytes absorb the soft gamma radiations from ^{125}I (E=0.035 MeV) to a markedly greater extent than that from ^{131}I (E=0.36 MeV).

Reviews of the properties and synthesis of these and similar nucleosides have been presented by MICHELSON (1963), ZORBACH and TIPSON (1968, 1973), KOCHETKOV and BUDOVSKII (1972), BLOCH (1973), TS'O (1974), and WATANABE et al. (1974).

V. Metabolism

A. Catabolism

Metabolic studies of the catabolic fate of IdUrd were performed in mice by PRUSOFF et al. (1960). Swiss female mice bearing the Ehrlich ascites carcinoma were administered four doses of IdUrd (12 μmol) labeled with ^{131}I at 12 h intervals. Following the last injection, 3 h later the ascites cells were collected, extracted with $HClO_4$ and subjected to ion exchange chromatography. Two radioactive substances were found in the acid soluble fraction of which 5% was 5-iodouracil and 95% iodide.

The rate of urinary excretion in Swiss mice was studied following an intraperitoneal injection of a single dose of [^{131}I]-IdUrd. Within 4 h approximately 74%

of the administered radioactivity appeared in the urine, and maximum excretion (91%) within 24 h (PRUSOFF et al., 1960). Chromatographic analysis of the urinary metabolic derivatives of IdUrd showed a minimum of seven radioactive peaks. Three major ^{131}I-containing peaks were identified as IdUrd (6.6%), iodouracil (3.8%), and iodide (83%). Because large amounts of free iodide formed following administration of [^{131}I]-IdUrd, it was of interest to identify the deiodinated reaction products. Thus, in a similar experiment with ^{3}H-IdUrd, seven radioactive substances in the urine were located by column chromatography. The only radioactive compound which had UV-absorption characteristics was identified as uracil. The other radioactive substances were not characterized. A minimum of four products contained both ^{3}H and ^{131}I, however they were not characterized either.

Other studies are in agreement with these findings, and show that the initial degradation product of IdUrd is 5-iodouracil which is catabolized subsequently to uracil and iodide, not only in mouse and rat, but also in man; iodide is the major radioactive metabolic product that occurs in blood, as well as in urine (COMMERFORD et al., 1960; WELCH and PRUSOFF, 1960; CALABRESI et al., 1961; HAMPTON and EIDINOFF, 1961; KRISS et al., 1962).

Studies in man by CALABRESI et al. (1961) showed that intravenous infusion of [^{131}I]-IdUrd (100–120 mg/kg) during periods of 2 to 3 h daily for 5 or 6 days maintained significant blood levels of IdUrd for about 4 h. Of the injected radioactivity 4 h after completion of the infusion 44% was in the urine and within 24 h about 90% had been excreted. After termination of the infusion of IdUrd about one-third of the radioactivity excreted within a 2 h interval was IdUrd, and thereafter very little IdUrd was excreted, iodouracil and iodide being the major urinary excretion products. Thus IdUrd is rapidly destroyed in man to iodouracil and iodide.

In an attempt to decrease the rate of catabolism as well as to obviate the marked instability to heat and the insolubility of IdUrd, CHANG and WELCH (1961) synthesized 5-iodo-2′-deoxycytidine (IdCyd) (Fig. 1). Studies in mice by BAKHLE et al. (1964a) revealed that 5-iodocytosine exerted a lethal effect in mice in dosages at which the corresponding ribonucleoside, deoxyribonucleoside (IdCyd), or the analogous derivatives or uracil were inocuous. The toxicity could be prevented by 5-methylcytosine but not by uracil or thymine. The biologic studies of IdCyd were disappointing in man (CRAMER et al., 1962; CALABRESI, 1963; CALABRESI et al., 1963), because it is a poor substrate for mammalian deoxycytidine kinase and a good substrate for the deaminase. Thus an inadequate amount is converted to 5-iodo-2′-deoxycytidylate which is essential in order to protect IdCyd from deamination to IdUrd and subsequent cleavage to 5-iodouracil. Hence, the activity of IdCyd as an antineoplastic agent is not greater than that of IdUrd (CRAMER et al., 1961, 1962; PRUSOFF, 1963; CALABRESI, 1963), and may in some instances have been less (CRAMER et al., 1962).

It is of interest that IdCyd is under investigation as an antiviral agent against herpes simplex virus (SCHILDKRAUT et al., 1975). Whereas IdCyd, as indicated above, is a poor substrate for mammalian deoxycytidine kinase, it, as well as 5-bromo-2′-deoxycytidine (DOBERSON et al., 1976), is a good substrate for the herpes simplex virus induced pyrimidine deoxyribonucleoside kinase. In order to protect uninfected cells that have deaminase activity and hence could form IdUrd, tetrahydrouridine, which is a potent inhibitor of this enzyme, has been used effectively.

The incorporation of labeled thymidine and IdUrd into DNA is used for measurement of cell kinetics in animal tumors or cell culture (CLEAVER, 1957; VAN ROOIJEN, 1975; LEE et al., 1976; HECK et al., 1977). An advantage of IdUrd is its greater susceptibility to enzyme degradation relative to thymidine. Although both thymidine and IdUrd are used for this purpose (for review see PRUSOFF and GOZ, 1975), reutilization of thymidine derived from DNA may be as high as 60%. IdUrd, in comparison to thymidine, is preferentially attacked by nucleoside phosphorylase (PONTIS et al., 1961; ZIMMERMAN, 1962; BIRNIE et al., 1963; FOX and PRUSOFF, 1965) and hence is subject to considerably less reutilization, which is an important characteristic for its use as a marker.

The mechanism involved in the dehalogenation of iodouracil which is formed by catabolism (enzymic phosphorolysis) of IdUrd is still under investigation. Dehalogenation of iodouracil may involve NADPH-linked dihydrouracil dehydrogenase-catalyzed reduction of the 5,6 double bond to form 5-iodo-5,6-dihydrouracil (IH_2Ura) with subsequent spontaneous elimination of HI to form uracil. Evidence supporting an enzymic involvement in the reduction step was presented by COOPER and GREER (1970). KIM et al. (1976) however support an enzymic involvement in the subsequent dehalogenation step rather than a spontaneous dehalogenation of the reduced iodouracil based on the rate of a spontaneous elimination of the halide being too slow. These investigators (KIM et al., 1976) believe that the dehalogenation of IH_2Ura in a soluble rat liver preparation is a two-step process, the first being an enzymic hydrolysis of the reduced pyrimidine ring to yield acyclic 2-iodo-3-ureidopropionate, and

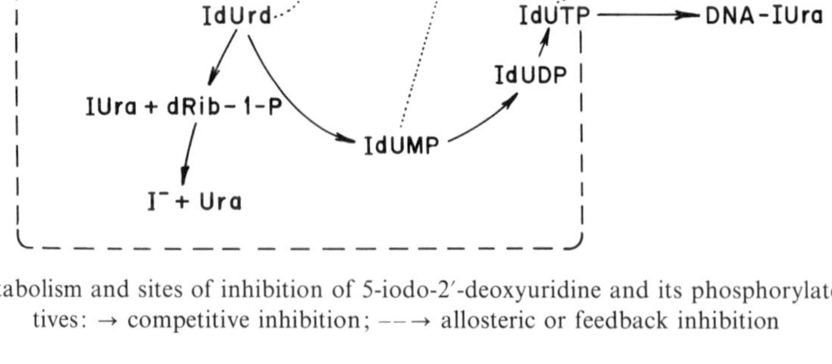

Fig. 2. Metabolism and sites of inhibition of 5-iodo-2′-deoxyuridine and its phosphorylated derivatives: → competitive inhibition; - - → allosteric or feedback inhibition

the second being a nonenzymic cyclization with release of iodide ion and formation of 2-amino-2-oxazoline-5-carboxylate. Under these conditions only small amounts of uracil were found.

Although all previous reports support the formation of iodide from IdUrd only after phosphorolysis to iodouracil, WATAYA and SANTI (1975) found that thymidylate synthetase could catalyze the dehalogenation of both 5-bromo- and 5-iodo-2′-deoxyuridylate. Of relevance is also the ability of sulfhydryl compounds (cysteine, glutathione) to dehalogenate BrdUrd under conditions that are nearly physiologic (WATAYA et al., 1973). The importance of these dehalogenation reactions for the degradation of halogenated nucleoside analogs remains to be established.

B. Anabolism

The steric and electronic similarities of IdUrd to thymidine allow the utilization of IdUrd and its phosphorylated derivatives as substrates for the various enzymes concerned with the biosynthesis of DNA (Fig. 2). Thus, IdUrd is incorporated into the DNA, but not RNA or protein of mammalian cells, plant cells, bacterial cells, or phage and animal viruses.

For such biosynthesis there is a marked preference for the utilization of thymidine relative to IdUrd (PRUSOFF, 1960; HUGHES et al., 1964; FOX and PRUSOFF, 1965; BAUGNET-MAKIEW and GOUTIER, 1968). Comparison of the relative uptake of equimolar amounts of radioactive thymidine and IdUrd into the DNA of Ehrlich ascites cells in vivo found a 40 times greater utilization of thymidine (PRUSOFF, 1960). Furthermore, the uptake of thymidine, relative to IdUrd, into DNA was found by BAUGNET-MAKIEW and GOUTIER (1968) to vary from tissue to tissue: by a factor of 2 in bone marrow, thymus, and normal liver, by a factor of 3.8 in spleen, and by a factor of 5 to 6 in regenerating rat liver. A direct correlation was found by DETHLEFSEN (1969) between the amount of IdUrd incorporated into the tumor DNA and the amount administered. Similarly, PRUSOFF (1960) had found an augmented uptake of IdUrd into DNA of Ehrlich ascites cells in vivo when the amount of IdUrd and the frequency of its administration were increased. Because thymidine and IdUrd use the same anabolic pathways (Fig. 2), it is not unexpected that thymidine can decrease the utilization of IdUrd for the biosynthesis of DNA.

VI. Mode of Inhibition

Although the similarities in physical and chemical characteristics of thymidine and IdUrd are sufficient to allow utilization of both compounds and their phosphorylated derivatives by the same enzymes (Fig. 2), there are differences in consequence of their respective incorporation into DNA. IdUrd and its phosphorylated derivatives are alternate substrates and hence kinetics of inhibition are of the competitive type. In addition, the triphosphate of IdUrd exerts, as does dTTP, a feedback inhibition of thymidine kinase, dCMP deaminase, and ribonucleoside diphospho-reductase. These interrelationships are depicted in Fig. 2. Incorporation of IdUrd into the DNA of neoplastic and plant cells or bacteria and viruses results in inhibition of replication; and similar uptake into normal cells also may cause inhibition of replication or death, and unless repaired by replacement with normal cells we see toxicity. Thus replacement of the methyl group in the 5-position of thymidine with an iodine atom is responsible for the specific physical and biologic properties of IdUrd.

Sterically there is little difference between thymidine and IdUrd since the size of the iodine atom, as defined by its van der Waals radius, is 2.15 Å as compared to 2.00 for the methyl group. However in IdUrd the electron configuration of the pyrimidine moiety is altered because of the inductive effect of the iodine atom, and this results in a more acidic dissociation constant. The pKa of thymidine is 9.8, whereas that of IdUrd is 8.25. Since the N-1 position is substituted with the deoxyribose moiety, the proton on the N-3 position is the one to be dissociated.

X-ray diffraction analysis of crystalline IdUrd by CAMERMAN and TROTTER (1964) revealed an unusually short intermolecular distance of 2.96 Å between the iodine atom and the oxygen of a carbonyl group, whereas the calculated sum of their van der Waals radii is 3.55 Å. They postulated that the ability of iodine to form charge transfer bonds may cause an increased interchain attraction that could either prevent or delay the synthesis of virus DNA. The formation of a similar charge transfer complex between the iodine atom of IdUrd in DNA and an adjacent base in the same DNA strand may be responsible for the increase in stacking energy found in DNA substituted with halogenated uracil bases (STERNGLANZ and BUGG, 1975). Of concern are the findings of RAHMAN and WILSON (1970) who found in a study of the crystal and molecular structure of 5-iodouridine, the corresponding ribonucleoside, no shortening of the interatomic distances. STERNGLANZ and BUGG (1975) believe that the altered stacking interactions may primarily be responsible for the mispairing between 5-halogenated uracil and guanine bases in DNA, rather than either ionization or enol-keto tautomerism.

A consequence of the incorporation of IdUrd or BrdUrd into viral DNA is an increase in its fragility (EASTERBROOK and DAVERN, 1963; MCCREA and LIPMAN, 1967) as well as a decrease in the infectivity of the isolated DNA, which is proportional to the amount incorporated (BUETTNER and WERCHAU, 1973). KAN and PRUSOFF (1976) found a direct correlation between the growth of adenovirus 2 in media supplemented with IdUrd and the loss of infectivity of these particles, and similarly FISCHER and PRUSOFF (1977) found a relationship between the uptake of 5-iodo-5′-amino-2′,5′-dideoxyuridine into the DNA of herpes simplex virus type 1 and the decrease in the ability of this virus to replicate. These direct findings clearly relate incorporation of IdUrd into DNA as an essential feature of the inhibitory process.

The ability of IdUrd or BrdUrd to have specific effects on embryonic development and expression of differentiated cell functions in a variety of biologic systems (RUTTER et al., 1973; PRUSOFF and GOZ, 1975; BICK, 1977), as well as the induction or repression of specific enzymes in mammalian cells (STELLWAGEN and TOMKINS, 1971a; KOYAMA and ONO, 1972; GOZ, 1974; BICK and SOFFER, 1976; GOZ and WALKER, 1976; GURR et al., 1977), may be related to the finding of tracts of thymidine in DNA. If specific genes have varying amounts of thymidine clusters and random incorporation of IdUrd into DNA occurs, then those genes, which are rich in thymidine tracts, will have a greater probability of incorporation of IdUrd and hence be specifically affected. Those genes which are highly redundant would require considerably more uptake to achieve a similar effect. SCHWARTZ (1976, and references cited therein) compared the uptake of thymidine and BrdUrd, found a selective uptake of BrdUrd but not of thymidine into selective regions of DNA, and postulated that incorporation into a few critical regulatory sequences, which are responsible for the control of gene expression in animal cells, could account for the selectivity of action in induction, embryo formation, differentiation, etc. A similar selectivity of uptake was found by STROM and DORFMAN (1976).

However, in a study of the effect of BrdUrd on the methylation of DNA in rat hepatoma, SINGER and co-workers (1977) found the percentage of substitution relative to thymidine uptake into highly repetitive, moderately repetitive and single copy sequences of DNA to be the same in each repetition class irrespective of the extent of substitution with BrdUrd, which varied from 2.1% to 95%.

STELLWAGEN and TOMKINS (1971a, b) related the selective inhibition to a translation event based on differential labilities of certain messenger RNA transcribed from halogen-substituted DNA and the proteins formed therefrom. Those proteins with high turnovers would be affected initially even though all mRNA synthesis was affected.

Base pair errors in either replication of DNA or in transcription could result from IdUrd or BrdUrd existing in the anionic or enol form to a greater extent than would thymidine at physiologic pH. Thus, LAWLEY and BROOKES (1962) have calculated that 50 times more BrdUrd exists in the anionic form than does thymidine at neutral pH. This explanation has been questioned. Thus, STERNGLANZ and BUGG (1975) postulate that the increase in stacking energy found in DNA substituted with halogenated bases may be primarily responsible for the mispairing, rather than either ionization or enol-keto tautomerism. Furthermore, SHUGAR and his co-workers (SHUGAR, 1978; KULIKOWSKI and SHUGAR, 1978) have found that the proportion of the two tautomers do not change appreciably when a halogen is inserted into the 5-position of a nucleoside, and hence factors other than tautomerism per se appear to be responsible for mispairing. A recent study, by KAUFMAN and DAVIDSON (1978) on the basis for bromouracil mutagenesis in mammalian cells, found this phenomenon to be related not to the amount of incorporation into DNA, but rather to the concentration of BrdUrd to which the cells were exposed.

These physical effects have very important consequences for the normal biologic functions of DNA, which have been pointed out in earlier sections. That transcription is indeed affected is supported by the studies of JONES and DOVE (1972) who found a seven-fold reduction in the synthesis of RNA in

BrdUrd substituted *Escherichia coli*, and by HILL and BASERGA (1975) who found in a eukaryotic system that transcribed RNA from fibroblasts grown in the presence of BrdUrd had about a 30% increase in guanylate and a 30% decrease in adenylate. This obviously could affect the proteins to be translated, and the key question is: *The synthesis of which specific protein is primarily affected?* Studies by KAN and PRUSOFF (1976) referred to above with adenovirus 2, and by PENNINGTON (1976) with vaccinia virus did indeed find the synthesis of viral induced-specific proteins to be affected when the virus replication was inhibited by IdUrd and BrdUrd respectively. GILBERT and co-workers (1974) found BrdUrd administered to Drosophila melanogaster to cause the disappearance of several proteins normally synthesized, as well as the appearance of an abnormal protein. Transcriptional errors may not be involved, since BICK (1975) found *no* such errors in cell lines that had 0, 60%, or 100% substitution of DNA-thymidine with BrdUrd. Similarly, STAMBROOK and WILLIAMSON (1974) found no BrdUrd induced transcriptional errors. Perhaps this is because of a more efficient repair excision during replication.

In addition to base errors, biologic consequence of incorporation of IdUrd or BrdUrd into DNA may be related to a greater binding affinity of substituted DNA to specific protein. LIN and RIGGS (1972) found a 10 times greater binding of the lac repressor to BrdUrd-substituted lac operator relative to the unsubstituted lac operator. Thus a tighter binding of substituted DNA to chromosomal or regulatory proteins in cells could result in the inhibition of expression of differentiated cell functions (GORDON et al., 1976; S.Y. LIN et al., 1976), and a tighter binding of specific regions of substituted DNA to RNA polymerase could affect not only the rate of RNA formation (JONES and DOVE, 1972; PAWLOWSKI, 1976) but also the relative amount of the various RNAs normally transcribed (GRADY and CAMPBELL, 1974; PRICE, 1976; LYKKESFELDT, 1977; PALAYOOR, 1977), as well as the composition or properties of the transcripts (HILL and BASERGA, 1975). These findings may be related to the alteration in conformation found during circular dichroism spectrums analysis of normal and BrdUrd substituted DNA. Although the spectrum of the DNA differed only slightly, the corresponding chromatin showed marked differences (LAPEYRE and BEKLOR, 1974; SIMPSON and SEARLE, 1974). Chromatin extensively substituted with BrdUrd has been characterized by SIMPSON and SEARLE (1974), and no difference from control chromatin was found in the composition of proteins, histones and nonhistones as well as the ability of the proteins to be dissociated by sodium phosphate in urea. Thus if differences in binding were present, they were not detected by the techniques used.

Although considerable information has been gleaned about a number of specific biologic and physical consequences that result from incorporation of 5-bromo- or 5-iodo-2′-deoxyuridine into DNA of a number of different biologic systems, much is contradictory and the penultimate event responsible for the biologic effect is yet to be elucidated.

References

Aamodt, L., Goz, B.: An immunological study of an enzyme made by phage containing 5-iodo-2'-deoxyuridine-substituted deoxyribonucleic acid. Biochem. Pharmacol. *19*, 2400 (1970)
Aaronson, S.A., Todaro, G.T., Scolnick, E.M.: Induction of murine C-type viruses from clonal lines of virus-free BALB/3T3 cells. Science *174*, 157 (1971)
Albert, D.A., Percy, D.H., Puliafito, C.A., Fritsch, E., Pavan-Langston, D., Lin, T.S., Ward, D.C., Prusoff, W.H.: AIU: An antiherpetic drug with low neonatal toxicity in mice Adv. Ophthalmol. *38*, in press
Albert, D.M., Lahav, M., Bhatt, P., Reid, T.W., Ward, R.E., Cykiert, R.C., Lin, T.S., Ward, D.C., Prusoff, W.H.: Successful therapy of herpes hominis keratitis in rabbits by 5-iodo-5'-amino-2', 5'-dideoxyuridine (AIU). J. Invest. Opthalmol. *15*, 470 (1976)
Bagshaw, M.A., Doggett, R.L.S.: A clinical study of chemical radiosensitization. Front. Radiat. Ther. Oncol. *4*, 164 (1969)
Bagshaw, M.A., Doggett, R.L.S., Smith, K.C., Kaplan, H.S., Nelson, T.S.: Intra-arterial 5-bromodeoxyuridine and x-ray therapy. Am. J. Roentgenol. Radium. Ther. Nucl. Med. *99*, 886 (1976)
Bakhle, Y.S., Creasey, W.A., Sartorelli, A.C., Prusoff, W.H.: Some biological and biochemical properties of 5-iodocytosine. Biochem. Pharmacol. *13*, 1249 (1964a)
Bakhle, Y.S., Prusoff, W.H., McCrea, J.F.: Precaution in the use of iodine-125 as a radioactive tracer. Science *143*, 799 (1964b)
Baugnet-Maniew, L., Goutier, R.: Mechanisms responsible for the low incorporation into DNA of the thymidine analogue, 5-iodo-2'-deoxyuridine. Biochem. Pharmacol. *17*, 1017 (1968)
Berry, R.J., Andrews, J.R.: Modification of the radiation effect on the reproductive capacity of tumor cells in vivo with pharmacological agents. Radiat. Res. *16*, 82–88 (1962a)
Berry, R.J., Andrews, J.R.: Modification of radiation effect on mammalian tumour cells by pharmacological agents. Nature (London) *196*, 185–186 (1962b)
Bick, M.D.: Misincorporation of GTP during transcription of poly dAT-dAT and poly dABU-dABU. Nucleic Acid Res. *2*, 1513 (1975)
Bick, M.D.: Bromodeoxyuridine inhibition of Friend leukemia cell induction. Biochim. Biophys. Acta *476*, 279 (1977)
Bick, M.D., Soffer, M.: Altered glucose-6-phosphate dehydrogenase in bromodeoxyuridine-substituted cells. Nature (London) *260*, 788 (1976)
Birnie, G.D., Kroeger, H., Heidelberger, C.: Studies of fluorinated pyrimidines. XVIII. The degradation of 5-fluoro-2'-deoxyuridine and related compounds by nucleoside phosphorylase. Biochemistry *2*, 566 (1963)
Bloch, A.: The design of biologically active nucleosides. In: Drug design. Ariens, E.J., (ed.), Vol. IV, p. 286. New York: Academic Press 1973
Booth, B.A., Sartorelli, A.C.: Growth inhibition of a spectrum of transplanted mouse tumors by combinations of inhibitors of nucleic acid biosynthesis and alkylating agents. Cancer Res. *23*, 1762 (1963)
Boston Interhospital Virus Study Group and the NIAID-sponsored Cooperative Antiviral Clinical Study. N. Engl. J. Med. *292*, 599 (1975)
Breeden, C.J., Hall, T.C., Tyler, H.R.: Herpes simplex encephalitis treated with systemic 5-iodo-2'-deoxyuridine. Ann. Intern. Med. *65*, 1050 (1966)
Brockman, R.W., Anderson, E.P.: Pyrimidine analogues. In: Metabolic inhibitors. Hochster, R.M., Quastel, J.H., (eds.), Vol. I, p. 239. New York: Academic Press 1963
Brownstone, A.D.: A simple preparation of 5-iodo-2'-deoxyuridine labelled with iodine-131 using iodine monochloride. Nature (London) *199*, 1285 (1963)
Buettner, W., Werchau, H.: Incorporation of 5-iodo-2'-deoxyuridine (IUdR) into SV40 DNA. Virology *52*, 553 (1973)
Bui, N.M., Gillett, R., Dumont, P.: An improved synthesis of 5-iodo-2'-deoxyuridine-I^{131} and 5-ioduracil-I^{131}. Int. J. Appl. Radiat. Isot. *16*, 337 (1965)
Bulmer, D., Stocco, D., Morrow, J.: Bromodeoxyuridine induced variations in the level of alkaline phosphatase in several human heteroploid cell lines. J. Cell. Physiol. *87*, 357 (1976)
Burchenal, J.H., Oettgen, H.F., Reppert, J.A., Coley, V.: Studies on the synergism of fluorinated pyrimidines and certain pyrimidine and purine derivatives against transplanted mouse leukemia. Cancer Chemother. Rep. *6*, 1 (1960)

Buthala, D.A.: Cell culture studies on antiviral agents. I. Action of cytosine arabinoside and some comparisons with 5-iodo-2-deoxyuridine. Proc. Soc. Exp. Biol. Med. *115*, 69 (1964)

Calabresi, P.: Regional protection in cancer chemotherapy. I. Infusions of thymidine into external carotid artery of patients receiving systemic 5-iodo-2′-deoxyuridine. J. Clin. Invest. *41*, 1484 (1962)

Calabresi, P.: Current status of clinical investigations with 6-azauridine, 5-iodo-2′-deoxyuridine, and related compounds. Cancer Res. *23*, 1260 (1963)

Calabresi, P., Cardoso, S.C., Finch, S.C., Kligerman, M.M., von Essen, C.F., Chu, M.Y., Welch, A.D.: Initial clinical studies with 5-iodo-2′-deoxyuridine. Cancer Res. *21*, 550 (1961)

Calabresi, P., Creasey, W.A., Prusoff, W.H., Welch, A.D.: Clinical and pharmacological studies with 5-iodo-2′-deoxycytidine. Cancer Res. *23*, 583 (1963)

Calothy, G., Hirai, K., Defendi, V.: 5-Bromodeoxyuridine incorporation into simian virus 40 deoxyribonucleic acid. Effects on simian virus 40 replication in monkey cells. Virology *55*, 329 (1973)

Camerman, N., Trotter, J.: 5-iodo-2′-deoxyuridine: relation of structure to its antiviral activity. Science *144*, 1348 (1964)

Chang, P.K., Welch, A.D.: Preparation of 5-iodo-2′-deoxycytidine. Biochem. Pharmacol. *8*, 327 (1961)

Chang, P.K., Welch, A.D.: Iodination of 2′-deoxycytidine and related substances. J. Med. Chem. *6*, 428 (1963)

Chaube, S., Murphy, M.L.: Teratogenic effects of 5-chlorodeoxyuridine on the rat fetus; protection by physiological pyrimidines. Cancer Res. *24*, 1986 (1964)

Chen, M.S., Prusoff, W.H.: Kinetic, photochemical studies, and alteration of ultraviolet sensitivity of *E. coli* thymidine kinase by halogenated allosteric regulators and substrate analogs. Biochemistry *16*, 3310 (1977)

Chen, M.S., Chang, P.K., Prusoff, W.H.: Photochemical studies and ultraviolet sensitization of *E. coli* thymidylate kinase by various halogenated substrate analogs. J. Biol. Chem. *251*, 6555 (1976a)

Chen, M.S., Ward, D.C., Prusoff, W.H.: Specific herpes simplex virus induced incorporation of 5-iodo-5′-amino-2′,5′-dideoxyuridine into deoxyribonucleic acid. J. Biol. Chem. *251*, 4833 (1976b)

Cheng, Y.-C., Goz, B., Neenan, J.P., Ward, D.C., Prusoff, W.H.: The selective inhibition of herpes simplex virus by 5′-amino-2′,5′-dideoxy-5-iodouridine. J. Virol. *15*, 1284 (1975)

Cheong, L., Rich, M.A., Eidinoff, M.L.: Introduction of the 5-halogenated uracil moiety into deoxyribonucleic acid of mammalian cells in culture. J. Biol. Chem. *235*, 1441 (1960)

Cleaver, J.E.: Thymidine metabolism and cell kinetics, Amsterdam: North-Holland 1957

Coggin, J.H., Larson, V.M., Hilleman, M.R.: Prevention of SV_{40} virus tumorigenesis by irradiated, disrupted and iododeoxyuridine trated tumor cell antigens. Proc. Soc. Exp. Biol. Med. *124*, 774 (1967)

Commerford, S.L., Gitlin, D., Hughes, W.L.: Inhibitory effect of small doses of x-radiation on incorporation of iododeoxyuridine (IDU) into DNA. Fed. Proc. *19*, 359 (1960)

Cooper, G.M., Greer, S.: Irreversible inhibition of dehalogenation of 5-iodouracil by 5-diazouracil and reversible inhibition by 5-cyanouracil. Cancer Res. *30*, 2937 (1970)

Cramer, J.W., Morris, N.R.: Absence of DNA synthesis in one-half of a population of mammalian tumor cells inhibited in culture by 5-iodo-2′-deoxyuridine. Mol. Pharmacol. *2*, 363 (1966)

Cramer, J.W., Prusoff, W.H., Welch, A.D.: 5-Bromo-2′-deoxycytidine (BCDR) II. Studies with murine neoplastic cells in culture and *in vitro*. Biochem. Pharmacol. *8*, 331 (1961)

Cramer, J.W., Prusoff, W.H., Welch, A.D., Sartorelli, A.C., Delamore, I.W., von Essen, C.F., Chang, P.K.: Studies on the biochemical pharmacology of 5-iodo-2′-deoxycytidine *in vitro* and *in vivo*. Biochem. Pharmacol. *11*, 761 (1962)

Cysyk, R., Prusoff, W.H.: Alteration of ultraviolet sensitivity of thymidine kinase by allosteric regulators, normal substrates, and a photoaffinity label, 5-iodo-2′-deoxyuridine, a metabolic analog of thymidine. J. Biol. Chem. *247*, 2522 (1972)

Davidson, R.L., Bick, M.D.: Bromodeoxyuridine dependence – a new mutation in mammalian cells. Proc. Natl. Acad. Sci. *70*, 138 (1973)

Dawber, R.: Idoxuridine in herpes zoster: further evaluation of intermittent topical therapy. Br. Med. J. *2*, 526 (1974)

Dethlefsen, L.A.: Tumor radioactivity from ^{125}I or ^{3}H-labeled IUdR. Cancer Res. *29*, 1717 (1969)
Djordjevic, B., Szybalski, W.: Genetics of human cell lines. III. Incorporation of 5-bromo- and 5-iododeoxyuridine into the deoxyribonucleic acid of human cells and its effect on radiation sensitivity. J. Exp. Med. *112*, 509 (1960)
Dobersen, M.J., Jerkofsky, H., Greer, S.: Enzymatic studies on the basis for selective inhibition of herpes simplex virus and varicella-zoster virus by 5-bromo-deoxycytidine. Fed. Proc. *35*, 1689 (1976)
Dubbs, D.R., Kit, S., De Torres, R.A., Anken, M.: Virogenic properties of bromodeoxyuridine-sensitive and bromodeoxyuridine-resistant simian virus 40-transformed mouse kidney cells. J. Virol. *1*, 968 (1967)
Dunn, D.B., Smith, J.D.: Incorporation of halogenated pyrimidines into the deoxyribonucleic acids of *Bacterium coli* and its bacteriophages. Nature (London) *174*, 305 (1954)
Dunn, D.B., Smith, J.D.: Effects of 5-halogenated uracils on the growth of *E. coli* and their incorporation into deoxyribonucleic acids. Biochem. J. *67*, 494 (1957)
Easterbrook, K.B., Davern, C.I.: The effect of 5-bromodeoxyuridine on the multiplication of vaccinia virus. Virology *19*, 509 (1963)
Eidinoff, M.L., Rich, M.A.: Incorporation of unnatural pyrimidine bases into deoxyribonucleic acid of mammalian cells. Science *129*, 1550 (1959)
Erikson, R.L., Szybalski, W.: Molecular radiobiology of human cell lines. I. Comparative sensitivity to x-rays and ultraviolet light of cells containing halogen-substituted DNA. Biochem. Biophys. Res. Commun *4*, 258 (1961)
Ey, R.C., Hughes, W.F., Holmes, A.W.: Clinical and laboratory evaluation of idoxuridine (IDU) therapy in herpes simplex keratitis. Arch. Ophthalmol. *71*, 325 (1964)
Fischer, P.H., Chen, M.S., Prusoff, W.H.: A relationship between the antiviral activity of 5-iodo-5′-amino-2′,5′-dideoxyuridine (AIdUrd) and its incorporation into herpes simplex virus DNA. Pharmacologist *19*, 209 (1977)
Fox, B.W., Prusoff, W.H.: The comparative uptake of I^{125} labeled 5-iodo-2′-deoxyuridne and thymidine-H^{3} into tissues of mice bearing hepatoma-129. Cancer Res. *25*, 234 (1965)
Friedkin, M., Roberts, D.: The enzymatic synthesis of nucleosides. II. Thymidine and related pyrimidine nucleosides. J. Biol. Chem. *207*, 257 (1954)
Fujiwara, Y., Oki, T., Heidelberger, C.: Fluorinated pyrimidines. XXXVII. Effect of 5-trifluoromethyl-2′-deoxyuridine on the synthesis of deoxyribonucleic acid of mammalian cells in culture. Mol. Pharmacol. *6*, 273 (1970)
Geeraets, W.J., Wong, G., Guerry, D., III: The effect of idoxuridine (IDU) on corneal stromal cells in tissue culture. Med. College Virginia Quart., p. 30 (1965)
Gilbert, E.F., Pitot, H.C., Bruyere, H.J., Jr., Cheung, A.L.: Abnormal proteins in *drosophila melanogaster* subsequent to 5-bromodeoxyuridine administration. Comp. Biochem. Physiol. *47B*, 229 (1974)
Goldin, A., Venditti, J.M., Kline, I., Mantel, N.: Evaluation of antileukemic agents employing advanced leukemia L1210 in mice IV. Cancer Res. *21*, CS 27 (1961)
Gollin, F.F., Ansfield, F.J., Vermund, H.: Behandlung inoperabler Bronchialkarzinome durch Kombination von Chemotherapie und Bestrahlung. Dtsch. Med. Wochenschr. *45*, 2140 (1964)
Gordon, D.M., Karnofsky, D.A.: Chemotherapy of herpes simplex keratitis. Am. J. Ophthal. *55*, 229 (1963)
Gordon, J.S., Bell, G.I., Martinson, H.C., Rutter, W.J.: Selective interaction of 5′-bromodeoxyuridine substituted DNA with different chromosomal proteins. Biochemistry *15*, 4778 (1976)
Goz, B.: The induction of alkaline phosphatase activity in HeLa cells by 5-iodo-2′-deoxyuridine. Cancer Res. *34*, 2393 (1974)
Goz, B., Prusoff, W.H.: The ability of phage containing 5-iodo-2′-deoxyuridine-substituted DNA to induce enzymes. J. Biol. Chem. *243*, 4750 (1968)
Goz, B., Prusoff, W.H.: The relation of antiviral activity of IUdR to gene function in phage. Ann. N.Y. Acad. Sci. *173*, 379 (1970a)
Goz, B., Prusoff, W.H.: Pharmacology of viruses. Annu. Rev. Pharmacol. *10*, 143 (1970b)
Goz, B., Walker, K.P.: The incorporation of 5-iodo-2′-deoxyuridine into the DNA of HeLa cells and the induction of alkaline phosphatase activity. Cancer Res. *36*, 4480 (1976)
Grady, L.J., Campbell, W.P.: The distribution of 5-bromodeoxyuridine in the DNA of polyoma-transformed mouse cells and some apparent effects on transcription. Exp. Cell Res. *87*, 127 (1974)

Greer, S.: Studies on ultraviolet irradiation of *Escherichia coli* containing 5-bromouracil in its DNA. J. Gen. Microbiol. *22*, 618 (1960)

Greer, S., Zamenhof, S.: Effect of 5-bromouracil in deoxyribonucleic acid of *E. coli* on sensitivity to ultraviolet radiation. Abstr. papers 131st Meet. Am. Chem. Soc. 3C (1957)

Gunther, H.L., Prusoff, W.H.: Studies on the mechanism of resistance to pyrimidines in Streptococcus faecalis. I. An unusual effect of 5-iodouracil and 5-iodo-2′-deoxyuridine. J. Biol. Chem. *238*, 1091 (1963)

Gurr, J.A., Becker, J.E., Potter, V.R.: The diverse effects of 5′-bromodeoxyuridine on enzyme activities in cultured H35 hepatoma cells. J. Cell Physiol. *81*, 271 (1977)

Gurwith, M.J., Harman, C.E., Merigan, T.C.: Approach to diagnosis and treatment of herpes simplex encephalitis. Calif. Med. *115*, 63 (1971)

Hakala, M.T.: Tissue culture studies on mechanisms of action of some purine and thymine analogs. Fed. Proc. *17*, 236 (1958)

Hakala, M.T.: Mode of action of 5-bromodeoxyuridine on mammalian cells in culture. J. Biol. Chem. *234*, 3072 (1959).

Hampton, E.G., Eidinoff, M.L.: Administration of 5-iododeoxyuridine-I^{131} in the mouse and rat. Cancer Res. *21*, 345 (1961)

Handschumacher, R.E., Welch, A.D.: Agents which influence nucleic acid metabolism. In: The nucleic acids. Chargaff, E., Davidson, J.N. (eds.), Vol. III, p. 453. New York: Academic Press 1960

Hanna, C.: Effect of several analogs of idoxuridine on the uptake of tritium labeled thymidine in the rabbit cornea infected with herpes simplex. Exp. Eye Res. *5*, 164 (1966)

Heck, H.D'A., McReynolds, J.H., Anbar, M.: A stable isotope method for measurement of thymidine incorporation into DNA. Cell Tissue Kinet. *10*, 111 (1977)

Heidelberger, C., Griesbach, C., Ghobar, A.: The potentiation by 5-iodo-2′-deoxyuridine (IDUR) of the tumor-inhibitory activity of 5-fluoro-2′-deoxyuridine (FUDR). Cancer Chemother. Rep. *6*, 37 (1960)

Herrmann, E.C., Jr.: Plaque inhibition test for detection of specific inhibitors of DNA containing viruses. Proc. Soc. Exp. Biol. N.Y. *107*, 142 (1961)

Hill, B.T., Baserga, R.: Effect of 5-bromodeoxyuridine on the transcriptional properties of the genome W1-38 human diploid fibroblasts. Chem. Biol. Interact. *10*, 363 (1975)

Hirt, B.: Evidence for semiconservative replication of circular polyoma DNA. Proc. Natl. Acad. Sci. USA *55*, 997 (1966)

Hitchings, G.H., Elion, G.B.: Purine analogues. In:Metabolic inhibitors. Hochstern, R.M., Quastel, J.H., (eds.), Vol. I, p. 215. New York: Academic Press 1963

Hitchings, G.H., Falco, E.A., Sherwood, M.B.: The effects of pyrimidines on the growth of lactobacillus casei. Science *102*, 251 (1945)

Hoshino, T., Sano, K.: Radiosensitization of malignant brain tumors with bromouridine (thymidine analog). Acta Radiol. *8*, 15 (1969)

Hsu, T.C., Somers, C.E.: Effect of 5-bromodeoxyuridine on mammalian chromosomes. Proc. Natl. Acad. Sci. *47*, 396 (1961)

Hsu, T.C., Somers, C.E.: Properties of L cells resistant to 5-bromodeoxyuridine, Exp. Cell. Res. *26*, 404 (1962)

Hsu, T.C., Billen, D., Levan, A.: Mammalian chromosomes *in vitro*. XV Patterns of transformation. J. Natl. Cancer Inst. *27*, 515 (1961)

Hughes, W.L., Commerford, S.L., Gitlin, D., Krueger, R.C., Schultze, B., Shah, V., Reilly, P.: Deoxyribonucleic acid metabolism *in vivo*. I. Cell proliferation and death as measured by incorporation and elimination of iododeoxyuridine. Fed. Proc. *23*, 640 (1964)

Humphrey, R.M., Hsu, T.C.: Further studies on biological properties of mammalian cell lines resistant to 5-bromodeoxyuridne. Tex. Rep. Biol. Med. *23*, 321 (1965)

Itoi, M., Gefter, J.W., Kaneko, N., Ishii, Y., Ramer, R.M., Gasset, A.R.: Teratogenicities of ophthalmic drugs. I. Antiviral ophthalmic drugs. Arch. Ophthalmol. *93*, 46 (1975)

Izutsu, I., Biesele, J.J.: Effects on HeLa cell division of physiologic deoxyribonucleosides and deoxyribonucleotides. Cancer Res. *26*, 910 (1966)

Jaffee, J.J., Prusoff, W.H.: The effect of 5-iododeoxyuridine upon the growth of some transplantable rodent tumors. Cacer Res. *20*, 1383 (1960)

Johnson, T.B., Johns, C.O.: Researches on pyrimidines; some 5-iodo pyrimidine derivatives; 5-iodocytosine. J. Biol. Chem. *1*, 305 (1905–06)

Jones, P.A., Benedict, W.F., Baker, M.S., Mondal, S., Rapp, U., Heidelberger, C.: Oncogenic transformation of C3H/10T 1/2 clone 8 mouse embryo cells by halogenated pyrimidine nucleosides. Cancer Res. *36*, 101 (1976)
Jones, T.C., Dove, W.F.: Photosensitization of transcription by bromodeoxyuridine substitution. J. Mol. Biol *64*, 409 (1972)
Juel-Jensen, B.E.: Herpes simplex and zoster. Br. Med. J. *1*, 406 (1973)
Juel-Jensen, B.E.: Virus diseases. Practitioner *213*, 508 (1974)
Juel-Jensen, B.E., MacCallum, F.O.: Idoxuridine in herpes zoster. Br. Med. J. *2*, 41 (1974)
Juel-Jensen, B.E., MacCallum, F.O., MacKenzie, A.M.R., Pike, M.C.: Treatment of zoster with idoxuridine in dimethyl sulphoxide. Results of two double-blind controlled trials. Br. Med. J. *4*, 776 (1970)
Kajiwara, K., Mueller, G.C.: Molecular events in the reproduction of animal cells. III. Fractional synthesis of DNA with BUdR and its effect on cloning efficiency. Biochim. Biophys. Acta *91*, 486 (1964)
Kan, J., Prusoff, W.H.: Effect of iododeoxyuridine (IdUrd) on adenovirus 2. Fed. Proc. *35*, 624 (1976)
Kaplan, A.S., Ben-Porat, T.: Differential incorporation of iododeoxyuridine into DNA of pseudorabies virus-infected and noninfected cells. Virology *31*, 734 (1967)
Kaplan, A.S., Ben-Porat, T., Kamiya, T.: Incorporation of 5-bromodeoxyuridine and 5-iododeoxyuridine into viral DNA and its effect on the infective process. Ann. N.Y. Acad. Sci. *130*, 226 (1965)
Kaplan, H.S.: Radiosensitization by the halogenated pyrimidine analogues: Laboratory and clinical investigations. In: Radiation protection and sensitization. Moroson, H.L., Quintiliani, M. (eds.), p. 35. New York: Barnes and Noble 1970
Kaufman, E.R., Davidson, R.L.: Bromodeoxyuridine mutagenesis in mammalian cells: Mutagenesis is independent of the amount of bromouracil in DNA. Proc. Natl, Acad. Sci. *75*, 4982 (1978)
Kaufman, H.E.: Clinical cure of herpes simplex keratitis by 5-iodo-2′-deoxyuridine. Proc. Soc. exp. Biol. (N.Y.). *109*, 251 (1962)
Kaufman, H.E., Martola, E., Dohlman, C.: Use of 5-iodo-2′-deoxyuridine (IDU) in treatment of herpes simplex keratitis. Arch. Opthalmol. *68*, 235 (1962a)
Kaufman, H.E., Nesburn, A.B., Maloney, D.E.: IDU therapy of herpes simplex. Arch. Ophthalmol. *67*, 583 (1962b)
Kim, B.D., Keenen, S., Bodnar, J.K., Sander, E.G.: Role of enzymatically catalyzed 5-iodo-5,6-dihydrouracil ring hydrolysis on the dehalogenation of 5-iodouracil. J. Biol. Chem. *251*, 6909 (1976)
Kim, J.H., Gelbard, A.S., Perez, A.G., Eidinoff, M.L.: Effect of 5-bromodeoxyuridine on nucleic acid and protein synthesis and viability in HeLa cells. Biochim. Biophys. Acta *134*, 388 (1967)
Kit, S., Dubbs, D.R., Pierkarski, L.J., Hsu, T.C.: Deletion of thymidine kinase activity from L cells resistant to bromodeoxyuridine. Exp. Cell Res. *31*, 297 (1963)
Kit, S., Dubbs, D.R., Frearson, P.M.: HeLa cells resistant to bromodeoxyuridine and deficient in thymidine kinase activity. Int. J. Cancer *1*, 19 (1966)
Klement, V., Nicolson, M.O., Huebner, R.J.: Rescue of the genome of focus forming virus from rat non-productive lines by 5-bromodeoxyuridine. Nature New Biol. *234*, 12 (1971)
Kochetkov, N.K., Budovskii, E.I., (eds.): Organic chemistry of nucleic acids, Vols. 1 and 2. London, New York: Plenum Press 1972
Koyama, H., Ono, T.: Further studies on the induction of alkaline phosphatase by 5-bromodeoxyuridine in a hybrid line between mouse and Chinese hamster in culture. Biochim. Biophys. Acta *264*, 497 (1972)
Kriss, J.P., Tung, L., Bond, S.: The distribution and fate of bromodeoxyuridine in the mouse and rat. Cancer Res. *22*, 1257 (1962)
Ku, K.Y., Prusoff, W.H.: A comparative study of the effect of normal substrates and 5-iodo-2′-deoxyuridine triphosphate, a metabolic analog of thymidine triphosphate on the inactivation of *Escherichia coli* DNA polymerase I and II. J. Biol. Chem. *249*, 1239 (1974)
Kulikowski, T., Shugar, D., Nucleic Acid Res. Sp. Publ. *4*, 7–10 (1978)
Landolt, A.M.: Resultate der postoperativen Behandlung des Glioblastoma multiforme mit einer strahlensensibilisierenden Substanz (5-bromo-2′-deoxyuridine). Acta Neurochir. *24*, 263 (1971)
Langen, P.: Antimetabolites of nucleic acid metabolism. New York: Gordon and Breach 1975

Lapeyre, J.N., Bekhor, I.: Effects of 5-bromo-2′-deoxyuridine and dimethyl sulfoxide on properties and structure of chromatin. J. Mol. Biol. *89*, 137 (1974)

Lauter, C.B., Bailey, E.J., Lerner, A.M.: Absence of idoxuridine and persistence of herpes simplex virus in brains of patients being treated for encephalitis. Proc. Soc. Exp. Biol. Med. *150*, 23 (1975)

Lawley, P.D., Brookes, P.: Ionization of DNA bases or base analogues as a possible explanation of mutagenesis, with special reference to 5-bromodeoxyuridine. J. Mol. Biol. *4*, 216 (1962)

Lazar, A., Schlesinger, M., Horowitz, A.T., Heller, E.: Induction of a carcinogenic oncornavirus in C57BL/6 mouse embryo cells by 5-iododeoxyuridine. Nature (London) *255*, 648 (1975)

Lee, D.-J., Prensky, W., Krause, G., Hughes, W.L.: Blood thymidine level and iododeoxyuridine incorporation and reutilization in DNA in mice given long-acting thymidine pellets. Cancer Res. *36*, 4577 (1976)

Lin, S.Y., Riggs, A.D.: *Lac* operator analogues: bromodeoxyuridine substitution in the *lac* operator affects the rate of dissociation of the *lac* repressor. Proc. Natl. Acad. Sci. *69*, 2574 (1972)

Lin, S.Y., Lin, D., Riggs, A.D.: Histones bind more tightly to bromodeoxyuridine-substituted DNA than to normal DNA. Nucleic Acid Res. *3*, 2183 (1976)

Lin, T.S., Neenan, J.P., Cheng, Y.-C., Prusoff, W.H., Ward, D.C.: Synthesis and antiviral activity of 5- and 5′-substituted thymidine analogs. J. Med. Chem. *19*, 495 (1976)

Littlefield, J.W.: Studies on thymidine kinase in cultured mouse fibroblasts. Biochim. Biophys. Acta *95*, 14 (1965)

Loddo, B., Colla, P.L.: Resistance and dependence in viral chemotherapy. In: Drug resistance and selectivity: Biochemical and cellular basis. Mihich, E. (ed.), p. 221. New York: Academic Press 1973

Loo, T.L., Michael, M.E., Garceau, A.J., Reid, J.C.: 6-Thiouric acid – a metabolite of 6-mercaptopurine. J. Am. Chem. Soc. *81*, 3039 (1959)

Lowy, D.R., Rowe, W.P., Teich, N., Hartley, J.W.: Murine leukemia virus; high-frequency activation *in vitro* by 5-iododeoxyuridine and 5-bromodeoxyuridine. Science *174*, 155 (1971)

Lykkesfeldt, A.E., Andersen, H.A.: Preferential inhibition of rDNA transcription by 5-bromodeoxyuridine. J. Cell Sci. *25*, 95 (1977)

Maass, G., Haas, R.: Über die Bildung von virusspezifischem SV-40 Antigen in Gegenwart von 5-Jod-2′-deoxyuridin. Arch. Ges. Virusforsch. *18*, 253 (1966)

Maichuk, Y.F., Pozdnyakov, V.L., Galegov, G.A., Bikbulatov, R.M.: Antiviral activity of 5-bromouridine in an experiment and its therapeutic effectiveness in herpesvirus infection of the eyes. Vop. Virusol. *18*, 408 (1973)

Mark, J.B.D., Calabresi, P.: Regional protection in cancer chemotherapy. II. Preliminary studies with hypogastric artery infusion of thymidine during treatment with 5-iodo-2′-deoxyuridine. Cancer Chemother. Rep. *16*, 545 (1962)

Mathias, A.P., Fischer, G.A.: The metabolism of thymidine by murine leukemic lymphoblasts (L5178Y). Biochem. Pharmacol. *11*, 57 (1962)

Mathias, A.P., Fischer, G.A., Prusoff, W.H.: Inhibition of the growth of mouse leukemia cells in culture by 5-iodo-deoxyuridine. Biochim. Biophys. Acta *36*, 560 (1959)

McCrea, J.R., Lipman, M.B.: Strand-length measurements of normal and 5-iodo-2′-deoxyuridine treated vaccinia virus deoxyribonucleic acid released by the Kleinschmidt method. J. Virol. *1*, 1037 (1967)

McGill, J., Williams, H., McKinnon, J., Holt-Wilson, A.D., Jones, B.R.: Reassessment of idoxuridine therapy of herpetic keratitis. Trans. Ophthal. Soc. U.K. *94*, 542 (1974)

Michelson, A.M.: The chemistry of nucleosides and nucleotides. New York: Academic Press 1963

Mohler, W.C., Elkind, M.M.: Radiation response of mammalian cells grown in culture. III. Modification of x-ray survival of Chinese hamster cells by 5-bromodeoxyuridine. Exp. Cell. Res. *30*, 481 (1963)

Morris, N.R., Cramer, J.W.: DNA synthesis by mammalian cells inhibited in culture by 5-iodo-2′-deoxyuridine. Mol. Pharmacol. *2*, 1 (1966)

Morris, N.R., Cramer, J.W.: 5-Iodo-2′-deoxyuridine and DNA synthesis in mammalian cells. Exp. Cell Res. *51*, 555 (1968)

North, R.D., Pavan-Langston, D., Geary, P.: Herpes simplex virus types 1 and 2: therapeutic response to antiviral drugs. Arch. Ophthal. *94*, 1019 (1976)

Palayoor, T.: Transcriptional effects of 5-bromo-2′-deoxyuridine in postimplantation mouse embryos. Experientia *33*, 448 (1977)

Palmer, C.G.: 5-bromodeoxyuridine-induced constrictions in human chromosomes. Cand. J. Genet. Cytol. *12*, 816–830 (1970)

Papac, R.E., Jacobs, E.C., Wong, F., Collom, A., Skoog. W., Wood, D.A.: Clinical evaluation of the pyrimidine nucleosides 5-fluoro-2′-deoxyuridine and 5-iodo-2′-deoxyuridine. Cancer Chemother. Rep. *20*, 143 (1962)

Pawlowski, P.J.: Effect of 5-bromodeoxyuridine on the appearance of cytoplasmic poly-A containing RNA. J. Cell Physiol. *89*, 19 (1976)

Pennington, T.H.: Effect of 5-bromodeoxyuridine on vaccinia virus-induced polypeptide synthesis: Selective inhibition of the synthesis of some post-replicative polypeptides. J. Virol. *18*, 1131 (1976)

Percy, D.H.: Teratogenic effects of the pyrimidine analogues 5-iododeoxyuridine and cytosine arabinoside in late fetal mice and rats. Teratology *11*, 103 (1975)

Percy, D.H., Albert, D.M.: Developmental defects in rats treated postnatally with 5-iododeoxyuridine (IUdR). Teratology *9*, 275 (1974)

Percy, D.H., Albert, D.M., Amemiya, T.: Oscular defects in newborn rats treated with 5-iododeoxyuridine. Proc. Soc. Exp. Biol. Med. *14*, 1272 (1973)

Perkins, E.S., Ward, R.M., Sears, M.L., Prusoff, W.H., Welch, A.D.: Antiviral activities of several iodinated pyrimidine deoxyribonucleosides. Nature (London) *194*, 985 (1962)

Pontis, H., Degerstedt, G., Reichard, P.: Uridine and deoxyuridine phosphorylases from Ehrlich ascites tumor. Biochim. Biophys. Acta *51*, 138 (1961)

Price, P.M.: The effect of 5-bromodeoxyuridine on messenger RNA production in cultured cells. Biochim. Biophys. Acta *447*, 304 (1976)

Prusoff, W.H.: Effect of 5-bromouracil on utilization of thymidine by *Streptococcus faecalis*. Proc. Soc. Exp. Biol. Med. *85*, 564 (1954)

Prusoff, W.H.: Synthesis and biological activities of iododeoxyuridine, an analog of thymidine. Biochim. Biophys. Acta *32*, 295 (1959)

Prusoff, W.H.: Incorporation of iododeoxyuridine into the deoxyribonucleic acid of mouse Ehrlich ascites tumor cells *in vivo*. Biochim. Biophys. Acta *39*, 327 (1960)

Prusoff, W.H., Goz, B.: Chemotherapy – molecular aspects. In: The herpes-viruses. Kaplan, A.S., (ed.), p. 641. New York: Academic Press 1973

Prusoff, W.H., Goz, B.: Halogenated pyrimidine deoxyribonucleosides. In: Antineoplastic and immunosuppressive agents. Sartorelli, A.C., Johns, D.G., (eds.), Vol. II, p. 272. Berlin, Heidelberg, New York: Springer 1975

Prusoff, W.H., Ward, D.C.: Nucleoside analogs with antiviral activity. Biochem. Pharmacol. *25*, 1233 (1976)

Prusoff, W.H., Jaffe, J.J., Gunther, H.: Studies in the mouse of the pharmacology of 5-iododeoxyuridine, an analogue of thymidine. Biochem. Pharmacol. *3*, 110 (1960)

Prusoff, W.H., Bakhle, Y.S., McCrea, J.R.: Incorporation of 5-iodo-2′-deoxyuridine into the deoxyribonucleic acid of vaccinia virus. Nature (London) *199*, 1310 (1963)

Prusoff, W.H., Bakhle, Y.S., Sekely, L.: Cellular and antiviral effects of halogenated deoxyribonucleosides. Ann. N.Y. Acad. Sci. *130*, 135 (1965)

Puliafito, C.A., Robinson, N.L., Albert, D.M., Pavan-Langston, D., Lin, T.S., Ward, D.C., Prusoff, W.H.: Therapy of experimental herpes simplex keratitis in rabbits with 5-iodo-5′-amino-2′, 5′-dideoxyuridine. Proc. Soc. Exp. Bio. Med. *156*, 92 (1977)

Rahman, A., Wilson, H.R.: The crystal and molecular structure of 5-iodouridine. Acta Crystallogr. Sect. B *26*, 1765 (1970)

Rapp, F., Vanderslice, D.: Spread of zoster virus in human embryonic lung cells and the inhibitory effect of iododeoxyuridine. Virology *22*, 321 (1964)

Rapp, F., Butel, J.S., Feldman, L.A., Kitakara, T., Melnick, J.L.: Differential effects of inhibitors on the steps leading to the formation of SV40 tumor and virus antigens. J. Exp. Med. *121*, 935 (1965)

Renis, H.E.: Chemotherapy of genital herpes simplex virus type 2 infections of female hamsters. Antimicrob. Agents Chemother. *11*, 701 (1977)

Roizman, B., Aurelian, L., Roane, P.R., Jr.: The multiplication of herpes simplex virus. I. The programming of viral DNA duplication in HEp-2 cells. Virology *21*, 482 (1963)

Ruffolo, P.R., Ferm, V.H.: The embryocidal and teratogenic effects of 5-bromodeoxyuridine in the pregnant hamster. Lab. Invest. *14*, 1547 (1965)
Rupp, W.D., Prusoff, W.H.: Incorporation of 5-iodo-2′-deoxyuridine into bacteriophage T1 as related to ultraviolet-sensitization or -protection. Nature (London) *202*, 1288 (1964)
Rupp, W.D., Prusoff, W.H.: Photochemistry of iodouracil. I. Photoproducts obtained in water. Biochem. Biophys. Res. Commun. *18*, 145 (1965a)
Rupp, W.D., Prusoff, W.H.: Photochemistry of iodouracil. II. Effects of sulfur compounds, ethanol and oxygen. Biochem. Biophys. Res. Commun. *18*, 158 (1965b)
Rutter, W., Pictet, R., Morris, P.W.: Toward molecular mechanisms of developmental processes. Annu. Rev. Biochem. *42*, 601 (1973)
Sano, K., Sato, F., Hoshino, T., Nagai, M.: Experimental and clinical studies of radiosensitizers in brain tumors, with special reference to BUdR-antimetabolite continuous regional infusion-radiation therapy (BAR therapy). Neurol. Med. Chir. *7*, 51 (1965)
Sano, K., Hoshino, T., Nagai, M.: Radiosensitization of brain tumor cells with a thymidine analogue (bromouridine). J. Neurosurg. *28*, 530 (1968)
Schiek, W., Schiek, E.: Untersuchung über infektiöses bromdesoxyuridinhaltiges Herpes Virus Hominis, Bestimmung der Dichte und der Sedimentationskonstanten im CsCl-H_2O-Dichtegradienten. Arch. Ges. Virusforsch. *28*, 229 (1969)
Schildkraut, I., Cooper, G.M., Greer, S.: Selective inhibition of the replication of herpes simplex virus by 5-halogenated analogues of deoxycytidine. Mol. Pharmacol. *11*, 153 (1975)
Schwartz, S.A.: Enzymatic determination of nonrandom incorporation of 5-bromodeoxyuridine in rat DNA. Biochemistry *15*, 3097 (1976)
Shugar, D.: In: Antimetabolites in biochemistry, biology and medicine. FEBS Symp., July 10–12, Praque, Czechoslovakia, 1978
Silvester, D.J., White, W.D.: Preparation of very high specific activity IUdR, IUR and iodouracil labelled with iodine 125, 131, 132. Nature (London) *200*, 65 (1963)
Simon, E.H.: Effect of 5-bromodeoxyuridine on cell division and DNA replication HeLa cells. Exp. Cell. Res. *9*, 263 (1963)
Simpson, R.T., Searle, R.L.: Characterization of chromatin extensively substituted with 5-bromodeoxyuridine. Biochemistry *13*, 4609 (1974)
Singer, J., Stellwagen, R.H., Roberts-Ems, J., Riggs, A.D.: 5-Methylcytosine content of rat hepatoma DNA substituted with bromodeoxyuridine. J. Biol. Chem. *252*, 5509 (1977)
Skalko, R.G., Packard, D.S., Jr.: The teratogenic response of the mouse embryo to 5-iododeoxyuridine. Experientia *29*, 198 (1973)
Skalko, R.G., Packard, D.S., Jr., Schwerdmann, R.N., Raggio, J.F.: The teratogenic response of mouse embryos to 5-bromodeoxyuridine. Teratology *4*, 87 (1971)
Skalko, R.G., Packard, D.S., Jr., Caniano, D.A., Sax, R.D.: Incorporation of 5-iododeoxyuridine into the DNA of mouse embryos: Its relation to embryotoxicity. Teratology *12*, 157 (1975)
Smith, J.D., Freeman, G., Vogt, M., Dulbecco, R.: The nucleic acid of polyoma virus. Virology *12*, 185 (1960)
Smith, K.O.: Some biological aspects of herpes virus-cell interactions in the presence of 5-iodo-2′-deoxyuridine (IDU); demonstrations of a cytotoxic effect by herpes virus. J. Immunol. *91*, 582 (1963)
Smith, K.O., Dukes, C.D.: Effect of 5-iodo-2′-deoxyuridine (IDU) on herpes virus synthesis and survival in infected cells. J. Immunol. *92*, 550 (1964)
Stambrook, P., Williamson, R.: Error frequency in 5 S RNA from cells grown in S-bromodeoxyuridine. Europ. J. Biochem. *48*, 297 (1974)
Stellwagen, R.H., Tomkins, G.M.: Preferential inhibition by 5-bromodeoxyuridine of the synthesis of tyrosine aminotransferase in hepatoma cell cultures. J. Mol. Biol. *56*, 167 (1971a)
Stellwagen, R.H., Tomkins, G.M.: Differential effect of 5-bromodeoxyuridine on the concentrations of specific enzymes in hepatoma cells in culture. Proc. Natl. Acad. Sci. *68*, 1147 (1971b)
Sternglanz, H., Bugg, C.E.: Relationship between the mutagenic and base-stacking properties of halogenated uracil derivatives. The crystal structures of 5-chloro- and 5-bromouracil. Biochim. Biophys. Acta *378*, 1 (1975)
Stewart, S.E., Kasnic, G., Jr., Draycott, C., Feller, W., Golden, A., Mitchell, E., Ben, T.: Activation *in vitro*, by 5-iododeoxyuridine, of a latent virus resembling C-type virus in a human sarcoma cell line. J. Natl. Cancer. Inst. *48*, 273 (1972)

Strom, C.M., Dorfman, A.: Distribution of 5-bromodeoxyuridine and thymidine in the DNA of developing chick cartilage. Proc. Natl. Acad. Sci. *73*, 1019 (1976)
Suarez, H.G., Morris, A.G., Lavialle, C., Cassingena, R.: Enhanced SV40-virus replication in Chinese hamster kidney cells pretreated with 5-iodo-2′-deoxyuridine. Arch. Virol. *50*, 249 (1976)
Thompson, R.L., Wilkin, M.L., Hitchings, G.H., Elion, G.B., Falco, E.A., Russell, P.B.: The effects of antagonists on the multiplication of vaccinia virus *in vitro*. Science *110*, 454 (1949)
Ts'o, P.O.P. (ed.): Basic principles in nucleic acid chemistry, Vols. 1 and 2. New York: Academic Press 1974
Van Rooijen, N.: A comparative study on the uptake in vitro of [^{3}H]thymidine, [^{131}I]5-iodo-2′-deoxyuridine and [^{3}H]deoxycytidine in mouse spleen cells using double isotope autoradiography. J. Immunol. Methods *8*, 151 (1975)
Vermund, H.: Enhancement of radiation effects by chemotherapy. Acta Radiol. Suppl. *311* (1971)
Visser, D.W., Lagerborg, D.L., Pearson, H.E.: Inhibition of mouse encephalomyelitis virus, *in vitro*, by certain nucleoprotein derivatives. Proc. Soc. Exp. Biol. Med. *79*, 571 (1952)
Visser, D.W., Frisch, D.M., Huang, B.: Synthesis of 5-chlorodeoxyuridine and a comparative study of 5-halodeoxyuridines in *E. coli*. Biochem. Pharmacol. *5*, 157 (1960)
Voytek, P.: Purification of thymidine phosphorylase from *Escherichia coli* and its photoinactivation in the presence of thymine, thymidine, and some halogenated analogs. J. Biol. Chem. *250*, 3660 (1975)
Voytek, P., Chang, P.K., Prusoff, W.H.: Kinetic and photochemical studies of 3-N-methyl-5-iodo-2′-deoxyuridine. J. Biol. Chem. *247*, 567 (1972)
Watanabe, K.A., Hollenberg, D.H., Fox, J.J.: Nucleosides LXXXV, On mechanisms of nucleoside synthesis by condensation reactions. J. Carb. Nucleosides Nucleotides *1*, 1 (1974)
Wataya, Y., Santi, D.V.: Thymidylate synthetase catalyzed dehalogenation of 5-bromo- and 5-iodo-2′-deoxyuridylate. Biochem. Biophys. Res. Commun. *67*, 818 (1975)
Wataya, Y., Negishi, K., Hayatsu, H.: Debromination of 5-bromo-2′-deoxyuridine by cysteine. Formation of deoxyuridine and S-[5-(2′-deoxyuridyl)] cysteine. Biochemistry *12*, 3992 (1973)
Welch, A.D., Prusoff, W.H.: A synopsis of recent investigations of 5-iodo-2′-deoxyuridine. Cancer Chemother. Rep. *6*, 29 (1960)
Welch, A.D., Jaffe, J.J., Cardoso, S.S., Finch, S.C., Calabresi, P., Liebow, A.A., Prusoff, W.H.: Studies on the pharmacology of 5-iododeoxyuridine in animals and man. Proc. Am. Assoc. Cancer Res. *3*, 161 (1960)
Wigand, R., Klein, W.: Properties of adenovirus substituted with iododeoxyuridine. Arch. Gesamte Virusforsch. *45*, 298 (1974)
Wilkof, L.J., Lloyd, H.H., Dulmadge, E.A., Dixon, G.J.: Kinetic evaluation of the effect of hydroxyurea on viability of replicating cultured leukemia L1210 cells. J. Natl. Cancer Inst. *44*, 201 (1970)
Yoshikura, H., Zajdela, F.: Induction du virus endogene, type C, par la 5-iododeoxyuridine; augmentation de cette induction par des hydrocarbures polycycliques. C.R. Acad. Sci. *282*, 1383 (1976)
Yoshikura, H., Zajdela, F., Perin, F., Perin-Roussel, O., Jacquignon, P., Latarjit, R.: Enhancement of 5-iododeoxyuridine-induced endogenous C-type virus activation by polycyclic hydrocarbons: apparent lack of parallellism between enhancement and carcinogenicity. J. Natl. Cancer Inst *58*, 1035 (1977)
Zamenhof, S., De Giovanni, R., Rich, K.: *Escherichia coli* containing unnatural pyrimidines in its deoxyribonucleic acid. J. Bacteriol. *71*, 60 (1956)
Zimmerman, M.: The possible identity of thymidine phosphorylase and pyrimidine deoxyribosyl transferase of rat liver. Biochem. Biophys. Res. Commun. *8*, 169 (1962)
Zorbach, W.W., Tipson, R.S., (eds.): Synthetic procedures in nucleic acid chemistry, Vols. 1 and 2. New York: Interscience Publisher 1968, 1969

Neocarzinostatin

I.H. GOLDBERG

The antitumor antibiotic neocarzinostatin (NCS), isolated from the culture filtrates of *Streptomyces carzinostaticus* variant F-14 (ISHIDA et al., 1965), is an acidic single-chain polypeptide with a molecular weight of 10,700 (MEIENHOFER et al., 1972a). The protein has been purified to homogeneity and its amino acid sequence (Fig. 1) (MEIENHOFER et al., 1972a, b; MAEDA et al., 1974; SAMY et al., 1977) and physical properties (MAEDA et al., 1973; SAMY and MEIENHOFER, 1974) have been determined. There are high degrees of homology of some regions of NCS and the protein antibiotic actinoxanthin (KHAKHLOV et al., 1969, 1976). NCS exists in a tight proteolysis-resistant conformation with an antiparallel β-pleated sheet structure (SAMY et al., 1974). It possesses two reduction-resistant disulfide bridges and lacks methionine and histidine. The positions of the disulfides have not yet been unambiguously assigned. NCS contains two tryptophan residues in positions 46 (buried) and 79 and one buried tyrosine residue at position 32. Oxidation of tryptophan 79 does not result in loss of biological activity (SAMY et al., 1974). Similarly, acylation of the amino groups (alanine 1 and lysine 20) does not affect the activity of NCS (MAEDA, 1974; SAMY, 1977). In the other hand, modification of the carboxyl groups results in loss of activity (SAMY, 1977). Further, spontaneous deamidation of asparagine

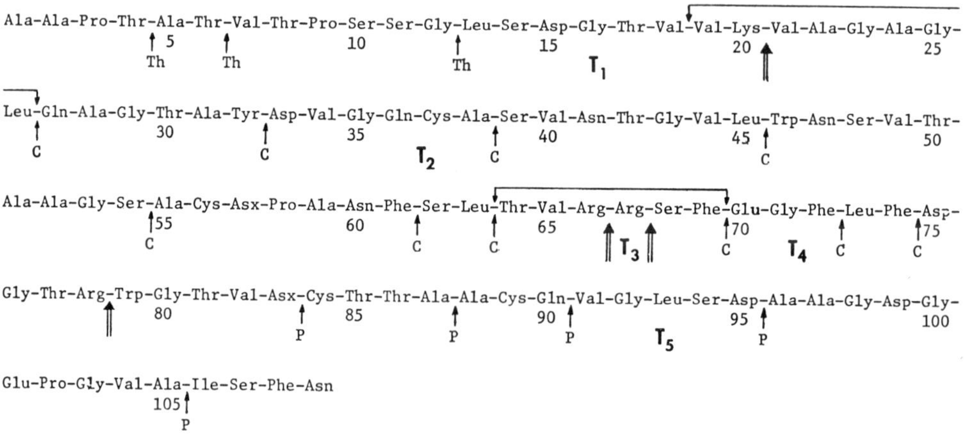

Fig. 1. Structure of neocarzinostatin. *Double arrows* indicate tryptic cleavage; *small arrows* show some of the subsequent cleavages by thermolysis (Th), chymotrypsin (C), or pepsin (P). Overlap peptides are indicated by a *bridged arrow* (MEIENHOFER et al., 1972)

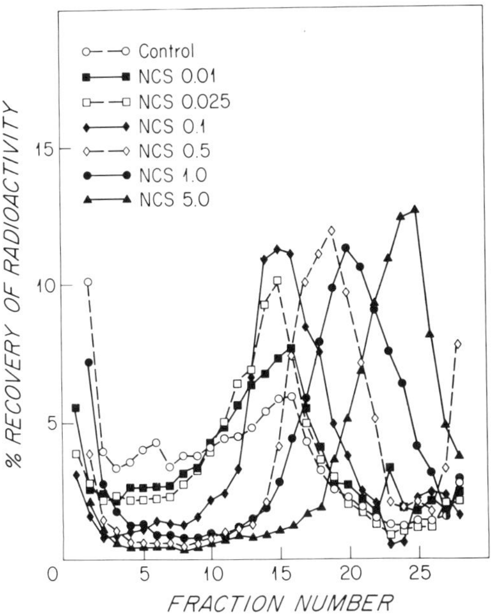

Fig. 2. Alkaline sucrose gradient analysis of DNA of HeLa cells treated with NCS. HeLa cells were labeled with [^{14}C]thymidine, treated with NCS, and analyzed by alkaline sucrose gradients. Centrifugation is *from right to left*. The peak of marker T4 DNA (71.1S) was in fraction number 24 (HATAYAMA and GOLDBERG, 1979)

83 at a weakly acidic pH generates "preneocarzinostatin" which lacks biological activity (MAEDA and KUROMIZU, 1977). The chemically deamidated compound is thought to be the same as the material isolated from culture filtrates that antagonizes NCS activity (KIKUCHI et al., 1974). NCS is readily inactivated by exposure to long wave length U.V. light (ISHIDA et al., 1965; KOHNO et al., 1974; BURGER et al., 1978; M. NAPIER and I.H. GOLDBERG, unpublished data), and this is presumably due to chromophoric absorption in the region of 360 nm (SAMY et al., 1974; M. NAPIER and I.H. GOLDBERG, unpublished data).

NCS is cytotoxic for gram-positive bacteria (ISHIDA et al., 1965) and a variety of experimental tumor cells (ISHIDA et al., 1965; BRADNER and HUTCHISON, 1966; KUMAGAI et al., 1966; SAKAMOTO et al., 1973; SASADA et al., 1976; HATAYAMA and GOLDBERG, 1979). There have been reports from Japan of its effectiveness in the treatment of solid tumors and acute leukemia in man (TAKAHASHI et al., 1969; HIRAKI et al., 1973; ANEHA et al., 1974; KITAJIMA et al., 1974, 1975; KINANI et al., 1975; MASAOKA et al., 1977). Phase 1 studies with NCS in the U.S. have recently been reported (GRIFFIN et al., 1977).

Considerable evidence has accumulated to show that DNA is an important target in the action of NCS. Thus, low levels of NCS selectively inhibit DNA in sensitive bacteria and mammalian cells (ONO et al., 1966; HOMMA et al., 1970; SAWADA et al., 1974; BEERMAN and GOLDBERG, 1977; HATAYAMA and GOLDBERG, 1979), induce degradation of existing DNA in bacteria (ONO et

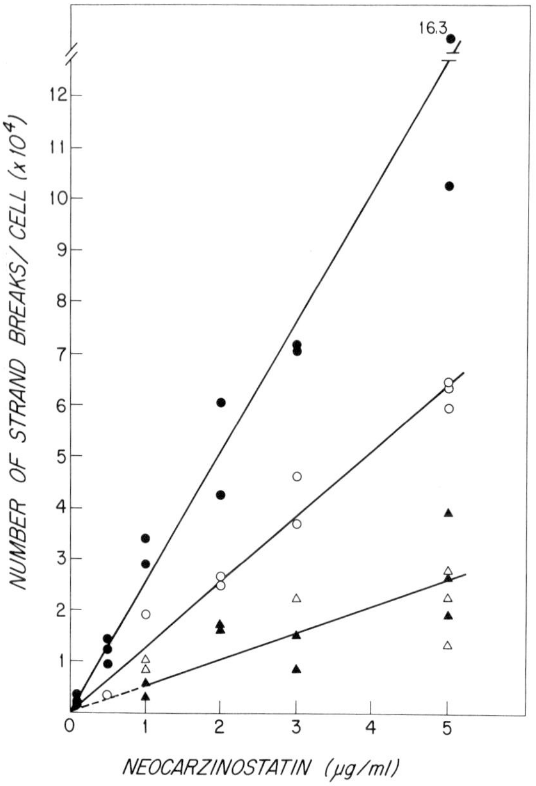

Fig. 3. Damage of HeLa cell DNA caused by NCS and its repair. ●——● Total number of single-strand breaks per cell immediately after treatment with NCS; ▲——▲ total number of double-strand breaks per cell immediately after treatment with NCS; *open symbols* represent respective breaks after 5 h reincubation without NCS. The regression lines were determined by the method of least squares (HATAYAMA and GOLDBERG, 1979)

al., 1966; OHTSUKI and ISHIDA, 1975a), and produce breaks in the DNA of mammlian cells (BEERMAN and GOLDBERG, 1974; SAWADA et al., 1974; TATSUMI et al., 1974; OHTSUKI and ISHIDA, 1975b; BEERMAN and GOLDBERG, 1977; BEERMAN et al., 1977; HATAYAMA and GOLDBERG, 1979). Under the cell lysis and centrifugation conditions employed in Fig. 2, the DNA of control HeLa cells sediments in alkaline sucrose gradients as a broad band with the main peak at 205S (fraction numbers 14–16) in addition to more rapidly sedimenting material. At the NCS concentrations of 0.01–0.025 μg/ml, only DNA of the 205S size is produced under this condition; the 205S material increases at the expense of the more rapidly sedimenting material, presumably due to single-strand nicks. NCS at 0.1 μg/ml produces not only more 205S DNA but also induces the single-strand scission of this size DNA, as represented by the small, more slowly sedimenting shoulder of the main peak in the gradient pattern. NCS concentrations of 0.5 μg/ml and above show clearly the dose-dependent, single-strand cleavage of DNA. A correlation exists between the ability of NCS to induce

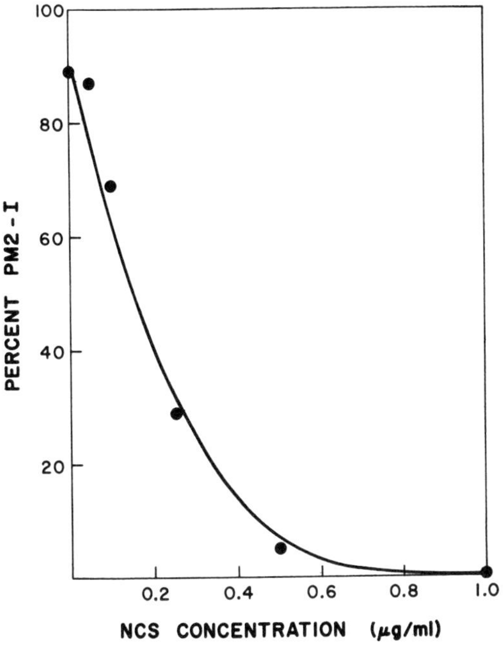

Fig. 4. Single strand scission of superhelical PM2 (Form I) DNA by NCS. The conversion of superhelical PM2 DNA (Form I) to the singly nicked circular duplex form (Form II) was followed on alkaline sucrose gradients (BEERMAN et al., 1977)

breakage of cellular DNA in HeLa cells and its inhibition of DNA replication and cell growth (BEERMAN and GOLDBERG, 1977; BEERMAN et al., 1977). NCS-induced single-strand breaks in HeLa cells can be repaired to a considerable extent but repair of double-strand breaks is less efficient (HATAYAMA and GOLDBERG, 1979) and the latter may account for the cell-killing activity of the antibiotic. As shown in Fig. 3, the number of single-strand breaks remaining after a 5-h repair period is about twice that of the double-strand breaks not repaired at the relatively high doses of NCS required to detect double strand breaks. Extrapolating from the number of double-strand breaks produced at drug levels of 1–5 μg/ml we find that there are about 55–60 double-strand breaks per cell at the mean lethal dose (at which there is 37% survival of cells) of 0.01 μg/ml NCS. Thus it appears that a small number of such breaks in a critical region of the genome may be the lethal event. Further, the so-called "DNA complex" consisting of DNA, lipid, and protein is disrupted by NCS treatment of HeLa cells and this is accompanied by the release within the cell of free DNA (HATAYAMA and GOLDBERG, 1979). DNA repair synthesis is activated by NCS-induced DNA damage as revealed by the induction of unscheduled DNA synthesis in treated lymphocytes (TATSUMI et al., 1975) and by the marked stimulation of thymidine incorporation into parental (but not newly made replicative) DNA in HeLa cells and isolated nuclei (KAPPEN and GOLDBERG, 1978a). Further, low levels of NCS cause a block in the G_2 phase of the cell cycle (EBINA

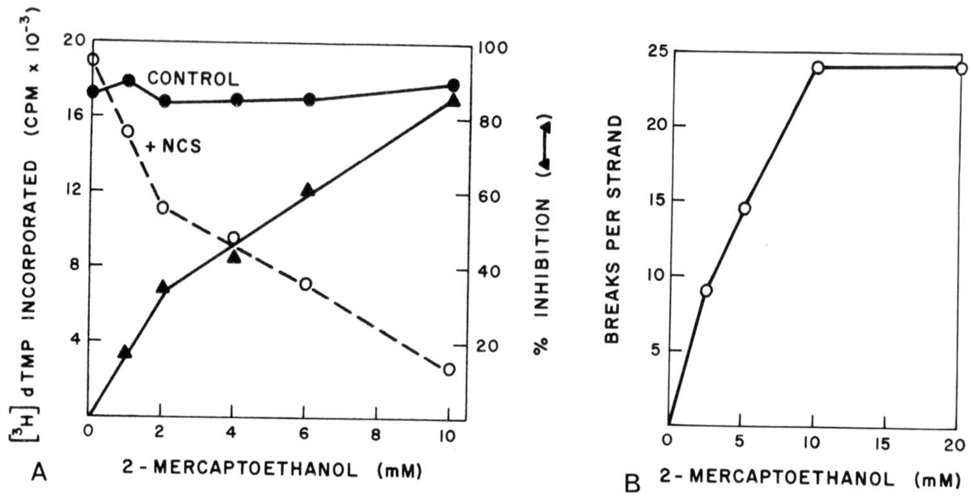

Fig. 5A and B. Influence of 2-mercaptoethanol on NCS-induced inhibition of DNA polymerase I and breakage of DNA. **A** DNA synthesis by DNA polymerase I. **B** Quantitation of NCS-induced strand breaks in λDNA by alkaline sucrose gradient analysis (KAPPEN and GOLDBERG, 1977)

et al., 1975; RAO and RAO, 1976) and chromosomal abberrations in mammalian cells (KUMAGAI et al., 1966; RAO and RAO, 1976).

Strong evidence for the involvement of DNA in NCS action comes from experiments showing that NCS is a mutagen for *Escherichia coli* and that mutagenicity and cell killing are affected in inverse ways by a recA mutation (TATSUMI and NISHIOKA, 1977). We have also found NCS to be mutagenic for *Salmonella typhimurium*, especially in strains bearing the plasmid pKM101 which has been implicated in error-prone repair (EISENSTADT et al., 1978). Finally, the lethal effect of NCS in L-1210 cells has been found to be potentiated by caffeine, an inhibitor of postreplication repair (SASADA et al., 1976).

NCS causes single-strand nicks in superhelical (Fig. 4) and linear duplex DNA in vitro and this reaction is stimulated at least 1000-fold by the presence of a mercaptan (BEERMAN and GOLDBERG, 1974; TATSUMI et al., 1974; ISHIDA and TAKAHASHI, 1976; BEERMAN et al., 1977; KAPPEN and GOLDBERG, 1977; POON et al., 1977; ISHIDA and TAKAHASHI, 1978; KAPPEN and GOLDBERG, 1978b; SIM and LOWN, 1978). At higher doses of NCS double-strand breaks are produced, presumably as the result of the random placement of single-strand breaks within a small number of base-pairs of one another.

NCS-treated DNA is a much poorer primer for *E. coli* DNA polymerase I than untreated DNA (Fig. 5) (TSURUO et al., 1971; KAPPEN and GOLDBERG, 1977), and the enzyme has been shown to bind to the site of DNA damage in a nonfunctional form (Fig. 6) (KAPPEN and GOLDBERG, 1977). The degree of inhibition of DNA synthesis by NCS depends on the concentrations of NCS and of 2-mercaptoethanol during preincubation (Fig. 5A). In the control containing no drug, [³H]dTMP incorporation is not affected to any significant extent by concentrations of 2-mercaptoethanol up to 10 mM in the preincubation reaction (4 mM in the final polymerization reaction), whereas in the presence

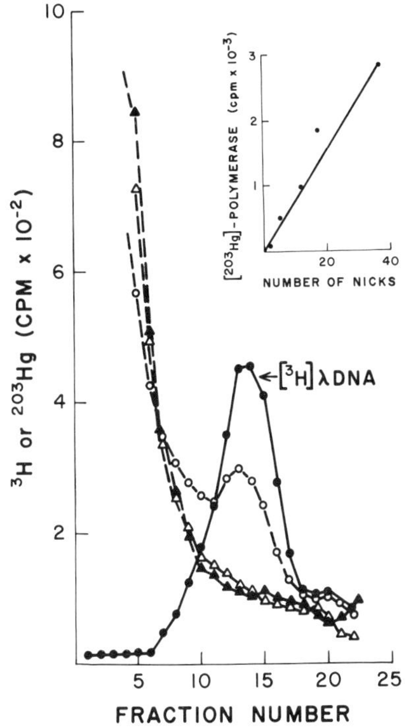

Fig. 6. Effect of NCS treatment of λ[^{3}H]DNA on [^{203}Hg]DNA polymerase I binding. Binding was determined by neutral sucrose gradient analysis, with sedimentation *from left to right*. The number of strand breaks was determined by alkaline sucrose gradient analysis. △ control; ▲ +NCS in the absence of 2-mercaptoethanol; ○ +NCS in the presence of 2-mercaptoethanol (KAPPEN and GOLDBERG, 1977)

of NCS the inhibition increases with increasing concentrations of 2-mercaptoethanol with maximal inhibition being obtained at 10 mM. The NCS-induced inhibition of DNA polymerase I activity, as described by the concentration of 2-mercaptoethanol, is related to the number of single-strand breaks in the DNA. As shown in Fig. 5A, the maximal inhibition of dTMP incorporation by NCS occurs under conditions of maximal strand scission (Fig. 5B), suggesting that there is a connection between the two effects of the drug. That NCS-induced strand breakage generates inactive binding sites for DNA polymerase I is shown in experiments in which either untreated DNA or excess enzyme are able to overcome the inhibition in a competitive way. Further, [^{203}Hg]DNA polymerase I bound to NCS-treated DNA (Fig. 6) and binding correlates with the extent of nicking (Fig. 6 insert). It appears that one molecule of enzyme binds to each break introduced by NCS.

The breaks possess both 3′- and 5′-phosphoryl termini, indicative of the existence of a gap of one or more nucleotides (POON et al., 1977; KAPPEN and GOLDBERG, 1978c). As expected, generation of a 3′-OH group by treatment of NCS-nicked DNA with alkaline phosphatase converts the DNA into a much better primer for DNA polymerase I than DNA unexposed to the antibiotic.

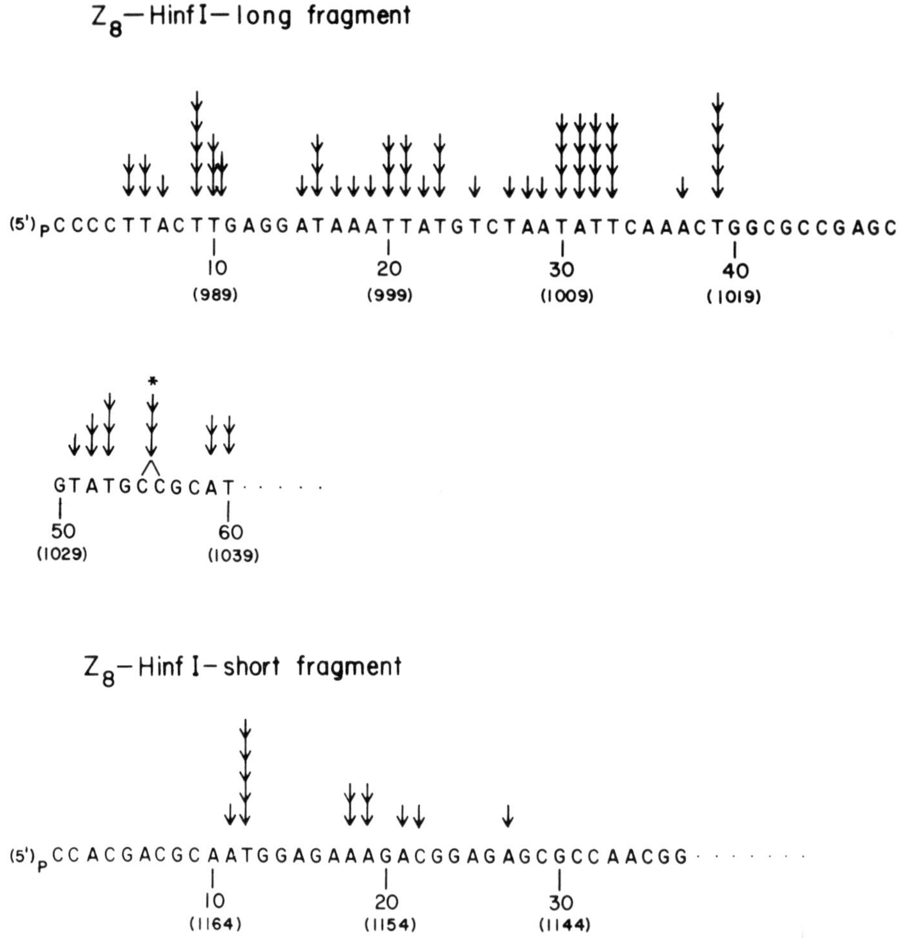

Fig. 7. NCS cleavage sites in two restriction enzyme fragments of duplex ΦX174 DNA as determined by the DNA sequencing technique of MAXAM and GILBERT (1977). The *number of arrows* indicates the relative intensity of the bands on the autoradiograms. Very faint bands deserving significantly less than one arrow are not shown. * Position attacked by neocarzinostatin in the single-stranded fragment. The nucleotide position in the Sanger map is indicated *within parentheses*. The sequence of the short fragment is the complement of that in the Sanger map (HATAYAMA and GOLDBERG, 1978)

Recent studies have shown that a damaged sugar fragment (carbons 1′, 2′, and 3′) can be released from NCS-treated DNA in the form of a material behaving like malondialdehyde, especially after alkaline treatment (HATAYAMA and GOLDBERG, unpublished data), suggesting that sugar fragment release is incomplete without additional treatment. DNA strand cleavage is also accompanied by the release of the bases thymine (ISHIDA and TAKAHASHI, 1976; POON et al., 1977) and adenine (POON et al., 1977). Only about 15% as much adenine is released as is thymine. The requirement for thymidylic and deoxyadenylic acids in the scission reaction was also revealed by experiments in which various synthetic

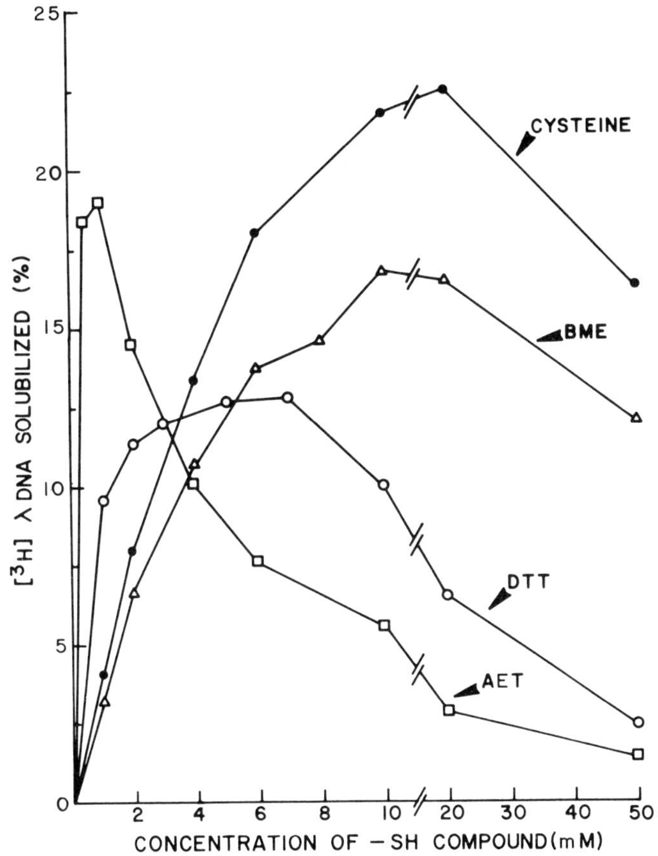

Fig. 8. Effect of different sulfhydryl compounds on the activity of NCS (100 µg/ml). The concentrations of the -SH agents (BME, β-mercaptoethanol; DTT, dithiothreitol) were varied as indicated. The trichloroacetic acid solubility of [^{3}H]λDNA was measured at 20 min (Kappen and Goldberg, 1978b)

and natural DNA's of different base composition were tested for their ability to protect against the cutting of radioactive lambda virus DNA (Poon et al., 1977). The amount of thymine released correlated well with the number of strand scissions. Further, using the DNA sequencing technique of Maxam and Gilbert (1977) NCS was shown in the presence of 2-mercaptoethanol to cleave double-stranded ΦX174 DNA restriction fragments almost exclusively at deoxythymidylic and deoxyadenylic acid residues (Hatayama et al., 1978). Overall, deoxythymidylic acid residues are attacked much more frequently than are deoxyadenylic acid residues (Fig. 7), although there is variability in the attack rate for both nucleotides at different locations in the DNA molecule. While all deoxythymidylic acid residues are sites of scission, not all deoxyadenylic acid residues are cleavage sites, but there appears to be no clear-cut nucleotide sequence specificity in determining cleavage frequency. In agreement with the protection experiments, single-stranded DNA is a very poor substrate for NCS-

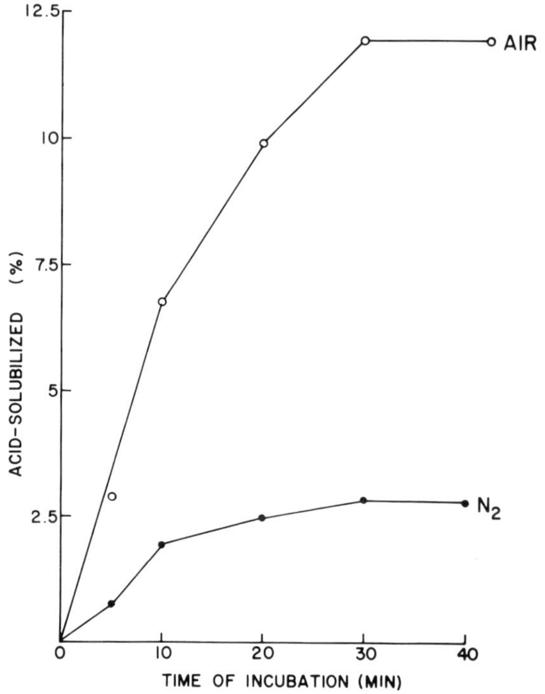

Fig. 9. Time course of activity of NCS in air or in N_2. Air or N_2 was bubbled through the reaction mixture containing 100 μg/ml NCS and 7.5 mM β-mercaptoethanol. The acid-solubilization of [^{3}H]λDNA was measured (KAPPEN and GOLDBERG, 1978b)

induced scission. It is of interest that both members of a base pair, deoxythymidylic and deoxyadenylic acids, are the main targets for NCS, for the chances of producing double-strand breaks in AT-poor or homopolymeric regions will be significantly increased over that caused by the otherwise random placement of single-strand scissions. Since double- and not single-strand breaks are considered to be lethal events (FREIFELDER, 1966; LEENHOUTS and CHADWICK, 1978), this action of NCS may be important in determining its cytotoxicity. NCS attack sites at thymidylic and deoxyadenylic acid residues in DNA have also been found by D'ANDREA and HASELTINE (1978). Further, these results are in agreement with the earlier finding with DNA polymerase I that DNA synthesis directed by poly[d(A-T)] is much more sensitive to NCS than that by poly[d(G-C)] (KAPPEN and GOLDBERG, 1977).

While NCS-induced cutting of DNA in vitro is markedly stimulated by the presence of a mercaptan, high levels of the mercaptan inhibit the reaction (Fig. 8) (KAPPEN and GOLDBERG, 1978b). This latter effect is seen especially clearly with the radiation-protector (and free radical scavenger) S,2-aminoethylisothiuronium bromide · HBr (AET). Since AET rearranges rapidly when neutralized to form 2-mercaptoethylguanidine, it is likely that the latter is the active form. While less active than a mercaptan, we have found that sodium borohydride can also activate the reaction. In addition, preincubation of NCS with

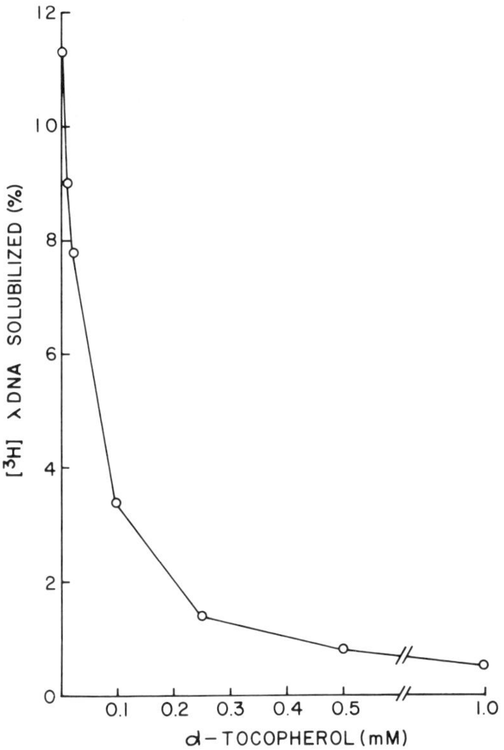

Fig. 10. Inhibition of NCS activity by α-tocopherol. NCS (100 μg/ml)-induced acid-solubilization of [^{3}H]λDNA was measured at 30 min in a reaction similar to that in Fig. 9 (KAPPEN and GOLDBERG, 1978b)

a mercaptan results in its rapid inactivation (ISHIDA and TAKAHASHI, 1978; KAPPEN and GOLDBERG, 1978b). These data suggested that reduction of the disulfide(s) of NCS was necessary to generate an active form of the drug and that a free radical mechanism may be involved in the DNA cutting reaction. The former was also suggested by experiments in which NCS activation was obtained by photoreduction of the disulfides in the presence of sodium hypophosphite (SIM and LOWN, 1978). Support for involvement of radical mechanism comes from the requirement for O_2 in the DNA scission reaction (Fig. 9) (BURGER et al., 1978; KAPPEN and GOLDBERG, 1978b; SIM and LOWN, 1978) and its inhibition by low concentrations of the potent peroxyl free radical scavenger α-tocopherol (Fig. 10) (KAPPEN and GOLDBERG, 1978b). Acid-solubilization of DNA by NCS was blocked 50% at 50 μM α-tocopherol. On the other hand, exogenous metals have yet to be implicated in the reaction since various metal chelators (EDTA, 8-hydroxyquinoline, deferoxamine, diethyldithiocarbamate, neocuproine, cuprizone) do not block the reaction (KAPPEN and GOLDBERG, 1978b and unpublished data). Similarly, superoxide dismutase does not inhibit the reaction. Unexpectedly, various alcohols and organic solvents have been found to stimulate the mercaptan-dependent reaction significantly (KAPPEN and

GOLDBERG, 1978b). It is of interest that, like the mercaptans, these solvents inactivate NCS in a preincubation; it is possible that they facilitate the generation of an active, labile (presumably containing free sulfhydryls) form of the antibiotic. As of this writing, the precise mechanism whereby NCS cuts DNA is not known. The generation of sulfhydryls in NCS and their possible oxidation to free radical forms may be responsible, but further experimentation is required. A possible role for a non-protein chromophore in the mechanism of NCS action is under investigation (M.A. NAPIER and I.H. GOLDBERG, unpublished data).

It also remains to be demonstrated conclusively that the mechanism for DNA damage discovered in the in vitro system pertains in the intact cell. Mechanisms for cell killing not involving direct effects on DNA have also been proposed. Thus, studies using NCS covalently bound to Agarose or Sepharose suggest the possibility that the cytotoxic effect may be a membrane-mediated event (NAKAMURA and ONO, 1974; LAZARUS et al., 1977). Also, very high levels of NCS inhibit the vinblastine-induced formation of microtubular paracrystals (EBINA and ISHIDA, 1975) and cap formation and cell spreading in mammalian cells (EBINA et al., 1977), but these effects are probably not responsible for cell killing. Definitive evidence for DNA as a primary target for NCS in cells and for the base specificity existing under in vitro conditions being involved in cellular DNA damage must come from genetic experiments and DNA-sequencing studies in intact cells.

Acknowledgment. This work was supported by U.S. Public Health Service Research Grant GM 12573 from the National Institutes of Health.

References

Aneha, Y., Kikuchi, K., Kanno, H.: Administration of an antineoplastic agent of high molecular weight, neocarzinostatin, in cases of gastric cancer. Jpn. J. Clin. Med. *32*, 870–874 (1974)

Beerman, T.A., Goldberg, I.H.: DNA strand scission by the antitumor protein neocarzinostatin. Biochem. Biophys. Res. Commun. *59*, 1254–1261 (1974)

Beerman, T.A., Goldberg, I.H.: The relationship between DNA strand-scission and DNA synthesis inhibition in HeLa cells treated with neocarzinostatin. Biochim. Biophys. Acta *475*, 281–293 (1977)

Beerman, T.A., Poon, R., Goldberg, I.H.: Single-strand nicking of DNA *in vitro* by neocarzinostatin and its possible relationship to the mechanism of drug action. Biochim. Biophys. Acta *475*, 294–306 (1977)

Bradner, W.T., Hutchison, D.J.: Neocarzinostatin (NCS-69856): an antitumor antibiotic effective against ascitic leukemia L1210 in mice. Cancer Chemother. Rep. *50*, 79–84 (1966)

Burger, R.M., Peisach, J., Horwitz, S.B.: Effect of light and oxygen on neocarzinostatin stability and DNA-cleaving activity. J. Biol. Chem. *253*, 4830–4832 (1978)

D'Andrea, A.D., Haseltine, W.A.: Sequence specific cleavage of DNA by the antitumor antibiotics neocarzinostatin and bleomycin. Proc. Natl. Acad. Sci. USA *75*, 3608–3612 (1978)

Ebina, T., Ishida, N.: Inhibition of formation of microtubular paracrystals in HeLa-S_3 cells by neocarzinostatin. Cancer Res. *35*, 3705–3709 (1975)

Ebina, T., Ohtsuki, K., Seto, M., Ishida, N.: Specific G2 block in HeLa-S_3 cells by neocarzinostatin. Eur. J. Cancer *11*, 155–158 (1975)

Ebina, T., Satski, M., Ishida, N.: Inhibition of surface immunoglobulin central capping of Daudi cells and cell spreading of HeLa-S_3 cells by neocarzinostatin. Cancer Res. *37*, 4423–4429 (1977)

Eisenstadt, E., Wolf, M., Goldberg, I.H.: Mutagenicity of neocarzinostatin in *Escherichia coli* and *Salmonella typhimurium*. Abstract for the Tenth Annual Meeting of the Environmental Mutagen Society, in press (1978)

Freifelder, D.: DNA strand breakage by X-irradiation. Radiation Res. *29*, 329–338 (1966)

Griffin, T., Comis, R.L., Lokich, J., Canellos, G.: Neocarzinostatin: phase I study. Proc. Am. Assoc. Cancer Res. and ASCO *18*, 302 (1977)

Hatayama, T., Goldberg, I.H.: DNA damage and repair in relation to cell killing in neocarzinostatin-treated HeLa cells. Biochim. Biophys. Acta, in press (1979)

Hatayama, T., Goldberg, I.H., Takeshita, M., Grollman, A.P.: Nucleotide specificity in DNA scission by neocarzinostatin. Proc. Natl. Acad. Sci. USA *75*, 3603–3607 (1978)

Hiraki, K., Kamimura, O., Takahashi, I., Nagao, T., Kitajima, K., Irino, S.: Neocarzinostatin: Une approche nouvelle dans la chimiotherapie des leucemies aigues. Rev. Fr. d'Hémat. *13*, 29–35 (1973)

Homma, M., Koida, T., Saito-Koide, T., Kamo, I., Seto, M., Kumagai, K., Ishida, N.: Specific inhibition of the initiation of DNA synthesis in HeLa cells by neocarzinostatin. Prog. Antimicrob. Anticancer Chemother. Proc. 6th Int. Congr. Chemother. *2*, 410–415 (1970)

Ishida, R., Takahashi, T.: *In vitro* release of thymine from DNA by neocarzinostatin. Biochem. Biophys. Res. Commun. *68*, 256–261 (1976)

Ishida, R., Takahashi, T.: Role of mercaptoethanol in *in vitro* DNA degradation by neocarzinostatin. Cancer Res. *38*, 2617–2620 (1978)

Ishida, N., Miyazaki, K., Kumagai, K., Rikimaru, M.: Neocarzinostatin, an antitumor antibiotic of high molecular weight. J. Antibiot. *18*, 29–37 (1965)

Kappen, L.S., Goldberg, I.H.: Effect of neocarzinostatin-induced strand scission on the template activity of DNA for DNA polymerase I. Biochemistry *16*, 479–485 (1977)

Kappen, L.S., Goldberg, I.H.: Neocarzinostatin induction of DNA repair synthesis in HeLa cells and isolated nuclei. Biochim. Biophys. Acta *520*, 481–489 (1978a)

Kappen, L.S., Goldberg, I.H.: Activation and inactivation of neocarzinostatin-induced cleavage of DNA. Nucleic Acids Res. *5*, 2959–2967 (1978b)

Kappen, L.S., Goldberg, I.H.: Gaps in DNA induced by neocarzinostatin bear 3′- and 5′-phosphoryl termini. Biochemistry *17*, 729–733 (1978c)

Khokhlov, A.S., Cherches, B.Z., Reshetov, P.D., Smirnova, G.M., Sorokina, I.B., Prokoptzeva, T.A., Koloditskaya, T.A., Smirnov, V.V., Navashin, S.M., Fomina, I.P.: Physico-chemical and biological studies on actinoxanthin, an antibiotic from *Actinomyces globisporus* 1131. J. Antibiot. *22*, 541–544 (1969)

Khokhlov, A.S., Reshetov, P.D., Chupova, L.A., Cherches, B.Z., Zhigis, L.S., Stoyachenko, I.A.: Chemical studies on actinoxanthin. J. Antibiot. *29*, 1026–1034 (1976)

Kikuchi, M., Shoji, M., Ishida, N.: Pre-neocarzinostatin, a specific antagonist of neocarzinostatin. J. Antibiot. *27*, 766–774 (1974)

Kinami, Y., Miyazaki, H., Koyama, F.: The treatment of pancreatic carcinoma with neocarzinostatin. J. Jpn. Soc. Cancer Ther. *10*, 502–508 (1975)

Kitajima, K., Kamimura, O., Hiraki, K.: Neocarzinostatin: a new chemotherapeutic approach to acute leukemia. Acta Haematol. Jpn. *37*, 316–323 (1974)

Kitajima, K., Kaminura, O., Nagao, T.: Neocarzinostatin: a new agent active in the treatment of acute leukemia. Bibl. Haematol. *40*, 751–752 (1975)

Kohno, M., Haneda, I., Koyama, Y., Kikuchi, M.: Studies on the stability of antitumor protein, neocarzinostatin. I. Stability of solution of neocarzinostatin. Jap. J. Antibiot. *27*, 707–714 (1974)

Kumagai, K., Ono, Y., Nishikawa, T., Ishida, N.: Cytological studies on the effect of neocarzinostatin on HeLa cells. J. Antibiot. *19*, 69–74 (1966)

Lazarus, H., Raso, V., Samy, T.S.A.: *In vitro* inhibition of human leukemic cells (CCRF-CEM) by agarose-immobilized neocarzinostatin. Cancer Res. *37*, 3731–3736 (1977)

Leenhouts, H.P., Chadwick, K.H.: The crucial role of DNA double-strand breaks in cellular radiobiological effects. Adv. Radiat. Biol. *7*, 55–101 (1978)

Maeda, H.: Chemical and biological characterization of succinyl neocarzinostatin. J. Antibiot. *27*, 303–311 (1974)

Maeda, H., Kuromizu, K.: Spontaneous deamidation of a protein antibiotic, neocarzinostatin, at weakly acidic pH. J. Biochem. *81*, 25–35 (1977)

Maeda, H., Shiraishi, H., Onodera, S., Ishida, N.: Conformation of antibiotic protein, neocarzinostatin, studied by plane polarized infrared spectroscopy, circular dichroism and apitcal rotatory dispersion. Int. J. Peptide Protein Res. *5*, 19–26 (1973)

Maeda, H., Glaser, C.B., Czombos, J., Meienhofer, J.: Structure of the antitumor protein neocarzinostatin. Purification, amino acid composition, disulfide reduction, and isolation and composition of tryptic peptides. Arch. Biochem. Biophys. *164*, 369–378 (1974)

Masaoka, T., Hasegawa, Y., Yoshitake, J., Ueda, T., Takubo, T., Shibata, H., Nakamura, H., Senda, N.: Mode of decrease of leukemic cells and leukocytes during neocarzinostatin treatment. Cancer Treat. Rep. *61*, 73–75 (1977)

Maxam, A.M., Gilbert, W.: A new method for sequencing DNA. Proc. Natl. Acad. Sci. USA *74*, 560–564 (1977)

Meienhofer, J., Maeda, H., Glaser, C.B., Czombos, J., Kuromiz, K.: Primary structure of neocarzinostatin, an antitumor antibiotic. Science *178*, 875–876 (1972a)

Meienhofer, J., Maeda, H., Glaser, C.B., Czombos, J.: Structural studies on neocarzinostatin, an antitumor polypeptide antibiotic. In: Progress in peptide research. Lande, S. (ed.), Vol. 2, pp. 295–306. New York: Gordon and Breach 1972b

Nakamura, H., Ono, K.: Growth inhibition of leukemic cells by neocarzinostatin-sepharose. Proc. Jpn. Cancer Assoc. 33rd Annual Meeting, p. 112 (1974)

Ohtsuki, K., Ishida, N.: Mechanism of DNA degradation induced by neocarzinostatin in *Bacillus subtilis*. J. Antibiot. *28*, 229–236 (1975a)

Ohtsuki, K., Ishida, N.: Neocarzinostatin-induced breakdown of deoxyribonucleic acid in HeLa-S_3 cells. J. Antibiot. *28*, 143–148 (1975b)

Ono, Y., Watanabe, Y., Ishida, N.: Mode of action of neocarzinostatin: Inhibition of DNA synthesis and degradation of DNA in *Saccina lutea*. Biochim. Biophys. Acta *119*, 46–58 (1966)

Poon, R., Beerman, T.A., Goldberg, I.H.: Characterization of DNA strand breakage *in vitro* by the antitumor protein neocarzinostatin. Biochemistry *16*, 486–492 (1977)

Rao, A.P., Rao, P.N.: The cause of G2 arrest in CHO cells treated with anticancer drugs. J. Natl. Cancer Inst. *57*, 1139–1143 (1976)

Sakamoto, K., Endo, N., Sakka, M.: Effect of neocarzinostatin on V-79 Chinese hamster cells *in vitro*. Eur. J. Cancer *9*, 725–728 (1973)

Samy, T.S.A.: Neocarzinostatin: effect of modification of side chain amino and carboxyl groups on chemical and biological properties. Biochemistry *16*, 5573–5578 (1977)

Samy, T.S.A., Meienhofer, J.: Chemical modification and physical studies of the antitumor protein neocarzinostatin. In: Proc. Int. Workshop Hormones and Proteins, San Francisco, 1974. Bewley, T.A., Lin, M., Ramachandran, J. (eds.), pp. 143–156. Hong Kong: The Chinese University of Hong Kong 1974

Samy, T.S.A., Atreyi, M., Maeda, H., Meienhofer, J.: Selective tryptophan oxidation in the antitumor protein neocarzinostatin and effects on conformation and biological activity. Biochemistry *15*, 1007–1013 (1974)

Samy, T.S.A., Hu, J-M., Meienhofer, J., Lazarus, H., Johnson, R.K.: A facile method of purification of neocarzinostatin, an antitumor protein. J. Natl. Cancer Inst. *58*, 1765–1768 (1977)

Sasada, M., Sawada, H., Nakamura, T., Uchino, H.: Caffeine potentiation of lethality of L-1210 cells treated with neocarzinostatin. Gann *67*, 447–449 (1976)

Sawada, H., Tatsumi, K., Sasada, M., Shirakawa, S., Nokamura, T., Wakisaka, G.: Effect of neocarzinostatin on DNA synthesis in L1210 cells. Cancer Res. *34*, 3341–3346 (1974)

Sim, S-K., Lown, J.W.: The mechanism of the neocarzinostatin-induced cleavage of DNA. Biochem. Biophys. Res. Commun. *81*, 99–105 (1978)

Takahashi, M., Toriyama, K., Maeda, H., Kikuchi, M., Kumagai, K., Ishida, N.: Clinical trials of a new antitumor polypeptide: neocarzinostatin (NCS). Tohoku J. Exp. Med. *98*, 273–280 (1969)

Tatsumi, K., Nishioka, H.: Effect of DNA repair systems on antibacterial and mutagenic activity of an antitumor protein, neocarzinostatin. Mutat. Res. *48*, 195–204 (1977)

Tatsumi, K., Nakamura, T., Wakisaka, G.: Damage of mammalian cell DNA *in vivo* and *in vitro* induced by neocarzinostatin. Gann *65*, 459–461 (1974)

Tatsumi, K., Sakane, T., Sawada, H., Shirakawa, S., Nakamura, T., Wakisaka, G.: Unscheduled DNA synthesis in human lymphocytes treated with neocarzinostatin. Gann *66*, 441–444 (1975)

Tsuruo, T., Satoh, H., Ukita, T.: Effect of the antitumor antibiotic neocarzinostatin on DNA synthesis *in vitro*. J. Antibiot. *24*, 423–429 (1971)

Nitracrine

M. GNIAZDOWSKI, J. FILIPSKI, and M. CHORĄŻY

In 1954 LEDÓCHOWSKI and his co-workers at the Department of Chemistry of Drugs, Polytechnical University of Gdańsk, undertook a research project on the synthesis and chemical properties of new acridine derivatives (cf. LEDÓCHOWSKI, 1976). These compounds were subsequently tested for their cytostatic and antitumor activity.The derivatives with programed structural changes were synthetized to enable the study on their structure–activity relationship. Some of the compounds with the dialkylaminoalkylamino side chain at C_9 of the acridine ring exhibited cytostatic activity. This activity was particularly pronounced in the compound coded C-283 (RADZIKOWSKI et al., 1976a). It was tested in a number of biologic, biochemical, and clinical investigations. A common nonproprietary name of the drug, nitracrine has been recently adopted. The drug has been referred to under its original code C-283 or its trade name Ledakrin in most of the papers published until now.

Chemistry

Major steps in chemical synthesis of nitracrine are shown in Fig. 1. Nitracrine, 1-nitro-9-(3-dimethyl-aminopropylamino)acridine dihydrochloride monohydrate (chemical formula $C_{18}H_{20}N_4O_2 \cdot 2HCl \cdot H_2O$, molecular weight 415.3 daltons) forms orange-colored crystals, easily soluble in water, methanol, and ethanol,

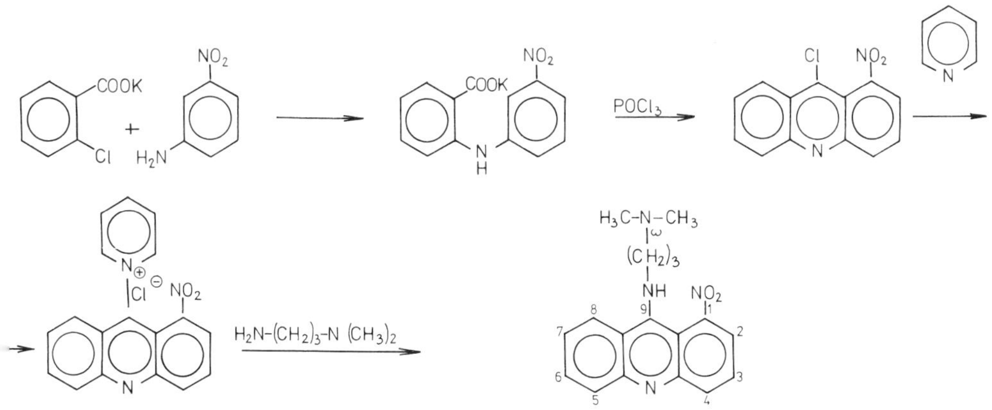

Fig. 1. Synthesis of nitracrine (LEDÓCHOWSKI, 1976)

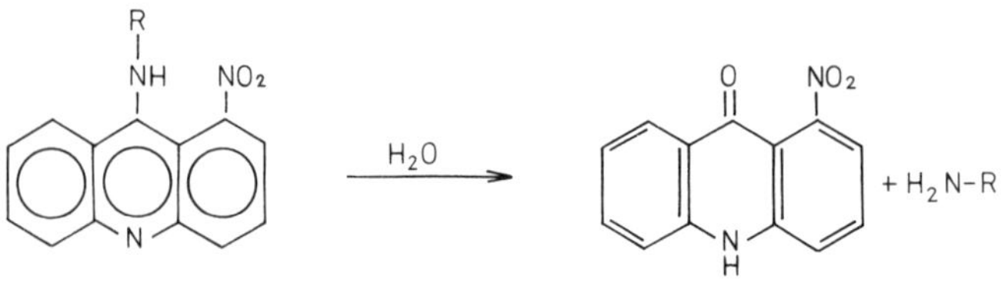

Fig. 2. Hydrolysis of 1-nitro-9-alkylaminoacridine

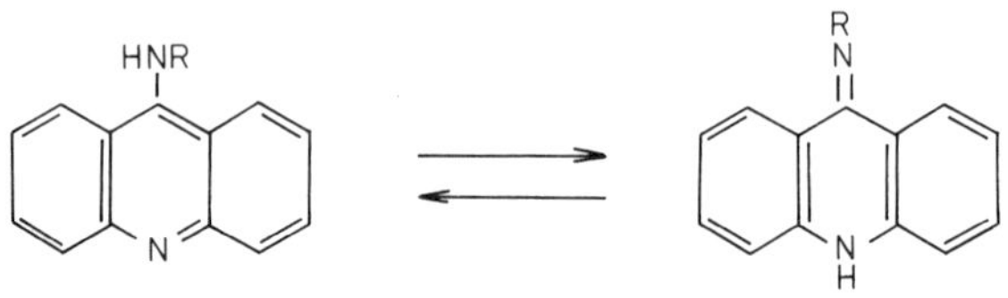

Fig. 3. 9-alkylaminoacridine–alkyliminoacridan

slightly in benzene, diethyl ether, etc. Concentrated solutions of nitracrine in water are acidic (pH 4). The free base is poorly soluble in water but easily in organic solvents (LEDÓCHOWSKI, 1974). Its dissociation constants are: $pKa_1 = 6.45$ (dissociation of the proton at N_{10}), and $pKa_2 = 8.8$ (dissociation of the proton at the terminal nitrogen of the side chain, FILIPSKI et al., 1975). The drug obeys the law of LAMBERT and BEER over a broad range of concentration (BIEDRZYCKI et al., 1977). Crystalline nitracrine exposed to light decomposes, giving a mixture of unidentified products. Nitracrine hydrolyses in aqueous solution (Fig. 2) to 1-nitroacridone (LEDÓCHOWSKI and SKONIECZNY, 1975, 1976; LEDÓCHOWSKI et al., 1976). The kinetics of the hydrolysis suggests that there is an equilibrium between aminoacridine and iminoacridan. Theoretical calculations (DAUTER et al., 1976) confirmed that nitracrine dissolved in water exists predominantly in the imino form (Fig. 3). This conclusion was supported by the results of the crystallographic X-ray studies (DAUTER et al., 1975). The

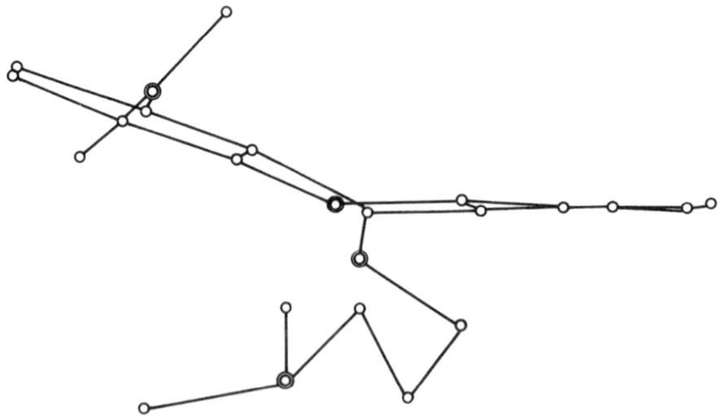

Fig. 4. Conformation of nitracrine molecule as determined by X-ray studies of nitracrine monoiodide crystals (DAUTER et al., 1975)

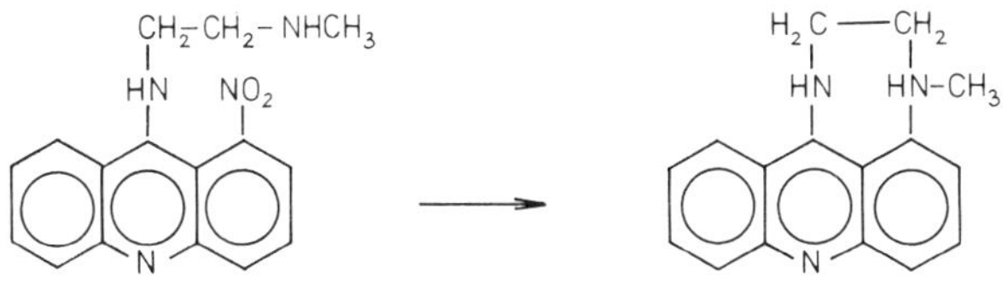

Fig. 5. Intramolecular nucleophilic substitution of 1-nitro group in the molecule of 1-nitro-9-(2-methylaminoethylamino)acridine (SKONIECZNY and LEDÓCHOWSKI, 1977)

conformation of the molecule of nitracrine monoiodide in the crystal form is shown in Fig. 4.

The nitro group of nitracrine is susceptible to reduction. The polarographic half-wave potential of nitracrine is low as compared to other less biologically active isomers, bearing nitro group at position 2, 3, and 4 of the acridine ring (CHODKOWSKI et al., 1970; CHODKOWSKI and KIWAK, 1973). Sulfhydryl compounds added to solutions of nitracrine change its spectral properties, which is probably due to the reduction of the nitro group (GNIAZDOWSKI et al., 1975). As recently shown by SKONIECZNY and LEDÓCHOWSKI (1977), the homolog of nitracrine, 1-nitro-9-(2-methylaminoethylamino)acridine, has the interesting property of intramolecular nucleophilic substitution of the nitro group (Fig. 5).

Cytotoxic and Cytostatic Activity in Screening Tests

Several hundreds of acridine derivatives synthesized by LEDÓCHOWSKI and his co-workers were routinely examined by means of the Miyamura test and checked on their properties of inhibiting the germination of *Lepidium sativum* and the growth of sarcoma 180 in mice (cf. LEDÓCHOWSKI, 1976). Nitracrine and some selected derivatives were also tested in cell cultures. KB, ELD, HeLa, FAF 28G3, human amnion cells, and *Euglena gracilis* cultures were used in these extensive studies (RADZIKOWSKI et al., 1967a, b, c; KONOPA et al., 1969; CHOTKOWSKA and KONOPA, 1972). The experiments showed that nitracrine generated the largest zone of inhibition of dehydrogenases activity in the Miyamura test as compared to other compounds under research. The drug reduced the germination of *Lepidium sativum* to 27% of the control. The cytostatic effects in the cell culture were evaluated on the basis of cell growth, changes of morphology, and mitotic activity. It was found that the ID_{50} (concentration inhibiting the growth of the cell culture to 50%) was approximately 10^{-9} g/ml. The administration of nitracrine to tumor-bearing rats and mice caused prolongation of the survival time of the animals and decrease of the tumor mass (Table 1). Prolongation by 95% of the survival time of the rats bearing the line of Yoshida ascitic sarcoma, resistant to the alkylating agents, was particularly interesting (KWAŚNIEWSKA and WINKLER, 1969). Some tumors (e.g., L1210 leukemia) were resistant to nitracrine (Table 1). The drug was recently tested at the U.S. National Cancer Institute (coded as NSC 247561) in a number of screening systems. The lack of activity towards L1210 ascitic leukemia was confirmed. Slight prolon-

Table 1. Results of screening tests in model systems

Tumor	Administration	Daily dose (mg/kg)	Criteria of effect evaluation	Effect of the optimal dose[b]
Solid sarcoma 180	i.p.[a]	0.125–0.5	Mean tumor weight	60%–80%
Ascitic Ehrlich	i.p.	0.125–0.375	Mean survival time	55%
Ascitic NK leukemia	i.p.	0.125–0.375	Mean survival time	60%
Ascitic L1210 leukemia	i.p.	0.125–0.375	Mean survival time	0%
Walker solid carcinoma 256	i.p.	0.125–0.375	Mean survival time	0%
Walker solid carcinoma 256	Intramuscular perfusion	0.1–20 min	Mean survival time	Total remission
Yoshida ascitic sarcoma	i.p.	0.0675–0.25	Mean survival time	60%
Yoshida ascitic refractory sarcoma	i.p.	0.15–0.3	Mean survival time	95%
Ascitic leukemia P 388	i.p.	0.65–0.125	Mean survival time	0%

[a] Intraperitoneally (from RADZIKOWSKI, 1976).
[b] In percent of the decrease of the mean tumor weight or the increase of the mean survival time as indicated.

gation of the mean survival time was observed in the case of ascitic leukemia P388 and Lewis lung carcinoma in mice. The drug significantly prolonged the survival of albino rats with Walker carcinosarcoma 256 (cf. RADZIKOWSKI, 1976) and also showed strong antimycotic and bacteriostatic activity (KURNATOWSKA and KADŁUBOWSKI, 1977).

Structure–Activity Relationship

The dimethylaminopropylamino side chain at position 9 and the nitro group at position 1 of the acridine ring are the characteristic features of the molecule of nitracrine. Comparison of the biologic properties of a great number of acridines, synthetized by the group formerly led by ZYGMUNT LEDÓCHOWSKI and recently by ANDRZEJ LEDÓCHOWSKI, allows to draw the following conclusions (cf. LEDÓCHOWSKI, 1976). (a) The lack of the nitro group or its replacement at different positions of the acridine ring by methyl or methoxyl (RADZIKOWSKI et al., 1969a), halogen (RADZIKOWSKI et al., 1967c), or dimethylamino group (RADZIKOWSKI et al., 1969b) reduces the activity of the compound. (b) The translocation of the nitro group to other positions in the ring results in the decrease of activity. (c) The length of the side chain within the range of three to five carbon atoms between the amino groups has no influence on the biologic effect of the compounds. Similarly, branching of the chain does not decrease the biologic activity. The derivative containing two ethyl groups at the terminal nitrogen atom instead of two methyl groups exhibits the same cytostatic effect (KONOPA et al., 1969). Similar observations concerning the influence of the chain length and structure on the antimalarial properties of acridine derivatives were reported by ALBERT (1966). (d) The derivatives with a higher degree of structural modifications exhibit a significant cytostatic effect as long as the nitro group is at position 1 and acridine molecules bear the dialkylaminoalkyl side chain. The translocation of the chain to position 10 with simultaneous oxidation of the molecule to acridone (RADZIKOWSKI et al., 1971), or the oxidation of either terminal or N_{10} nitrogen to N-oxide, produce compounds of biologic activity comparable to that of nitracrine (HRABOWSKA et al., 1976). (e) The introduction of an additional methyl group in position 4, a methoxyl group in position 4 or 7, or halogen in position 6 of the acridine ring results in highly active compounds as well (HRABOWSKA et al., 1970).

The role of the aminoalkyl chain and the position of the nitro group deserve some comment. Nitroaminoacridines without chains are less active than nitracrine. A 100-fold higher LD_{50} of 1-nitro-9-aminoacridine for mice was reported by ALBERT (1966). The corresponding nitro isomers display different biologic activity. The differences, however, are not as distinct as those observed for nitracrine and its isomers, and exhibit other structure–activity relationship. The highest biologic activity was observed by ALBERT et al. (1945) for 3-nitro-9-aminoacridine. 3-nitro (C-257) and 4-nitro isomers (C-265) of nitracrine show lower effect than the drug and its 2-nitro isomer (C-264) is practically inactive (KONOPA et al., 1969, 1976a). Apparently, the introduction of the side chain into the molecule of nitroaminoacridine changes substantially the mechanism of its biologic activity.

Clinical Application

Positive response of some transplanted tumors to nitracrine, lack of bone marrow toxicity and its distinct cytostatic effect justified clinical trials of the drug in human cancer.

The first stage of clinical investigations was carried out at the Institute of Oncology in Gliwice. They were continued in other medical centers in Poland. In a number of different human cancers nitracrine exhibited encouraging effects. In patients suffering from ovarian carcinoma with intraperitoneal or intrapleural exudate, a single dose of nitracrine administered intracavitally after the evacuation of the exudate resulted in the lack of fluid increase lasting several months in 40 out of 52 patients (KWAŚNIEWSKA-ROKICIŃSKA, 1976). The inhibition of the accumulation of exudate after nitracrine treatment was confirmed by PIOTROWSKA-SOWIŃSKA (1976) in 14 out of 21 patients with different cancers.

In the case of tumors that do not derive from the epithelium, such as mesothelioma, myosarcoma, and peritoneal pseudomyxoma, remissions were observed (JABŁOŃSKI and GERBER, 1974; PIOTROWSKA-SOWIŃSKA, 1976; PAWLICKI et al., 1977). In the case of colon carcinoma the administration of nitracrine after surgical treatment in 14 cases out of 30 resulted in remissions lasting from 1 to 5 years (BRATKOWSKA-SENIÓW et al., 1976b). Clinical trials were undertaken in patients with lung carcinoma. In 3 out of 5 cases partial regression was observed (KWAŚNIEWSKA-ROKICIŃSKA et al., 1976). The results of the treatment of other 19 patients with advanced lung carcinoma confirmed its effectiveness (KWAŚNIEWSKA-ROKICIŃSKA, unpublished observation). The results of combination treatment were encouraging as well. Out of 55 patients with bronchial carcinoma, to whom nitracrine was administered after lobectomy, 43 survived at least one year (ROGALSKI et al., 1976).

Nitracrine was applied intravenously in mammary carcinoma. Improvement in 4 out of 14 cases was reported (KWAŚNIEWSKA-ROKICIŃSKA, 1974). A review of therapy results of other human cancers was published by RADZIKOWSKI (1974). Administration of nitracrine did not result in impairment of erythrocytes, leukocytes, and blood platelets. The level of hemoglobin and the hematocrit remained unchanged during nitracrine treatment. However, transient lymphocytopenia was observed in patients after administration of the drug. This effect was accompanied by the diminished ability of lymphocytes for phytohemagglutinine-induced blastoid transformation (BRATKOWSKA-SENIÓW et al., 1976a).

Toxicity

The LD_{50} and maximal tolerated dose (MTD) of nitracrine for mice and rats are shown in Table 2. The difference between toxic doses of the drug after intravenous and intragastric administration suggests that either the drug is unstable, or its absorption from the gastro-intestinal tract is low. Cats and rabbits responded to nitracrine with a short-lasting fall of blood pressure and ECG changes appearing 3–15 min after the administration of 10–20 mg of the drug per kg of body weight. Administration of 5 mg of nitracrine per kg exerted a spasmolytic activity in rabbits and a dose close to LD_{50} evoked paralytic ileus in rats. In vitro spasmolytic action of nitracrine on the small intestine was observed in guinea pigs and rats. In a small dose (10% of LD_{50}) the drug stimulated the central nervous system, diminishing the duration of the thiopental-evoked sleep. Higher doses of nitracrine had an opposite effect, prolonging the duration of sleep. Slight inhibition of antibody production in rabbits was found after administration of nitracrine in a dose close to one LD_{50}. No changes in the creatinine clearance were observed. In animals treated with nitracrine slight but evident pathologic changes were found, particularly in liver and kidney, heart muscle, lymph node cortex, and intestinal epithelium. Degenerative changes of the seminiferous epithelium in the rabbit were observed, but the reproductive function of animals was not impaired. Blood coagulation after administration of the drug decreased (GIEŁDANOWSKI et al., 1971, 1972a

Table 2. Acute toxicity of nitracrine (mg/kg). (From GIEŁDANOWSKI, 1976)

	Intraveneous administration		Intragastric administration	
	LD_{50}	MTD	LD_{50}	MTD
Rats	1	0.7	34	18
Mice	0.72	0.52	26	8

b; GIEŁDANOWSKI, 1974, 1976). Preliminary pharmacokinetic experiments were done with nitracrine labeled with ^{14}C in the side chain and ^{3}H at the acridine ring. Of the total radioactivity administered to rats 30%–40% was excreted with urine and feces during two days, and 50%–60% during ten days. After that time the animals were killed. Of the input 5%–7% was found in the liver and kidneys. The other organs contained smaller amounts of radioactivity (JERZYKOWSKI et al., 1976).

Ultrastructural Changes in the Cell

Nitracrine induces distinct changes in the ultrastructure of the cell. They are especially significant in the cell nucleus and consist in the condensation and margination of chromatin around the nuclear membrane, the segregation of nucleolar components, and the aggregation of the interchromatinic granules. These changes were observed in liver cell nuclei as early as 15 min after the drug administration to rats, and were fully reversible if the dose was not too high (10 mg/kg). Similar changes were observed in ascites cells of human ovarian carcinoma (VORBRODT, 1970a; KRZYŻOWSKA-GRUCA et al., 1973) and nuclei of L1210 mouse leukemia ascites cells (KULCZYCKA, personal communication). Autoradiography and biochemical analysis showed that the ultrastructural changes in the nucleus are accompanied by an inhibition of RNA synthesis. Similar ultrastructural alterations in the cell nucleus can be induced by several other chemical agents and are considered a reflection of the inhibition of transcription (STENRAM and WILLEN, 1968).

None of the nuclear changes described was observed in rats or mice treated with C-264, the 2-nitro isomer of nitracrine (KULCZYCKA and KRZYŻOWSKA-GRUCA, unpublished data). The appearance of helical forms of polysomes was the first noticeable change in the cytoplasm observed in hepatocytes 15 min after the drug injection. Helical polysomes disappeared after 2 h. In nitracrine-treated cells ribosomes detached from the rough endoplasmic reticulum which converted into a smooth form (VORBRODT, 1970b).

Effect on Macromolecular Biosynthesis

Significant inhibition of incorporation of ^{32}P into RNA (70%–80%) was observed by MENDECKI et al. (1969) in the regenerating rat liver after administration of nitracrine. Addition of the drug at a concentration of 10^{-8} g/ml to KB cell culture resulted in 80% of inhibition of RNA synthesis after a few hours of incubation. At the drug concentration of 10^{-6} g/ml both RNA and DNA synthesis were completely inhibited after 30 min of incubation, while only a partial (50%) inhibition of incorporation of labeled phenylalanine occurred (FILIPSKI et al., 1975). Similar results were obtained by KONOPA et al., (1972; 1976a) on the incorporation of labeled thymidine into DNA, uridine into RNA, and leucine into proteins of HeLa cells. Comparable effects on macromolecular syntheses at 10–50 times higher concentration of the 3-nitro isomer of nitracrine (C-257) were observed, but no inhibition of RNA synthesis occurred in the presence of the 2-nitro isomer (C-264) (KONOPA et al., 1976a). Strong effects, comparable to nitracrine, of the homologs with two (C-337) and five (C-609) carbon atoms in the side chain on the incorporation of the labeled uridine in KB cells were shown by FILIPSKI et al. (1975). Nitracrine exhibited strong inhibition of DNA and RNA synthesis in synchronous cultures of *Euglena gracilis* (CHOTKOWSKA and KONOPA, 1973).

These results suggest that inhibition of nucleic acids synthesis may be the primary effect of nitracrine and point to DNA as the target of the drug in the cell.

Reversible Complexes with DNA

Interactions of nitracrine with DNA causes a metachromatic shift in the visible absorption spectrum of the drug and enables one to follow the formation of complexes by spectrophotometric titration (FILIPSKI et al., 1970). The formation of complexes of acridines with nucleic acids depends on the positive charges of dye molecules (LÖBER, 1967). Protonation of the molecules is an important factor, limiting the application of the titration method to certain pH ranges. The interpretation of the Scatchard plots of the titration data is ambiguous when the protonated and unprotonated forms of the dye, displaying different molar extinction coefficients, coexist in solution at a given pH and both interact with DNA, forming different complexes.

Availability of the analogs of nitracrine afforded the study of the acid-base properties of the drugs and their effect on the interaction with DNA. The dissociation constant for the proton at N_{10} of the acridine ring changes with the length of the carbon chain in the dimethylaminoalkyl group. pKa_1 values of the derivatives with the number of carbon atoms in the chain equal to two (C-337), three (nitracrine, C-283), four (C-205), and five (C-609) are 4.75; 6.45; 7.2 and 7.4, respectively (FILIPSKI et al., 1970, 1975). These differences among the pKa_1 values are due to the electron-withdrawing effect of the terminal protonated amino group, transmitted through the alkyl chain: the longer the chain, the higher the pKa_1 value. On the other hand, pKa_2 values relating to the terminal tertiary amino group remain rather unchanged (8.6–8.8) for these derivatives. The increase in pKa_1 is observed when the acridines are bound to DNA (FILIPSKI et al., 1975).

Binding curves of DNA with nitracrine at pH 4.55 (bivalent cation form prevailing at this pH) and with C-337 at pH 7.0 (monovalent cation) were determined (Fig. 6). During titration of DNA with both dyes, biphasic curves were observed, which indicates that either at least two types of binding sites or two types of dye–DNA or dye–dye interactions exist. Surprisingly, the positive charge on the acridine ring does not influence significantly the complex formation (FILIPSKI et al., 1975).

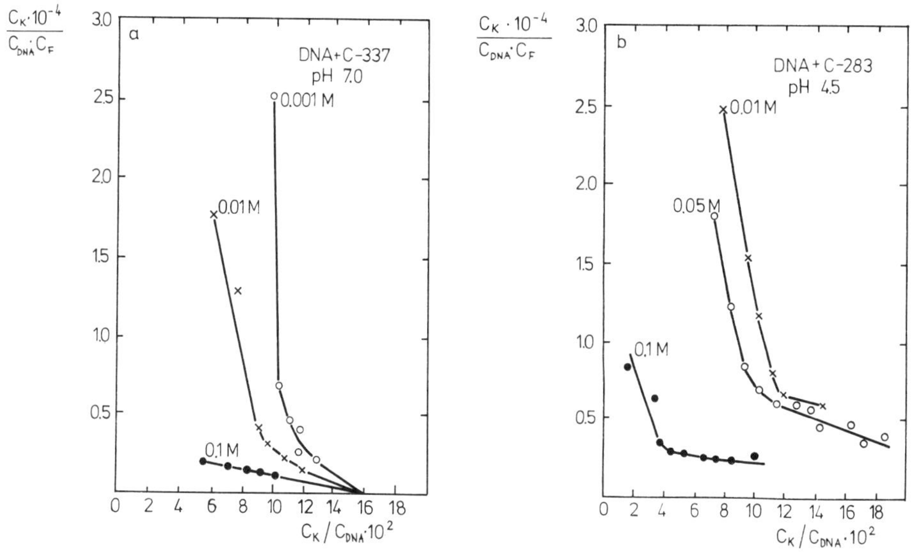

Fig. 6a and b. Binding of acridine derivatives in monovalent cation form (**a** C-337, pH 7.0) and bivalent cation form (**b** nitracrine, pH 4.55). The experimental data were plotted according to Scatchard (FILIPSKI et al., 1975)

The only difference between nitracrine and its biologically inactive 2-nitro isomer (C-264), detected by means of spectrophotometric titration, was that the latter dye gives one type of complex with DNA in its doubly charged positive form. Binding constants for the "stronger" binding of nitracrine and its 2-nitro-isomer fall into the same range of values (MARCZYŃSKI, 1975; FILIPSKI et al., 1977). Similar conclusions were drawn by KONOPA et al. (1976a). Complexes of DNA with nitracrine and its 2-nitro (C-264), 3-nitro (C-257), and 4-nitro (C-265) isomers did not differ markedly in their constants of the "stronger" binding. Paradoxically, a lower number of binding sites was found for nitracrine than for its biologically less active isomers.

Neither DNA nor nitracrine and its 2-nitro isomer (C-264) show Cotton effects at 300–400 nm. There is no optical activity of the DNA-C-264 complex, while that of nitracrine exhibits a strong negative Cotton effect in the visible wavelength range (MARCZYŃSKI, 1975). Addition of nitracrine to the preformed DNA-C-264 complex does not induce Cotton effects. It may be assumed that both nitroacridines compete for similar sites in DNA.

Nitroacridines increase stability of the double-stranded DNA during thermal denaturation. There is a correlation between protonation of acridines and their effect on T_m (FILIPSKI et al., 1975). This fact can be ascribed to a decrease of the electrostatic repulsion between negatively charged DNA phosphates by the protonated molecules (Table 3).

Preference of nitracrine for AT-rich sequences was shown. Cesium chloride gradient ultracentrifugation of the total yeast DNA in the presence of the drug gives a better separation of mitochondrial DNA (83% AT) from nuclear DNA (60% AT) than does ethidium bromide (MARCZYŃSKI, 1975).

Table 3. Increased stability of the secondary structure of DNA after complexing of acridine derivatives

Acridine	r	r′	ΔTm
C-337	0.04	0.004	0.6
Nitracrine	0.05	0.045	3.5
C-609	0.06	0.06	4.7

Tm was determined in 0.01 M phosphate buffer, pH 7.0. Values of pKa_1s were estimated by spectrophotometric titration. r = the number of dye molecules per nucleotide, and r′ = the number of dye molecules charged in the ring per nucleotide. (From FILIPSKI et al., 1975).

Steric properties of the complex of SV40 DNA with nitracrine were characterized by FILIPSKI et al. (1977). They applied the technique of CRAWFORD and WARING (1967), and BAUER and VINOGRAD (1968). Centrifugation of the supercoiled closed circular SV40 DNA shows that the binding of nitracrine or its 2-nitro isomer first decreases the DNA sedimentation constant (Fig. 7), then, after the minimum (equivalence point) is reached, an increase of the sedimentation constant is observed. These changes are due to the unwinding of the superhelix and to the subsequent reversal of supercoiling (WARING, 1971, 1975). The effect of nitracrine and its biologically inactive 2-nitro isomer (C-264) on supercoiled DNA (Fig. 7) justifies the conclusion that both dyes form intercalative complexes with DNA, and that intercalation alone is not responsible for the biologic activity of the drug.

The inhibitory effect of nitracrine on calf thymus DNA transcription with *E. coli* RNA polymerase depends on sulfhydryl compounds (GNIAZDOWSKI et al., 1972). In the absence of thiols, nitracrine and some of its 1-nitro derivatives

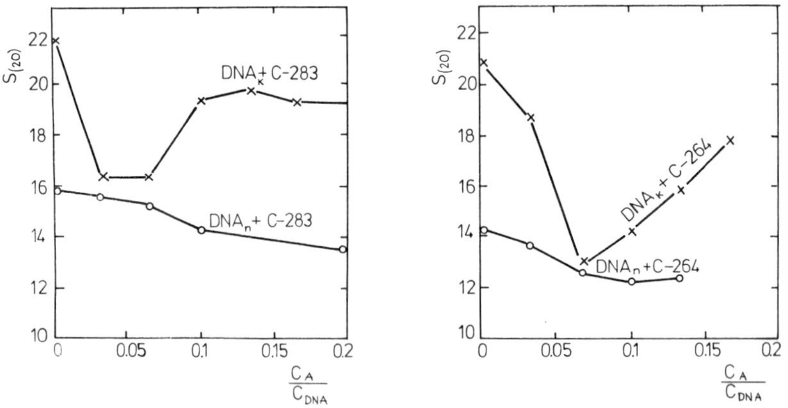

Fig. 7. Effect of nitracrine or C-264 on sedimentation constants of SV40 DNA supercoiled form (DNA_K) and nicked form (DNA_n). C_A/C_{DNA}-acridine derivative to DNA input ratio (FILIPSKI et al., 1977)

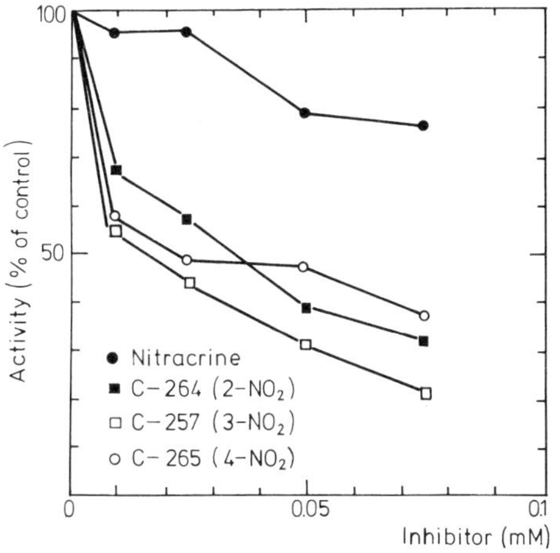

Fig. 8. Effect of nitracrine and its nitro isomers on RNA synthesis in vitro in the absence of thiols. Calf thymus DNA and *E. coli* RNA polymerase were used (SZMIGIERO et al., 1977)

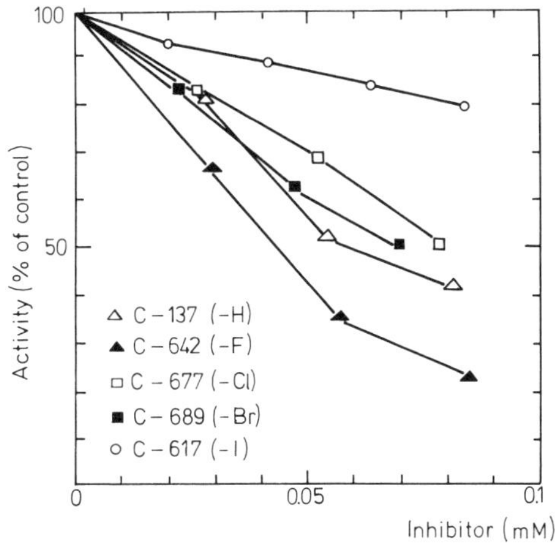

Fig. 9. Effect of 1-halogenated 9-aminopropylacridines on RNA synthesis in vitro (SZMIGIERO et al., 1977)

display a surprisingly low inhibition of RNA synthesis (GNIAZDOWSKI et al., 1972, 1975; SZMIGIERO et al., 1977).

To explain this phenomenon, it was assumed that between 1-nitro and 9-aminoalkyl groups of nitracrine a steric hindrance occurs which causes the nitro group to be twisted round the carbon–nitrogen bond. A part of the nitracrine molecule may, therefore, be too large to be accomodated between two adjacent base pairs in the DNA double helix (GNIAZDOWSKI et al., 1974; SZMIGIERO et al., 1977). In fact, roentgenographic studies of DAUTER et al. (1975) proved that there is a 60° twist of the nitro group of nitracrine around the carbon–nitrogen bond and a butterfly-like arrangement of its phenylene rings (Fig. 4).

To check the model of the "disturbed" or "imperfect" intercalation, the 2-nitro (C-264), 3-nitro (C-257) and 4-nitro (C-265) isomers of nitracrine and its analogs, containing different substituents at position 1, were tested for their effects on transcription (Fig. 8). The steric hindrance discussed above cannot be ascribed to the 2-, 3-, or 4-nitro isomers of nitracrine. They can, therefore, be more easily inserted into DNA than 1-nitro-9-aminoalkylacridines. Their effect on RNA synthesis was considerably higher than that of nitracrine in the absence of thiols (Fig. 8). Further support for the proposed explanation comes from experiments on analogs with different substituents at position 1 (Fig. 9). As predicted by this model, a decrease in the inhibitory effect was observed when the size of the group at position 1 increased (Szmigiero et al., 1977). Although substitutions in the ring modify acid properties of acridine, this does not seem to explain the observed correlation.

Low inhibitory effects of nitracrine were shown in other model systems in vitro. DNA synthesis in HeLa cell homogenates was relatively insensitive to nitracrine, while its nitro isomers displayed higher effect (Konopa et al., 1974, 1976a). Similarly, low inhibition of transcription was observed in rat liver nuclei and the possibility of a lack of activity, due to a low drug uptake by the nucleus, was excluded (Marczyński, 1975).

The comparison of physicochemical properties with the template toxicity for DNA of nitracrine and its biologically inactive analog does not satisfactorily explain the potent biologic effect of the drug, nor its mechanism of action.

Thiol-Dependent Reaction of Nitracrine with DNA

The incubation of nitracrine with DNA in the presence of thiol, prior to the addition of the enzyme, leads to a significant inhibition of transcription. Quantitatively, the level of inhibition depends on temperature (Gniazdowski et al., 1972), thiol concentration (Szmigiero et al., 1977), and time (Gniazdowski et al., 1975). A considerably greater inhibition is observed with dithiothreitol than with β-mercaptoethanol or α-thioglycerol (Fig. 10).

Among several DNA-interacting dyes only analogs of nitracrine, belonging to the 1-nitro-9-aminoalkylacridine series, and one 1-nitro-10-aminoalkylacridone derivative (C-492) exhibited the thiol-dependent inhibitory effect (Gniazdowski et al., 1975; Szmigiero et al., 1977). Neither the unsubstituted and halogenated analogs of nitracrine, nor its 2-, 3- or 4-nitro isomers showed any enhancement of the inhibition in the presence of thiols (Szmigiero et al., 1977).

In the absence of DNA, nitracrine reacts with thiols giving inactive product(s) (Gniazdowski et al., 1972, 1975). As shown by infrared spectrophotometry, the product is devoid of the nitro group (Gniazdowski et al., 1975). This suggests that the reduction of the nitro group is involved in the reaction of nitracrine with DNA in the presence of thiols. Cain et al. (1976) suggested that thiolysis of the 9-aminoalkyl group during the reaction might also occur.

Several substitution products of nitracrine in the presence of hydrogen sulfide were identified by Weltrowski and Ledóchowski (1977). Extraction with isobu-

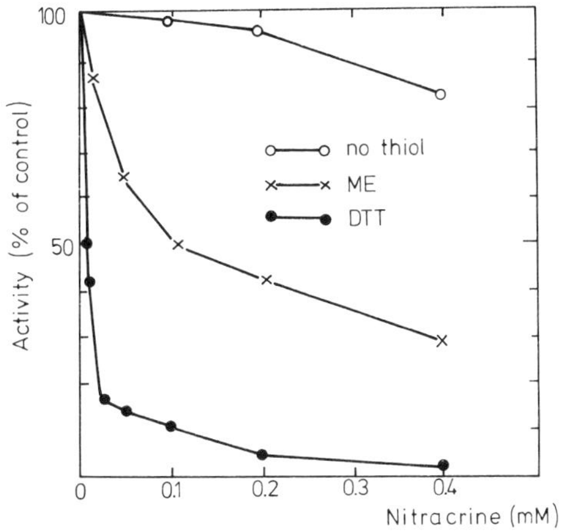

Fig. 10. Effect of nitracrine on RNA synthesis in vitro. Nitracrine was incubated with DNA without thiols, at 12 mM mercaptoethanol (ME) or 2 mM dithiothreitol (DTT) prior to the addition of the enzyme (GNIAZDOWSKI et al., 1975)

Table 4. Comparison of the stability of complexes of nitracrine, its analogs and related compounds with DNA

Conditions of complex formation		Template activity (% of control)	
	Dye/DNA (mol/mol)	Direct estimation	Estimation after extraction and dialysis
+Nitracrine	0.10	21	5
+C-337	0.10	62	57
+C-205	0.10	38	5
+C-609	0.10	29	8
+C-137	0.50	12	94
+Ethidium bromide	0.45	2	98
+Actinomycin D	0.03	5	78

Inhibitory effects of the dyes were examined after exposure of DNA to a dye and 5 mM dithiothreitol at the ratio dye to DNA (mol of dye per mol of DNA phosphate). The template activity of DNA preparations was examined either directly or after extraction with isobutyl alcohol and dialysis. (From GNIAZDOWSKI et al., 1975; SZMIGIERO et al., 1977).

tyl alcohol and dialysis restored entirely or almost completely the template activity of DNA, previously complexed with noncovalently bound dyes (ethidium bromide, actinomycin, or the nitro group–lacking derivative of nitracrine, C-137). Nitracrine-DNA complexes formed in the presence of thiols are resistant to similar treatment and remain inactive (Table 4). To explain the thiol-dependent enhancement of the inhibition, it was suggested that during the nitracrine-thiol reaction a by-product may be transiently formed, binding presumably covalently to DNA and affecting DNA-dependent RNA synthesis. Dependence of the template activity on the amount of ^{3}H-nitracrine, bound to calf thymus DNA,

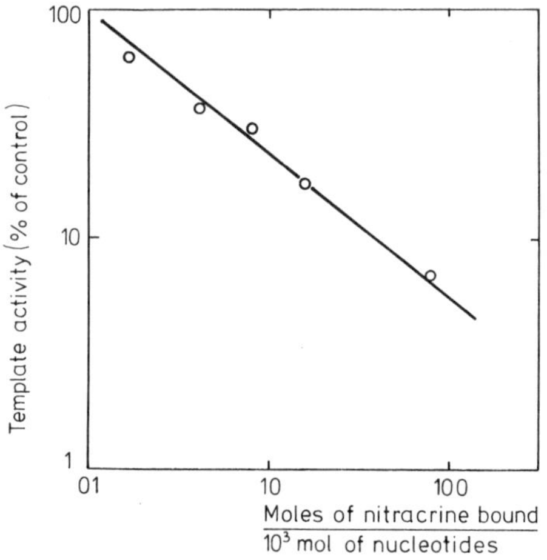

Fig. 11. Relationship between the amount of nitracrine molecules bound to DNA in the presence of dithiothreitol and the template activity of the complex. The number of the drug molecules bound per 1000 nucleotides in DNA was determined after extraction with isobutanol and dialysis. The template activity was examined with *E. coli* RNA polymerase (GNIAZDOWSKI et al., unpublished results)

Table 5. Effect of nitracrine-DNA complex on the transcription of free DNA

Preincubation conditions (8 min at 38° C)	Additions at 8 min	^{14}C-GMP incorporated (90 s, 37° C) c.p.m.
Enzyme, DNA^F	DNA^L, NTP, Rif	587
Enzyme, DNA^F, DNA^L	NTP, Rif	340
Enzyme, DNA^L	DNA^F, NTP, Rif	31
Enzyme, DNA^L	NTP, Rif	19

Irreversible complexes of nitracrine-DNA (DNA^L) were prepared as described in the legend to Table 4. Either free DNA (DNA^F, 4 μg) or DNA^L was incubated with the enzyme in 0.05 ml for 8 min. Then, the synthesis was initiated by addition of nucleoside triphosphates (NTP), rifampicin (Rif., 1 μg) and DNA^L or DNA^F as indicated. The samples (final volume 0.1 ml) were treated with trichloroacetic acid (Gniazdowski et al., unpublished results).

is shown in Fig. 11. The complexes were formed in the presence of dithiothreitol, using the drug labeled in the ring. If the assumption that the acridine ring is attached integrally to DNA as well as the determined stoichiometry are correct, only a few dye molecules can cause a potent damage to the DNA template function. The nature of the nitracrine binding to DNA in the presence of sulfhydryl compounds remains unknown. The intercalating dye, ethidium bromide, competes with nitracrine for the template and at high concentration prevents nitracrine from binding (WILMAŃSKA et al., 1977).

In the transcription system with *E. coli* RNA polymerase the amount of the enzyme bound to the irreversible nitracrine-DNA complex is comparable to that bound to free DNA (Table 5). Kinetics of the enzyme binding and

Table 6. Effect of nitracrine on the average chain length

Nitracrine mM	Nucleotide incorporation (in pmol)				Average chain length
	γ-^{32}P-ATP	γ-^{32}P-GTP	^{14}C-AMP	^{14}C-GMP	
0.00	6.5	6.9	7,050	9,450	2,460
0.05	5.6	4.1	3,960	5,590	1,970
0.10	5.8	4.9	3,480	4,455	1,480
0.20	5.8	4.2	2,350	3,500	1,170
0.40	5.0	2.9	1,760	2,815	1,160

Calf thymus DNA (40 µg/assay) was incubated with nitracrine, substrates, and 12 mM mercaptoethanol at 20° C for 1 hour before the addition of *E. coli* RNA polymerase (for further details see GNIAZDOWSKI et al., 1975). The enzyme (0.1 ml) was added to the incubation mixture, and the samples (final volume 0.25 ml) were incubated for 10 min at 37° C. Then, the reaction was terminated with trichloroacetic acid. Initiation assay (γ-^{32}P-ATP and γ-^{32}P-GTP) and assay of total RNA synthesis (^{14}C-AMP and ^{14}C-GMP) were performed in separate samples. The average chain length was calculated according to the following equation:

$$\frac{(^{14}\text{C-AMP}+{}^{14}\text{C-GMP})\times 2}{\gamma\text{-}^{32}\text{P-ATP}+\gamma\text{-}^{32}\text{P-GTP}}$$ (ŚLASKA et al., in preparation).

dissociation at a low ionic strength are similar for both types of templates. The enzyme bound to the template treated with nitracrine seems to be more susceptible to higher ionic strength (GNIAZDOWSKI et al., unpublished observation). The analysis of the transcript synthesized on DNA with apparently low amount of the attached drug indicates a decrease in the number of synthesized chains measured by γ-^{32}P-ATP and γ-^{32}P-GTP incorporation. The average chain length also decreases in the presence of DNA treated with the drug (Table 6). A shift to a lower molecular weight of RNA, synthesized on nitracrine-DNA complex, is observed (results not shown).

The results of the experiments described above indicate that binding of nitracrine to DNA does not significantly inhibit the association of the enzyme with the template but affects subsequent steps of RNA synthesis, initiation, and elongation, or induces premature termination.

Mechanism of the Drug Action in the Cell

The availability of radioactively labeled samples of nitracrine enabled to search for the sites of drug action in the cell.

After injection of ^{3}H-nitracrine into rats, a considerable amount of radioactivity was detected in polysomes, cytoplasmic sap, and in the nuclei of hepatocytes. From the components of chromatin a significant amount of the label was recovered in DNA (Table 7). DNA isolated from Ehrlich ascites tumor treated with ^{3}H-nitracrine contained the radioisotope coprecipitating with DNA in the presence of trichloroacetic acid (KONOPA et al., 1976a). Under similar conditions, the nitracrine–DNA complexes prepared in vitro can be completely

Table 7. Distribution of radioactivity in hepatocyte subcellular components after intraperitoneal administration of ^{3}H-nitracrine to rats (FILIPSKI and GRÖBNER, unpublished results)

Fractions		% of recovered radioactivity
Nuclear fractions	Non-histone protein	7
	histones	1
	RNA	2
	DNA	11
Post mitochondrial fractions	Polysomes	36
	supernatant	30

(over 99%) dissociated. The label, co-isolated with DNA, was insensitive to ribonuclease or pronase. Incubation with deoxyribonuclease rendered over 70% of the radioactivity acid-soluble (KOŁDEJ, 1976).

A DNA preparation with coprecipitating radioactivity was subjected to hydrolysis with deoxyribonuclease, venom phosphodiesterase, and alkaline phosphatase. The digest was analyzed by means of column (KONOPA et al., 1976b) and thin layer chromatography (KOŁDEJ, 1976). Several peaks on the radiochromatogram were detected but none corresponded to the original nitracrine (Fig. 12).

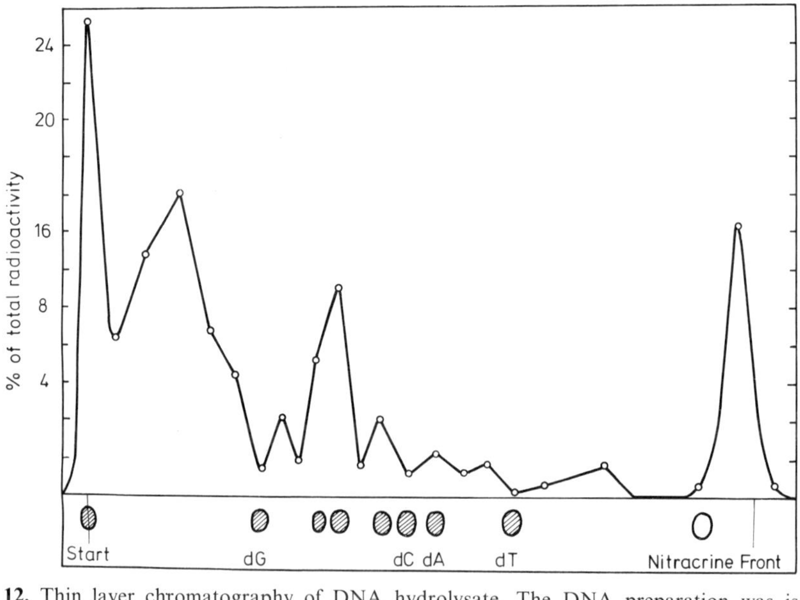

Fig. 12. Thin layer chromatography of DNA hydrolysate. The DNA preparation was isolated from Ehrlich ascites tumor cells following exposition of the mice to ^{14}C-nitracrine and hydrolyzed with deoxyribonuclease, venom phosphodiesterase and alkaline phosphatase. dG, dC, dA and dT correspond to spots of deoxyguanosine, deoxycytidine, deoxyadenosine and deoxythymidine respectively (KOŁDEJ, 1976)

Table 8. The amount of nitracrine molecules bound to Ehrlich ascites tumor cells DNA after injection of ^{14}C-nitracrine

	Time after injection (in h)				
	1.5	3	4	5	24
Number of nitracrine molecules per 1000 DNA nucleotides	0.21	0.28	1.00	0.56	0.09
Number of determinations	1	7	7	2	1
Number of animals in the single experiments	2	3–10	10	4	4

Mice bearing Ehrlich ascites tumor were injected intraperitoneally with ^{14}C-nitracrine (30 mg/kg). After the time indicated the animals were sacrificed and DNA was isolated from ascites cells according to Kay et al. (1952) with minor modifications. The acid-insoluble radioactivity bound to DNA was determined after precipitation with trichloroacetic acid and washing with ethanol and ether. (From KOŁDEJ, 1976; see also KONOPA et al., 1976a).

Up to one molecule of the drug or its metabolite per one thousand nucleotides of DNA, isolated from Ehrlich ascites tumor (KONOPA and KOŁDEJ, 1974; KONOPA et al., 1976b) or L1210 leukemia cells (FILIPSKI et al., 1977) was found after administering to mice nitracrine labeled in the acridine ring. It should be mentioned that the former tumor is sensitive, while the latter resistant to the drug. The maximum binding was observed 3 h after injection of the drug (Table 8). Radioactivity could also be detected in cellular DNA when nitracrine labeled in the alkyl chain was injected to the animals (KOŁDEJ, 1976; FILIPSKI et al., 1977), although somewhat different amounts of the drug were found in DNA. Independent attachment of both parts of the drug molecule, repair mechanisms or differences in the experimental model used may be responsible for this discrepancy.

DNA isolated from ascites cells of mice treated with nitracrine exhibited an enhanced tendency to spontaneous renaturation as was shown spectrophotometrically (Fig. 13) or by hydroxyapatite chromatography (KOŁDEJ, 1976). It was shown that none of the biologically inactive isomers increased the spontaneous denaturation significantly. This observation suggests that cross-links are introduced by the drug into DNA. This conclusion was recently confirmed by FILIPSKI et al. (1977).

A satellite component of DNA, isolated from mouse L1210 leukemia cells, can be separated in an alkaline cesium chloride gradient into the "light" and "heavy" strand, When such satellite DNA was isolated from the nitracrine-treated cells, it gave, in the alkaline gradient, only one band corresponding to the cross-linked strands (Fig. 14).

Evidence that binding of DNA with nitracrine in vivo affects its template properties has been recently obtained by KRAWCZYK (personal communication). The nuclei of the hepatocytes isolated from drug-treated rats are inactive in RNA synthesis in vitro system. The inhibition was due to template inactivation since the addition of exogenous DNA restored the activity.

A decrease of the activity of glycolytic enzymes after exposition of Ehrlich ascites tumor cells to nitracrine was reported by GUMIŃSKA (1973). According to the author the effect may be caused by repression of the corresponding

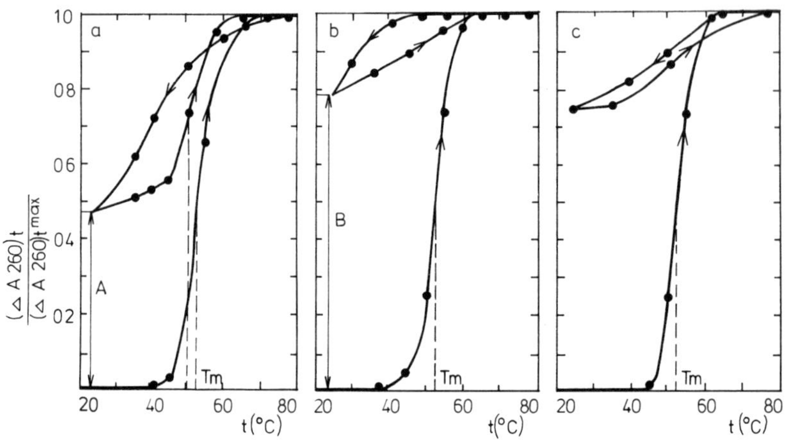

Fig. 13a–c. Profiles of thermal denaturation and renaturation of DNA from Ehrlich ascites tumor cells. **a** Nitracrine-DNA complex isolated following in vivo exposition to the drug; **b** control DNA: **c** nitracrine-DNA complex (1:1000) formed in vitro (KOLDEJ, 1976)

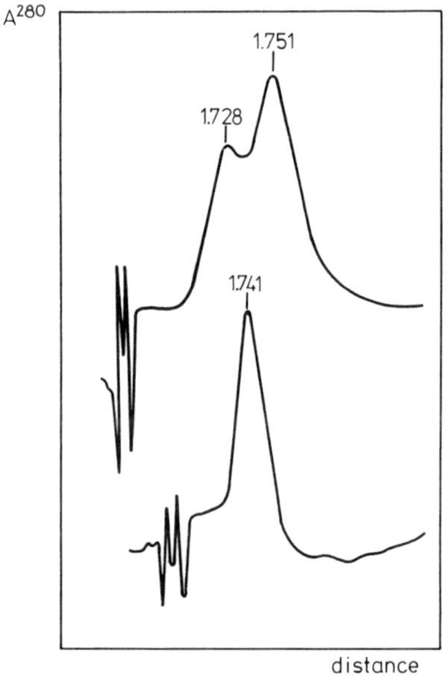

Fig. 14. Alkaline gradient centrifugation of satellite DNA fraction isolated from L-1210 mouse leukemia cells after administration of the drug to the animals (FILIPSKI et al., 1977)

genes. Binding of nitracrine to DNA in the cell is probably the crucial phenomenon responsible for the biologic effect of the drug. However, DNA does not seem to be the only target of nitracrine. As can be inferred from Table 7, large amounts of the label can be detected in postnuclear fractions. Liver polyribosomes, isolated from rats after injection of ^{3}H-nitracrine, contained radioactivity in the polysomal fraction. Pretreatment of polysomes with ribonuclease shifted the radioactivity to the top gradient. It was shown that both proteins and RNA contained the presumptive metabolite(s) of nitracrine (GRÖBNER and FILIPSKI, unpublished observation).

The nature of the reactions leading to the cross-link formation in DNA and to the covalent binding of nitracrine to macromolecules remains unknown. Several facts concerning the chemical reactivity of the drug and its changes in biologic systems could stimulate further investigations. SKONIECZNY and LEDÓCHOWSKI (1977) pointed out the high reactivity of the nitro group in substituted 1-nitro-9-aminoacridines (Fig. 5). They suggested that similar nucleophilic substitution, purines or/and pyrimidines acting as nucleophilic reagents, might be responsible for the covalent binding. The presence of the nitro group at position 1 potentially enhances the reactivity of C_2 and C_9. As recently shown by LEDÓCHOWSKI and KONIECZNY (1977), 1-nitro-9-phenoxyacridine, in the presence of ferric chloride, reacts with piperidine yielding 1-nitro-2, 9-dipiperidylacridine and 1-nitro-9-aminopiperidylacridine. Acridines are excreted as their 2-hydroxyderivatives (cf. ALBERT, 1966).

Recently PAWLAK and KONOPA (1979) studied the irreversible binding of ^{14}C-nitracrine to proteins during incubation of the drug with the postmitochondrial supernatant, cytosol, and microsomes of rat liver and HeLa cells. According to their results, hydrolysis and oxidation of the 9-aminoalkyl side chain occur and there are two possible pathways leading to the formation of other active centers in the acridine ring. Under anaerobic conditions the nitro group can be reduced by subcellular fractions to a highly reactive hydroxylamine derivative. Alternatively, the formation of an epoxide intermediate which could bind to protein was suggested. The inhibition of epoxide hydratase, which could inactivate the intermediate, enhances significantly binding of nitracrine to protein (PAWLAK and KONOPA, 1979).

Chemical and biochemical experiments indicate that there is a number of "hot" centers in the molecule of nitracrine. The terminal dimethylamino group can be hydrolyzed and oxidized to N-alkylhydroxylamine. The 9-alkylamino group can undergo hydrolysis and thiolysis. The 1-nitro group is susceptible to reduction and/or to substitution by heterocyclic amines. Nucleophilic substitution of the hydrogen atom at position 2 can occur and a double bond between C_2 and C_3 in the acridine ring can be oxidized giving a highly reactive epoxide. These centers might be taken into consideration to account for the attachment of the drug to macromolecules.

General Conclusions

Nitracrine is a compound of complex metabolism when compared to other acridines (WOLFE, 1975, rev.). Activation of nitracrine in the cell leads to the formation of metabolites. As in some model systems the reduction of the nitro group seems to be one of the activation steps. The metabolites can bind to several cellular components affecting their functions. Best known is their effect on DNA. Covalent binding of the drug is an event at the molecular level which is responsible for the change of DNA properties. Although the nature of the adduct is not fully understood, there are probably at least two centers in the drug molecule, reacting with DNA and inducing cross links. The drug affects template properties of DNA. The experimental data indicate that there are other possible binding sites of nitracrine in the cell. Further research is needed to elucidate their significance for the biologic activity of the drug.

Acknowledgments. The authors are grateful for the discussion of the manuscript and for permission to quote their unpublished results to the following persons: J. Konopa, Z. Krawczyk, C. Kwaśniewska-Rokicińska, A. Ledóchowski, C. Radzikowski, S. Skonieczny, J. Święcki. A large part of the experimental work reviewed in this chapter was supported by the Pharmaceutical Industry "Polfa."

The work of authors' laboratories has been supported in part by grant No 1301 of the Polish National Cancer Program (J.F. and M.C.) and by the Polish Academy of Sciences under project 09.7.1 (M.G.).

References

Albert, A.: The acridines. London: Arnold Ltd. 1966

Albert, A., Rubbo, S.D., Goldacre, R.J., Davey, M.E., Stone, J.D.: The influence of chemical constitution on antibacterial activity. Part II: A general survey of the acridine series. Br. J. Exp. Pathol. *26*, 160–192 (1945)

Bauer, W., Vinograd, J.: The interaction of closed circular DNA with intercalative dyes. I. The superhelix density of SV40 DNA in the presence and absence of dye. J. Mol. Biol. *33*, 141–171 (1968)

Biedrzycki, J., Błażejewski, J., Ledóchowski, A., Szychliński, J.: Research on tumour inhibiting compounds. Part LIII. Preliminary investigation on spectroscopic and photochemical behaviour of 1-nitro-9-(3′-dimethylaminopropylamino) acridine and its isomers. Rocz. Chem. *51*, 379–384 (1977)

Bratkowska-Seniów, B., Dziedzic, J., Fengler, I., Steuden, W., Szymaniec, S., Wysocka, M.: Morphologic blood pattern in patients treated with Ledakrin. Mater. Med. Pol. *8*, 295–301 (1976a)

Bratkowska-Seniów, B., Oleszkiewicz, L., Kozak, E., Krizar, T.: Ledakrin in treatment of colon carcinoma. Mater. Med. Pol. *8*, 323–330 (1976b)

Cain, B.F., Wilson, W.R., Baguley, B.C.: Structure activity relationship for thiolytic cleavage rates of antitumor drugs in the 4′-(9-acridinylamino) methanesulfaniline series. Mol. Pharmacol. *12*, 1027–1035 (1976)

Chodkowski, J., Kiwak, W.: Polarographic investigation on acridine derivatives. Part V. 1-Nitro-9-alkylaminoacridines. Rocz. Chem. *47*, 1401–1408 (1973)

Chodkowski, J., Kiwak, W., Walczak, E.: Polarographic investigation on acridine derivatives. Part I. Preliminary communication. Rocz. Chem. *44*, 1603–1606 (1970)

Chotkowska, E., Konopa, J.: Cytotoxic properties of nitro derivatives of 9-aminoacridine in cultures of *Euglena gracilis*. Arch. Immunol. Ther. Exp. *20*, 289–294 (1972)

Chotkowska, E., Konopa, J.: The influence of 1-nitro-9-(3′-dimethylaminopropylamino) acridine on biosynthesis of DNA, RNA and protein in synchronized cultures of *Euglena gracilis*. Arch. Immunol. Ther. Exp. *21*, 767–774 (1973)

Crawford, L.V., Waring, M.J.: Supercoiling of polyoma virus DNA measured by its interaction with ethidium bromide. J. Mol. Biol. *25*, 23–30 (1967)

Dauter, Z., Bogucka-Ledóchowska, M., Hempel, A., Ledóchowski, A., Kosturkiewicz, Z.: Crystal and molecular structure of 1-nitro-9-(3-dimethylaminopropylamino)-acridine (C-283) monoiodide. Rocz. Chem. *49*, 859–861 (1975)

Dauter, Z., Bogucka-Ledóchowska, M., Hempel, A., Ledóchowski, A., Kosturkiewicz, Z.: X-ray investigation on acridine derivatives. Part I. Crystal and molecular structure of 1-nitro-9-(3-dimethylaminopropylamino)-acridine hydroiodide. Rocz. Chem. *50*, 1573–1583 (1976)

Filipski, J., Chorąży, M., Mendecki, J.: Investigations of complex formation between some derivatives of 9-aminoacridine and nucleic acids. Stud. Biophys. *24/25*, 249–256 (1970)

Filipski, J., Marczyński, B., Chorąży, M.: Complexes of derivatives of 1-nitro-9-aminoacridine with DNA. Acta Biochim. Pol. *22*, 119–129 (1975)

Filipski, J., Marczyński, B., Sadzińska, L., Chałupka, G., Chorąży, M.: Interactions of some nitro-derivatives of substituted 9-aminoacridine with DNA. Biochim. Biophys. Acta *478*, 33–43 (1977)

Giełdanowski, J.: Basic and developed pharmacological investigation of compound C-283. In: Compound C-283. Radzikowski, C. (ed.), pp. 115–148. Warszawa: United Pharmaceutical Industry "Polfa" 1974

Giełdanowski, J.: Studies of pharmacological activity of several acridine derivatives with cytostatic and oncostatic properties. Mater. Med. Pol. *8*, 252–257 (1976)

Giełdanowski, J., Szaga, B., Patkowski, J., Pelczarska, A.: Immunosuppressive properties of acridine and acridone derivatives. Arch. Immunol. Ther. Exp. *19*, 465–483 (1971)

Giełdanowski, J., Patkowski, J., Szaga, B., Teodorczyk, J.: Preclinical pharmacologic studies in 1-nitro-9-(dimethylaminopropylamino)acridine and its N-oxide. I Acute and subchronic action. Arch. Immunol. Ther. Exp. *20*, 399–418 (1972a)

Giełdanowski, J., Patkowski, J., Szaga, B., Teodorczyk, J.: Preclinical pharmacologic studies on 1-nitro-9-(dimethylaminopropylamino)-acridine and its N-oxide. II Chronic action. Arch. Immunol. Ther. Exp. *20*, 419–444 (1972b)

Gniazdowski, M., Ślaska, K., Szmigiero, L., Jaros-Kamińska, B.: Effect of the 1-nitro-9-aminoacridine derivative (C-283) on the DNA transcription by *E. coli* polymerase *in vitro*. Stud. Biophys. *31/32*, 417–425 (1972)

Gniazdowski, M., Szmigiero, L., Ślaska, K., Jaros-Kamińska, B., Ciesielska, E.: Relation between chemical structure of acridines and their effect on the RNA synthesis *in vitro*. 9th Meet. FEBS Abstr. Commun., p. 117. Budapest 1974

Gniazdowski, M., Szmigiero, L., Ślaska, K., Jaros-Kamińska, B., Ciesielska, E.: Influence of thiols on inhibition of ribonucleic acid synthesis in vitro by a 1-nitro-9-aminoacridine derivative, C-283. Mol. Pharmacol. *11*, 310–318 (1975)

Gumińska, M.: The effect of 1-nitro-9-aminoacridine on respiration and glycolysis in Ehrlich ascites tumor cells. Acta Biochim. Pol. *20*, 333–341 (1973)

Hrabowska, M., Ledóchowski, A., Horowska, B., Bogucka, M., Onoszko, K.: A search for antitumor compounds. VII Biologic studies. Antitumor properties of 10 new 1-nitro-9-aminoacridine derivatives. Arch. Immunol. Ther. Exp. *18*, 230–238 (1970)

Hrabowska, M., Ledóchowski, A., Onoszko, K.: A search for antitumor compounds. XI Biologic studies. Antitumor properties of 19 new 9-aminoacridine and 1-or 3-nitro-9-aminoacridine derivatives. Arch. Immunol. Ther. Exp. *24*, 249–258 (1976)

Jabłoński, K., Gerber, J.: Results of treatment of cancer patients with C-283 at the Gynecological Clinics of the Obstetrics and Gynecology Institute of the Medical Academy Wrocław. In: Compound C-283. Radzikowski, C. (ed.), pp. 185–220. Warszawa: United Pharmaceutical Industry "Polfa" 1974

Jerzykowski, T., Szalsza-Kuśnierczyk, M., Chałupka, G., Chorąży, M.: Excretion and organ distribution of the cytostatic preparation Ledakrin (preparation C-283) in rat. Acta Med. Pol. *17*, 169–174 (1976)

Kay, E.R.H., Simmons, N.S., Dounce, A.: An improved preparation of sodium desoxyribonucleate. J. Am. Chem. Soc. *74*, 1724–1726 (1952)

Kołdej, K.: On interactions of Ledakrin with deoxyribonucleic acid. Doctor's thesis. Gdańsk Polytechnic, Gdańsk Poland, 1976 (in Polish)

Konopa, J., Kołdej, K.: Studies on the mechanism of action of antitumor agent 1-nitro-9-(3-dimethylaminopropylamino) acridine C-283. In: Progress in chemotherapy. Daikos, G.K. (ed.), Vol. 3, pp. 705–708. Athens: 1974

Konopa, J., Ledóchowski, A., Matuszkiewicz, A., Jereczek-Morawska, E.: *In vitro* studies on the cytotoxic properties of 9-amino-nitroacridine derivatives. Neoplasma *16*, 171–179 (1969)

Konopa, J., Matuszkiewicz, A., Kołdej, K.: Studies on the mode of action of nitro derivatives of 9-aminoacridine with antitumor activity. Symposium on mechanism of cytostatic agents, p. 10. Budapest Oct. 26–28, E.A.C.R. Abstr. Budapest Akad. Kiado 1972

Konopa, J., Chotkowska, E., Kołdej, K., Matuszkiewicz, A., Pawlak, J.W., Woynarowski, J.M.: Studies on the mechanism of antitumour activity of Ledakrin. Mater. Med. Pol. *8*, 258–265 (1976a)

Konopa, J., Kołdej, K., Pawlak, J.W.: Covalent binding of 1-nitro-9-(3′-dimethyl-n-propylamino) acridine, a new antitumor drug to DNA of Ehrlich ascites tumor cells *in vivo*. Chem. Biol. Interact. *13*, 99–103 (1976b)

Krzyżowska-Gruca, S., Gruca, S., Kwaśniewska-Rokicińska, C., Vorbrodt, A.: Nuclear and nucleolar ultrastructural lesions induced by 1-nitro-9-aminoacridine (C-283) in human ovarian carcinoma cells. Eur. J. Cancer *9*, 785–788 (1973)

Kurnatowska, A., Kadłubowski, R.: Bacteriostatic, antimycotic and trichomonicidal effect of new anticancer drug, Ledakrin, Polfa. Polski Tygodnik Lekarski *32*, 1767–1769 (1977) (in Polish)

Kwaśniewska-Rokicińska, C.: Results of C-283 in the treatment of patients at the Oncology Institute (Gliwice). In: Compound C-283. Radzikowski, C. (ed.), pp. 149–184. Warszawa: United Pharmaceutical Industry "Polfa" 1974

Kwaśniewska-Rokicińska, C.: Evaluation of the effectiveness of Ledakrin in ovarian and breast cancer. In: Ledakrin. Radzikowski, C. (ed.), pp. 7–41. Wrocław: Instytut Immunologii i Terapii Doświadczalnej 1976 (in Polish)

Kwaśniewska-Rokicińska, C., Winkler, A.: The effect of 1-nitro-9-aminoacridine on Yoshida sarcoma sensitive and resistant to alkylating agents. Arch. Immunol. Ther. Exp. *17*, 376–379 (1969)

Kwaśniewska-Rokicińska, C., Święcki, J., Drosik, K.: Preliminary observations on the Ledakrin effects in treatment of patients with lung carcinoma. Mater. Med. Pol. *8*, 289–294 (1976)

Ledóchowski, A.: 1-nitroacridines: a new group of antitumor compounds. In: Compound C-283. Radzikowski, C. (ed.), pp. 35–63. Warszawa: United Pharmaceutical Industry "Polfa" 1974

Ledóchowski, A.: Ledakrin – anticancerous medicine 1-nitro-9(3-dimethylaminopropylamino)-acridine·2 HCl·H_2O. Mater. Med. Pol. *8*, 237–251 (1976)

Ledóchowski, A., Konieczny, M.T.: Nucleophilic substitution in position 2 of 1-nitroacridine derivative – a new suggestion of antitumour action of Ledakrin. Rocz. Chem. *51*, 1561–1563 (1977)

Ledóchowski, A., Skonieczny, S.: Reactions at C-9 of acridine derivatives. Part XI. A new interpretation of the mechanism of nucleophilic substitution in 9-phenoxyacridine in phenol. Rocz. Chem. *49*, 891–897 (1975)

Ledóchowski, A., Skonieczny, S.: Reaction at C-9 of acridine derivatives. Part XII. Hydrolysis of some derivatives of 1-nitro-9-aminoacridine and their N-oxides. Rocz. Chem. *50*, 415–422 (1976)

Ledóchowski, A., Sobczyk, Z., Kunikowski, A., Kowalewska, C.: Reactions at C-9 of acridine derivatives. Part XIII. Hydrolysis of derivatives of 9-aminoacridine. Rocz. Chem. *50*, 1257–1273 (1976)

Löber, C.: Über die Komplexbindung von Acridinfarbstoffen mit DNA. Stud. Biophys. *2*, 79–86 (1967)

Marczyński, B.: Investigations on the complexes of DNA with nitro-9-aminoacridine derivatives. Doctor's thesis. Silesian University, Katowice, Poland, 1975 (in Polish)

Mendecki, J., Więckowska, Z., Chorąży, M.: Inhibition of RNA synthesis by 9-aminoacridine in regenerating rat liver and cell culture. Acta Biochim. Pol. *16*, 253–262 (1969)

Pawlak, J.W., Konopa, J.: Irreversible binding of ^{14}C-Ledakrin (nitracrine) with rat liver and HeLa cells subcellular fractions *in vitro*. Biochem. Pharmacol. (submitted for publication, 1979)

Pawlicki, M., Migdał, K., Żukowska-Vogelgesang, B., Mitus, J.: Assessment of the effectiveness of Ledakrin in treatment of patients with malignant effusions in serous cavities. Nowotwory *27*, 135–139 (1977) (in Polish)

Piotrowska-Sowińska, J.: Clinical observations of the Ledakrin effects in treatment of patients with malignant neoplasma. Mater. Med. Pol. *8*, 266–272 (1976)

Radzikowski, C.: The antitumor effect of C-283 in human patients. In: Compound C-283. Radzikowski, C. (ed.), pp. 9–18. Warszawa: United Pharmaceutical Industry Polfa 1974

Radzikowski, C.: Antineoplastic activity of C-283 preparation (Ledakrin) in model experiments. Mater. Med. Pol. *8*, 345–349 (1976)

Radzikowski, C., Więckowska, Z., Woźniakowska, Z., Chorąży, M.: Cytotoxic and cytostatic effect of the derivative of 1-nitro-9-aminoacridine in tissue culture. Neoplasma *14*, 121–134 (1967a)

Radzikowski, C., Ledóchowski, Z., Ledóchowski, A., Peryt, J., Hrabowska, M., Konopa, J., Balk, M., Jereczek, E.: A search for new antitumor compounds. Biological studies. Part III. Antitumor properties of 14 new acridine derivatives. Arch. Immunol. Ther. Exp. *15*, 233–240 (1967b)
Radzikowski, C., Ledóchowski, Z., Ledóchowski, A., Bogucka, M., Hrabowska, M., Konopa, J., Balk, M., Jereczek, E.: A search for new antitumor compounds. Biological studies. Part IV. Antitumor properties of 21 new acridine derivatives. Arch. Immunol. Ther. Exp. *15*, 241–248 (1967c)
Radzikowski, C., Ledóchowski, A., Hrabowska, M., Horowska, B., Stefańska, B., Konopa, J., Morawska, E.: A search for antitumor compounds. V. Biologic studies. Antitumor properties of 41 new acridine derivatives. Arch. Immunol. Ther. Exp. *17*, 86–98 (1969a)
Radzikowski, C., Ledóchowski, A., Hrabowska, M., Stefańska, B., Horowska, B., Konopa, J., Morawska, E., Urbańska, M.: A search for antitumor compounds. VI Biologic studies. Antitumor properties of 29 new acridine derivatives of group XVII-XVIII. Arch. Immunol. Ther. Exp. *17*, 99–110 (1969b)
Radzikowski, C., Wysocka-Skrzela, B., Hrabowska, M., Konopa, J., Jereczek-Morawska, E., Onoszko, K., Ledóchowski, A.: A search for antitumor compounds. IX Biologic studies. Antitumor properties of 17 new acridine derivatives. Arch. Immunol. Ther. Exp. *19*, 219–228 (1971)
Rogalski, E., Domagała, J., Kołodziej, J.: Results of combined treatment with lung tissue resection and simultaneous administration of Ledakrin in bronchial carcinoma. Mater. Med. Pol. *8*, 311–315 (1976)
Skonieczny, S., Ledóchowski, A.: Intramolecular substitution of the nitro group of 1-nitro-9-alkylaminoethylamino acridine. Rocz. Chem. *51*, 2279–2281 (1977)
Stenram, U., Willén, R.: Effects of proflavine on ultrastructure and RNA and protein synthesis in the liver of rats. Exp. Cell Res. *50*, 505–514 (1968)
Szmigiero, L., Ślaska, K., Ciesielska, E., Jaros-Kamińska, B., Gniazdowski, M.: Structure of acridines and their effect on RNA synthesis *in vitro*. Acta Biochim. Pol. *24*, 35–44 (1977)
Vorbrodt, A.: Ultrastructural nuclear and nucleolar lesions induced by 1-nitro-9-aminoacridine in rat liver cells. Folia Histochem. Cytochem. *8*, 248–254 (1970a)
Vorbrodt, A.: Ultrastructural lesions induced by 1-nitro-9-aminoacridine in the cytoplasm of rat liver cells. Folia Histochem. Cytochem. *8*, 255–259 (1970b)
Waring, M.J.: Binding of drugs to supercoiled circular DNA: evidence for and against intercalation. Prog. Mol. Subcell. Biol. Hahn, F.E. (ed.), Vol. 2, pp. 216–231. Berlin, Heidelberg, New York: Springer 1971
Waring, M.J.: Ethidium and Propidium. In: Antibiotics. Corcoran, J.W., Hahn, F.E. (eds.) Vol. III, pp. 141–163. Berlin, Heidelberg, New York: Springer 1975
Weltrowski, M., Ledóchowski, A.: Reaction of 1-nitro-9-amino(3-dimethylaminopropylamino)-acridine with hydrogen sulphide. Rocz. Chem. submitted for publication (1977)
Wilmańska, D., Szmigiero, L., Małagocka, E., Jaros-Kamińska, B., Gniazdowski, M.: Effect of 1-nitro-9-aminoalkylacridine (Ledakrin, C-283) binding with chromatin on DNA template activity. Medycyna Doświadczalna Mikrobiologia *29*, 147–152 (1977) (in Polish)
Wolfe, A.D.: Quinacrine and other acridines. In: Antibiotics. Corcoran, J.W., Hahn, F.E. (eds.), Vol. III, pp. 203–233. Berlin, Heidelberg, New York: Springer 1975

Phleomycin

Ch.F. Earhart, Jr.

I. Discovery and Structure

MAEDA et al. reported the isolation of phleomycin in 1956. It is a broad spectrum antibiotic with unusually high specific activity against *Mycobacterium phlei* and its name is derived from this latter property (MAEDA, 1965). Phleomycin is isolated from the water-soluble, basic fraction of the culture fluid of *Streptomyces verticillus*. As initially isolated, phleomycin is a copper-containing blue powder (TAKITA, 1959); treatment with hydroxyquinoline removes the copper, leaving a white powder which, except for a slight reduction in activity against mycobacteria, has undiminished antibacterial properties. In 1964 IKEKAWA et al. demonstrated that copper-containing phleomycin is a mixture of approximately 12 related components. These compounds, A, B, C, D_1, D_2, E, F, G, H, I, J, and K, were resolved by Sephadex column chromatography. Unless otherwise indicated, "phleomycin" will continue to refer to this complex of antibiotics for the remainder of this review.

It is necessary to state at the outset that different lots of phleomycin vary in the relative proportions of their components. This fact has apparently been responsible for conflicting reports regarding the ability of phleomycin to (1) specifically block DNA synthesis and (2) to prevent RNA virus replication. It may also account for the variations reported for the minimal concentrations of phleomycin necessary to inhibit growth of various cell types. Lastly, several groups (MAEDA et al., 1956; SLEIGH and GRIGG, 1976) have reported phleomycin to be stable in weakly alkaline and neutral solutions, but unstable below pH 7. However, the antimicrobial activity of one batch was enhanced by exposure to pH 1 (PIETSCH and ENG, 1969). PIETSCH (1969a), PIETSCH (1975) and POST and PRICE (1975) have discussed variations in phleomycin lots.

The structures of several components of the phleomycin complex have been determined in conjunction with bleomycin structural studies. This work has been summarized in a previous volume in this series (UMEZAWA, 1975) and elsewhere (KERSTEN and KERSTEN, 1974). The phleomycins are glycopeptides with molecular weights of approximately 1,400–1,500 (Fig. 1). Figure 1 also serves to emphasize the similarities in structure among the compounds comprising phleomycin, and between phleomycin and bleomycin. Phleomycinic acid and bleomycinic acid, which are probably common to all phleomycins and bleomycins, respectively, differ only in that bleomycin contains one additional carbon-carbon double bond. Phleomycins D_2, F and G′ are identical to bleomy-

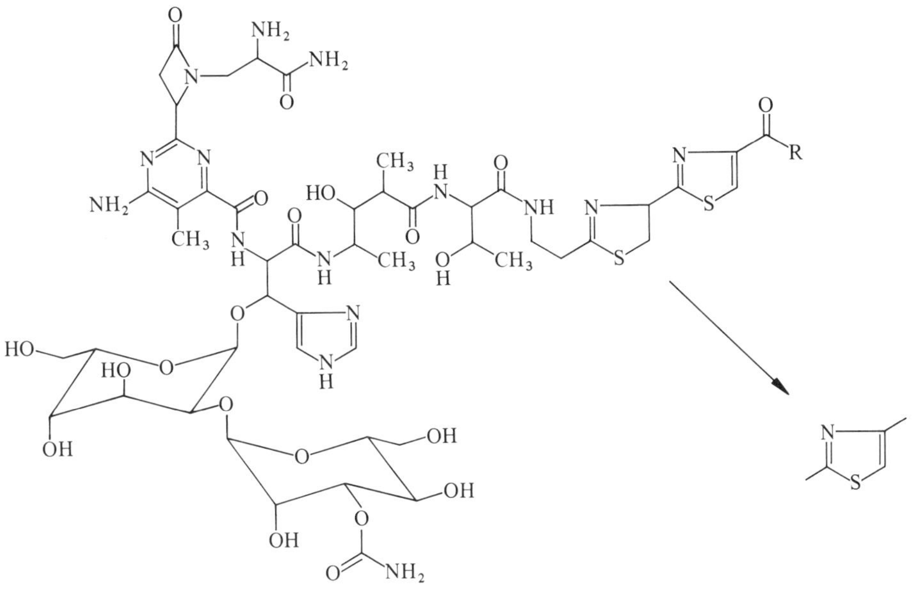

	R
Phleomycinic acid	$-OH$
D_1	$-NH-(CH_2)_4-NH-C(=NH)-NH_2$
E	$-NH-(CH_2)_4-NH-C(=NH)-NH-(CH_2)_4-NH-C(=NH)-NH_2$

Fig. 1. Structures of phleomycinic acid and phleomycins D_1 and E. The arrow indicates the difference between phleomycinic acid, which contains a dihydrothiazole moiety, and bleomycinic acid, which contains a conjugated dithiazole ring system

cins B_2, B_4 and B_6 and phleomycins D_1, E, and G are dihydrobleomycins B_2, B_4, and B_6, respectively.

In a search for antibiotics similar to phleomycin, the bleomycins were discovered (UMEZAWA et al., 1966; UMEZAWA, 1975). More recently, additional related antibiotics have been found; these include zorbamycin and zorbonomycin (ARGOUDELIS et al., 1971), YA-56X and Y (ITO et al., 1971; YA-56X is identical to zorbamycin [OHASHI et al., 1973]), victomycin (TAKASAWA et al., 1975a), and platomycin A and B (TAKASAWA et al., 1975b). Together, these antibiotics comprise the phleomycin–bleomycin group.

II. Growth Inhibitory Properties

Much of the interest in phleomycin stems from its antitumor activity (see Sect. II.A) and its ability to arrest DNA synthesis without greatly affecting RNA and protein synthesis (TANAKA et al., 1963; GRIGG, 1969; REITER et al.,

1972; FARRELL and REITER, 1973). These properties have led to studies with a variety of living systems, including prokaryotic, fungal, plant, and animal; the resultant findings demonstrate that phleomycin has an extremely broad range of biologic activity (summarized in PIETSCH, 1975). Values reported for the phleomycin sensitivity of a given cell type vary considerably. These variations occur not only because of differences in phleomycin batches (see Sect. I) but also because of differences in (1) methods of testing for growth inhibitory activity and (2) factors affecting cell sensitivity, which in the case of prokaryotes is influenced by the growth medium and the growth stage of the culture (GRIGG, 1969), and which in eukaryotes varies with stages in the cellular growth cycle (see Sect. II.A). [PIETSCH and CLAPPER (1969) have suggested that bacterial cells, like eukaryotic cells, display differences in phleomycin receptivity during their division cycle, but the definitive experiments, in which synchronized cell populations would be employed, have not been performed.]

A. Anticellular Activity

Phleomycin inhibits the growth of gram-negative and gram-positive bacteria and mycobacteria (MAEDA et al., 1956) and has antitumor activity (BRADNER and PINDELL, 1962; ISHIZUKA et al., 1966). Tables describing the antibacterial and antitumor activities of individual phleomycin components are available (ISHIZUKA et al., 1966). Approximate values for minimal growth inhibitory concentrations of copper-free phleomycin for several common bacteria are as follows: *Staphylococcus aureus*, 0.025–0.1 μg/ml; *Bacillus subtilis*, 0.0001 μg/ml; *Escherichia coli*, 0.1 μg/ml; and *Mycobacterium phlei*, 0.0004–0.002 μg/ml (MAEDA, 1965; ISHIZUKA et al., 1966). BRADNER and PINDELL (1962) demonstrated that doses of 1–4 mg phleomycin/kg/day for seven days resulted in significant inhibition of several types of tumors, including transplanted carcinomas and a sarcoma, in mice. Similar but more comprehensive tests were conducted by ISHIZUKA et al. (1966) and similar results were obtained. Daily doses of 0.025–5.0 mg phleomycin/kg were effective in inhibiting ascites type of Ehrlich carcinoma and a sarcoma in mice. Large doses were required if the treatment did not start promptly after the mice were injected with tumor cells.

B. Antiviral Activity

Replication of the following DNA viruses is inhibited by 25–50 μg phleomycin/ml; vaccinia, SV40, equine herpes type 2, simian adenovirus, herpes simplex, and polyoma (TEVETHIA and RAPP, 1969; IWATA and CONSIGLI, 1971). TEVETHIA and RAPP pointed out the good, although not absolute, correspondence between the extent of viral inhibition by phleomycin and the percentage of AT base pairs in the viral DNA.

There are several reports of phleomycin-induced inhibition of viruses with RNA genomes. However, this area has not been extensively studied, and some reservations regarding the validity of the existing work seem justified. HECHT and SUMMERS (1970) reported that phleomycin inhibited poliovirus-specified RNA synthesis in HeLa cells, provided the drug was added during the first 90 min after infection. A 95%–100% inhibition was reported at a phleomycin concentration (100 μg/ml) which resulted in less than 20% inhibition of HeLa cell DNA, RNA, or protein synthesis. However, the relative absence of effects on host cell macromolecular syntheses by the very high concentrations (33–200 μg/ml) of phleomycin used is not consistent with the work of others (KAJIWARA et al., 1966; DVORDJEVIC and KIM, 1967). Also, TEVETHIA and RAPP (1969) found no inhibition of poliovirus replication at a phleomycin concentration of 50 μg/ml.

The significance of a subsequent study (KOCH, 1971) on the effect of phleomycin on poliovirus replication is complicated by the fact that the phleomycin used was from a lot (616) known to be contaminated with conjugated nitriles. In these experiments, phleomycin clearly interfered with the cellular functions required for viral replication. Interestingly, a 5-min exposure of single-stranded poliovirus RNA to 2 μg phleomycin/ml reduced the infectivity of the RNA by 99%, whereas intact virions were unaffected by 200 μg/ml of the antibiotic. WATANABE and AUGUST (1968) showed that phleomycin from lot 616 can increase the T_m of reovirus RNA, which is double-stranded.

The effect of phleomycin on the replication of bacteriophage has been studied in relatively few systems. Addition of phleomycin soon after infection with PBS2, a *B. subtilis* phage whose DNA contains uracil in place of thymine, inhibits phage DNA synthesis (POST and PRICE, 1975). Two other DNA phages, T7 (SHIVE and EARHART, 1976) and ϕX174 (PITTS and SINSHEIMER), are similarly inhibited. Interestingly, the T-even phage (T2, T4, and T6) are able to replicate, albeit to a reduced extent, in the presence of 20 μg phleomycin/ml (SHIVE and EARHART, 1976). This unexpected result probably arises because infection with these phage blocks phleomycin-stimulated solubilization of intracellular DNA (bacterial and phage) (FARRELL and REITER, 1973; SHIVE and EARHART, 1976). This inhibition can occur even after the drug-mediated solubilization of bacterial DNA has begun (FARRELL and REITER, 1976). The mechanism by which the inhibition of phleomycin-induced solubilization occurs is not understood; some phage-specified proteins must be synthesized, however, as the inhibition does not take place if cells are infected with phage ghosts or if cells are infected in the presence of chloramphenicol (FARRELL and REITER, 1976). The well-documented envelope alterations which occur following T-even phage infection (MATHEWS, 1971) are apparently not responsible for the insensitivity to phleomycin; these modifications are complete with respect to their physiologic consequences 5 min after infection whereas phleomycin resistance develops throughout the infective cycle (SHIVE and EARHART, 1976). It should be mentioned that one lot of phleomycin (no. 616) inhibits the multiplication of RNA phage R23 (WATANABE and AUGUST, 1968), and MS2 (PIETSCH, 1969a), and of DNA phage T2 (WATANABE and AUGUST, 1968) as well. This is the lot which has been shown to contain a nitrile contaminant in sufficient concentrations to inhibit cellular respiration (PIETSCH, 1969a); addition of 4 μg/ml of phleomycin from this lot to a culture of *E. coli* immediately stops further increase in cellular mass.

C. Toxicity

The toxicity of phleomycin to mice, rats, rabbits, and guinea pigs was studied by ISHIZUKA et al. (1966). Phleomycin displayed delayed toxicity. For mice and rats 25 mg phleomycin/kg is lethal, and the lethal dose for rabbits and guinea pigs is 12.5 mg/kg. The manner of delivery of the dose, that is, intravenous, intraperitoneal, or subcutaneous, has little effect on the LD_{50} value. (Orally administered phleomycin, however, has remarkably low toxicity, which is probably indicative of poor absorption and/or inactivation and modification at the low pH which exists in the stomach.) In another set of experiments, the localization of phleomycin in various organs of tumor-bearing mice was determined 5 h after the antibiotic was subcutaneously injected. (Mice bearing one of two types of tumors, either the solid form or the ascites form of Ehrlich carcinoma, were used in these studies.) In both cases, phleomycin was found to be concentrated preferentially in the kidney and tumors, although significant concentrations were also present in the blood, spleen, and lungs. Studies with dogs indicated that phleomycin causes irreversible kidney malfunction. (Administration of 0.5 mg/kg every 3 days was lethal.) Autopsy also disclosed hemorrhaging in the gastrointestinal tract; specifically, hemorrhagic spots were noted in the pylorus and the duodenum, and hemorrhaging and ulcers were observed in the colon mucosa. Twice weekly doses of 0.3 mg phleomycin/kg were used successfully to treat a lymphosarcoma.

UMEZAWA (1975) has suggested that the irreversible renal toxicity caused by phleomycins may be due to their terminal amine moieties. All phleomycins give a positive Sakaguchi reaction (despite initial reports [MAEDA et al., 1956] to the contrary), whereas the bleomycin A complex gives a negative Sakaguchi reaction (UMEZAWA et al., 1966) and does not cause kidney damage (ISHIZUKA et al., 1967).

Phleomycin has repeatedly been shown to inhibit cell division and DNA synthesis in eukaryotic cells. TANAKA et al. (1963) reported a 99% inhibition of DNA synthesis in HeLa cells after the addition of 4 μg phleomycin/ml and 2 μg/ml were found completely to inhibit mitosis. In subsequent studies (see below) the concentration of phleomycin necessary to inhibit DNA synthesis was invariably much higher than that necessary to block cell division. Cells are most sensitive to blockage of cell division immediately following completion of DNA synthesis (KAJIWARA et al., 1966). Similarly, phleomycin affects cellular viability, as measured by colony-forming ability, maximally in the G-2 phase (DJORDJEVIC and KIM, 1967). The effect of phleomycin (0.5–5 μg/ml) on mitotic lily cells in culture was studied by HOTTA and STERN (1969). Entry into meiosis as well as mitosis was prevented by the antibiotic and cells in any stage of meiosis were also inhibited. These authors documented the ability of phleomycin to inhibit chromosomal organization changes, whether from the condensed to the extended form or vice versa, and stated that this action on chromosomal structure is the principal observable effect of phleomycin. That phleomycin affects chromosomal structure was first reported by MATTINGLY (1967) and later by KIHLMAN et al. (1967), who studied phleomycin toxicity in another plant system, *Vicia faba* (bean) root tips. G-2 phase cells were most sensitive to phleomycin and, after recovery from mitotic inhibition, numerous chromosomal aberrations were observed in metaphase cells. Freshly-prepared phleomycin solutions at concentrations as low as 0.03–0.1 μg/ml caused subchromatid, chromatid, and chromosome defects.

Exposure to low concentrations (0.1–1.0 μg/ml) of phleomycin for 24 h also causes chromosomal abnormalities in cultured human leucocytes (JACOBS et al., 1969) and the incidence of aberrations is concentration-dependent. At 25 μg phleomycin/ml, the chromosomes were so badly fragmented that the number of abnormalities per metaphase could not be determined. Exposure to 20 μg phleomycin/ml for 15 min was sufficient to cause the DNA of T cells and SV40-transformed normal and xeroderma pigmentosum cells to migrate in alkaline sucrose gradients as if a nonrandom breakdown of the DNA had occurred (KLEIJER et al., 1973).

An approach to bypass the potential toxicity of phleomycin was suggested by the observation that compounds such as caffeine (GRIGG, 1970), coumarin, Pyronin Y, and several nontoxic thiopurines (GRIGG et al., 1971) act synergistically with phleomycin to bring about DNA breakdown and cell death in *E. coli*. The potentiating effect of these compounds, termed "amplifiers" by GRIGG, is similar in some cases to increasing the phleomycin concentration 100-fold. The basic strategy, then, is to find a relatively nontoxic amplifier which is either unaltered in animals or modified to a metabolite which retains amplifying activity. Administration of such an amplifier in conjunction with a low level of phleomycin could conceivably be useful against kidney and urinary tract infections, if the therapeutic index were determined by the amplifier and not phleomycin. With this in mind, a large number of substituted purines have been prepared and screened by GRIGG and his collaborators (ANGYAL et al., 1974; BROWN and STEPHANSON, 1974; BHUSHAN et al., 1975; BROWN and STEPHANSON, 1976; BROWN et al., 1977); more that 30 purines have been identified as amplifiers. The most recent study (GRIGG et al., 1977) demonstrated that a wide range of aromatic compounds can also act as amplifiers and suggested that at least three structural features are required if a compound is to potentiate the antibacterial effects of phleomycin. All amplifiers (1) are cationic or have a nitrogen which can be readily protonated, (2) have areas greater than those of simple bicyclic molecules, and (3) contain six-membered carbocyclic or heterocyclic aromatic rings.

That many substances, with varying abilities to be taken up and accumulated in different organisms and tissues, have been identified as amplifiers has led to an expanded goal for this research. It is now being proposed that a *series* of amplifier–phleomycin regimes be developed.

III. Interaction with Membranes

A. Permeability

Cellular membranes and envelopes of all cell types appear to be remarkably permeable to phleomycin. The toxicity studies described above (ISHIZUKA et al., 1966) demonstrated a very rapid uptake and loss of phleomycin in the various tissues of mice. After 12 h of being administered, all traces of phleomycin were absent from the blood and urine of mice. In similar studies with rabbits, blood and urine were free of phleomycin after 12 and 24 h, respectively.

Pietsch et al. (1969) used two types of assays, bioassay and neutron activation analysis (which is feasible because of the copper in phleomycin), to study phleomycin permeability in mouse membranes. By both assay procedures, clearance of phleomycin appeared to occur by simple diffusion. Phleomycin (500 μg) had a 22 min body half-life in mice. Although this same high permeability is apparently true for microorganisms, as evidenced by the low doses required for bacteriostatic and bactericidal effects, no quantitative studies have been carried out. Sleigh and Grigg (1977), in order to explain the effects of simultaneous addition of sulfhydryl compounds and phleomycin (see Sect. IV.A), have suggested that entry of phleomycin into *E. coli* is a "relatively slow process". They are considering time intervals of only a few minutes, however, and their suggestion is not inconsistent with the idea that phleomycin readily penetrates cells. This property of phleomycin is particularly interesting in the case of gram-negative species, where the outer membrane has been shown to be a general permeability barrier to saccharides and saccharide-like molecules with molecular weights of 600 and greater (Decad and Nikado, 1976).

B. Effect on the Association of DNA with Membrane

A quite different type of interaction between phleomycin and membrane has been suggested by Reiter et al. (1972). Addition of phleomycin (20 μg/ml) to cultures of *Bacillus subtilis* resulted in drug-induced solubilization of cellular DNA and, importantly, the release of DNA from membrane. It was not possible, however, to determine in this system if this release process was a secondary effect resulting from nicks and double strand breaks introduced into the DNA or was, in fact, a distinct specific activity of phleomycin. That a low level of nuclease activity can result in the release of DNA from membrane has been documented in other systems (McIntosh and Earhart, 1975). Suggestive evidence for a phleomycin-induced release of cellular DNA from membrane also comes from studies of T4-infected *E. coli* B (Farrell and Reiter, 1976). In uninfected and, with the exception of mutants of one phage gene, T4-infected cells release of bacterial DNA from membrane occurs after addition of phleomycin. However, in the absence of a functional T4 *denA* gene product (which is endonuclease II, an enzyme thought to be the first phage-coded enzyme to attack host DNA), no release of bacterial DNA occurs, either in the presence or absence of phleomycin, and no phleomycin-induced solubilization takes place. However, unlike other T4 strains, infection with *denA* mutants subsequent to phleomycin addition, at a time when release from membrane must have already taken place, does not inhibit further solubilization. The authors argue that T4 has two different mechanisms for inhibiting phleomycin induced solubilization; in the absence of endonuclease II this inhibition is attributed to interference by an unknown mechanism with the phleomycin-induced release of DNA from membrane. Unfortunately, the procedure used to assay DNA-membrane attachments in these interesting experiments is not well characterized, particularly with respect to components of the rapidly-sedimenting fraction, which presumably contains membrane as well as single-stranded DNA. Also, the procedure is unusual in that alkaline, not neutral, sucrose gradients are employed and the centrifugal forces and time of centrifugation are much greater than those typically used in DNA-membrane assays.

Stationary cultures are ten times more resistant to phleomycin-induced DNA breakdown than are exponentially-growing cultures (GRIGG, 1969). SLEIGH and GRIGG (1976) have evoked naturally-occurring changes in the extent of cellular DNA attachment to membrane as a possible explanation for this phenomenon. The bacterial chromosome reportedly becomes attached to cell membrane at initiation of replication and is released on termination (WORCEL and BURGI, 1974); SLEIGH and GRIGG postulate that only membrane-attached DNA is sensitive to phleomycin damage. There is a possibility, however, that the results of WORCEL and BURGI are in error due to the poor recovery of DNA from starved cells that is obtained with their DNA-membrane assay procedure. RYDER and SMITH (1974) modified the procedure used by WORCEL and BURGI such that excellent DNA recoveries resulted and found no release of the chromosome from the cell envelope at the termination of DNA replication. The phleomycin resistance exhibited by cells which have completed DNA synthesis may be related to DNA conformation, as RYDER and SMITH observed that membrane-associated nucleoids sediment much more rapidly when isolated from cells which have completed DNA synthesis than from exponentially-growing cells.

IV. Mode of Action

A. Binding of Phleomycin to DNA

Phleomycin has been shown to bind to DNA by gel filtration (PIETSCH, 1973) and by ultraviolet and circular dichroism difference spectrum (KRUEGER et al., 1973). The initial data for such an association resulted from studies by FALASHI and KORNBERG, which provided two types of evidence that phleomycin binds to DNA. (1) The thermal denaturation of DNA is affected by the presence of phleomycin (45 μg/ml); phleomycin increases both the melting temperature (T_m) and the breadth of transition (σ_t), which is defined as the temperature range in which 30.8% to 69.2% of the transition occurs. [The increase in σ_t is not as pronounced in the absence of Mg^{2+}; Mg^{2+} is not a normal component of buffers for DNA melting studies (MANDEL and MARMUR, 1968) and, in fact, no effect of phleomycin on σ_t has been observed in subsequent studies in which buffers lacking Mg^{2+} were used (see below).] (2) FALASHI and KORNBERG also determined that DNA polymerase is inhibited by phleomycin. This inhibition is independent of enzyme concentration and dependent on the concentration of DNA and its adenine + thymine content.

The ability of phleomycin to increase the T_m of DNA has been confirmed several times. NAGAI et al. (1969) demonstrated such an increased T_m for *E.*

coli B DNA and noted that the increase was independent of the presence of 2-mercaptoethanol. This latter point is of interest because, in similar experiments with bleomycin, the presence of mercaptoethanol resulted in decreased T_m values. An additional peculiarity of the effect of phleomycin on T_m values is that the antibiotic has no significant effect on DNA samples with T_m values of 80° C or higher (Falashi and Kornberg). It was suggested that this was either because there is poor binding of phleomycin to DNA with low AT contents or that phleomycin dissociates from DNA at higher temperatures. The former explanation has recently been excluded by Shive and Earhart (1976), who studied the effect of phleomycin on the T_ms of T4 DNA, nonglucosylated T4 DNA, and calf thymus DNA. The DNA samples were each dissolved in two different buffers; in one (SSC; Mandel and Marmur, 1968) each DNA had a T_m greater than 80° C and, in the other (0.2 SSC) the T_ms were reduced to approximately 70° C. In agreement with the findings of Falashi and Kornberg, phleomycin had no effect on the T_ms of DNA in SSC buffer, whereas in 0.2 SSC phleomycin caused an increase in T_m in each case. Clearly, it is the effect of temperature on the binding of phleomycin to DNA and not AT content which is the crucial factor in the failure of phleomycin to influence T_ms at high temperature. It should be noted, however, that elevated temperatures may have a structural effect on phleomycin. Friedman et al. (1974) reported that incubation of phleomycin for 1 h at 90° C reduces the effectiveness of the drug by 60%.

Pietsch and coworkers have provided evidence that phleomycin interacts with AT base pairs. Analysis of infrared spectra of phleomycin–DNA complexes indicated that phleomycin binds to a carbonyl group on DNA (Pietsch and Garrett, 1968). In vitro (Pietsch and Garrett, 1968) and in vivo (Pietsch and Corbett, 1968) data suggest that the binding site is the carbonyl oxygen at the 2 position of thymidine. Experiments in which Hg^{2+}, an ion which reacts preferentially with TT pairs (Yamane and Davidson, 1960), and phleomycin were used in competitive binding and growth inhibition studies yielded results indicating that Hg^{2+} and phleomycin attack the same sites in the cell. The phleomycin–DNA interaction is believed to involve hydrogen bonding. Further, electron micrographs show that nodules appear at irregular intervals on replicating *E. coli* chromosomes after phleomycin treatment. Pietsch and Garrett (1969a, 1969b) have interpreted these observations as suggesting that phleomycin receptors are homogeneous sequences of poly AT and that the nodules are clusters of phleomycin on DNA. The finding that phleomycin binds equally well to naked DNA and deoxyribonucleoprotein indicates that the drug is located within the minor groove while associated with DNA (Pietsch, 1969b). This location is also thought to explain the sparing effect on transcription exhibited by phleomycin.

Pietsch, on the basis of these extensive studies on the binding of phleomycin to DNA, has suggested several means by which phleomycin could act. (1) The presence of phleomycin clusters at homogeneous sequences of poly AT, which would normally be unstable regions of DNA, may stabilize these regions to such an extent that strand dissociation, and hence replication, is prevented (Pietsch and Garrett, 1969a). (2) Studies with molecular models suggest that, with phleomycin bound to T and in the minor groove, thymine would be sterically prevented from assuming the configuration necessary for it to perform its template function. If the receptor site for phleomycin were at the origin of replication, initiation would be prevented. If a replicating fork were to come upon a phleomycin cluster, it is suggested that DNA synthesis would be interrupted and that at least one of the new strands would be cleaved and degraded (PIETSCH, 1975).

B. Postulated Mechanisms

At this time there is no scheme which is able completely to explain the action of phleomycin. Any such mechanism will have to be consistent with the following observations: (1) phleomycin binds to DNA, (2) phleomycin has affinity for AT base pairs, (3) eukaryotic cells in different phases of the cell cycle and cultures of prokaryotic cells in different growth phases exhibit altered sensitivities, (4) phleomycin induces DNA breakdown, and (5) in at least some cases phleomycin damage is inhibited by the presence of energy poisons. Two rather general mechanisms for phleomycin action proposed by PIETSCH were presented earlier (see Sect. IV.A).

SLEIGH (1976), and SLEIGH and GRIGG (1977) have proposed a very plausible mechanism for the in vitro and in vivo DNA breakage brought about by low levels ($\leqq 2\ \mu$g/ml) of phleomycin. The proposed reaction mechanism, which does not involve nucleases but which does require the presence of sulfhydryl compounds, is presented immediately below and the supporting evidence is then detailed. Briefly, sulfhydryl compounds are oxidized to the free radical form $RS^{\cdot}$ by a reaction catalyzed by metal ions in the presence of oxygen. The free radical form reacts with phleomycin; phleomycin bound to DNA is activated and DNA damage occurs whereas the free radicals convert unbound phleomycin to an inactive form.

STERN et al. (1974) demonstrated that low concentrations of phleomycin can act in vitro on adenovirus type 2 DNA and on phage lambda DNA to produce single-strand breaks. [More precisely, these authors demonstrated that phleomycin acts either to cause nicks in DNA or the formation of alkali-labile sites, as DNA degradation was examined using alkaline sucrose gradients. The same caveat applies to the results of SLEIGH and GRIGG (see below).] A reducing agent was required for this reaction and 20 mM dithiothreitol was routinely used. Both native and denatured DNA were cleaved but no activity against RNA was detected. SLEIGH (1976) studied the in vitro breakage of phage T2 DNA by phleomycin and established that, in addition to sulfhydryl compounds, oxygen and metal ions are required as well. Oxidation of thiols is known to require oxygen and a metal ion catalyst (JOCELYN, 1972). [Neither STERN et al. (1974) nor SLEIGH (1976) detected any DNA breakage in the presence of reducing agent alone. This is an important control, as thiols such as 2-mercaptoethanol and dithiothreitol under certain conditions can cause single-strand scissions (LOWN and SIM, 1977).] The oxygen requirement was determined by noting the absence of DNA damage when the incubation was carried out under nitrogen. That catalysts such as Fe^{2+} or Cu^{2+} are involved was demonstrated by adding EDTA, which is known to abolish the catalytic oxidation of thiols; EDTA inhibited phleomycin-induced DNA damage. Similarly, DNA breakage was inhibited by removing Cu^{2+} from phleomycin with 8-hydroxyquinoline. The latter observation suggests that metal ions must be associated with phleomycin and hence in close proximity to DNA in order to bring about DNA damage.

That sulfhydryl-mediated DNA cleavage is a significant mechanism in vivo is suggested by the following results obtained with *E. coli* cells (SLEIGH and GRIGG, 1977). The effect of phleomycin on intact cells was inhibited by the chelating agents EDTA and 8-hydroxyquinoline, by the sulfhydryl blocking agent N-ethylmaleimide, and by the antioxidant KI. In spheroplasts, DNA degradation was augmented by the addition of dithiothreitol which increased the intracellular concentration of free thiol groups and, conversely, decreasing the intracellular concentration of sulfhydryl groups by genetic means reduced phleomycin-induced DNA breakage.

The observation that simultaneous addition of mercaptoethanol and phleomycin inhibits drug-induced killing (NAKAYAMA, 1975) and that dithiothreitol in combination with phleomycin decreases DNA damage in whole cells (SLEIGH and GRIGG, 1977) is apparently inconsistent with the postulated mechanism. However, if permeation of phleomycin into *E. coli* is a relatively slow process, the results can be explained by thiol inactivation of phleomycin before it can associate with DNA (SLEIGH and GRIGG, 1977).

Several reports (TAKITA, 1959; ISHIZUKA et al., 1966) have shown that the in vivo activity of phleomycin is not significantly altered by the removal of its copper. This can be reconciled with the free radical hypothesis by assuming that phleomycin rapidly regains a trace metal under the experimental conditions used. Another observation which requires explanation is evidence that phleomycin induced strand breakage is apparently energy-dependent. Thus, CCCP (*m*-chlorophenylcarbonylcyanide hydrazone) inhibited DNA cleavage in *Bacillus subtilis* (REITER et al., 1972) and *E. coli* (FARRELL and REITER, 1973). The latter observation was confirmed with sodium cyanide by NAKAYAMA (1975). Possibly, however, the energy poisons form complexes with Cu^{2+} and Fe^{2+} such that thiol oxidation is prevented; that cyanide can inhibit the thiol oxidation reaction is known (HARRISON, 1924). Lastly, inhibition of protein synthesis either by amino acid starvation or chloramphenicol addition has been shown to suppress both phleomycin-induced killing and strand breakage (NAKAYAMA, 1975). This phenomenon could be related to the observation that stationary-phase cells are relatively resistant to phleomycin. The suggestion (see Sect. III) that DNA is in a different, more phleomycin resistant, conformation under these nonreplicating conditions may be responsible for this finding.

A second mechanism for phleomycin-induced chromosome breakage has been postulated to operate at high ($\geqq 20\ \mu g/ml$) phleomycin concentrations. In this scheme, phleomycin is believed to produce local sites of denaturation in DNA which are subsequently acted on by endonucleases specific for single-stranded regions. Evidence for this second mechanism comes from a variety of approaches. Thus, at high phleomycin concentrations DNA cleavage occurs in glutathione-deficient cells and in the presence of KI (SLEIGH and GRIGG,

1977). Initial evidence for a phleomycin-induced enzymic degradation of DNA mechanism was the finding that expression of the bactericidal effects of phleomycin in *E. coli* B was dependent on the presence of a functional excision repair system (GRIGG, 1969). Correspondingly, phleomycin-resistant mutants were all found to be UV sensitive. In a subsequent study (GRIGG, 1970) degradation of the DNA of *E. coli* B cells lacking an excision endonuclease was indistinguishable from that of wild-type *E. coli* B when caffeine was added with phleomycin. In *E. coli* K-12 NAKAYAMA (1975) determined that phleomycin-induced DNA breakage occurred whether or not the strains were excision defective (Uvr) or defective in recombinational repair (Rec). The only difference found was in cell survival, where Rec^+ strains were observed to be more resistant to phleomycin than Rec^- strains. Endonuclease I has been eliminated as being responsible for phleomycin-induced DNA damage (SHIVE and EARHART, 1975). SLEIGH and GRIGG (1974) demonstrated that both phleomycin and caffeine, singly or together, can sufficiently denature DNA in vitro to permit a single-strand specific endonuclease from *Neurospora crassa* to act.

On the basis of available evidence it seems premature to conclude that two distinct mechanisms for phleomycin-induced DNA damage exist. In fact, the distinction between the nonenzymic and enzymic mechanisms may be artificial. If, for instance, phleomycin bound to DNA acted to increase the rate at which free bases are lost from DNA, i.e., in the manner of alkylating agents, the single-strand breaks observed in in vitro experiments would occur as a result of exposure to alkaline conditions (LINDAHL and LJUNGQUIST, 1975). In fact, ROSS and MOSES (personal communication) have evidence that bleomycin treatment produces alkali-labile sites, not single-strand breaks. In vivo the apurinic sites would be acted on by endonucleases, such as endonuclease IV of *E. coli* (LJUNGQUIST, 1977), which specifically catalyze the formation of single-strand breaks at apurinic and apyrimidic sites in DNA. Such enzymes have been found in all cell types investigated. It could be postulated that in the presence of phleomycin repair of apurinic sites, the first step of which is presumably carried out by endonuclease IV-like enzymes, is inhibited and/or the number of such sites formed overwhelms the rate at which subsequent steps in repair can occur.

References [1]

Angyal, A.M., Grigg, G.W., Badger, R.J., Brown, D.J., Lister, J.H.: Purines as amplifiers of the antibiotic activity of phleomycin against *Escherichia coli* B. J. Gen. Microbiol. *85*, 163–168 (1974)

Argoudelis, A.D., Bergey, M.E., Pyke, T.R.: Zorbamycin and related antibiotics. I. Production, isolation, and characterization. J. Antibiot. *24*, 543–557 (1971)

Bhushan, K., Brown, D.J., Lister, J.H., Stephanson, L.G., Yoneda, F.: Purine studies. XVII. The synthesis of 2-substituted 6,9-di-and 6, 8, 9-tri-methylpurines as amplifiers of phleomycin. Aust. J. Chem. *28*, 2553–2559 (1975)

Bradner, W.T., Pindell, H.M.: Antitumour properties of phleomycin. Nature (London) *196*, 682–683 (1962)

1 The literature review for this article was completed in Sept. 1977.

Brown, D.J., Stephanson, L.G.: Purine studies. XIII. The metabolism of 2,9-dimethyl-8-methylthiopurine and 2-carbamoylmethylthio-6,9-dimethylpurine in mice. Aust. J. Chem. *27*, 1371–1375 (1974)

Brown, D.J., Stephanson, L.G.: Purine studies. XIX. Rodential metabolism of 2-(6′,8′,9′-trimethylpurin-2′-ylthio) propionamide and related purines. Aust. J. Chem. *29*, 1031–1037 (1976)

Brown, D.J., Dunlap, W.C., Grigg, G.W., Kelly, J.: Thiazolo[5,4-*d*] pyrimidine derivatives as amplifiers of phleomycin against *E. coli*. Aust. J. Chem. *30*, 1775–1783 (1977)

Decad, G.M., Nikaido, H.: Outer membrane of gram-negative bacteria. XII. Molecular sieving function of cell wall. J. Bacteriol. *128*, 325–336 (1976)

Djordjevic, B., Kim, J.: Lethal effects of phleomycin in different stages of the division cycle of HeLa cells. Cancer Res. *27*, 2255–2260 (1967)

Falaschi, A., Kornberg, A.: Phleomycin, an inhibitor of DNA polymerase. Fed. Proc. *23*, 940–945 (1964)

Farrell, L.D., Reiter, H.: Phleomycin-stimulated degradation of deoxyribonucleic acid in *Escherichia coli*. Antimicrob. Agents Chemother. *4*, 320–326 (1973)

Farrell, L.D., Reiter, H.: Phleomycin-stimulated solubilization of deoxyribonucleic acid in *Escherichia coli*. II. Inhibition of solubilization by bacteriophage T4. Can J. Microbiol. *22*, 645–653 (1976)

Friedman, R.M., Stern, R., Rose, J.A.: Phleomycin stimulation of thymidine triphosphate incorporation by animal cell nuclei. J. Natl. Cancer Inst. *52*, 693–697 (1974)

Grigg, G.W.: Induction of DNA breakdown and death in *Escherichia coli* by phleomycin. Its association with dark repair processes. Mol. Gen. Genet. *104*, 1–11 (1969)

Grigg, G.W.: Amplification of phleomycin induced death and DNA breakdown by caffeine in *Escherichia coli*. Mol. Gen. Genet. *107*, 162–172 (1970)

Grigg, G.W., Edwards, M.J., Brown, D.J.: Effects of coumarin, thiopurines, and pyronin Y on amplification of phleomycin-induced death and deoxyribonucleic acid breakdown in *Escherichia coli*. J. Bacteriol. *107*, 599–609 (1971)

Grigg, G.W., Gero, A.M., Hughes, J.M., Sasse, W.H.F., Bliese, M., Hart, N.K., Johansen, O., Kissane, P.: Amplifications of phleomycin and bleomycin-induced antibiotic activity in *Escherichia coli* by aromatic cationic compounds. J. Antibiot. *30*, 870–878 (1977)

Harrison, D.G.: CXXXIV. The catalytic action of traces of iron on the oxidation of cysteine and glutathione. Biochem. J. *18*, 1009–1022 (1924)

Hecht, T.T., Summers, D.F.: The effect of phleomycin on poliovirus RNA replication. Virology *40*, 441–447 (1970)

Hotta, Y., Stern, H.: The action of phleomycin on meiotic cells. Cancer Res. *29*, 1699–1703 (1969)

Ikekawa, T., Iwami, F., Hiranka, H., Umezawa, H.: Separation of phleomycin components and their properties. J. Antibiot. *17A*, 194–199 (1964)

Ishizuka, M., Takayama, H., Takeuchi, T., Umezawa, H.: Studies on antitumor activity, antimicrobial activity and toxicity of phleomycin. J. Antibiot. *19A*, 260–271 (1966)

Ishizuka, M., Takayama, H., Takeuchi, T., Umezawa, H.: Activity and toxicity of bleomycin. J. Antibiot. *20A*, 15–24 (1967)

Ito, Y., Ohashi, Y., Egawa, Y., Yamaguchi, T., Furumai, T., Enomoto, K., Okuda, T.: Antibiotic YA 56, a new family of phleomycin-bleomycin group antibiotics. J. Antibiot. *24*, 727–731 (1971)

Iwata, A., Consigli, R.A.: Effect of phleomycin on polyoma virus synthesis in mouse embryo cells. J. Virol. *7*, 29–40 (1971)

Jacobs, N.F., Neu, R.L., Gardner, L.I.: Phleomycin-induced mitotic inhibition and chromosomal abnormalities in cultured human leucocytes. Mutat. Res. *7*, 251–253 (1969)

Jocelyn, P.C.: Biochemistry of the SH group. London: Academic Press Inc. 1972

Kajiwara, K., Kim, U., Mueller, G.: Phleomycin, an inhibitor of replication of HeLa cells. Cancer Res. *26*, 233–236 (1966)

Kersten, H., Kersten, W.: Inhibitors of nucleic acid synthesis. Berlin, Heidelberg, New York: Springer 1974

Kihlman, B.A., Odmark, G., Hartley, B.: Studies on the effects of phleomycin on chromosome structure and nucleic acid synthesis in *Vicia faba*. Mutat. Res. *4*, 783–790 (1967)

Kleijer, W.J., Hoeksema, J.I., Sluyter, M.L., Bootsma, D.: Effects of inhibitors on repair of DNA in normal human and xeroderma pigmentosum cells after exposure to X-rays and ultraviolet irradiation. Mutat. Res. *17*, 385–394 (1973)

Koch, G.: Differential effect of phleomycin on the infectivity of poliovirus and poliovirus-induced ribonucleic acids. J. Virol. *8*, 20–34 (1971)
Krueger, W.C., Pschigoda, L.M., Reusser, F.: Interactions of DNA with zorbamycin, phleomycin, and bleomycin; ultraviolet absorption and circular dichroism measurements. J. Antibiot. *26*, 424–428 (1973)
Lindahl, T., Ljungquist, S.: Apurinic and apyrimidinic sites in DNA. In: Molecular mechanisms for repair of DNA, Part A. Hanawalt, P.C., Setlow, R.B., (eds.), pp. 31–38. New York: Plenum Press 1975
Ljungquist, S.: A new endonuclease from *Escherichia coli* acting at apurinic sites in DNA. J. Biol. Chem. *252*, 2808–2814 (1977)
Lown, J.W., Sim, S-K.: The mechanism of the bleomycin-induced cleavage of DNA. Biochem. Biophys. Res. Commun. *77*, 1150–1157 (1977)
Maeda, K.: Streptomyces products inhibiting mycobacteria. New York: John Wiley and Sons Inc. 1965
Maeda, K., Kosaka, H., Yagishita, K., Umezawa, H.: A new antibiotic, phleomycin. J. Antibiot. *9A*, 82–85 (1956)
Mandel, M., Marmur, J.: Use of ultraviolet temperature profile for determining the guanine plus cytosine content of DNA. In: Methods in enzymology. Grossman, L.D, Moldave, K., (eds.), Vol. 12b, pp. 195–206. New York: Academic Press Inc. 1968
Mathews, C.K.: Bacteriophage biochemistry. New York: Van Nostrand Reinhold Co. 1971
Mattingly, E.: Induction of chromosome and chromatid-type aberrations by phleomycin. Mutat. Res. *4*, 51–57 (1967)
McIntosh, M.A., Earhart, C.F.: Effect of ribonuclease on the association of deoxyribonucleic acid with the membrane in *Escherichia coli*. J. Bacteriol. *122*, 592–598 (1975)
Nagai, K., Yamaki, H., Suzuki, H., Tanaka, N., Umezawa, H.: The combined effects of bleomycin and sulfhydryl compounds on the thermal denaturation of DNA. Biochem. Biophys. Acta *179*, 165–171 (1969)
Nakayama, H.: Phleomycin-induced lethality and DNA degradation in *Escherichia coli* K12. Mutat. Res. *29*, 21–33 (1975)
Ohashi, Y., Abe, H., Kawabe, J., Ito, Y.: The constitutional amine of antibiotic YA-56. Agric. Biol. Chem. *37*, 2387–2391 (1973)
Pietsch, P.: Phleomycin: biological and chemical variations in different batches. Microbios *1*, 387–392 (1969a)
Pietsch, P.: Structural events in DNA in transcription and replication: the influence of histones on *in vitro* reactions of actinomycin-D and phleomycin-909. Cytobios *4*, 375–391 (1969b)
Pietsch, P.: Biopolymers in drug technology: the use of DNA in purifying phleomycin. Biotechnol. Bioeng. *15*, 1039–1044 (1973)
Pietsch, P.: Phleomycin and bleomycin. In: Handbook of experimental pharmacology, Part 2. Sartorelli, A.C., Johns, D.G., (eds.), Vol. 38, pp. 850–876. Berlin, Heidelberg, New York: Springer 1975
Pietsch, P., Clapper, G.: Receptivity of DNA to phleomycin. Cytobios *1*, 145–152 (1969)
Pietsch, P., Corbett, C.: Competitive effects of phleomycin and mercuric chloride in vivo. Nature (London) *219*, 933–934 (1968)
Pietsch, P., Eng, R.: Phleomycin: enhancement of properties by treatment with acid. Microbios *1*, 213–223 (1969)
Pietsch, P., Garrett, H.: Primary site of reaction in the in vitro complex of phleomycin in DNA. Nature (London) *219*, 488–489 (1968)
Pietsch, P., Garrett, H.: Phleomycin: evidence of *in vivo* binding to DNA. Cytobios *1A*, 7–15 (1969a)
Pietsch, P., Garrett, H.: Phleomycin-induced changes in the ultrastructure of DNA. Biophys. J. *9A*, 126 (1969b)
Pietsch, P., Corbett, C., Briden, D.W., Jewett, G.: Diffusability of phleomycin studied by means of neutron activation analysis. Physiol. Chem. Phys. *1*, 232–236 (1969)
Pitts, J.D., Sinsheimer, R.L.: Effects of phleomycin upon replication of bacteriophage ϕX174. J. Mol. Biol. *15*, 676–680 (1965)
Post, L., Price, A.R.: Inhibition of bacteriophage PBS2 replication in *Bacillus subtilis* by phleomycin. J. Virol. *15*, 363–371 (1975)

Reiter, H., Milewskiy, M., Kelley, P.: Mode of action of phleomycin on *B. subtilis*. J. Bacteriol. *111*, 586–592 (1972)

Ryder, O.A., Smith, D.W.: Isolation of membrane-associated folded chromosomes from *Escherichia coli*: effect of protein synthesis inhibition. J. Bacteriol. *120*, 1356–1363 (1971)

Shive, K., Earhart, C.: Phleomycin-induced solubilization of deoxyribonucleic acid in uninfected and T bacteriophage-infected *Escherichia coli* B. Antimicrob. Agents Chemother. *10*, 150–156 (1976)

Sleigh, M.J.: The mechanism of DNA breakage by phleomycin *in vitro*. Nucl. Acids Res. *3*, 891–901 (1976)

Sleigh, M.J., Grigg, G.W.: Induction of local denaturation in DNA *in vitro* by phleomycin and caffeine. FEBS Lett. *39*, 35–38 (1974)

Sleigh, M.J., Grigg, G.W.: The mechanism of sensitivity to phleomycin in growing *Escherichia coli* cells. Biochem. J. *155*, 87–99 (1976)

Sleigh, M.J., Grigg, G.W.: Sulphydryl-mediated DNA breakage by phleomycin in *Escherichia coli*. Mutat. Res. *42*, 181–189 (1977)

Stern, R., Rose, J.A., Friedman, R.M.: Phleomycin-induced cleavage of deoxyribonucleic acid. Biochemistry *13*, 307–312 (1974)

Takasawa, S., Kawamoto, I., Okachi, R., Kohakura, M., Yahashi, R., Nara, T.: A new antibiotic victomycin (XK 49-1-B-2). II. Isolation, purification and physiochemical and biological properties. J. Antibiot. *28A*, 366–371 (1975a)

Takasawa, S., Kawamoto, I., Sato, S., Yahashi, R., Okachi, R., Yamamoto, M., Sato, T., Nara, T.: Platomycins A and B. II. Physiochemical properties. J. Antibiot. *28A*, 662–667 (1975b)

Takita, T.: Studies on purification and properties of phleomycin. J. Antibiot. *12A*, 285–289 (1959)

Tanaka, N., Yamaguchi, H., Umezawa, H.: Mechanism of action of phleomycin, a tumour-inhibitory antibiotic. Biochem. Biophys. Res. Commun. *10*, 171–174 (1963)

Tevethia, S.S., Rapp, F.: The effect of phleomycin on the replication of papovavirus SV40 and other DNA viruses in simian cells. Cancer Res. *29*, 912–917 (1969)

Umezawa, H.: Bleomycin. In: Antibiotics. Corcoran, J., Hahn, F., (eds.), Vol. III, pp. 21–33. New York: Springer 1975

Umezawa, H., Maeda, K., Takeuchi, T., Okami, Y.: New antibiotics, bleomycin A and B. J. Antibiot. *19A*, 200–209 (1966)

Watanabe, M., August, J.T.: Replication of RNA bacteriophage R23. II. Inhibition of phage-specific RNA synthesis by phleomycin. J. Mol. Biol. *33*, 21–33 (1968)

Worcel, A., Burgi, E.: Properties of a membrane-attached form of the folded chromosome of *Escherichia coli*. J. Mol. Biol. *82*, 91–105 (1974)

Yamane, T., Davidson, N.: On the complexing of deoxyribonucleic acid (DNA) by mercuric ion. J. Am. Chem. Soc. *83*, 2599–2607 (1960)

Polyene Antibiotics: Nystatin, Amphotericin B, and Filipin

R.W. HOLZ

I. Introduction

The polyene antibiotics comprise a class of molecules that are toxic to fungi but not to bacteria. They are produced by the bacteria *Streptomyces*. Although there are many polyene antibiotics (KINSKY, 1967) only three are used clinically to treat fungal infections – nystatin, amphotericin B, and candicidin. All three are used in the treatment of topical infections, while only amphotericin B is used against systemic infections. Nystatin and amphotericin B are most frequently used clinically, and have been extensively studied experimentally. This review will focus mainly on these two polyene antibiotics with special emphasis given to their mechanism of action. Filipin, another well-studied polyene antibiotic will also be discussed. Reviews about the polyene antibiotics are available concerning general information (LAMPEN, 1966; KINSKY, 1967; KINSKY, 1970; HAMILTON-MILLER, 1973) and clinical use and toxicity (BENNETT, 1974, 1976; APPEL and NEU, 1977).

II. Chemical Structure

The polyene antibiotics have molecular weights of approximately 1,000. They possess large lactone rings which contain a nonpolar transconjugated double bond system and a polar polyhydroxylic portion. The antibiotics differ in: (1) the size of the ring, (2) the number of conjugated double bonds, and (3) the number and type of substituents attached to the ring (HAMILTON-MILLER, 1973).

MECHLINSKI and SCHAFFNER (1974) have shown with high speed liquid chromatography that nystatin consists of at least three components; the major component is a tetraene. The two minor components consist of another tetraene and a heptaene and represent over 15% of the polyene present. Amphotericin B, on the other hand, is essentially one single compound with only trace amounts of two minor components. It is the only polyene antibiotic whose absolute structure has been determined by X-ray crystallography (MECHLINSKI and SCHAFFNER, 1970). Amphotericin B contains a heptaene unit, many hydroxyls,

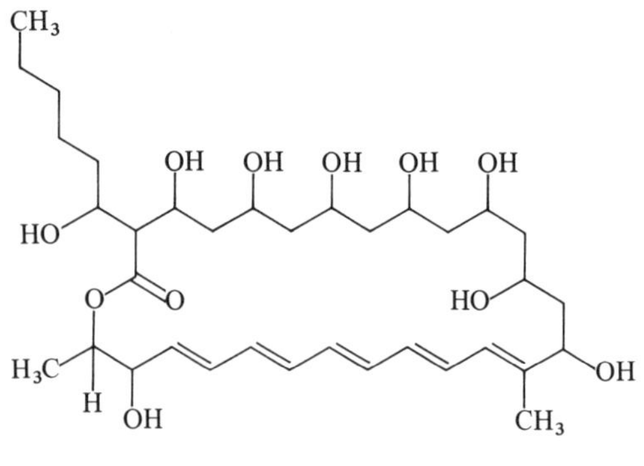

Filipin, $C_{35}H_{58}O_{11}$

a

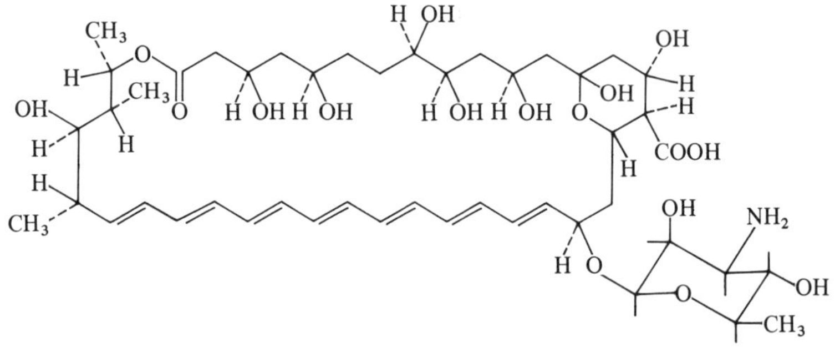

Amphotericin B, $C_{47}H_{73}O_{17}N$

b

Fig. 1a and b. Chemical structures of **a** filipin III and **b** amphotericin B. The structure of filipin III was obtained by chemical means (PANDEY and RINEHART, 1970). The structure of amphotericin B was determined by X-ray crystallography (MECHLINSKI and SCHAFFNER, 1970). Nystatin differs from amphotericin B in that it contains a tetraene and diene in place of the heptaene; in other respects the molecules are very similar (CHONG and RICKARDS, 1970)

a carboxyl group, and an amino sugar (Fig. 1). At neutral pH, amphotericin B is a zwitterion. It is poorly soluble in both water and strongly nonpolar solvents. Because of its amphipathic nature, one suspects that it would interact at a water–lipid interface.

At the time that the structure of nystatin was determined (CHONG and RICKARDS, 1970), the heterogeneity of the preparation was unknown. Nonetheless, a structure was assigned that was very similar to that of amphotericin B except that it contained a tetraene and a diene unit. The solubility characteristics of the nystatin mixture are similar to those of amphotericin B (DUTCHER et al., 1955).

Filipin is a mixture of four–five species similar in structure (PANDEY and RINEHART, 1970). They are all pentaenes and none contain the polar carboxyl group or amino sugar that is found in amphotericin B and nystatin. Filipin III constitutes 53% of the filipin complex and is shown in Fig. 1.

It must be remembered in this review that most of the effects attributed to nystatin and filipin are actually being attributed to mixtures. A further discussion of the structure of these molecules will be deferred until the mechanism of action is considered below.

III. Biologic Effects and the Interaction with Membrane Sterol

It was early noted that the polyene antibiotics were toxic to fungi but not to bacteria (HAZAN and BROWN, 1951). It took many years, however, before the mechanism underlying this specificity was understood. KINSKY (1961) showed that the polyenes alter membrane permeability in *Neurospora crassa*. He observed that the polyenes caused a rapid fall in mycelial dry weight which was accompanied by the release of cellular components (inorganic salts, amino acids, sugars, nucleotides) into the growth medium. The same polyene concentration that caused this leakage in whole cells (approximately 10^{-6} M) caused shrinkage of protoplasts in isotonic sucrose and lysis in isotonic saline. These observations together with the inability to demonstrate any effect on known enzyme systems in vitro (LAMPEN, 1966) strongly suggested that the primary action of the polyenes was to increase cell membrane permeability.

The striking biologic specificity of action of the polyene antibiotics is based upon a requirement for sterol in the membrane (see LAMPEN, 1966). The polyene antibiotics are lethal to fungi, higher algae, flatworms, snails, and they lyse red blood cells in isotonic saline; the membranes of all these organisms or cells contain sterol. The polyenes have no effect on bacteria and blue-green algae, both of which are sterol-free. Furthermore, sterol added to the medium protects the former group from the harmful action of the polyene antibiotics (GOTTLIEB et al., 1958). Direct evidence for a sterol requirement was obtained by WEBER and KINSKY (1965) in their study of the sensitivity of *Acholeplasma laidlawii* to filipin. *Acholeplasma*, although it does not synthesize sterol, is able to incorporate sterol into the membrane if sterol is present in the growth medium. It was found that filipin inhibited growth and caused lysis of cells grown in the presence of cholesterol, but had no effect on cells grown in its absence. Hence, sterol was necessary for polyene toxicity.

The effects of a number of polyene antibiotics were investigated by DEKRUIJFF et al. (1974a, b). Instead of measuring toxicity, they measured specific permeability increases of the membranes of *Acholeplasma* induced by the antibiotics. Permeability increases were induced by filipin, nystatin and amphotericin B only if sterol was present in the membrane. The identity of the sterol was important, with at least two structural requirements being evident: (1) a 3β-hydroxyl group was required. Cholesterol and cholestanol, each with a 3β-hydroxyl group, were active whereas epicholesterol and epicholestanol, each with a 3α-hydroxyl group, were inactive; (2) the steroid nucleus must be planar. Coprostanol with a bent (cis) A/B ring was inactive whereas the active sterols all had coplanar rings. With the same sterols, results on liposomes (see below) were virtually identical with those on *Acholeplasma* (DEKRUIJFF et al., 1974a, b). In addition, steroids that could not be investigated with *Acholeplasma* could be investigated with liposomes. A keto group cannot substitute for the 3β-hydroxyl (cholestane-4-6-diene-3-one and cholesten-3-one were ineffective). Absence of a hydrocarbon tail at C-17 partially reduces the effects.

In two other model membrane systems, monolayers (DEMEL et al., 1965) and planar bilayer membranes (VAN ZUTPHEN et al., 1966; ANDREOLI and MONAHAN, 1968; CASS et al., 1970) the sterol requirement for polyene antibiotic interaction has also been demonstrated.

The universality of the sterol requirement is impressive.[1] The sensitivity of organisms and cells to the polyenes follows the phylogenetic occurrence of sterol in the membrane. In addition, the sensitivity to the polyene antibiotics of *Acholeplasma* and model membrane systems where lipid composition can be controlled are directly dependent upon the presence of sterol. Hence, on the strength of all these investigations, one concludes that the *biologic specificity of polyene antibiotic action is based upon the presence of membrane-bound sterol.* This fact has obvious implications for the clinical effectiveness and toxicity of the polyene antibiotics. These considerations will be discussed below.

IV. The Polyene Antibiotic–Sterol Interaction: Spectroscopic and Calorimetric Studies

The demonstration of a sterol requirement for the action of the polyene antibiotics and the subsequent demonstration that nystatin and amphotericin B create molecular size pores as a result of this interaction (see below) prompted a number of spectroscopic studies of the interaction between the polyene antibiotics and sterol. Most of these studies take advantage of the strong chromophore of the extended conjugated double bond system of the polyenes. Ultraviolet, fluorescent and Raman spectroscopy have been used.

Filipin, amphotericin B, and nystatin all show similar UV spectroscopic changes induced by *free cholesterol* dispersed in aqueous solution (NORMAN et al., 1972a, b). The absorption maxima characteristic of the polyenic group change in relative intensity but not in energy (wavelength). This suggests that there is a relatively weak interaction with perhaps some conformational restriction of the polyenic moiety. The steroid structural requirements for interaction

1 There is a report (HSUCHEN and FEINGOLD, 1973) that liposomes composed of lecithin with saturated hydrocarbon chains (dipalmitoyl and distearoyl lecithins) are sensitive to nystatin and amphotericin B and that cholesterol decreases this sensitivity. The lipids were in the gel state (below the transition temperature) and it was suggested that the rigidity of the hydrocarbon tails was the important characteristic which allowed interaction with the antibiotics. However, selective permeability changes characteristic of the action of nystatin and amphotericin B (see Sect. V) were not demonstrated. It is possible that detergent effects of the polyene antibiotics may explain the findings. More information concerning the interaction of the polyene antibiotics with saturated phospholipids is necessary to evaluate these effects.

with filipin were studied in detail and found to be minimal. Filipin interacts with steroids containing an ester linkage, a 3-keto, or 3α-hydroxyl group as well as with steroids containing a 3β-hydroxyl group. Planarity of the steroid nucleus and presence of a C-17 side chain are also not required. However, there is some specificity since interactions do not occur with lecithin, cetyl alcohol or with molecules with a ruptured steroid nucleus. The interaction appears to be hydrophobic and not dependent upon hydrogen bond formation, since salts and urea have little effect whereas detergents and low polarity solvents prevent the interaction. There is no evidence for covalent bond formation.

When steroid is incorporated into liposomes, the structural requirements become much more stringent and closely resemble those necessary for the biologic and physiologic actions of the polyenes. For interaction with filipin the 3β-hydroxyl and planar steroid nucleus are required. The interaction is weakened if the C-17 side chain is absent. Amphotericin B preferentially interacted with liposomes containing 3β-hydroxyl, planar sterols although significant but smaller interactions were obtained with 3α-hydroxy, 3-keto, esterified, and nonplanar steroids. In addition, cetyl alcohol gave significant interaction. Characteristic changes in the UV spectrum also occur when filipin or amphotericin B interact with red blood cells or with *Acholeplasma laidlawii* containing cholesterol. Changes do not occur if *Acholeplasma laidlawii* does not contain sterol in the membrane. Nystatin did not show U.V. spectral evidence for interaction with lecithin-cholesterol liposomes or with cholesterol-containing membranes of *Acholeplasma laidlawii*.

The fluorescence of filipin, amphotericin B, and nystatin changes in the presence of sterol dispersions (SCHROEDER et al., 1971; BITTMAN and FISCHKOFF, 1972). Excitation spectrums of filipin and nystatin are altered in intensity but not in wavelength. The partial quantum efficiency of the filipin fluorescence decreases (SCHROEDER et al., 1971). Increases in fluorescence polarization of filipin and amphotericin B (BITTMAN and FISCHKOFF, 1972) suggest that the antibiotic molecules are bound. Methanol reverses the fluorescence polarization of filipin induced by cholesterol, which is further evidence for a hydrophobic interaction.

Raman spectroscopy also demonstrates polyene antibiotic–sterol interaction (BUNOW and LEVIN, 1977). Both dimyristoyl lecithin and dimyristoyl lecithin–cholesterol single walled vesicles have a gel to liquid crystalline phase transition at 24° C. The intensity of the C=C stretching mode emission of amphotericin B decreases four fold over the transition range only if cholesterol is present. Cholesterol presumably allows amphotericin B to penetrate into the hydrocarbon interior of the bilayer.

A potentially powerful method has been devised to determine the orientation of amphotericin B in the membrane. Polarized absorption spectrums have been obtained of amphotericin B interacting with monolayers composed of pure egg lecithin, pure cholesterol, and equimolar egg lecithin and cholesterol. There are cholesterol-dependent shifts of the positions and intensities of specific absorption peaks. The data are consistent with a cholesterol-dependent insertion into the monolayer of part of the amphotericin B molecule with its long axis (parallel with the polyene moiety) perpendicular to the plane of the monolayer.

In summary, the spectroscopic data directly demonstrate interaction of filipin, amphotericin B, and nystatin with sterol. Although the correlations are generally good, there are some discrepancies between the spectroscopic data and the physiologic effects. For example, although there is spectroscopic evidence for nystatin interaction with cholesterol dispersions, there was a lack of UV spectroscopic evidence for cholesterol-dependent nystatin interaction with liposomes (see above). In contrast, nystatin did induce cholesterol-dependent increases in permeability of liposomes and other membrane systems (DEKRUIJFF et al., 1974a, b). In addition, nystatin binds preferentially to cholesterol-containing rather than cholesterol-free membranes from *Acholeplasma laidlawii*. Thus, spectroscopy may sometimes not monitor the physiologically relevant interaction of the antibiotics with the membrane.

Differential scanning calorimetry has illuminated some aspects of the polyene antibiotic interaction with cholesterol-containing membranes (DEKRUIJFF et al., 1974a, b). The energy content of the transition from the liquid-crystalline to the gel state of dielaidoyl lecithin is reduced by cholesterol. This is qualitatively explained as resulting from a liquifying effect of cholesterol on the gel state. Filipin, amphotericin B, and nystatin partially or completely reverse this decrease in energy content of the transition. They have no effect on the transition energy in the absence of sterol. Therefore, filipin, amphotericin B, and nystatin appear to have a common mode of action to reduce the cholesterol interaction with lecithin.

The greater structural requirements of the steroid for interaction with the polyenes in lecithin–cholesterol liposomes compared to pure steroid dispersions suggest that an important factor for the membrane effects of the polyene antibiotics is the bilayer configuration. This undoubtedly adds steric restrictions to the interaction. It creates requirements for a 3β-hydroxyl group, a planar steroid nucleus, and a C–17 side chain to maximize the polyenes antibiotic–sterol interaction. These same structural characteristics maximize sterol–lecithin interaction in model membranes (DEMEL et al., 1972a, b; DEKRUYFF et al., 1972). Thus, the polyene–sterol interaction has characteristics in common with the lecithin–sterol interaction. The effect of the polyene antibiotics to reverse the sterol effect on the transition temperature of lecithin suggests, in addition, that there is competition between the polyene antibiotics and the phospholipid for sterol.

V. Mechanism of Action

Because the biologic evidence strongly suggested that the site of action of the polyene antibiotics was the plasma membrane, the mechanism of action of the polyenes has been extensively investigated in model membrane systems. These studies will be considered below. *The data strongly suggest that nystatin and amphotericin B interact with sterol to create molecular-size aqueous channels in membranes.*

A. Monolayer and Liposome Studies

Filipin and nystatin in subphase concentrations of approximately 10^{-8}M are able to penetrate monolayers of pure cholesterol above the collapse presence of monolayers of the antibiotics alone. They are unable to penetrate pure phospholipid monolayers (DEMEL et al., 1965).

Aqueous phospholipid dispersions form closed concentric lamellar structures, called liposomes, with aqueous phases between the lamellas. KINSKY et al. (1968) found that filipin (10^{-5}M) released glucose from the aqueous phases of cholesterol containing liposomes; the greater the amount of cholesterol present in the liposomes the greater the sensitivity to filipin. Amphotericin B and nystatin also showed preferential interaction with cholesterol containing liposomes (WEISSMAN and SESSA, 1967; KINSKY et al., 1968). Subsequent liposome studies by DEKRUIJFF et al. (1974a) demonstrated that both nystatin and amphotericin B caused a selective permeability change in cholesterol-containing liposomes with the membranes becoming more permeant to K^+ than to glucose. The permeability characteristics of amphotericin B-treated liposomes were more fully investigated; K^+, Cl^-, and erythritol were very permeant whereas glucose and Mg^{2+} were relatively impermeant. Filipin, on the other hand, released K^+ and glucose at comparable rates and, therefore, did not appear to cause a selective permeability increase. There is considerable evidence from a variety of sources (CASS et al., 1970; DEKRUIJFF et al., 1974a) that filipin interacts with sterol containing membranes grossly to alter the membrane. This action is distinct from the more subtle effects of nystatin and amphotericin B on sterol-containing membranes to cause selective permeability increases.

KINSKY et al. (1966) demonstrated with negative-staining electron microscopy that filipin creates 125 Å diameter pits in cholesterol-containing liposomes and red blood cell membranes but not in cholesterol-free liposomes. Subsequent freeze-etch electron microscopy showed that these pits do not traverse the membrane and, therefore, are not aqueous pores (VERKLEIJ et al., 1973; TILLACK and KINSKY, 1973); instead, they are probably filipin–cholesterol complexes in the hydrocarbon interior of the bilayer (DEKRUIJFF and DEMEL, 1974).

B. Studies on Planar Bilayer Membranes

The planar bilayer membrane (MUELLER and RUDIN, 1969; MONTAL and MUELLER, 1972) is the lipid bilayer incarnate of both the Davson–Danielli bimolecular leaflet model and the more current, fluid mosaic model of the plasma membrane. The membrane can be made of phospholipids and sterol and has a thickness comparable to that of biological membranes (approximately 50 Å). Unmodified, it is a homogeneous structure with the properties that one would predict for a 50 Å low-dielectric hydrocarbon layer. It is highly permeable to lipophilic solutes, moderately permeable to water, and virtually impermeable to hydrophilic solutes and ions (MUELLER and RUDIN, 1969). Because electric, tracer permeability, and osmotic permeability measurements can be readily performed on these membranes, they are powerful tools for investigating the mechanism of action of membrane active substances. They have been extremely useful in investigating the mechanism of action of nystatin and amphotericin B. The studies show that nystatin and amphotericin B act almost identically to create molecular size aqueous channels in membranes.

1. Electrical Effects

Both nystatin and amphotericin B cause large conductance increases when added to one or both sides of a bilayer membrane. The conductance is enormously potentiated when added to both sides of the membrane. The one-sided effects that are especially pertinent to the biologic action of the antibiotics will be considered first.

MARTY and FINKELSTEIN (1975) found that nystatin at concentrations that are effective on biologic membranes (5–100 μg/ml) caused the conductance to increase several orders of magnitude from 10^{-8} to $10^{-4} \Omega^{-1}$ cm^{-2}. The conductance increased supralinearly with antibiotic concentration. Quantitatively the effects were extremely variable. Similar concentrations of nystatin on different membranes could give conductances that varied over 100-fold. The conductances were strongly but not completely cation selective (50 mV for a tenfold KCl activity gradient). The presence of ergosterol in the membrane but not of cholesterol greatly enhanced the one-sided effects. Amphotericin B on one side of a cholesterol-containing membrane also caused cation selective conductance increases.

With nystatin or amphotericin B on both sides of the membrane, the concentration necessary to achieve a given conductance was $^1/_{10}$ to $^1/_{1,000}$ of that necessary to achieve the same conductance with the antibiotic on only one side of the membrane (MARTY and FINKELSTEIN, 1975). The conductance with the antibiotics on both sides of the membrane was strongly but not completely *anion* selective (approximately 50 mV for a tenfold KCl activity gradient), in contrast to the *cation* selectivity induced by the one-sided effects. Although there may be a small conductance increase with nystatin or amphotericin B on both sides without sterol in the membrane, it is insignificant compared to the large conductance increase obtained with either cholesterol or ergosterol present. Ergosterol-containing membranes were more sensitive than cholesterol-containing membranes to the two-sided effects of nystatin and amphotericin B.

With the antibiotics on both sides of the membrane the conductances were reproducible and could increase from $10^{-8} \Omega^{-1}$ cm^{-2} (unmodified membrane) to larger than $10^{-2} \Omega^{-1}$ cm^{-2} in 0.1 M NaCl (CASS et al., 1970). The conductance was proportional to the antibiotic concentration (when equal on both sides of the membrane) raised to the fourth to twelfth power. The exact power depended upon the lipid. When the antibiotic was removed from the aqueous phase, the conductance fell to that of the unmodified membrane. Hence, the effects are reversible.

Thus, with nystatin or amphotericin B on one or both sides of the membrane, one can obtain conductance increases. With the antibiotics on both sides, the conductances are much larger, less variable, are anion selective and are almost completely sterol dependent. With the antibiotic on only one side, not only are the conductances smaller and more variable, but they are cation selective, and do not exhibit so strong a sterol requirement. The supralinearity of the conductance with antibiotic concentration for both the one- and two-sided effects, suggests that numerous antibiotic molecules interact to cause the conductance effects. The reversibility of the effects implies that a dynamic equilibrium of antibiotic molecules exists between the aqueous and lipid phases.

Even on the basis of these dramatic electric effects on bilayers, little can be said about the mechanism of action of the polyenes. A critical question is whether there are changes in the water and nonelectrolyte permeability associated with the large conductance increase. Because of the large and reproducible conductance effects of nystatin or amphotericin B, when present on both sides of the membrane, the water and nonelectrolyte permeability changes were determined with the antibiotics present in both aqueous phases. The results of these studies indicate that aqueous channels or pores are formed by nystatin and amphotericin B.

2. Water and Nonelectrolyte Permeability

The water and nonelectrolyte permeabilities of polyene-treated membranes were determined by measuring both the flux of labeled species in the absence of an osmotic gradient and by measuring bulk water flow in the presence of a concentration gradient of the material studied (ANDREOLI et al., 1969; HOLZ and FINKELSTEIN, 1970).

a) Results. A crucial result in these experiments was that at a given salt concentration, pH, and temperature, the values for the tracer permeability coefficient (P_d) of water and of solute increased linearly with membrane conductance (HOLZ and FINKELSTEIN, 1970). It was, therefore, possible to normalize any value of P_d to that of a membrane with an arbitrary conductance. For analysis in Table 1 the results were normalized to a conductance of $10^{-2}\Omega^{-1}\cdot cm^{-2}$ in 0.1 M NaCl. It is evident that the permeabilities of water, urea, ethylene glycol, and glycerol decreased sharply with increasing molecular size. Glycerol was only 1% as permeant as water. For membranes at the same conductance the absolute values of P_d's of amphotericin B-treated membranes were approximately 50% smaller than those of nystatin-treated membranes. However, the relative selectivity among neutral species was similar.[2]

P_f, the water permeability determined in an osmotic experiment, also increased linearly with membrane conductance. Thus, in Table 1, the P_f's were also normalized to $10^{-2}\Omega^{-1}\cdot cm^{-2}$ and compared. At a given conductance, maximal and identical bulk water flow was obtained with sucrose, glucose,

2 On a molecular level the interaction of nystatin and amphotericin B on bilayers must be virtually identical since two-sided electric effects are obtained with nystatin on one side and amphotericin B on the other side of the membrane (FINKELSTEIN and HOLZ, 1973).

Table 1. Permeability of thin lipid membranes in the presence of nystatin or amphotericin B

	Nystatin		Amphotericin B	
	Relative P_d	σ	Relative P_d	σ
Water	100 (12.0×10^{-4} cm/s)	0	100 (6.0×10^{-4} cm/s)	0
Urea	7.9	0.55	11	0.57
Ethylene glycol	3.8	0.67	–	–
Glycerol	1.0	0.78	1.3	–
Glucose	–	1.0	–	1.0
Sucrose	–	1.0	–	–
NaCl	–	1.0	–	1.0
	$\frac{P_f}{(P_d)\text{water}} = 3.3$		$\frac{P_f}{(P_d)\text{water}} = 3.0$	

Comparisons are made by first normalizing the P_d's and the P_f's to those of membranes of conductance $10^{-2}\,\Omega^{-1}\,\text{cm}^{-2}$ in 0.1 M NaCl. The permeabilities are expressed relative to the water permeability induced by nystatin or amphotericin B. The values of the tracer water permeability are given in parentheses. (Adapted from HOLZ and FINKELSTEIN, 1970).

or NaCl as the impermeant solutes. With the smaller molecules, glycerol, ethylene glycol, and urea, less than maximal water flows were obtained. σ, the ratio of the actual flow with these smaller solutes to the maximal flow determined with an impermeant solute, is inversely related to the permeability (KEDEM and KATCHALSKY, 1958). In Table 1 one finds that for the smallest solute, urea, bulk water flow was approximately 50% of the maximal flow ($\sigma = 0.55$ on a nystatin-treated membrane), and with increasing molecular size the bulk water flow reached the limiting value obtained with glucose, sucrose, and NaCl.

There are several important points to be made from the tracer and osmotic data:

b) Existence of Aqueous Pores. If water and hydrophilic solutes cross the membrane by first dissolving in the lipid phase on one side and then diffusing across to the other side where they return to an aqueous phase, one expects the following: (1) $P_f = (P_d)_{water}$ because the same forces and mechanism (solubility–diffusion) cause water transport in an osmotic experiment and in a tracer experiment. (2) The P_ds of even small hydrophilic solutes would be very small because of their very low lipid solubility. (3) $\sigma = 1$ for all hydrophilic solutes because of the absence of interaction of solute and water in the membrane. These characteristics are precisely those of the unmodified thin lipid membrane (FINKELSTEIN and CASS, 1968), and one concludes, therefore, that water crosses the unmodified membrane by a solubility-diffusion mechanism.

For the nystatin or amphotericin B-treated membrane the data are quite different. $P_f/(P_d)_w$ is significantly greater than 1 (~ 3). P_ds of hydrophilic solutes are relatively large and decrease inversely with molecular size. *The membrane acts as a sieve to distinguish between molecules on the basis of size.* And finally, σ is less than one for several hydrophilic solutes and increases with increasing molecular size. The evidence strongly suggests that nystatin and amphotericin B create aqueous pores in thin lipid membranes. The explanation for the inequality between P_f and $(P_d)_w$ in a porous membrane is that in an osmotic experiment water flows by a different mechanism (quasilaminar flow) from that in a tracer experiment. In other words, water molecules move in a cooperative manner during osmosis. Similarly, σ values significantly less than one[3] indicate that solutes interact with water molecules when they traverse the membrane; therefore, an aqueous pore denotes a local modification of such high water content that any molecule, including water itself, that passes through it interacts significantly with water.

c) Size of the Pores. σ for glycerol is approximately 0.8, and σ for glucose is 1.0; the membrane is quite tight to glycerol and essentially impermeable to glucose. On this basis, an effective pore radius of approximately 4 Å can be assigned.

The ability of a small hydrophilic solute to enter and pass through an aqueous pore is certainly dependent not only on its Stokes–Einstein radius but also on hydrogen bonding and van der Waals interactions between solute and pore. Therefore, a pore considerably larger than 4 Å in radius might still effectively exclude molecules of this size because of these other factors. Nevertheless, the permeabilities of small hydrophilic solutes through pores created by nystatin or by amphotericin B are (to a first approximation) inversely correlated with their Stokes–Einstein radiuses.

d) Area Occupied by Pores. If one assumes that water within a pore has approximately the same diffusion coefficient as in free solution, from the increase in water permeability caused by nystatin or amphotericin B one estimates that less than 0.01% of the membrane area is occupied by pores even when the antibiotic has increased the membrane conductance six orders of magnitude (HOLZ and FINKELSTEIN, 1970). Therefore, the nystatin- or amphotericin B-treated lipid bilayer membrane is a mosaic structure that contains a small number of aqueous pores (through which water, small hydrophilic solutes, and ions pass) in an expanse of unmodified membrane (through which mainly lipophilic molecules pass). This is not unlike the model of plasma membranes that is generally accepted by physiologists and that has its historical roots in the work of OVERTON and of COLLANDER. Nystatin and amphotericin B are, therefore, of interest not only because of their clinical importance but also because the pores they create are relevant models for pores that are thought to exist in biologic membranes.

3. Single Channel Electrical Measurements

Confirmation of the formation of aqueous channels by nystatin and amphotericin B has been obtained by independent means. ERMISHKIN et al. (1976) have observed discrete conductance jumps of 2–8 pmhos (depending upon the salt concentrations) induced in bilayer membranes by nystatin and amphotericin B (Fig. 2). From the size of the discrete events the rate at which ions cross

3 The σs for urea, ethylene glycol and glycerol are much lower than $1-[(P_d)_{solute}/P_f]\cdot(\bar{V}_{solute}/\bar{V}_w)$, which are the values σ would have if these solutes crossed the membrane through regions different from those crossed by water.

the membrane at 200 mV is calculated to be $2.5–10 \times 10^6$ ions/second. This is two–three orders of magnitude larger than the maximum transport rate (turnover number) for a known carrier, valinomycin (LÄUGER, 1972) whose rate is near the theoretical limit due to diffusion limitations across the membrane (STEIN, 1968). Because a channel of molecular dimensions can readily accommodate the passage of 10×10^6 ions/second (EHRENSTEIN and LECAR, 1972), the size of the discrete conductance jump strongly suggests that nystatin and amphotericin B create channels across the membrane.

The amphotericin B single channels were somewhat less than ideally anion selective and depended upon the presence of sterol (cholesterol) in the membrane. Thus, the characteristics of the single channels were similar to those of the high conductance membranes discussed above with the antibiotic present on both sides.

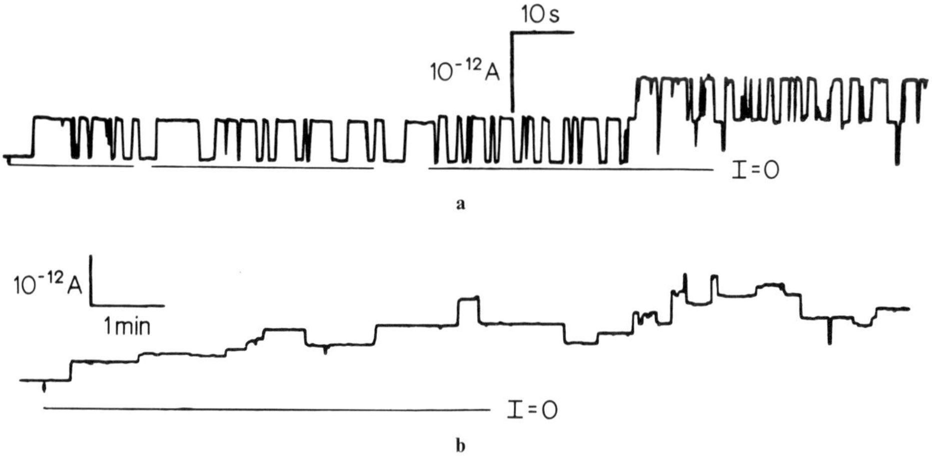

Fig. 2a and b. Discrete ionic channels created by **a** amphotericin B and **b** nystatin. The records show current fluctuations through bilayer membranes with 200 mV applied continuously across the membrane. The membranes were prepared from ox brain phospholipids and cholesterol (20:1). In record **a** the solution on both sides of the membrane contained 1×10^{-7} M amphotericin B and 2 M KNO_3. In record **b** the solution on both sides of the bilayer contained 1×10^{-7} M nystatin and 3 M KCl. Each discrete current increase or decrease is thought to result from an amphotericin B or nystatin channel opening or closing. (From ERMISHKIN et al., 1976)

C. Permeability Effects of Nystatin, Amphotericin B, and Filipin on Biological Membranes

A number of studies have been undertaken to characterize the permeability effects of the polyene antibiotics on biologic membranes. Because of inherent technical limitations of examining the biologic systems, the characterizations are generally not as detailed as on the planar bilayer membrane. However, a comparison of the effects on biologic membranes and the planar bilayer membranes can be made.

1. *Acholeplasma laidlawii*

The permeability effects of a number of polyene antibiotics including filipin, amphotericin B, and nystatin were examined on cholesterol-containing *Acholeplasma laidlawii* (DEKRUIJFF et al., 1974a, b). Nystatin and amphotericin B caused a net release of K^+ from the cells. K^+ release was not accompanied by release of the cytoplasmic enzyme glucose-6-phosphate dehydrogenase, which indicates that the integrity of the membrane was not compromised and that the cells were not lysed. Osmotic experiments demonstrated that with both amphotericin B and nystatin the membranes became permeant to univalent cations. Permeability decreased with increasing hydrated radius (permeability sequence, $Rb^+ > K^+ > Na^+ > Li^+$). The membranes also became permeable to chloride and were, therefore, neither strongly anion nor cation selective. The membranes were virtually impermeable to the divalent cations Ca^{2+} and Mg^{2+}. Hence, they selected for univalent over divalent cations. The amphotericin B and nystatin-treated cells had a graded permeability to nonelectrolytes (urea > erythritol > ribose > glucose > sucrose) that was also inversely related to size. Molecules smaller than glucose passed freely into the cells.

The permeability increases were, therefore, selective, and both in a series of cations and in a series of nonelectrolytes the permeabilities were inversely related to size. The sieving property of the permeability change, induced by amphotericin B and nystatin in cholesterol-containing *Acholeplasma laidlawii*, strongly suggests formation of aqueous channels. As with the bilayers, the cutoff in permeability at glucose among nonelectrolytes suggests an effective pore radius of 4 Å.

Filipin (2.5–20 μg/ml) increased K^+ leakage from *Acholeplasma laidlawii*. However, in contrast to nystatin and amphotericin B, filipin also released the cytoplasmic marker glucose-6-phosphate dehydrogenase, which suggests that cell lysis occurred. Turbidity measurements and microscopy showed that the cells had lysed. Thus, filipin acted in a nonselective manner in contrast to amphotericin B and nystatin. The effects of filipin on *Acholeplasma laidlawii* are consistent with the rupture of planar bilayer membranes caused by filipin (CASS et al., 1970).

2. Neurospora Protoplasts

Neurospora has ergosterol-containing membranes. The effects of nystatin, amphotericin B and filipin on protoplasts from *Neurospora crassa* (KINSKY, 1963) are similar to those on cholesterol-containing *Acholeplasma*. Nystatin and amphotericin B caused selective permeability increases wheras filipin caused a nonselective permeability increase. Nystatin and amphotericin B increased the permeability (measured osmotically) to sodium chloride and mannitol but not to sucrose. Filipin, on the other hand, increased the permeability to sodium chloride, mannitol and sucrose.

3. Human Red Blood Cell

On human red blood cells, nystatin (15–100 μM) caused a large reversible increase in monovalent ion permeability but not in divalent ion or sucrose permeability (CASS and DALMARK, 1973). The increase in monovalent ion permeability was strongly but not ideally cation selective and was proportional to the nystatin concentration raised to approximately the third power. These results are similar to those observed on planar bilayer membranes. The cation selectivity may be related to the one-sided effects that produce cation selectivity on planar bilayer membranes. This study on the red blood cell demonstrated the feasibility of using the reversible nystatin-induced permeability increase to dialyze cells with univalent salts to alter internal ion concentrations. The technique has become a useful experimental tool (see Sect. V.C.4)

4. Giant Neurons of *Aplysia californica*

The ability of the nystatin-induced membrane permeability to alter the internal salt concentrations of living cells has been utilized in studies on the giant neurons of the mollusc *Aplysia californica* (RUSSELL et al., 1977). Ion-sensitive microelectrodes were used to monitor the internal K^+ and Cl^- concentrations. Simultaneously, membrane electric properties were monitored by standard electrophysiologic techniques. Nystatin (15–30 μg/ml) reversibly increased the membrane conductance several times. The effect increases supralinearly with the nystatin concentration and was reversible within 30 min after the nystatin was removed from the bathing solution. The permeability to both univalent cations and chloride increased, although the membrane was more permeable to univalent cations. The permeability increase was relatively nonselective among the univalent cations (Cs^+, Rb^+, K^+, Na^+, Li^+). The membrane was impermeable to the divalent ions Ca^{2+} and Mg^{2+}. The permeability changes induced large and long-lasting (hours) alterations in the intracellular K^+ and Cl^- concentrations. After washing nystatin from the cells, one was able to follow the time course of the recovery of the cell to its initial state and examine parameters which are important in cell homeostasis. The technique of using nystatin-induced permeability changes of cell membranes to alter the intracellular milieu is a powerful tool and may have broad applications experimentally. It may also have clinical applications in combined drug therapies (see Sect. VI.E).

5. Isolated Lobster Axons

In isolated lobsters axons amphotericin B (10 μM) depolarized the membrane and increased the specific conductance fourfold. There was also a fourfold increase in the osmotic water permeability associated with these changes. As a result of the depolarization, the action potential was blocked but it could be restored by raising the temperature of the bathing solution from 10° C to 33° C. The ion selectivity of these conductance changes has not been satisfactorily investigated.

6. Fish Eggs

The effects of nystatin (10–50 μM) and amphotericin B (1–10 μM) were studied on a variety of fish eggs (ALBERT CASS, 1973, personal communication). Nystatin and amphotericin B reversibly increased the tracer water permeability of fertilized Fundulus (teleost) eggs that had undergone several cell divisions. Both these antibiotics also reversibly increased the conductance and depolarized Octopus, Loligo, and Sepia eggs (all cephalopods).

7. Comparison of Effects on Biological Membranes with Effects on Planar Bilayer Membranes

Table 2 compares the effects of nystatin and amphotericin B on planar bilayer membranes with those on biologic membranes. Where examined on both planar bilayer membranes and on biologic membranes there are a number of striking similarities:

1. 3β-hydroxyl sterol greatly enhances the effects.
2. Stoichiometry is supralinear.
3. Ion permeabilities increase.
4. Water and nonelectrolyte permeabilities increase.
5. Effective pore radius of 4 Å is estimated.

Similarities in the permeability effects of nystatin and amphotericin B on bilayer and biologic membranes suggest a common mode of action, the creation in the membrane of molecular-size aqueous channels or pores. The permeability changes occur in the ergosterol-containing membranes of *Neurospora* protoplasts as well as in cholesterol-containing membranes. The therapeutic fungistatic and fungicidal effects of nystatin and amphotericin B undoubtedly are consequences of pore formation in fungal membranes. Similarly, one suspects that the toxic effects of systemic amphotericin B are related to pore formation in cell membranes of the host. The events following pore formation and increased membrane permeability probably involve an altered intracellular milieu (perhaps similar to what was observed in the giant neurons of *Aplysia*), altered cell function and, ultimately, cell death.

Although in both biologic experiments and therapeutic use the polyene antibiotic is initially present only extracellularly, it is conceivable that the antibiotic could enter the cell and act on the membrane from two sides. An important question is whether the biologic effects of nystatin and amphotericin B are akin to the one- or two-sided effects on planar bilayer membranes. Bilayers are cation selective when the antibiotic is present on only one side of the

Table 2. Comparison of the permeability effects of nystatin and amphotericin B on planar bilayer membranes and cell membranes

	Planar bilayer membrane		*Acholeplasma laidlawii*[c] (cholesterol)	*Neurospora*[d] protoplasts	Red blood cells[e]	Aplysia giant neurons[f]	Lobster axon[g]	Fish eggs[h]
	One-sided[a] effect	Two-sided[b] effect						
Concentration of antibiotic (μM)	5–50 (N) 12 (A)	1–5 (N) 0.1–0.5 (A)	10–50 (N) 0.1–1.0 (A)	10 (A)	10–100 (N)	15–30 (N)	5–10 (A)	10–50 (N) 1–10 (A)
β-OH-Sterol greatly enhances effects	Yes	Yes	Yes	–	–	–	–	–
Antibiotic stoichiometry	Supralinear	Supralinear	–	–	Supralinear	Supralinear	–	–
Univalent ion permeability	Increases	Increases	Increases	Increases	Increases	Increases	Increases	Increases
Univalent ion selectivity	Cationic	Anionic	–	–	Cationic	Cationic	–	–
Divalent cation permeability	–	Unchanged	Unchanged	–	Unchanged	Unchanged	–	–
Water or nonelectrolyte permeability	–	Increases	Increases	Increases	Increases	–	Increases	Increases
Effective pore radius	–	4 Å	4 Å	4 Å	4 Å[i]	–	–	–

Concentrations are given for nystatin (N) and amphotericin B (A). When compared in the same system, the permeability effects of the two antibiotics are qualitatively very similar and no distinction need be made in the table.
[a] Marty and Finkelstein (1975); [b] Cass et al. (1970); Holz and Finkelstein (1970); [c] DeKruijff et al. (1974a); [d] Kinsky (1963); [e] Cass and Dalmark (1973); [f] Russell et al. (1977); [g] Holz and Freeman (1969); Freeman (1970); [h] A. Cass, personal communication (1973); [i] Based upon nystatin inducing a small permeability increase to glucose but no permeability increase to sucrose (A. Cass, personal communication, 1973).

membrane and anion selective when present on both sides of the membrane. In the two biologic systems where the selectivity was unambiguously determined (both with nystatin), the red blood cell and *Aplysia* giant neurons, the selectivities were cation selective. In addition, the concentrations generally necessary for the biologic effects are comparable to the higher concentrations necessary for the one-sided bilayer effects. The data, therefore, suggest that the biologic effects are similar to the one-sided bilayer effects.

D. Proposed Structure for the Amphotericin B and Nystatin Pore

Figure 3 is a CPK space-filling model of an amphotericin B molecule based upon the complete structural formula in Fig. 1. Also included in it for comparison is a model of lecithin. The following points should be noted:

1. The length of amphotericin B is equal to the length of lecithin. The long axis of the antibiotic is thus able to span one-half of the bilayer.
2. One end (the lower end in the figure) is especially polar; it contains the positively charged amino sugar and the negatively charged carboxyl group. Lecithin also contains a zwitterion polar end.

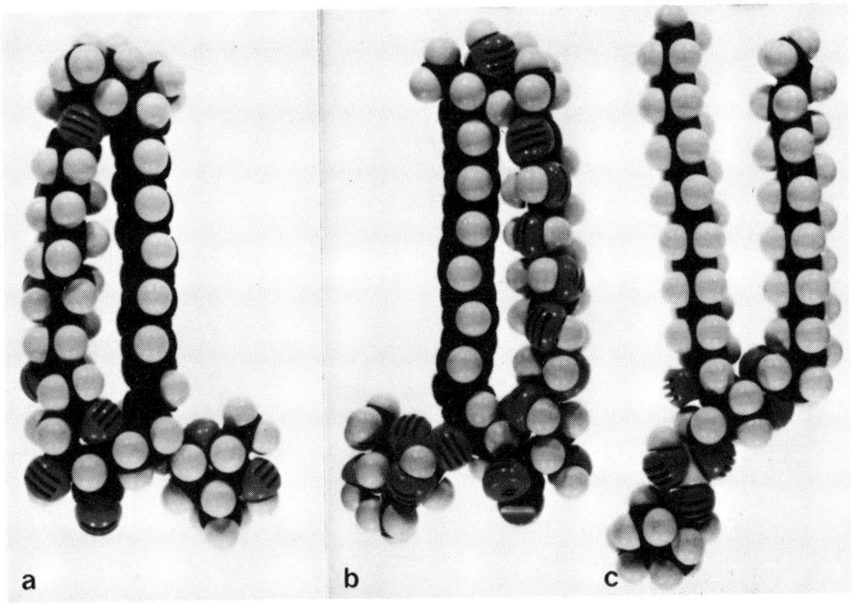

Fig. 3a–c. Molecular model (CPK) of amphotericin B. **a** The hydrophobic face of amphotericin B is seen. **b** The molecule has been rotated 180° about its long axis to reveal its opposite face with its many hydroxyl groups. At the bottoms of **a** and of **b** are the polar amino sugar and carboxyl groups; at the top is a single hydroxyl group which is seen most clearly in **b**. **c** A CPK space-filling model of lecithin is shown for comparison with amphotericin B. Note that amphotericin B consists of two chains: a polyene chain (seen on the right in **a** and on the left in **b**) and an amphipathic chain. The hydrophobic and hydrophilic sides of the amphipathic chain are seen on the left in **a** and on the right in **b**, respectively. (From FINKELSTEIN and HOLZ, 1973)

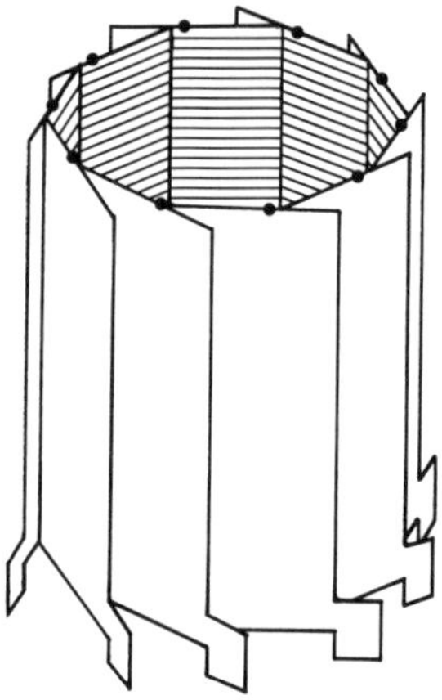

Fig. 4. Schematic drawing of a cylindrical micelle or half pore created by amphotericin B. Each amphotericin B molecule is represented as a plane with a protuberance at one end, the amino sugar, and a solid dot at the opposite end of the molecule, the single terminal hydroxyl group distinguished in Fig. 3. The *shaded portion* of each plane represents the polar hydroxyl side of the amphipathic chain. The *unshaded portion* of the plane represents the lipophilic faces of the molecule. At the *bottom* of the figure is the aqueous phase. At the *top* of the figure is either the other aqueous phase if a one-sided effect is considered, or the middle of the membrane if the two-sided effect is considered. One can see that the interior of the pore is polar, whereas the exterior is completely nonpolar. Between each pair of amphotericin B molecules around the exterior of the pore there is a wedge-shaped space that can accommodate a sterol molecule. The ring of hydroxyl groups at the top of the figure can interact with water in the amphotericin B-free aqueous phase for a one-sided pore which spans the membrane. Alternatively, with antibiotic on both sides of the membrane it can interact with an identical ring of hydroxyl groups from a cylindrical micelle from the other side. In the latter case, the interaction occurs in the middle of the membrane and two micelles are necessary to span the membrane. A nystatin half-pore is envisioned to have an almost identical structure. (From FINKELSTEIN and HOLZ, 1973)

3. The nonpolar end of amphotericin B (upper end in Fig. 2b) contains one conspicuous hydroxyl group.
4. The ring is collapsed making it unlikely that the pore is formed from the stacking of several open rings
5. One side of the collapsed ring (the right side in a and the left side in b) contains the hepaene and is lipophilic. The other side contains many hydroxyl groups and a hydrophilic face and lipophilic face.

Amphotericin B, thus, resembles a deviant membrane lipid. Instead of the two nonpolar hydrocarbon chains as in lecithin, it contains two rigid sides of the collapsed lactone ring, one of which is polyhydroxylic and amphipathic.

The structure of amphotericin B suggests a structure for the pore. Let us first consider the pore resulting from the effect of amphotericin B on both sides of a planar bilayer membrane. Half a pore is shown schematically in Fig. 4. Each amphotericin B molecule is anchored at the interface by its polar end and extends into the bilayer. The lipophilic sides of the compressed rings face outward to interact with the hydrocarbon of the membrane. Note that a single amphotericin B molecule would probably not exist with its long axis traversing the membrane because of the energetically unfavorable interaction of the hydroxyls with hydrocarbon. It is the interaction with the other amphotericin B molecules that allows penetration into the membrane and results in the formation of a cylindrical micelle. The perpendicular orientation of the antibiotic molecule is consistent with spectroscopic studies (OCKMAN, 1974). Half-pores may float independently in a sea of lipid, which is a concept consistent with the fluid mosaic model of biologic membranes. A full pore would, therefore, be formed when two half-pores (micelles) from each side of the membrane oppose and hydrogen bond to each other via the ring of end-hydroxyl groups from each micelle.

A full pore composed of 2 interacting micelles might be expected to be a more stable entity in the membrane than either micelle alone. This is supported by washout experiments in planar bilayer membranes (CASS et al., 1970). Conductance effects resulting from polyene on both sides of the membrane reverse slowly (half time of 20 min) when the antibiotic in the solution on one or both sides is removed. However, if the antibiotic is washed out after being only on one side of the bilayer for an extended time, and new antibiotic is added within 3 min to the other side, there is no conductance increase. In a separate experiment when antibiotic is added simultaneously to both sides, the conductance immediately begins to increase. Thus the full channel in the membrane is more stable than its precursors on both sides of the membrane.

It is possible to account for some of the properties of the amphotericin B-treated membrane by this model. By building a pore from CPK space-filling molecular models, one finds that cholesterol fits snugly between each pair of amphotericin B molecules (cf. DEKRUIJFF and DEMEL, 1974 for photograph). This allows hydrophobic interaction between amphotericin B and cholesterol, and helps to explain the sterol requirement. Such an interaction would be consistent with the results from differential scanning calorimetry that the polyene antibiotics remove sterol from its interaction with hydrocarbon chains of phospholipids. The internal radius of the constructed pore was approximately 7 Å, which is consistent with the experimental finding that molecules with Stokes–Einstein radii larger than 4 Å are excluded.

The number of antibiotic molecules per half-pore cannot be uniquely determined by such model building. By changing the angle of orientation one can produce pores with fewer or greater numbers of amphotericin B molecules than the ten shown in Fig. 3.

How then does one explain the one-sided effects on planar bilayer membranes and on biologic membranes? It was proposed for the channel created with antibiotic on both sides of the membrane that the ring of hydroxyls on one end of a micelle from one side would hydrogen bond within the membrane with the ring of hydroxyls from a micelle inserting from the other side. It is possible that for the one-sided effect the micelle alone fully spans the membrane and that this same ring of terminal hydroxyls interacts with the aqueous phase on the opposite side. It was noted that the length of the lactone ring is approximately one-half the length of the fully extended hydrocarbon chains of 2 phospholipid molecules. A micelle completely traversing the membrane must be unstable compared to two micelles interacting from opposite sides, as was proposed to explain the two-sided effect. It is suggested that the membrane might accommodate to pores of different lengths (Marty and Finkelstein, 1975). The hydrocarbon chain in the vicinity of a two-sided pore (composed of two micelles) could be stretched and in the vicinity of a one-sided pore (composed of one micelle) could be compressed to accommodate the structures. The variability of hydrocarbon thickness within the membrane might be accomplished by variable bending of the hydrocarbon chains and/or variable degrees of interdigitation of the hydrocarbon chains interacting from opposite sides. Nevertheless, one would expect single micelles to have a lower but finite probability of spanning the membrane compared to the complex of two micelles, and thus, higher antibiotic concentrations would be necessary for one-sided effects. Indeed, at least tenfold higher concentrations are necessary to obtain one-sided conductance effects than comparable two-sided effects. The concentrations necessary to obtain biologic effects are comparable to the concentrations necessary for one-sided effects on planar bilayer membranes (Table 2).

An important difference between channels formed with antibiotic on one or both sides of the membrane is the univalent ion selectivity. With antibiotic on both sides, the membrane becomes anion selective. With antibiotic on only one side, it is cation selective. One explanation for the anion selectivity would be that ions are interacting with the positively charged amino sugar. However, the derivative, N-acetyl amphotericin B, which not only does not have a positive charge, but is in fact negatively charged, still induces anion selectivity (Dennis et al., 1970; Finkelstein and Holz, 1973). The anion selectivity may be caused by the hydroxyl groups orienting their dipoles to substitute partially for the weak hydration sphere of the anion. This, of course, does not explain the cation selectivity when nystatin or amphotericin B is on one side of the membrane. The model proposes that the channel formed with nystatin or amphotericin B on both sides of the membrane is symmetrical while that formed with antibiotic only on one side is asymmetrical. In some unknown manner this difference in symmetry may play an important role in determining the ion selectivity.

It is also possible that the minor polyene components present together with nystatin and amphotericin B (see Sect. II) cause the one-sided conductance effects on the bilayers and biologic membranes. Four other polyene antibiotics, candicidin, fungimycin, trichomycin, and PA 150, all act on bilayers from one side to cause a cation selective conductance. It is conceivable that with nystatin or amphotericin B a small contamination of one of these other antibiotics or a related polyene antibiotic could account for the one-sided cation selective effects. The possibility that a contaminating species is responsible for the bilayer, biologic, and therapeutic effects is more likely for nystatin, which contains two minor components in significant amounts, than for amphotericin B which is very pure and has only trace contamination.

The polyene antibiotics do not all act in the same manner. Filipin, in contrast to nystatin and amphotericin B, lyses *Neurospora* protoplasts (Kinsky, 1962) and *Acholeplasma* (DeKruijff et al., 1974a) and breaks bilayers without causing selective permeability changes (Cass et al., 1970). Furthermore, filipin, but neither nystatin nor amphotericin B, creates structures within the membrane which can be seen by freeze-fracture electron microscopy (TILLACK and KINSKY, 1973; VERKLEIJ et al., 1973). The structures do not traverse the membrane. Filipin, which does not have a polar carboxyl or mycosamine moiety on one end of the molecule, probably does not have as strong a tendency as nystatin and amphotericin B to align itself perpendicular to the plane of the membrane. It has been suggested that filipin–cholesterol complexes occur within the hydrocarbon interior of the membrane and cause fragmentation of the membrane (DEKRUIJFF and DEMEL, 1974).

VI. Clinical Considerations

A. Clinical Uses

Nystatin and amphotericin B are frequently used in the treatment of fungal infections. As discussed above, they are toxic to fungi because of their ability to create aqueous pores in fungal plasma membranes, thereby increasing membrane permeability. The membranes become leaky and homeostasis can no longer be maintained. Nystatin is used to treat *Candida* infections of the skin, mucous membranes and the G.I. tract. Amphotericin B and another polyene antibiotic, candicidin, can also be used for treatment of superficial *Candida* infections.

Amphotericin B is the major drug used in the treatment of systemic mycosis. It is indicated in blastomycosis, histoplasmosis, cryptococcosis, candididiasis, torulopsosis, paracoccidioidomycosis, coccidioidomyosis, craniofacial mucormycosis, invasive aspergillosis, and extracutaneous sporotrichosis (BENNETT, 1974). It is generally administered intravenously as a colloidal suspension with sodium desoxycholate. Intra-articular injections of amphotericin B are sometimes used in mycotic infections of the joints. Intrathecal as well as intravenous administration of amphotericin B is used in coccidiodal and refractory cryptococcal meningitis. Neither amphotericin B nor nystatin is absorbed significantly from the G.I. tract. Successful treatment of a systemic mycosis depends upon the type and severity of the infection, the defense mechanisms of the patient and the control of the toxic effects of the antibiotic (see below) (BENNETT, 1976).

B. Toxicity

Infusion of amphotericin B invariably results in toxic side effects such as fever, chills, nausea, headache, anemia, and nephrotoxicity (BENNETT, 1976). At least in part, these toxic side effects probably result from amphotericin B interacting with the cholesterol-containing cell membranes of the host. The anemia is not hemolytic but probably results from a reversible suppression of the bone marrow (BRANDRISS et al., 1964).

By far the most serious complication is nephrotoxicity which has two major components – decreased glomerular filtration rate probably secondary to renal vasoconstriction, and impaired acid excretion coupled with hypokalemia (MCCURDY et al., 1968; APPEL and NEU, 1977). Nephrotoxicity invariably occurs with systemic administration and often limits the therapeutic dosage.

C. Resistance to the Polyene Antibiotics

The development of resistance to the polyene antibiotics during treatment is extremely rare. In vitro, however, resistant strains can be selected. The mechanisms of resistance are of interest because they relate to the mechanism of action of the polyenes. There are at least three types of resistance that have been described. Some strains of fungi are resistant because of reduced ergosterol content (ATHAR and WINNER, 1971; WOODS, 1971). These mutants strengthen the notion that sterol is required for the action of the polyenes. Resistance may occur because of the induction of an enzyme that degrades the polyene antibiotic (CAPEK and SIMEK, 1971). Finally, there are strains of *Candida albicans* which develop permeability changes due to nystatin and amphotericin B but remain viable in vitro (HSUCHEN and FEINGOLD, 1974). The mechanism of resistance in this latter case is not understood.

D. Selective Action of Nystatin and Amphotericin B on Fungal Rather Than Human Cell Membranes

There is evidence that ergosterol-containing membranes are more sensitive to nystatin and amphotericin B than cholesterol-containing membranes. Since fungal membranes contain ergosterol and mammalian membranes contain cholesterol, this might explain why at therapeutic dosages there are no overwhelming toxic effects to the host, although both fungal and human cell membranes contain β-hydroxyl sterol. In *Acholoplasma laidlawii* amphotericin B-induced K^+ release was approximately nine times faster with ergosterol-containing cells than with cholesterol-containing cells (DEKRUIJFF et al., 1974). Similar results were obtained with nystatin in experiments with sterol-requiring mutants of *Saccharomyces cerevisiae* (KARST and JUND, 1976). In cells preloaded with α-amino butyric acid, nystatin released the amino acid much more rapidly if the membranes contained ergosterol rather than an equal amount of cholesterol. Analogous observations have been made in model systems. The sensitivity of planar bilayer membranes to both the one-sided and the two-sided effects of nystatin and amphotericin is greater for ergosterol than for cholesterol-containing membranes (CASS et al., 1970; MARTY and FINKELSTEIN, 1975).

E. Synergism with Other Drugs

Because of the great toxicity of infused amphotericin B, one uses the lowest dosage possible to obtain therapeutic effects. A new approach to this problem was prompted by MEDOFF et al. (1971). They tested in vitro the toxicity to fungi of low concentrations of amphotericin B together with another antifungal agent, 5-fluorocytosine. They were able to obtain potentiating toxic effects – effects with both agents together that were greater than the sum of the effects of each alone. The rationale behind the use of a second agent with amphotericin B is that amphotericin B should increase the permeability of the membrane to the second drug. Because amphotericin B enhanced the incorporation of 5-fluorocytosine into the acid insoluble fraction (RNA) of *Candida albicans,* it is likely that amphotericin B increased the permeability of the membrane to the 5-fluorocytosine (MEDOFF et al., 1972). In vitro synergistic effects have also been obtained with amphotericin B and a variety of antibacterial drugs such as rifampin (MEDOFF et al., 1972) and tetracycline (KWAN et al., 1972). Nystatin can be used instead of amphotericin B (ASZALOS, 1975). Synergism has been demonstrated on a number of different fungi [i.e., *Cryptococcus neoformans, Candida tropicalis, Candida albicans, Saccharomyces cerevisiae* – MEDOFF et al. (1971), *Histoplasma capsulatum* – KOBAYASHI (1972), *Asperillus* – KITAHARA (1976)].

In vivo experiments have yielded variable results. Synergism has been demonstrated with amphotericin B and 5-fluorocytosine in the treatment of *Candida albicans* infection in mice (TITSWORTH and GRUNBERG, 1973; RABINOVICH et al., 1974). Additive, but not definite potentiating effects have been obtained with amphotericin B and 5-fluorocytosine in treatment of cryptococcosis in mice (BLOCK and BENNETT, 1973). Neither additive nor potentiating effects were obtained with amphotericin B and rifampin in the treatment of *Coccidiodes immitis* infection in mice (HUPPERT et al., 1976).

Experiments with animal cells in tissue culture have also demonstrated synergism between amphotericin B and rifampin or tetracycline (MEDOFF et al., 1973; MEDOFF et al., 1974). The specificities of the action of rifampin on RNA synthesis and of tetracycline on protein synthesis were maintained when their effects were potentiated by amphotericin B. HeLa cells which were impermeable to actinomycin D and resistant to it, took up actinomycin D and became sensitive to it in the presence of low concentrations of amphotericin B (MEDOFF et al., 1975).

At this time, there is little clinical information with humans concerning the potentiation of therapy with amphotericin B and a second drug in the treatment of systemic mycoses.

Amphotericin B and nystatin selectively increase membrane permeability by creating in membranes molecular size channels that exclude molecules the size of glucose (molecular weight 180) or larger. 5-Fluorocytosine (molecular weight 129) may be able to pass through the pore. Actinomycin D, molecular weight 1256, because of its large size, should not be permeable through the amphotericin B pore. However, as noted above, amphotericin B did, in fact, increase its intracellular uptake. Rifampin and tetracycline have molecular weights of 823 and 444 respectively, and they also should not be able to pass through the pore. Transport through the pores is undoubtedly influenced by factors other than just molecular size. Perhaps the significant organic solvent solubility of actinomycin D, rifampin, and tetracycline compared with glucose allows them to traverse the amphotericin B pore. However, there may be other mechanisms responsible for the increased uptake and synergism. For example, there must be a mechanism other than permeation through 4–7 Å radius pores that causes amphotericin B to enhance the uptake of *Escherichia coli* DNA into HeLa cells (KUMAR et al., 1974). Perhaps pinocytosis or endocytosis is increased by amphotericin B. In any event, it is likely that amphotericin B and nystatin have effects other than the creation of 4 Å radius pores that increase the permeation of large molecules in living cells. This issue is an important area for future investigations.

Summary

The polyene antibiotics nystatin and amphotericin B are clinically used antifungal agents which act by increasing the permeability of the plasma membrane. The biologic specificity of action of the polyene antibiotics is based upon the presence of a 3β-hydroxy sterol in the plasma membrane. The polyenes are active against fungi which have ergosterol-containing membranes and against mammalian cells which have cholesterol-containing membranes. They are inactive against bacteria which lack sterol. The sterol requirement for the action of the polyene antibiotics can also be demonstrated in model membrane systems. Spectroscopic studies and permeability studies in biologic and model membranes strongly suggest that nystatin and amphotericin B directly interact with membrane sterol to create 4 Å radius aqueous pores. The membrane permeability of small hydrophilic solutes and univalent ions increases with a resulting alteration in the intracellular milieu, and eventually cell death. Filipin, another polyene antibiotic, induces nonspecific permeability changes and cell lysis.

The structure of amphotericin B has been determined. It suggests that the pore consists of a cylindrical micelle of antibiotic and sterol molecules in the membrane. The structure explains some of the characteristics of the amphotericin B- (and nystatin-) induced permeability.

Nystatin and amphotericin B interact more strongly with ergosterol- than with cholesterol-containing membranes. The specificity suggests a selective action on fungal rather than human cell membranes and may account for the therapeutic usefulness of these agents.

Amphotericin B or nystatin have synergistic effects with other agents, i.e., 5-fluorocytosine, rifampin, actinomycin D or tetracycline. The synergism is probably due to an increased permeability to these second agents induced by the polyene antibiotic. However, the synergistic effect with drugs larger than 200 daltons molecular weight (i.e., rifampin, actinomycin D, tetracycline) may involve mechanisms other than the creation of 4 Å radius pores.

References

Andreoli, T.E.,Monahan, M.: The interactions of polyene antibiotics with thin lipid membranes. J. Gen. Physiol. **52**, 300–325 (1968)

Andreoli, T.E., Dennis, V.W., Weigl, A.M.: The effect of amphotericin B on the water and nonelectrolye permeability of thin lipid membranes. J. Gen. Physiol. **53**, 133–156 (1969)

Appel, G.B., Neu, H.C.: The nephrotoxicity of antimicrobial agents (third of three parts). N. Engl. J. Med. **296**, 784–787 (1977)
Aszalos, A.: Differential potentiation by nystatin of the effect of antibiotics on yeast and mammalian cells. Antimicrob. Agents Chemother. **7**, 754–757 (1975)
Athar, M.A., Winner, H.I.: The development of resistance by *Candida* species to polyene antibiotics *in vitro*. J. Med. Microbiol. **4**, 505–517 (1971)
Bennett, J.E.: Chemotherapy of systemic mycoses (first of two parts). N. Engl. J. Med. **290**, 30–32 (1974)
Bennett, J.E.: Review of amphotericin B. In: Chemotherapy. Williams, J.D., Geddes, A.M. (eds.), Vol. 6, pp. 105–106. New York: Plenum Press 1976
Bittman, R., Fischkoff, S.A.: Fluorescence studies of the binding of the polyene antibiotics filipin III, amphotericin B, nystatin, and lagosin to cholesterol. Proc. Natl. Acad. Sci. USA **69**, 3795–3799 (1972)
Block, E.R., Bennett, J.E.: The combined effect of 5-fluorocytosine and amphotericin B in the therapy of murine cryptococcosis. Proc. Soc. Exp. Biol. Med. **142**, 476–480 (1973)
Brandriss, M.W., Wolff, S.M., Moores, R., Stohlman, F.: Anemia induced by amphotericin B. J. Am. Med. Assoc. **189**, 663–666 (1964)
Bunow, M.R., Levin, I.W.: Vibrational Raman spectra of lipid systems containing amphotericin B. Biochim. Biophys. Acta **464**, 202–216 (1977)
Capek, A., Simek, A.: Antimicrobial agents XII. Relationship between biochemical resistance and microbial degradation of antimycotics. Folia Microbiol. **16**, 472–475 (1971)
Cass, A., Dalmark, M.: Equilibrium dialysis of ions in nystatin-treated red cells. Nature New Biol. **244**, 47–49 (1973)
Cass, A., Finkelstein, A., Krespi, V.: The ion permeability induced in thin lipid membranes by the polyene antibiotics nystatin and amphotericin B. J. Gen. Physiol. **56**, 100–124 (1970)
Chong, C.N., Rickards, R.W.: Macrolide antibiotic studies. XVI. The structure of nystatin. Tetrahedron Lett. **59**, 5145–5148 (1970)
De Kruijff B., Demel, R.A.: Polyene antibiotic-sterol interactions in membranes of *Acholeplasma laidlawii* cells and lecithin liposomes III. Molecular structure of the polyene antibiotic-cholesterol complexes. Biochim. Biophys. Acta **339**, 57–70 (1974)
De Kruijff, B., Demel, R.A., van Deenen, L.L.M.: The effect of cholesterol and epicholesterol incorporation on the permeability and on the phase transition of intact *Acholeplasma laidlawii* cell membranes and derived liposomes. Biochim. Biophys. Acta **255**, 331–347 (1972)
De Kruijff, B., Gerritsen, W.J., Oerlemans, A., Demel, R.A., van Deenen, L.L.M.: Polyene antibiotic-sterol interactions in membranes of *Acholeplasma laidlawii* cells and lecithin liposomes: I. Specificity of the membrane permeability changes induced by the polyene antibiotics. Biochim. Biophys. Acta **339**, 30–43 (1974)
De Kruijff, B., Gerritsen, W.J., Oerlemans, A., Van Dijck, P.W.M., Demel, R.A., Van Deenen, L.L.M.: Polyene antibiotic-sterol interactions in membranes of *Acholeplasma laidlawii* cells and lecithin liposomes: II. Temperature dependence of the polyene antibiotic-sterol complex formation. Biochim. Biophys. Acta **339**, 44–56 (1976)
Demel, R.A., van Deenen, L.L.M., Kinsky, S.C.: Penetration of lipid monolayers by polyene antibiotics: correlation with selective toxicity and mode of action. J. Biol. Chem. **240**, 2749–2753 (1965)
Demel, R.A., Bruckdorfer, K.R., van Deenen, L.L.M.: Structural requirements of sterols for the interaction with lecithin at the air water interface. Biochim. Biophys. Acta **255**, 311–320 (1972a)
Demel, R.A., Bruckdorfer, K.R., van Deenen, L.L.M.: The effect of sterol structure on the permeability of liposomes to glucose, glycerol, and Rb^+. Biochim. Biophys. Acta **255**, 321–330 (1972b)
Dennis, V., Stead, N.W., Andreloi, T.E.: Molecular aspects of polyene- and sterol-dependent pore formation in thin lipid membranes. J. Gen. Physiol. **55**, 375–400 (1970)
Dutcher, J.D., Walters, D.R., Wintersteiner, O.P.: Studies of the chemical properties and structure of nystatin (Mycostatin). In: Therapy of fungus diseases, an international symposium. Sternberg, T.H., Newcomer, V.D. (eds.), pp. 168–175. Boston, Mass.: Little, Brown and Company 1955

Ehrenstein, G., Lecar, H.: The mechanism of signal transmission in nerve axons. Annu. Rev. Biophys. Bioeng. **1**, 347–368 (1972)

Ermishkin, L.N., Kasumov, Kh.M., Potzeluyev, V.M.: Single ionic channels induced in lipid bilayers by polyene antibiotics amphotericin B and nystatine. Nature (London) **262**, 698–699 (1976)

Finkelstein, A., Cass, A.: Permeability and electrical properties of thin lipid membranes. J. Gen. Physiol. **52**, 145–172s (1968)

Finkelstein, A., Holz, R.: Aqueous pores created in thin lipid membranes by the polyene antibiotics nystatin and amphotericin B. In: Membranes. Eisenman, G. (ed.), Vol. 2, pp. 377–408. New York: Marcel Dekker Inc., 1973

Freeman, A.R.: Electrophysiological studies of polyene antibiotic effects on the lobster giant axon membrane. Fed. Proc. **29**, 795 (1970)

Ghosh, A., Ghosh, J.J.: Effect of nystatin and amphotericin B on the growth of *Candida albicans.* Ann. Biochem. Exp. Med. **23**, 29–41 (1963)

Gottlieb, D., Carter, H.E., Sloneker, J.H., Ammann, A.: Protection of fungi against polyene antibiotics by sterols. *Science.* **128**, 361 (1958)

Hamilton-Miller, J.M.T.: Chemistry and biology of the polyene macrolide antibiotics. Bacteriol Rev. **37**, 166–196 (1973)

Hazan, E.L., Brown, R.: Fungicidin, an antibiotic produced by a soil actinomycete. Proc. Soc. Exp. Biol. Med. **76**, 93–97 (1951)

Holz, R., Finkelstein, A.: The water and nonelectrolyte permeability induced in thin lipid membranes by the polyene antibiotics nystatin and amphotericin B. J. Gen. Physiol. **56**, 125–145 (1970)

Holz, R.W., Freeman, A.R.: Some effects of amphotericin B on isolated lobster walking limb axons. Biol. Bull. **137**, 404 (1069)

HsuChen, C.C., Feingold, D.S.: Polyene antibiotic action on lecithin liposomes: Effect of cholesterol and fatty acyl chains. Biochem. Biophys. Res. Commun. **51**, 972–978 (1973)

HsuChen, C.C., Feingold, D.S.: Two types of resistance to polyene antibiotics in *Candida albicans.* Nature (London) **251**, 656–659 (1974)

Huppert, M., Pappagianis, D., Sun, H., Gleason-Jordan, I., Colins, M.S., Vukovich, K.R.: Effect of amphotericin B and rifampin against *Coccidiodes immitis* in vitro and in vivo. Antimicrob. Agents Chemother. **9**, 406–413 (1976)

Karst, F., Jund, R.: Sterol replacement in *Saccharomyces cerevisiae.* Effect on cellular permeability and sensitivity to nystatin. Biochem. Biophys. Res. Commun. **71**, 535–534 (1976)

Kedem, O., Katchalsky, A.: Thermodynamic analysis of the permeability of biological membranes to nonelectrolytes. Biochim. Biophys. Acta. **27**, 229–246 (1958)

Kinsky, S.C.: Alterations in the permeability of *Neurospora crassa* due to polyene antibiotics. J. Bacteriol. **82**, 889–897 (1961)

Kinsky, S.C.: Effect of polyene antibiotics on protoplasts of *Neurospora crassa.* J. Bacteriol. **83**, 351–358 (1962)

Kinsky, S.C.: Comparative responses of mammalian erthrocytes and microbiol protoplasts to polyene antibiotics and vitamin A. Arch. Biochem. Biophys. **102**, 180–188 (1963)

Kinsky, S.C.: Polyene antibiotics. In: Antibiotics. Gottlieb, D., Shaw, P.D. (eds.), Vol. I, pp. 122–141. Berlin, Heidelberg, New York: Springer 1967

Kinsky, S.C.: Antibiotic interaction with model membranes. Annu. Rev. Pharmacol. **10**, 119–142 (1970)

Kinsky, S.C., Luse, S.A., van Deenen, L.L.M.: Interaction of polyene antibiotics with natural and artificial membrane systems. Fed. Proc. **25**, 1503–1510 (1966)

Kinsky, S.C., Haxby, J., Kinsky, C.G., Demel, R.A., van Deenen, L.L.M.: Effect of cholesterol incorporation on the sensitivity of liposomes to the polyene antibiotic filipin. Biochim. Biophys. Acta. **152**, 174–185 (1968)

Kitahara, M., Seth, V.K., Medoff, G., Kobayashi, G.S.: Activity of amphotericin B, 5-fluorocytosine, and rifampin against clinical isolates of *Aspergillus.* Antimicrob. Agents Chemother. **9**, 915–919 (1976)

Kobayashi, G.S., Medoff, G., Schlessinger, D., Kwan, C.N., Musser, W.E.: Amphotericin B potentiation of rifampin as an antifungal agent against the yeast phase of *Histoplasma capsulatum.* Science **177**, 709–710 (1972)

Kumar, V.K., Medoff, G., Kobayashi, G.S., Schlessinger, D.: Amphotericin B enhances uptake of *Escherichia coli* DNA into HeLa cells. Nature (London) **250**, 323–325 (1974)

Kwan, C.N., Medoff, G., Kobayashi, G.S., Schlessinger, D., Raskas, H.J.: Potentiation of the antifungal effects of antibiotics by amphotericin B. Antimicrob. Agents Chemother. **2**, 61–65 (1972)

Lampen, J.O.: Interference by polyenic antifungal antibiotics (especially nystatin and filipin) with specific membrane functions. In: Biochemical studies of antimicrobial drugs. Newton, B.A., Reynolds, P.E. (eds.), pp. 111–130. 16th Symp. Gen. Microbiol. Cambridge Univ. Press 1966

Läuger, P.: Carrier-mediated ion transport. Science. **178**, 24–30 (1972)

Marty, A., Finkelstein, A.: Pores formed in lipid bilayer membranes by nystatin. J. Gen. Physiol. **65**, 515–526 (1975)

McCurdy, D.K., Frederic, M., Elkinton, J.R.: Renal tubular acidosis due to amphotericin B. N. Engl. J. Med. **278**, 124–131 (1968)

Mechlinski, W., Schaffner, C.P.: Structure and absolute configuration of the polyene macrolide antibiotic amphotericin B. Tetrahedron Lett. **44**, 3873–3876 (1970)

Mechlinski, W., Schaffner, C.P.: Separation of polyene antifungal antibiotics by high-speed liquid chromatography. J. Chromatogr. **99**, 619–633 (1974)

Medoff, G., Comfort, M., Kobayashi, G.: Synergistic action of amphotericin B and 5-fluorocytosine against yeast-like organisims. Proc. Soc. Exp. Biol. Med. **138**, 571–574 (1971)

Medoff, G., Kobayashi, G.S., Kwan, C.N., Schlessinger, D., Venkov, P.: Potentiation of rifampicin and 5-fluorocytosine as antifungal antibiotics by amphotericin B. Proc. Natl. Acad. Sci. **69**, 196–199 (1972)

Medoff, G., Kwan, C.N., Schlessinger, D., Kobayashi, G.S.: Potentiation of rifampicin, rifampicin analogs, and tetracycline against animal cells by amphotericin B and polymyxin B. Cancer Res. **33**, 1146–1149 (1973)

Medoff, G., Schlessinger, D., Kobayashi, G.S.: Sensitivity of transformed and nontransformed cells to amphotericin B and several rifamycin derivatives. Cancer Res. **34**, 823–826 (1974)

Medoff, J., Medoff, G., Goldstein, M.N., Schlessinger, D., Kobayashi, G.S.: Amphotericin B-induced sensitivity to actinomycin D in drug-resistant HeLa cells. Cancer Res. **34**, 2548–2552 (1975)

Montal, M., Mueller, P.: Formation of bimolecular membranes from lipid monolayers and a study of their electrical properties. Proc. Natl. Acad. Sci. USA **69**, 3561–3566 (1972)

Mueller, P., Rudin, D.O.: Translocators in bimolecular lipid membranes: their role dissipative and conservative bioenergy transductions. Current Topics Bioenerg. **3**, 157–249 (1969)

Norman, A.W., Demel, R.A., de Kruyff, B., Geurts van Kessel, W.S.M., van Deenen, L.L.M.: Studies on the biological properties of polyene antibiotics: comparison of other polyenes with filipin in their ability to interact specifically with sterol. Biochim. Biophys. Acta. **290**, 1–14 (1972a)

Norman, A.W., Demel, R.A., de Kruyff, B., van Deenen, L.L.M.: Studies on the biological properties of polyene antibiotics: evidence for the direct interaction of filipin with cholesterol. J. Biol. Chem. **247**, 1918–1929 (1972b)

Ockman, N.: Interaction of amphotericin B with monolayers of egg lecithin and cholesterol: polarized absorption spectra. Biochim. Biophys. Acta. **345**, 253–282 (1974)

Pandey, R.C., Rinehart, K.L.: Polyene antibiotics. V. Characterization of components of the filipin complex. J. Antibiot. **23**, 414–417 (1970)

Rabinovich, S., Shaw., B.D., Bryant, T., Donta, S.T.: Effect of 5-fluorocytosine and amphotericin B on *Candida albicans* infection in mice. J. Infect. Dis. **130**, 28–31 (1974)

Russell, J.M., Eaton, D.C., Brodwick, M.S.: Effects of nystatin on membrane conductance and internal ion activities in *Aplysia* neurons. J. Memb. Biol. **37**, 137–156 (1977)

Schroeder, F., Holland, J.F., Bieber, L.L.: Fluorometric evidence for the binding of cholesterol to the filipin complex. J. Antibiot. **24**, 846–849 (1971)

Stein, W.D.: Turnover numbers of membrane carriers and the action of the polypeptide antibiotics. Nature (London) **218**, 570–571 (1968)

Tillack, T.W., Kinsky, S.C.: A freeze-etch study of the effects of filipin on liposomes and human erythrocyte membranes. Biochim. Biophys. Acta. **323**, 43–54 (1973)

Titsworth, E., Grunberg, E.: Chemotherapeutic activity of 5-fluorocytosine and amphotericin B against *Candida albicans* in mice. Antimicrob. Agents Chemother. **4**, 306–308 (1973)

Verkleij, A.J., De Kruijff, B., Gerritsen, W.F., Demel, R.A., van Deenen, L.L.M., Ververgaert, P.H.J.: Freeze- etch electron microscopy of erythrocytes, *Acholeplasma laidlawii* cells and liposomal membranes after the action of filipin and amphotericin B. Biochim. Biophys. Acta. **291**, 577–581 (1973)

Weber, M.M., Kinsky, S.C.: Effect of cholesterol on the sensitivity of *Mycoplasma laidlawii* to the polyene antibiotic filipin. J. Bacteriol. **89**, 306–312 (1965)

Weissmann, G., Sessa, G.: The action of polyene antibiotics on phopholipid cholesterol structures. J. Biol. Chem. **242**, 616–625 (1967)

Woods, R.A.: Nystatin resistant mutants of yeast: alterations in sterol content. J. Bacteriol. **108**, 69–73 (1971)

Zutphen, H. van, van Deenen, L.L.M., Kinsky, S.C.: The action of polyene antibiotics on bilayer lipid membranes. Biochem. Biophys. Res. Commun. **22**, 393–398 (1966)

Protein and Glycoprotein Toxins That Inactivate the Eukaryotic Ribosome

D. Vázquez

Introduction

An increasingly large number of protein and glycoprotein compounds (Table 1), including diphtheria toxin, toxin PA, abrin, ricin, crotins, curcins, PAP, alpha sarcin, enomycin and phenomycin, have been reported to block protein synthesis in both eukaryotes and eukaryotic microorganisms (for a review see Vázquez, 1979). Although these toxins all act catalytically, they differ in their mechanisms of action. Thus diphtheria toxin and toxin PA, in the presence

Table 1. Glycoprotein and protein toxins that block translation by eukaryotic systems

Toxins	Producer organisms	Chemical structure	Mode of action
Diphtheria toxin	*Corynebacterium diphtheria* β^{tox+}	Protein (MW = 62,000)	ADP-ribosylation of elongation factor EF-2
PAP toxin	*Pseudomonas aeroginosa*	Protein (MW = 54,000)	ADP-ribosylation of elongation factor EF-2
Ricin	Seeds of *Ricinus communis*	Glycoprotein (MW = 66,000)	Catalytic inactivation of the 60S ribosomal subunit
Abrin	Seeds of *Abrus Precatorius*	Glycoprotein (MW = 65,000)	Catalytic inactivation of the 60S ribosomal subunit
Crotin II	Seeds of *Croton tiglium*	Protein? or glycoprotein?	Catalytic inactivation of the 60S ribosomal subunit
Curcin II	Seeds of *Jatropha cursus*	Protein? or glycoprotein?	Catalytic inactivation of the 60S ribosomal subunit
PAP	Leaves of *Phytolacca americana*	Protein (MW = 27,000)	Catalytic inactivation of the 60S ribosomal subunit
Alpha sarcin	*Aspergillus giganteus*	Protein (MW = 16,000)	Enzymic degradation of the larger rRNA of the 60S ribosomal subunit
Enomycin	*Streptomyces mauvecolor*	Protein (MW = 11,000)	Catalytic inactivation of the 60S ribosomal subunit
Phenomycin	*Streptomyces fervens* var. *phenomyceticus*	Protein (MW = 10,000)	Catalytic inactivation of the 60S ribosomal subunit

Table 2. The effects of glycoprotein and protein toxins on model reactions to study some steps of the elongation cycle

	EF-1-dependent		EF-2-dependent			Non-enzymic trans-location
	Binding of aminoacyl-tRNA	GTP hydrolysis	Formation of the EF-2-GTP-ribosome complex	Uncoupled GTP hydrolysis	Translocation	
Ricin A-chain	Inhibition	Inhibition	Inhibition	No effect or inhibition	No effect or stimulation	No effect
Abrin A-chain	Inhibition	Inhibition	Inhibition	No effect or inhibition	No effect or stimulation	No effect
Alpha sarcin	Inhibition	Inhibition	Inhibition	Inhibition	No effect	–
PAP	Inhibition	Inhibition	Inhibition	No effect or stimulation	No effect or stimulation	–
Crotin II	Inhibition	Inhibition	Inhibition	No effect	No effect or inhibition	–
Enomycin	Inhibition	–	No effect	Inhibition	No effect	–

Data taken from different references as indicated in the text.

of NAD, enzymically modify elongation factor EF-2 forming ADP-ribosyl-EF-2 which functions less efficiently in translocation than does EF-2. Furthermore, the former complex is more stable than that formed with EF-2 under physiologic conditions and therefore recycling of the factors in the elongation cycle is drastically affected (VÁZQUEZ, 1979; review). In contrast, ricin A chain, abrin A chain, PAP, alpha sarcin, crotin II, curcin II, enomycin, and phenomycin act directly on ribosomes, inactivating catalytically 60S ribosomal subunits, apparently without a requirement for any additional cofactor (for a review see VÁZQUEZ, 1979). Such toxins are considered in detail in the present communication. Although they have a similar or related mechanism of action (Table 2) in that they inactivate catalytically 60S ribosomal subunits, the compounds not only have different chemical structures but also have different origins (Table 1).

Ricin and Abrin

An extensive review (OLSNES and PIHL, 1977) has already covered the toxic properties, chemical structures, functions and modes of action of ricin, abrin, and the related lectins *Ricinus communis* agglutinin and *Abrus precatorius* agglutinin. Ricin is a glycoprotein of molecular weight 66,000 isolated from seeds of *Ricinus communis*. It has also been equated with ricin D, ricin RCA_{60}, ricin II, RCA_{11} and ricin toxin (NICOLSON et al., 1974; OLSNES and PHIL, 1977), although some workers do not agree that these are one and the same compound

(LUGNIER and DIRHEIMER, 1973). Ricin, in chemical structure and mode of action, is very similar to abrin which is a glycoprotein of molecular weight 65,000 isolated from the seeds of *Abrus precatorius* (OLSNES and PIHL, 1973a). Abrin forms crystalline tetrameric structures (total molecular weight 260,000) detectable by X-ray diffraction studies (MCPHERSON and RICH, 1973). Neither ricin nor abrin cause appreciable cell agglutination, although such an effect is marked with both *Ricinus communis* agglutinin (also known as RCA_{120} and ricin I) and *Abrus precatorius* agglutinin, which have molecular weights of 120,000 and 134,000 respectively and are rich in carbohydrates (OLSNES and PIHL, 1972a; LUGNIER et al., 1974; NICOLSON et al., 1974; OLSNES et al., 1974a, 1975a). The high toxicity of ricin and abrin on eukaryotic cells results from their action in specifically blocking protein synthesis. The toxins have no effect on RNA synthesis and their inhibitory action on DNA synthesis is a secondary consequence of their specific blockade of protein synthesis (LIN et al., 1970; LIN et al., 1971). Accordingly, both ricin and abrin are potent antitumor drugs in mice bearing Ehrlich ascites cells (LIN et al., 1970; OLSNES et al., 1974b). Specific inhibition of protein synthesis by ricin and abrin has also been confirmed with other eukaryotic systems including HeLa cells (OLSNES and PIHL, 1972a), plasmacytoma cells (KO and KAJI, 1975), mouse myeloma cells (ONOZAKI et al., 1975), normal- and virus-transformed fibroblasts (NICOLSON et al., 1975) and a number of eukaryotic microorganisms, although intact yeast cells are impermeable to the drugs. In all these cases there is a lag period of 30–60 min before protein synthesis is halted by the toxins (GROLLMAN et al., 1974; REFSNES et al., 1974; KO and KAJI, 1975; NICOLSON et al., 1975; ONOZAKI et al., 1975). Mutants of Chinese hamster ovary cells and baby hamster kidney fibroblasts, both resistant to ricin, have also been isolated. However, although some of these mutants bind ricin only poorly, others bind ricin as efficiently as do normal sensitive cells (GOTTLIEB et al., 1974; MEAGER et al., 1976). A further inhibitory effect of ricin is related to the interaction of the B subunit with the cell membrane (NOMOTO et al., 1975). Thus the drug has been reported to decrease the level of cyclic AMP normally enhanced by preincubation of Yoshida ascites sarcoma with prostaglandin E_1.

Although both ricin and abrin contain two polypeptide chains joined by a S-S bond (Fig. 1) (FUNATSU, 1972; NICOLSON et al., 1974; OLSNES et al., 1974b), important differences exist between the chemical structures of the two drugs. Thus, abrin A chain (MW 30,000) does not contain carbohydrate whereas ricin A chain (MW 32,000) contains approximately 2.4% carbohydrate mainly in the form of four residues of mannose (OLSNES et al., 1974b, 1975a). However, both abrin B chain (MW 35,000) and ricin B chain (MW 34,000) contain some 7% carbohydrate which is in the form of 10–11 residues of mannose and 1–2 residues of glucosamine, the latter probably being present as acetyl glucosamine (OLSNES et al., 1974b, 1975a). There are also some differences in the amino acid composition of the two drugs (FUNATSU, 1972; NICOLSON et al., 1974; OLSNES et al., 1975a), which are in addition immunologically different (OLSNES et al., 1974c; EHRLICH, 1957) since the isolated A and B chains of each toxin do not crossreact. The heterologous chains abrin A/ricin B and ricin A/abrin B can easily be formed and are as toxic as ricin and abrin (OLSNES et al., 1974c).

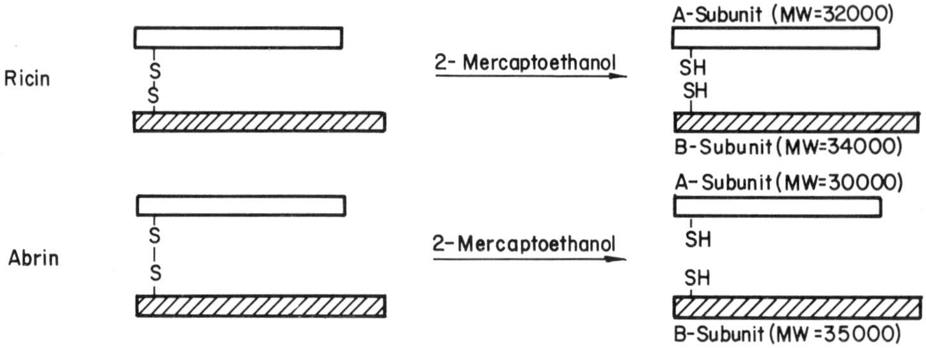

Fig. 1. Ricin and abrin structures

However, whereas anti-abrin or anti-ricin serum neutralizes only its homologous toxin, neither antitoxin can distinguish between the hybrid forms although antibodies specifically directed against determinants on A or B chains easily distinguish between the two hybrids (OLSNES et al., 1974c).

The treatment of ricin and abrin with 2-mercaptoethanol reduces the S-S bond joining their A and B chains and the subunits separate (Fig. 1). As a result, treatment of the toxins with 2-mercaptoethanol abolishes both their toxicity to animals and their inhibitory effect on protein synthesis in intact eukaryotic cells (OLSNES and PIHL, 1972b), although if the 2-mercaptoethanol is removed, the disulfide bonds reform and toxicity is restored (OLSNES et al., 1974b). In contrast, separation of the A and B chains by treatment with 2-mercaptoethanol results in a considerable increase of the toxic activity in cell-free systems (OLSNES and PIHL, 1972b). Apparently the free A chain is a very active inhibitor in cell-free systems, whereas the B chain is essentially without effect (OLSNES and PIHL, 1973a, b). Indeed all the evidence suggests that A chains have to be separated from B chains to allow inhibition of protein synthesis since the intact toxins, even at high concentrations, do not block translation in cell-free systems in the absence of reducing agents (for a review see OLSNES and PIHL, 1977). This provides an explanation for the slow kinetics of inhibition shown for the toxins in cell-free systems (OLSNES and PIHL, 1972a, c; GROLLMAN et al., 1974). In addition, however, it has also been reported that a small tryptic peptide from ricin (MW 12,500) can block translation in rabbit reticulocyte cell-free systems (LUGNIER et al., 1974).

The B chains of ricin and abrin, but not the A chains, bind to erythrocytes (OLSNES and PIHL, 1973a, b). Furthermore, the B chains are retained by Sepharose 4B columns and can be eluted with buffers containing galactose (OLSNES and PIHL, 1973b; OLSNES et al., 1974b). Indeed, ricin and abrin bind to both free galactose and lactose with a single binding site for the sugars on their B chains. It has been shown that (^{125}-I)-labeled ricin and abrin bind reversibly to both HeLa cells and erythrocytes and again the interaction is prevented or reversed by galactose or lactose, these sugars drastically reducing the inhibitory effect of the toxins (ONOZAKI et al., 1972; GROLLMAN et al., 1974; OLSNES et al., 1974b). It is clear from these results that the B subunit is required for the attachment of the toxin to the cells in order to facilitate the entry of the A subunit. This subunit can be freed, by reduction of the toxin inside the cell, and is then able to block protein synthesis (REFSNES et al., 1974).

The A subunits of both ricin and abrin inhibit translation by inactivating ribosomes (OLSNES, 1972; OLSNES and PIHL, 1972b; MONTANARO et al., 1973; OLSNES et al., 1973; BENSON et al., 1975; ONOZAKI et al., 1975). The inactivated site is located on the 60S ribosomal subunit and the toxins have no effect on the 40S subunit (SPERTI et al., 1973; BENSON et al., 1975; ONOZAKI et al., 1975). Thus (^{3}H)-labeled ricin A subunits bind to both 80S ribosomes and their corresponding 60S subunits but associate with neither 40S subunits nor bacterial ribosomes (HEDBLOM et al., 1976). Ribosomes from the different eukaryotic cells tested, including plants, green algae, and yeast, are sensitive to the toxins, whereas bacterial ribosomes are not affected (OLSNES et al., 1973; GRECO et al., 1974). There are, however, conflicting reports concerning the effects of the toxins on mitochondrial ribosomes. Thus ricin has been reported to block endogenous protein synthesis in both *Neurospora crassa* and yeast mitochondria (LUGNIER et al., 1976a), but was found to be ineffective on poly U-directed polyphenylalanine synthesis by ribosomes from rat liver mitochondria (GRECO et al., 1974).

Inhibition of 60S ribosomal subunits by ricin and abrin is catalytic rather than stoichiometric since a single molecule of the toxin can inactivate a large number of ribosomes (OLSNES and PIHL, 1972a, c; MONTANARO et al., 1973; CARRASCO et al., 1975). The A subunits of the toxins can, in fact, inactivate ribosomes in buffer solutions at a rate of 1500 ribosomes per min per toxin A subunit (OLSNES et al., 1975b) and this result clearly shows that the A subunit acts enzymically. The nature of the enzymic activity has not been elucidated to date since modifications of neither the ribosomal proteins (NICOLSON et al., 1975; LUGNIER et al., 1976b) nor ribosomal RNA (MITCHELL et al., 1976) by the toxins or their A subunits have been demonstrated.

There are contradictory reports concerning which events in translation are inhibited by the toxins. Since polyribosome breakdown was observed in extracts from both rat-liver (LIN et al., 1972) and HeLa cells (GROLLMAN et al., 1974) after a certain period of toxin treatment, it was postulated that ricin inhibits initiation of protein synthesis (GROLLMAN et al., 1974). However, ricin and abrin have been reported to stabilize polyribosomes in both rabbit-reticulocyte lysates (OLSNES and PIHL, 1972a; NICOLSON et al., 1975) and in mouse myeloma cells (ONOZAKI et al., 1975), suggesting that in these systems the toxins prevent elongation of the polypeptide chain. Ricin and abrin do not, in fact, affect peptide bond formation, but inhibit both the EF-1-dependent binding of aminoacyl-tRNA (CARRASCO et al., 1975) and GTP hydrolysis (BENSON et al., 1975; SPERTI et al., 1975) without affecting the nonenzymic binding of aminoacyl-tRNA (CARRASCO et al., 1975). These results clearly suggest that the toxins inactivate one site on the 60S ribosomal subunit involved in the interaction or function of EF-1. This site appears to be identical or overlapping with the ribosomal binding site for EF-2 since the toxins also inhibit formation of an EF-2-GTP-ribosome complex with washed ribosomes (CARRASCO et al., 1975; MONTANARO et al., 1975; NOLAN et al., 1976). In certain cases the toxins were reported to inhibit

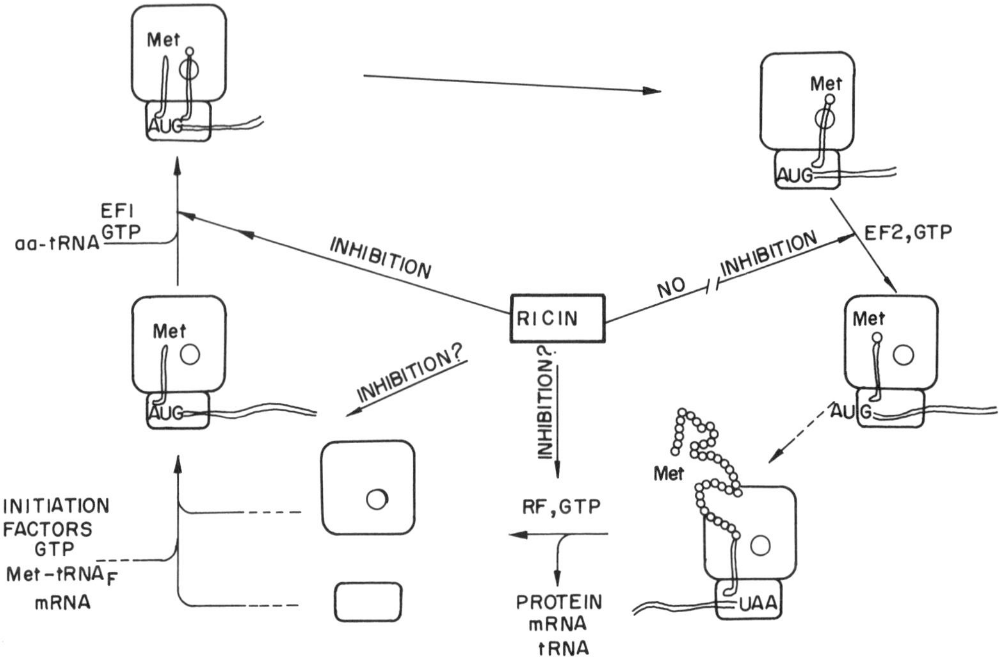

Fig. 2. The ribosome cycle showing the possible sites of inhibition by ricin

partially the EF-2-dependent uncoupled GTP hydrolysis (MONTANARO et al., 1973; BENSON et al., 1975; SPERTI et al., 1975), but other workers have observed that this reaction is stimulated by the toxins (SPERTI et al., 1976; FERNÁNDEZ-PUENTES and VÁZQUEZ, 1977). Nevertheless, inhibition of EF-2 binding by the toxins was confirmed by replacing GTP by either GDP or GMPPCP (CARRASCO et al., 1975), and prior attachment of EF-2 and aminoacyl-tRNA to ribosomes protects these particles from the inactivation that normally results from treatment with the toxins (FERNÁNDEZ-PUENTES et al., 1976a; MITCHELL et al., 1976). In addition, the inhibition of translation observed with toxin-treated ribosomes is obscured or abolished by increasing concentrations of EF-1, EF-2 or ribosomes (FERNÁNDEZ-PUENTES et al., 1976b). It appears therefore that the damage caused by ricin and abrin on the 60S ribosomal subunit does not totally inactivate the particle but causes a considerable decrease in the affinity between ribosomes and both EF-1-GTP and EF-2-GTP. Thus the toxins have no significant effect when an excess of either EF-1 or ribosomes is used (MONTANARO et al., 1975; SPERTI et al., 1975; FERNÁNDEZ-PUENTES et al., 1976b) although EF-1-dependent GTP hydrolysis and aminoacyl-tRNA binding are very sensitive to ricin and abrin when concentrations of EF-1 and ribosomes are limiting (BENSON et al., 1975; CARRASCO et al., 1975; SPERTI et al., 1975; FERNÁNDEZ-PUENTES et al., 1976b). Ricin and abrin inhibit neither EF-2-dependent translocation (MONTANARO et al., 1973; FERNÁNDEZ-PUENTES et al., 1976b; STIRPE et al., 1976) nor nonenzymic translocation induced by high concentration of K^+ (BARBACID et al., 1975; CARRASCO, personal communication), since the substrate bound to the acceptor site protects the ribosome from inactivation by the toxin (FERNÁNDEZ-PUENTES et al., 1976b). This explains why a large number of ribosomes derived from polysomes of drug treated cells escape inactivation by the toxin (FOODSTAD and OLSNES, 1977).

The results summarized above indicate that both ricin and abrin block aminoacyl-tRNA binding by preventing the attachment of EF-1-GTP-aminoacyl-tRNA complexes to ribosomes, thereby inhibiting elongation of polypeptide chains (Fig. 2). Common or overlapping sites located on 60S ribosomal subunits are involved in the attachment of GTP, itself bound to certain initiation, elongation, and termination factors (HASELKORN and ROTHMAN-DENES, 1973; TATE and CASKEY, 1974; JACKSON, 1975; MODOLELL and VÁZQUEZ, 1975; VÁZQUEZ, 1978; reviews). Inactivation of this ribosomal site by ricin and abrin might also result in inhibition of the initiation and termination processes (Fig. 2), although such effects remain to be demonstrated in suitable assay systems. Finally, it should be noted that a complex between ribosomal 5S RNA and a single ribosomal protein, sedimenting at 8S and derived from 60S ribosomal subunits, has low GTPase activity which is inhibited by both ricin and abrin A subunits. This complex might form the specific ribosomal target site for the toxins (BENSON et al., 1975; BENSON, 1977).

PAP, Alpha Sarcin, Crotins, Curcins, Enomycin, and Phenomycin

A number of proteins have recently been described, which appear to act in a way somehow related to that of the A subunits of ricin and abrin. Included in this group of proteins are the individual crotins, the individual curcins, alpha sarcin, enomycin, and probably phenomycin. All these proteins act selectively on eukaryotic systems and are similar to both ricin A chain and abrin A chain in that their inhibitory activity is rather low in intact cells probably because of cellular permeability barriers. However they are very active inhibitors in cell-free systems and much less than one molecule of each toxin per ribosome is required for inhibition of translation, suggesting that, as is the case for the A subunits of both ricin and abrin, all these proteins inactivate ribosomes enzymically. Indeed, in comparative studies with rabbit reticulocyte and yeast systems it has been shown that abrin, PAP, alpha sarcin and enomycin have in common an inhibitory effect on EF-1-dependent binding of aminoacyl-tRNA and do not inhibit EF-2-dependent translocation of peptidyl-tRNA (Table 2).

The crotins are proteins, extracted from the seeds of *Croton tiglium*, which are very active in blocking formation of EF-2-GTP-ribosome complexes while enhancing EF-2-dependent uncoupled GTP hydrolysis. The purified crotins, mainly crotin II, are very potent inhibitors of EF-1-dependent binding of aminoacyl-tRNA. It was proposed that croton II inhibited the translocation step in protein synthesis but the drug affects this reaction only poorly (SPERTI et al., 1976). Interaction of crotins with ribosomes may not be prevented by peptidyl-tRNA bound to the acceptor site, a situation which would contrast with that observed for both ricin and abrin A chain.

The curcins are proteins extracted from the seeds of *Jatropha curcas* and the compounds appear to have a mode of action similar to that of the crotins. It is of interest that the individual curcins are much less active than the curcin complex (SPERTI et al., 1976).

PAP is a basic protein, of MW 27,000 (TOMLINSON et al., 1974), extracted from the leaves of *Phytolacca americana* (WYATT and SHEPHERD, 1969). PAP blocks EF-1-dependent reactions involving both GTPase activity and binding of aminoacyl-tRNA to ribosomes (OBRIG et al., 1973; SUITS and IRVIN, 1976; FERNÁNDEZ-PUENTES and VÁZQUEZ, 1977). PAP also inhibits formation of the EF-2-GTP-ribosome complex but it has no effect on, and even enhances, EF-2-dependent GTP hydrolysis (OBRIG et al., 1973; FERNÁNDEZ-PUENTES and VÁZQUEZ, 1977). Cell-free systems from *Artemia Salina* are more sensitive to PAP than those from reticulocyte lysates, and this differential sensitivity appears to be related to differences in the EF-2 factor in each system (SUITS and IRVIN, 1976). PAP has an antiviral effect that probably results from its activity in preventing protein synthesis (TOMLINSON et al., 1974).

Alpha sarcin is a basic protein (MW 16,000) which contains the unusual amino acid sarcinine. It is produced in the fermentation broth of *Aspergillus giganteus*. Although it is a very active antitumor agent and is very cytotoxic it is hardly active against *E. coli* (OLSON and GOERNER, 1965; OLSON et al., 1965). Alpha sarcin blocks protein synthesis in extracts from wheat germ, yeast, rat liver, rabbit reticulocytes and Ehrlich ascites cells by inhibiting both EF-1-dependent GTP hydrolysis and binding of aminoacyl-tRNA to ribosomes but it has no effect on the nonenzymic binding of aminoacyl-tRNA to ribosomes (FERNÁNDEZ-PUENTES and VÁZQUEZ, 1977; SCHINDLER et al., 1977). Although alpha sarcin inhibits formation of EF-2-GTP-ribosome complexes and inhibits EF-2-dependent uncoupled GTP hydrolysis, it does not inhibit EF-2-dependent translocation (FERNÁNDEZ-PUENTES and VÁZQUEZ, 1977; SCHINDLER et al., 1977). Thus, alpha sarcin probably blocks translation by preventing functional interaction of EF-1-GTP-aminoacyl-tRNA complexes with ribosomes. Interaction of the toxin with ribosomes in the pretranslocated state does not appear to take place, as is also the case for abrin and ricin, and alpha sarcin does not, therefore, inhibit translocation. Catalytic inactivation of the 60S ribosomal subunit by alpha sarcin results from enzymic cleavage, by the protein, of 320 nucleotides from the 3′ terminal end of the larger ribosomal RNA of the 60S ribosomal subunit. This effect is fairly specific and was observed using preparations of ribosomes and 60S ribosomal subunits from both wheat germ and yeast, although rat liver polyribosomes did not respond (SCHINDLER and DAVIES, 1977). This lack of effect in rat liver polysomes was probably caused by the inability of the protein to gain access to ribosomes in the pretranslocated state. The larger RNA of the 50S ribosomal subunit of *E. coli* is also cleaved, although the toxin is a poor inhibitor of translation by *E. coli* ribosomes. However cleavage of *E. coli* ribosomes requires a rather high concentration of alpha sarcin (SCHINDLER and DAVIES, 1977).

Enomycin is a basic protein (MW 11,000), produced by *Streptomyces mauvecolor*, which is a potent inhibitor of polypeptide synthesis in cell-free systems from Ehrlich ascites carcinoma cells, rat liver (MIZUNO et al., 1967a), and yeast

(BATTANER and VÁZQUEZ, 1971). Enomycin inhibits binding of aminoacyl-tRNA to polyribosomes, and preliminary experiments suggest that it interacts with both 60S and 40S ribosomal subunits (MIZUNO et al., 1967b). In reticulocyte lysates enomycin allows formation of initiation complexes on 80S and 40S subunits. In fact, these complexes accumulate in the presence of the inhibitor (MIZUNO and UMEZAWA, 1976), since the EF-1-dependent binding of aminoacyl-tRNA is prevented (FERNÁNDEZ-PUENTES and VÁZQUEZ, 1977). Enomycin does not inhibit peptide bond formation in model systems, although the initial dipeptide (f-Met-val) is not formed in reticulocyte lysates in the presence of this inhibitor (MIZUNO and UMEZAWA, 1976). Furthermore, although enomycin also blocks the formation of the EF-2-GTP-80S-ribosome complex it does not affect translocation, suggesting that the toxin cannot interact with pretranslocated polyribosomes (FERNÁNDEZ-PUENTES and VÁZQUEZ, 1977).

Phenomycin is a basic protein (MW 10,000) produced by *Streptomyces fervens* that specifically prevents protein synthesis in eukaryotic cells (NISHIMURA, 1968a). In addition it blocks polypeptide synthesis in crude cell-free systems from both rabbit reticulocytes and rat liver (NISHIMURA, 1968b). In reticulocyte lysates phenomycin does not prevent formation of initiation complexes on 80S ribosomes and such complexes do in fact accumulate in the presence of the inhibitor. However, it has been reported that the drug blocks formation of the initial dipeptide (YAMAKI et al., 1974). This is compatible with an inhibitory effect of the toxin on EF-1-dependent binding of aminoacyl-tRNA; this possibility remains to be tested.

References

Barbacid, M., Fresno, M., Vázquez, D.: Inhibitors of polypeptide elongation on yeast polysomes. J. Antibiot. *28*, 453–462 (1975)

Battaner, E., Vázquez, D.: Inhibitors of protein synthesis by ribosomes of the 80S type. Biochim. Biophys. Acta *154*, 316–330 (1971)

Benson, S.C.: Correlation of inhibition of ribosomal GTPase and protein synthesis by abrin and ricin. Biochem. Biophys. Res. Commun. *75*, 845–850 (1977)

Benson, S., Olsnes, S., Pihl, A., Skorve, J., Abraham, K.A.: On the mechanism of protein synthesis inhibition by abrin and ricin. Inhibition of the GTP-hydrolysis. Site on the 60S ribosomal subunit. Eur. J. Biochem. *59*, 573–580 (1975)

Carrasco, L., Fernández-Puentes, C., Vázquez, D.: Effects of ricin on the ribosomal sites involved in the interaction of the elongation factors. Eur. J. Biochem. *54*, 499–503 (1975)

Ehrlich, P.: In: The collected papers of Paul Ehrlich. Vol. 2, pp. 21–44. London: Pergamon Press 1957

Fernández-Puentes, C., Vázquez, D.: Effect of some proteins that inactivate the eukaryotic ribosome. FEBS Lett. *78*, 143–146 (1977)

Fernández-Puentes, C., Benson, S., Olsnes, S., Pihl, A.: Protective effect of elongation factor 2 on the inactivation of ribosomes by the toxic lectins abrin and ricin. Eur. J. Biochem. *64*, 437–443 (1976a)

Fernández-Puentes, C., Carrasco, C., Vázquez, D.: Site of action of ricin on the ribosome. Biochemistry *15*, 4364–4369 (1976b)

Foodstad, O., Olsnes, S.: Studies on the accesibility of ribosomes to inactivation by the toxic lectins abrin and ricin. Eur. J. Biochem. *74*, 209–215 (1977)

Funatsu, M.: In: Proteins, structure and function. Funatsu, M., Hiromi, K., Imahori, K., Murachi, T., Narita, K., (eds.) pp. 103–139. John Wiley & Sons 1972

Gottlieb, C., Skinner, S.A.M., Kornfeld, S.: Isolation of a clone of chinese hamster ovary cells deficient in plant lectin-binding sites. Proc. Natl. Acad. Sci. USA *71*, 1078–1082 (1974)

Greco, M., Montanaro, L., Novello, F., Saccone, C., Sperti, S., Stirpe, F.: Inhibition of protein synthesis by ricin: experiments with rat liver mitochondria and nuclei and with ribosomes from *Escherichia coli*. Biochem. J. *142*, 695–697 (1974)

Grollman, A.P., Grunfeld, C., Brewer, C.F., Marcus, D.M.: Molecular pharmacology of plant lectins: studies on ricin and concanavalin A (NSC-143504). Cancer Chemother. Rep. *58*, 491–508 (1974)

Haselkorn, R., Rothman-Denes, L.B.: Protein synthesis. Annu. Rev. Biochem. *42*, 397–437 (1973)

Hedblom, M.L., Cawley, D.B., Houston, L.L.: The specific binding of ricin and its polypeptide chains to rat liver ribosomes and ribosomal subunits. Arch. Biochem. Biophys. *177*, 46–55 (1976)

Irvin, J.D.: Purification and partial characterization of the antiviral protein from *Phytolacca americana* which inhibits eukaryotic protein synthesis. Arch. Biochem. Biophys. *169*, 522–528 (1976)

Jackson, R.J.: In: MTP Int. Rev. Sci. Biochemistry. Synthesis of amino acids and proteins. Arnstein, H.R.V., (ed.), Vol. 7, pp. 89–135. Oxford: Medical and Technical Publishing Co. 1975

Ko, T.S., Kaji, A.: Effect of ricin on biosynthesis of myeloma protein (IgA) and general cellular proteins in MOPC-315 cells. Biochim. Biophys. Acta *414*, 155–160 (1975)

Lin, J.Y., Tserng, K.Y., Chen, C.C., Lin, L.T., Tung, T.C.: Abrin and ricin: new antitumor substances. Nature (London) *237*, 292–293 (1970)

Lin, J.Y., Liu, K., Chen, C.C., Tung, T.C.: Effect of crystalline ricin on the biosynthesis of protein, RNA and DNA in experimental tumors. Cancer Res. *31*, 921–923 (1971)

Lin, J.Y., Pao, C.C., Ju, S-T., Tung, T.C.: Polyribosome disaggregation in rat liver following administration of the phytotoxic proteins, abrin and ricin. Cancer Res. *32*, 943–947 (1972)

Lugnier, A.A.J., Dirheimer, G.: Differences between ricin and phytohemagglutinins from *Ricinus communis* seeds. FEBS Lett. *35*, 117–120 (1973)

Lugnier, A.A.J., Le Meur, M.A., Gerlinger, P., Dirheimer, G.: Inhibition of *in vitro* protein synthesis in a rabbit reticuloxyte cell-free system by toxic trypsic peptides from ricin. Biochimie *56*, 1287–1289 (1974)

Lugnier, A.A.J., Küntzel, H., Dirheimer, G.: Inhibition of *Neurospora crassa* and yeast mitochondrial protein synthesis by ricin, a toxic protein inactive on *E. coli* protein synthesis. FEBS Lett. *66*, 202–205 (1976a)

Lugnier, A.A.J., Dirheimer, G., Madjar, J.J., Reboud, J.P., Gordon, J., Howard, G.A.: Action of ricin from *Ricinus communis* L. seeds on eukaryote ribosomal proteins. FEBS Lett. *67*, 343–347 (1976b)

McPherson, A., Rich, A.: Studies on crystalline abrin: X-ray diffraction data, molecular weight, carbohydrate content and subunit structure. FEBS Lett. *35*, 257–261 (1973)

Meager, A., Ungkitchanukit, A., Hughes, R.C.: Variants of hamster fibroblasts to *Ricinus communis* toxin (ricin). Biochem. J. *154*, 113–124 (1976)

Mitchell, S.J., Hedblom, M., Cawley, D., Houston, L.L.: Ricin does not act as an endonuclease on L cells polysomal RNA. Biochem. Biophys. Res. Commun. *68*, 763–769 (1976)

Mizuno, S., Umezawa, H.: Inhibition of the initial dipeptide synthesis of globin chains by the antibiotic enomycin in the reticulocyte lysate. J. Antibiot. *29*, 309–315 (1976)

Mizuno, S., Nitta, K., Umezawa, H.: Mode of action of enomycin, an antitumor antibiotic of high molecular weight. I. Inhibition of protein synthesis. J. Biochem. *61*, 373–381 (1967a)

Mizuno, S., Nitta, K., Umezawa, H.: Mode of action of enomycin, an antitumor antibiotic of high molecular weight. II. Preferential binding of enomycin to mammalian ribosomes. J. Biochem. *61*, 382–387 (1967b)

Modolell, J., Vázquez, D.: In: MTP Int. Rev. Sci. Biochemistry. Synthesis of amino acids and proteins. Arnstein, H.R.V., (ed.), Vol. 7, pp. 137–178. Oxford: Medical and Technical Publishing Co. 1975

Montanaro, L., Sperti, S., Stirpe, F.: Inhibition by ricin of protein synthesis *in vitro*. Ribosomes as the target of the toxin. Biochem. J. *136*, 677–683 (1973)

Montanaro, L., Sperti, S., Mattioli, A., Testoni, G., Stirpe, F.: Inhibition by ricin of protein synthesis *in vitro*. Biochem. J. *146*, 127–131 (1975)

Nicolson, G.L., Blaustein, J., Etzler, M.E.: Characterization of two plant lectins from *Ricinus communis* and their quantitative interaction with a murine lymphoma. Biochemistry *13*, 196–204 (1974)

Nicolson, G.L., Lacorbiere, M., Hunter, T.R.: Mechanism of cell entry end toxicity of an affinity-purified lectin from *Ricinus communis* and its differential effects on normal and virus-transformed fibroblasts. Cancer Res. *35*, 144–155 (1975)
Nishimura, T.: Mechanism of action of phenomycin, a tumor-inhibitory polypeptide. J. Antibiot. *21*, 110–118 (1968a)
Nishimura, T.: Mechanism of action of phenomycin: comparative study with diphtheria toxin. J. Antibiot. *21*, 519–520 (1968b)
Nolan, R.D., Grasmuk, H., Drews, J.: The binding of tritiated elongation-factors 1 and 2 to ribosomes from Krebs II mouse ascites-tumor cells. The influence of various antibiotics and toxins. Eur. J. Biochem. *64*, 69–75 (1976)
Nomoto, A., Satoh, H., Ukita, T.: Effect of *Ricinus communis* toxin on cyclic adenosine 3′:5′-monophosphate metabolism in Yoshida ascites sarcoma cells. J. Biol. Chem. *250*, 2703–2708 (1975)
Obrig, T.G., Irvin, J.D., Hardesty, B.: The effect of an antiviral peptide on the ribosomal reactions of the peptide elongation enzymes, EF-I and EF-II. Arch. Biochem. Biophys. *155*, 278–289 (1973)
Olsnes, S.: Toxic proteins inhibiting protein synthesis. Naturwissenschaften *59*, 497–502 (1972)
Olsnes, S., Pihl, A.: Ricin a potent inhibitor of protein synthesis. FEBS Lett. *20*, 327–329 (1972a)
Olsnes, C., Pihl, A.: Treatment of abrin and ricin with β-mercaptoethanol. Opposite effects of their toxicity in mice and their ability to inhibit protein synthesis in a cell-free system. FEBS Lett. *28*, 48–50 (1972b)
Olsnes, S., Pihl, A.: Inhibition of peptide chain elongation. Nature (London) *238*, 459–461 (1972c)
Olsnes, S., Pihl, A.: Isolation and properties of abrin: a toxic protein inhibiting protein synthesis. Evidence for different biological functions of its two constituent-peptide chains. Eur. J. Biochem. *35*, 179–195 (1973a)
Olsnes, S., Pihl, A.: Different biological properties of the two constituent peptide chains of ricin, a toxic protein inhibiting protein synthesis. Biochemistry *12*, 3121–3126 (1973b)
Olsnes, S., Pihl, A.: Abrin, ricin and their associated agglutinins. In: Receptors and recognition, Ser. B. The specificity and action of animal, bacterial and plant toxins. Cuatrecasas, E., (ed.), Vol. 1, pp. 131–173. London: Chapman and Hall 1977
Olsnes, S., Heiberg, R., Pihl, A.: Inactivation of eukaryotic ribosomes by the toxic plant proteins abrin and ricin. Mol. Biol. Rep. *1*, 15–20 (1973)
Olsnes, S., Saltvedt, E., Pihl, A.: Isolation and comparison of galactose-binding lectins from *Abrus precatorius* and ricinus communis. J. Biol. Chem. *249*, 803–810 (1974a)
Olsnes, S., Refsnes, K., Pihl, A.: Mechanism of action of the toxic lectins abrin and ricin. Nature (London) *24* , 627–631 (1974b)
Olsnes, S., Pappenheimer, A.M., Meren, R.: Lectins from *Abrus precatorius* and *Ricinus communis*. II. Hybrid toxins and their interaction with chain-specific antibodies. J. Immunol. *113*, 842–847 (1974c)
Olsnes, S., Refsnes, K., Christensen, T.B., Pihl, A.: Studies on the structure and properties of the lectins from *Abrus precatorius* and *Ricinus communis*. Biochim. Biophys. Acta *405*, 1–10 (1975a)
Olsnes, S., Fernández-Puentes, C., Carrasco, L., Vázquez, D.: Ribosome inactivation by the toxin lecting abrin and ricin. I. Kinetics of the enzymic activity of the toxin A-chains. Eur. J. Biochem. *60*, 281–288 (1975b)
Olson, B.H., Goerner, G.L.: Alpha sarcin, a new antitumor agent. I. Isolation, purification, chemical composition, and the identify of a new amino acid. Appl. Microbiol. 13, 314–321 (1965)
Olson, B.H., Jennings, J.C., Roga, V., Junek, A.J., Schuurmans, D.M.: Alpha sarcin, a new antitumor agent. II. Fermentation and antitumor spectrum. Appl. Microbiol. *13*, 322–326 (1965)
Onozaki, K., Tomita, M., Sakurai, Y., Ukita, T.: The mechanism of the cytotoxicity of *Ricinus communis* phytoagglutinin toward rat ascites tumor cells. Biochem. Biophys. Res. Commun. *48*, 783–788 (1972)
Onozaki, K., Hayatsu, H., Ukita, T.: Inhibition of protein synthesis in mouse myeloma cells by *Ricinus communis* toxin. Biochim. Biophys. Acta *497*, 99–107 (1975)
Refsnes, K., Olsnes, S., Pihl, A.: On the proteins abrin and ricin. Studies of their binding to an entry into Ehrlich ascites cells. J. Biol. Chem. *249*, 3557–3562 (1974)
Schindler, D.G., Davies, J.E.: Specific cleavage of ribosomal RNA caused by alpha sarcin. Nucleic Acid Res. *4*, 1097–1110 (1977)

Schindler, D.G., Nolan, R.D., Davies, J.: Inhibition of eukaryotic protein synthesis by the antitumor protein alpha sarcin. Biochim. Biophys. Acta, in press (1977)

Sperti, S., Montanaro, L., Mattioli, A., Stirpe, F.: Inhibition of ricin of protein synthesis *in vitro*: 60S ribosomal subunit as the target of the toxin. Biochem. J. *136*, 813–815 (1973)

Sperti, S., Montanaro, L., Mattioli, A., Testoni, G.: Relationship between elongation factor 1 and elongation factor 2 dependent guanosine triphosphatase activities of ribosomes. Inhibition of both activities by ricin. Biochem. J. *148*, 447–451 (1975)

Sperti, S., Montanaro, L., Mattioli, A., Testoni, G., Stirpe, F.: Inhibition of protein synthesis *in vitro* by crotins and ricin. Effect on the steps of peptide elongation. Biochem. J. *156*, 7–13 (1976)

Stirpe, F., Pession-Brizzi, A., Lorenzoni, E., Strocchi, P., Montanaro, L., Sperti, S.: Studies on the proteins from the seeds of *Croton tiglium* and of *Jatropha curcas*. Biochem. J. *156*, 1–6 (1976)

Suits, J.P., Irvin, J.D.: The nature of the differential inhibition of polyphenylalanine synthesis in extracts from Artemia salina and rabbit reticulocytes by the *Phytolacca americana* protein. Mol. Biol. Rep. *2*, 363–367 (1976)

Tate, W.P., Caskey, C.T.: The mechanism of peptide chain termination. Mol. Cell. Biochem. *5*, 115–126 (1974)

Tomlinson, J.A., Walker, V.M., Flewett, T.H., Barclay, G.R.: The inhibition of infection by cucumber mosaic virus and influence virus by extracts from *Phytolocca americana*. J. Gen. Virol. *22*, 225–232 (1974)

Vázquez, D.: In: Inhibitors of protein biosynthesis. Berlin, Heidelberg, New York: Springer 1979

Wyatt, S., Shepherd, R.: Isolation and characterization of a virus inhibitor from *Phytolacca americana*. Phytopathology *59*, 1787–1794 (1969)

Yamaki, H., Nishimura, T., Kubota, K., Kinoshita, T., Tanaka, N.: Selective inhibition of initiation of globin synthesis by phenomycin. Biochem. Biophys. Res. Commun. *59*, 482–488 (1974)

Quinine

F.E. HAHN

Introduction

Quinine is the oldest chemotherapeutic drug still in use. The first recorded medical application of an infusion of the bark of the cinchona tree dates back to 1630 when Don Juan López de Cannizares was treated in Peru for an intermittent fever. Don Juan recommended the medication to the viceroy for the treatment of his wife, the Condesa de Chinchón. By 1639 the cinchona bark had reached Europe and became known as *Jesuits' powder*.

Quinine was isolated as an alkaloid from cinchona bark in 1820 by PELLETIER and CAVENTAU. The extensive chemical work on the elucidation of the structure and on the total synthesis of quinine has been reviewed by TURNER and WOODWARD (1953). The structure of quinine is shown in Fig. 1. Certain structure–activity relationships are discussed below.

The quinoline moiety of quinine has been incorporated into synthetic antimalarials such as the 8-aminoquinolines (SCHULEMANN, 1932), the 4-aminoquinolines (ANDERSAG et al., 1939) and a variety of experimental quinoline methanols (AINLEY and KING, 1938; WISELOGLE, 1946).

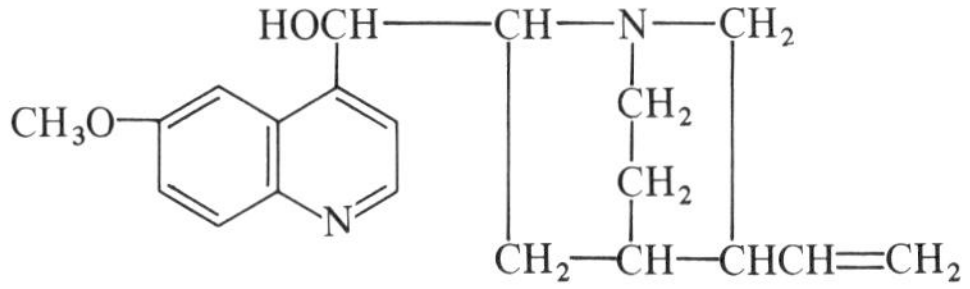

quinine: 6–methoxy–(5–vinyl–2–quinuclidyl)–4–quinolinemethanol

Fig. 1. Structure of quinine

Quinine as a Growth Inhibitor

Quinine is a highly active inhibitor of the erythrocytic forms of malarial parasites and, hence, an efficient drug for the clinical cure of malaria. The drug is also an effective gametocytocide in vivax and quartan malaria, but has little effect on the gametocytes of falciparum malaria. It is without effect

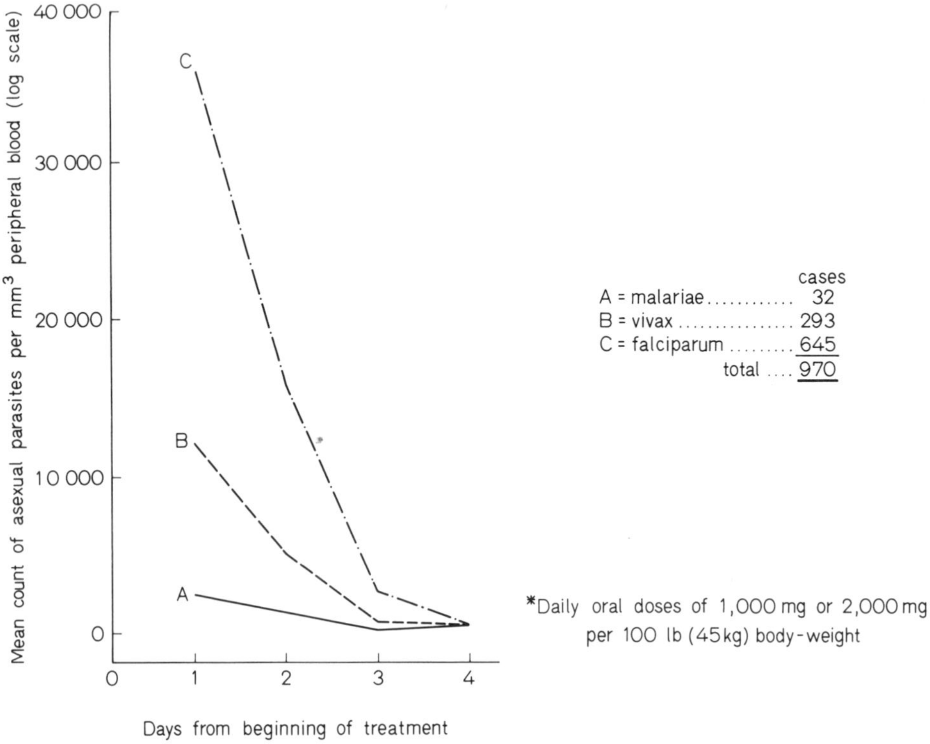

Fig. 2. Progressive disappearance of *Plasmodia* from erythrocytes of patients treated with quinine

on exoerythrocytic forms of plasmodia and on their sporozoites (GERBERG, 1971).

The progressive disappearance of plasmodia from the erythrocytes of patients, treated with 1 or 2 g of quinine per day, is shown in Fig. 2. This disappearance was first observed by ROMANOVSKY (1891) in cases of vivax malaria by using his newly developed histological stain. This is a matter of fundamental theoretical importance since it was the first demonstration of the *selective toxicity* of a chemotherapeutic drug for its target microorganism. The selective effect of quinine on intra-erythrocytic plasmodia is supported by the ability of parasitized red cells to accumulate the drug to 100–200 times the concentrations which are taken up by nonparasitized erythrocytes (POLET and BARR, 1968).

Depending upon the incubation temperature, quinine destroys the motility of the ciliate protozoan *Tetrahymena pyriformis*, at concentrations from $1.3\text{–}3.0 \times 10^{-4}$ M (CLANCY, 1968).

Little work has been reported on the effects of quinine on bacteria. At 10^{-3} M the drug inhibited the growth of *Escherichia coli*, an effect which could be partially reversed by supplying Ca^{2+} to the experimental medium (SILVERMAN, 1948). In a mass screening program quinine hydrobromide at concentrations between 10^{-3} and 10^{-4} M was found to inhibit by 50% the growth of the following microorganisms (FOLEY et al., 1959):

Lactobacillus fermenti
Lactobacillus casei
Streptococcus faecalis
Escherichia coli
Leuconostoc citrovorum
Candida albicans
Sacharomyces carlsbergensis

Since LAMBIN and BERNARD (1955) have shown that several alkaloids, including quinine, delay the onset of exponential growth of *Staphylococcus aureus* for up to 20 h, results of antibacterial screening should be viewed with caution. In fact, certain bacteria (*Pseudomonas aeruginosa* and *Bacillus anthracoides*) as well as several fungi utilize quinine as a nutrient (PRISELKOV et al., 1958). In the laboratory of this writer efforts at finding a quinine-sensitive bacterium have failed.

Quinine has been found to eliminate drug resistance genes from R-plasmids in bacteria without affecting bacterial growth at 10^{-4} M (HAHN and CIAK, 1971, 1976).

Quinidine, the diastereoisomer of quinine, decreased the number of pulsating heart muscle cells (in culture) and the frequency and magnitude of their contraction. Atrial cells were more sensitive to quinidine than ventricular cells (CAVANAUGH and CAVANAUGH, 1957).

Toxicity of Quinine

The toxic side reactions of quinine, collectively called "cinchonism", have been reviewed in great detail by FINDLAY (1951); subsequent writings are largely based upon his review. The oral LD_{50} of quinine sulfate in mice has been reported to be 1100 mg/kg (HILL, 1950), and the lethal dose of quinine dihydrochloride in rhesus monkeys is between 56 and 77 mg/kg. The lethal dose in rabbits upon i.v. injection is 208 mg/kg.

In man, the side effects of quinine are giddiness, deafness, ringing in the ears, tremors, and blurred vision. These symptoms usually disappear after the administration of the drug is discontinued, and are not serious.

The most serious toxic symptom is amblyopia which can follow excessively large doses such as from 6 to 10 g given over 2 days. This is a rare and unusual complication. The other important complication is hemoglobinuria, called "blackwater fever", which sometimes develops in patients treated with quinine for falciparum malaria.

Fatal collapse may occur as a result of intravenous injection, administered too quickly. This is produced by the ability of quinine to lower the blood pressure. Excessive doses may cause permanent impairment of sight or hearing. Recovery from single doses (orally) of 10 and 19.8 g has been reported but other patients died after single doses of 16 and 18 g. The maximal dose recommended for man is 2 g per day, i.e., 33 mg/kg for a person of 66 kg weight.

A chemotherapeutic index of ~10 would be quite unacceptable in newly developed drugs, but quinine has acquired renewed importance in the treatment of malaria caused by strains of *P. falciparum* which are resistant to 4-aminoquinolines.

Mode of Action of Quinine

Owing to the lack of a convenient test organism, mode of action studies of quinine have remained restricted to a relatively small volume of work on malarial parasites of animals. CLARKE (1952) reported that 10^{-5} M quinine dihydrochloride inhibited completely the incorporation of ^{32}P into the DNA of intra-erythrocytic *P. gallinaceum*. No dosage response correlation was established, and the author expressed her opinion that the action of quinine was "not direct, but is mediated by the host cell."

Similar experiments by SCHELLENBERG and COATNEY (1961) produced the dosage response curves shown in Fig. 3, and demonstrated that the incorporation of ^{32}phosphate into DNA was somewhat more sensitive to inhibition by quinine than its incorporation into RNA. The authors speculated that these inhibitions were "probably related more closely to inhibition of substrate utilization than to nucleic acid synthesis." However, the demonstration of typical log dosage–response curves indicates that the observed inhibitions were results of a reversible occupancy by quinine of a *drug receptor*, according to the law of mass action (HAHN, 1975).

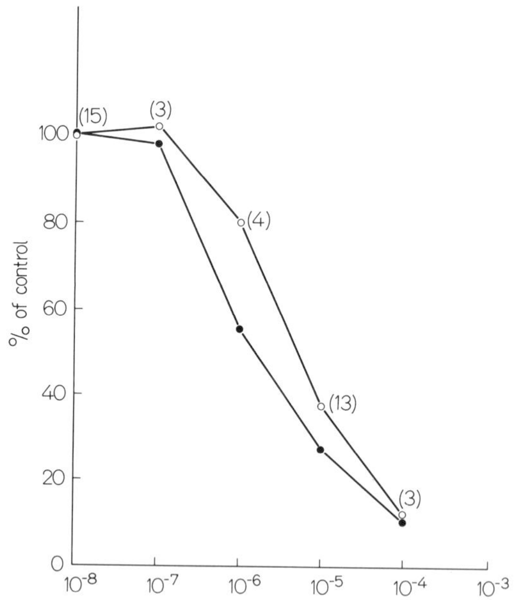

Fig. 3. Dosage–response curves of inhibitions of incorporation of ^{32}P into DNA ●, or RNA ○ of intra-erythrocytic *P. gallinaceum* (SCHELLENBERG and COATNEY, 1961)

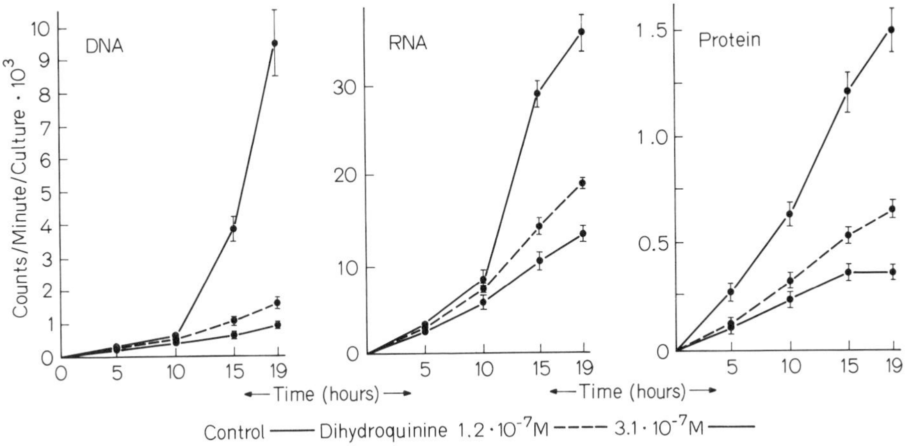

Fig. 4. Effects of quinine on biosyntheses of DNA, RNA, and protein in intra-erythrocytic *P. knowlesi* (POLET and BARR, 1968)

A more detailed and conclusive study of the effects of quinine on macromolecular biosyntheses was carried out by POLET and BARR (1968) on intra-erythrocytic *P. knowlesi* which undergoes *synchronous* schizogeny over a period of 20 hours. Dihydroquinine at 1.2 and 3.1×10^{-7} M inhibited the incorporation of tritiated orotic acid (a pyrimidine nucleotide precursor) into DNA much more strongly than into RNA. The drug also inhibited the incorporation of ^{14}C-isoleucine into the plasmodial proteins. These results are shown in Fig. 4. Citing studies from the laboratory of this writer (O'BRIEN et al., 1966) on the template toxicity of quinine in cell-free nucleic acid polymerization reactions, POLET and BARR postulated that the primary mechanism of action of quinine was an inhibition of plasmodial DNA synthesis.

The theory of HAHN et al. (1966) that quinine acts as a DNA template poison and, hence, inhibits DNA replication and RNA transcription, was also confirmed by VAN DYKE et al. (1969) in short-term experiments with *P. berghei* in rat erythrocytes. These plasmodia incorporated adenosine-8-^{3}H into their nucleic acids during 30 min incubation periods. This incorporation was inhibited by quinine, and the authors commented that the dosage response curves were "strikingly similar" to those from in vitro experiments of DNA and RNA polymerization reactions, catalyzed by bacterial enzymes and inhibited by quinine (O'BRIEN et al., 1966).

The work of VAN DYKE's group was extended to free *P. berghei* (LANTZ and VAN DYKE, 1971) which were shown to take up tritiated adenylic acid and to incorporate it into DNA and RNA. Quinine inhibited the incorporation into RNA somewhat more strongly than that into DNA but the dosage–response curves for these inhibitions indicated that higher concentrations of quinine were required than in previous experiments with intra-erythrocytic *P. berghei* (VAN DYKE et al., 1969). This is quite plausible in view of the fact that parasitized erythrocytes accumulate quinine (POLET and BARR, 1968) and, hence, provide a microculture environment in which the quinine concentration is considerably higher than in the surrounding experimental medium.

The action of quinine has also been studied in *T. pyriformis* in which cell division had been synchronized by a complicated heat treatment (CONKLIN et al., 1969). After cultures of the test organism had been subjected to seven temperature cycles, their synchronized cell division was inhibited by $2.5–5.0 \times 10^{-4}$ M quinine. Among incorporations of radioactive building blocks that of thymidine was most strongly inhibited by quinine, while incorporations of uracil, an amino acid mixture, or acetate, were considerably less affected. In a follow-up study CONKLIN and CHOU (1972) proposed that quinine inhibited the uptake of the precursors and that "this appeared to be one of the mechanisms ... for blocking precursor incorporation into DNA, RNA, and protein." The relationship between this work and the mode of action studies of quinine in plasmodia is difficult to evaluate since the determinants of permeability in plasmodia and *T. pyriformis* are not known.

Molecular Pharmacology and Structure–Activity Relationships of Quinine

Quinine inhibits the DNA-dependent DNA polymerase I and RNA polymerase reactions with calf thymus DNA as the template and enzymes, isolated from *E. coli* (O'BRIEN et al., 1966). The use of calf thymus DNA in these experiments and in other studies described in this section is justified because WALSH and SHERMAN (1968) have derived for the DNA of *P. berghei* a base composition of 40% [G+C] and 60% [A+T] which resembles the base composition of calf thymus DNA (CHARGAFF, 1955). The inhibitions could be represented by typical sigmoid-shaped log dosage–response curves with ED_{50}s of 9×10^{-4} M for DNA polymerase and 4×10^{-3} M for RNA polymerase.

Quinine shifts the melting profile of duplex DNA to higher temperatures: with 10^{-3} M quinine, the ΔT_m for calf thymus DNA was +8° (O'BRIEN et al. 1966). When the percent inhibition of the DNA polymerase reaction, caused by graded quinine concentrations, was diagrammatically represented as a function of log ΔT_m, caused by the same concentrations, the straight line in Fig. 5 was obtained (ESTENSEN et al., 1969). Since DNA synthesis requires the separation of the two companion strands of duplex DNA, the result of Fig. 5 can be interpreted to mean that the inhibition of DNA synthesis by quinine is a function of the stabilization of the double helix to forces which bring about strand separation.

Quinine gives a most general test for binding to DNA: it displaces methyl green from its complex with duplex DNA (KREY and HAHN, 1975). The formation of a DNA-quinine complex is also indicated by the hypochromic effect of DNA on the absorption spectrum of the drug. The general interpretation of such hypochromic effects is that the chromophore of a drug (in the case of quinine the quinoline moiety) is placed into a more hydrophobic molecular

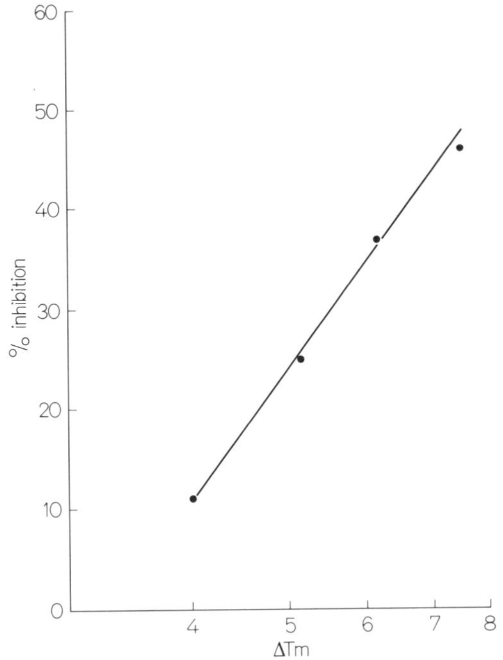

Fig. 5. Correlation between stabilization of duplex DNA to thermal strand separation (log ΔT_m) and percents inhibition of a cell-free DNA Polymerase I reaction (ESTENSEN et al., 1969)

environment which is the case for intercalation binding. The effect of DNA on the absorption spectrum of quinine is reversed by 6 M urea (O'BRIEN et al., 1966) as well as by 10^{-1} M NaCl or 10^{-2} M $MgCl_2$ (ESTENSEN et al., 1969). Evidently, ionic as well as nonpolar forces hold the DNA-quinine complex together.

By spectrophotometric indications, quinine does not interact with single-stranded DNA (ESTENSEN et al., 1969), i.e., with DNA which has been heat-denatured in the presence of formaldehyde and is unable to re-form the double-helical structure (STOLLAR and GROSSMAN, 1962). Poly dG:dC also produced a hypochromic shift in quinine's absorption spectrum but poly dA:dT and poly dI:dC had no such effect. Among polyribonucleotides only poly G caused hypochromicity in the absorption spectrum of quinine; poly G is known to possess extensive secondary structure. ESTENSEN et al. (1969) have interpreted these optical results as indications that double-strandedness and the presence of guanine are essential requirements for the binding of quinine to DNA.

The same authors have carried out spectrophotometric titrations of quinine with DNA and found that one molecule of the drug was bound per 40 base pairs of DNA with an apparent association constant of 1.5×10^5 M^{-1}. Additional quinine is bound by a weaker process to the extent of one drug molecule per 8 or 9 base pairs. At concentrations $>10^{-3}$ M, quinine precipitated DNA.

Quinine increases the viscosity but lowers the sedimentation rate of linear DNA (ESTENSEN et al., 1969). Such observations suggest that the drug is bound

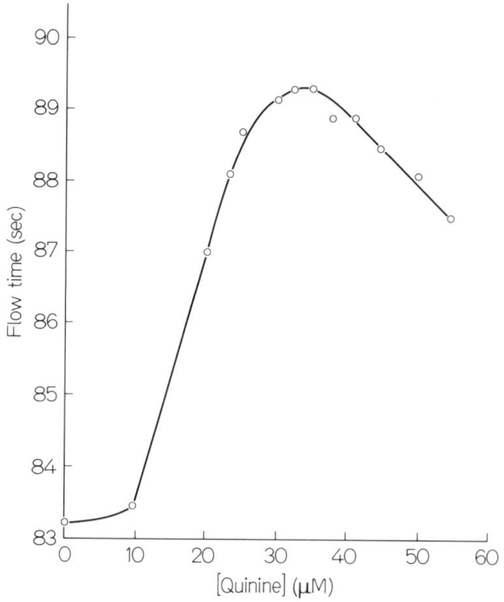

Fig. 6. Viscometric titration of circular supercoiled PM2 DNA with quinine (ALLISON and HAHN, 1977)

to DNA by intercalation. Conclusive evidence of intercalation binding has been furnished by ALLISON and HAHN (1977) who titrated closed circular supercoiled PM 2 DNA viscometrically with quinine. The results are shown in Fig. 6. The curve has the typical shape for a situation in which supercoils are progressively removed, an equivalence point is attained, and supercoils are reintroduced. Such systematic changes in superhelical density are proof of intercalation binding (WARING, 1970).

Relationships between the antimalarial activity and the structures of quinine derivatives have been reviewed by PINDER (1970). We shall discuss here only those structural features which may have a bearing on the ability of quinine to bind to DNA. Such a discussion has been published previously (HAHN and KREY, 1971).

The alcoholic hydroxyl group is probably essential for hydrogen bonding to DNA. Its elimination destroys antimalarial activity (COHEN and KING, 1938). Similarly, epimerization of this hydroxyl, yielding epiquinine, may introduce steric hindrance to hydrogen bond formation and does, in fact, result in a drastic reduction of antimalarial potency (COHEN and KING, 1938).
Changes in the distance and spatial relationship between the alcoholic hydroxyl group and the alicyclic amino nitrogen of the quinuclidine moiety should interfere with the bimodal (hydrogen and ionic) binding of quinine to DNA. In fact, breaking the bond between carbon atom 8 and the alicyclic nitrogen of the quinuclidine system destroys antimalarial activity (AINLEY and KING, 1938), while exchange of the entire quinuclidine system for -CH_2NR_2 which maintains a tertiary aliphatic amino group in the critical distance from the hydroxyl group yields compounds with significant activity (KING and WORK, 1942). Finally,

when this critical distance is provided by substituting piperidine for the quinuclidine system, a prototypical antimalarial quinoline methanol is obtained (AINLEY and KING, 1938).

In summary: studies on the molecular pharmacology of quinine and consideration of certain structure–activity relationships support the results of mode-of-action studies in plasmodia and strongly suggest that quinine acts as a DNA template poison and, hence, inhibits DNA replication and RNA transcription.

Resistance to Quinine

Experimental efforts to render various strains of animal malarias resistant to quinine have been reviewed in great detail by PETERS (1970). In the human malarias (POWELL and TIGERTT, 1968; PETERS, 1970; TIGERTT and CLYDE, 1976) genuine resistance has never been encountered. There are numerous reports, reviewed by the authors just cited, of differences in quinine sensitivity of different strains of plasmodia in different parts of the world. The continued importance of quinine as an antimalarial drug rests on its reliability, especially in cases in which infections have become resistant to synthetic antimalarials.

References

Ainley, A.D., King, H.: Antiplasmodial action and chemical constitution. II. Some simple synthetic analogs of quinine and cinchonine. Proc. R. Soc. **B 125**, 60–92 (1938)

Allison, R.G., Hahn, F.E.: Changes in superhelical density of closed circular deoxyribonucleic acid by intercalation of anti-R-plasmid drugs and primaquine. Antimicrob. Agents Chemother. **11**, 251–257 (1977)

Andersag, H., Breitner, S., Jung, H.: Verfahren zur Darstellung von in 4-Stellung basisch substituierte Aminogruppen enthaltenden Chinolinverbindungen. Ger. Pat. 683–692 (1939)

Cavanaugh, M.W., Cavanaugh, D.J.: Studies on the pharmacology of tissue cultures. I. The action of quinidine on cultures of dissociated chick-embryo heart cells. Arch. Int. Pharmacodyn. **110**, 43–55 (1957)

Chargaff, E.: Isolation and composition of the deoxypentose nucleic acids and of the corresponding nucleoproteins. In: The nucleic acids. Chargaff E., Davidson, J.N. (eds.), Vol. I. New York: Academic Press 1955

Clancy, C.F.: The lethal effect of certain antimalarial drugs on *Tetrahymena pyriformis*. Am. J. Trop. Med. Hyg. **17**, 359–363 (1968)

Clarke, D.H.: The use of phosphorus 32 in studies on Plasmodium gallinaceum. II. Studies on conditions affecting parasite growth in intact cells and in lysates. J. Exp. Med. **96**, 451–463 (1952)

Cohen, A., King, H.: Antiplasmodial action and chemical constitution. I. Cinchona alkaloidal derivatives and allied substances. Proc. R. Soc. **B 125**, 49–60 (1938)

Conklin, K.A., Chou, S.C.: The effects of antimalarial drugs on uptake and incorporation of macromolecular precursors by *Tetrahymena pyriformis*. J. Pharmacol. Exp. Ther. **180**, 158–166 (1972)

Conklin, K.A., Chou, S.C., Ramanathan, S.: Quinine: Effect on *Tetrahymena pyriformis*. I. Inhibition of synchronized cell division and site of action. Pharmacology **2**, 247–256 (1969)

Dyke, K., van, Szustkiewicz, C., Lantz, C.H., Saxe, L.H.: Studies concerning the mechanism of action of antimalarial drugs – Inhibition of the incorporation of adenosine-8-^{3}H into nucleic acids of *Plasmodium berghei*. Biochem. Pharmacol. **18**, 1417–1425 (1969)

Estensen, R.D., Krey, A.K., Hahn, F.E.: Studies on a deoxyribonucleic acid-quinine complex. Mol. Pharmacol. **5**, 532–541 (1969)

Findlay, G.M.: Toxic reactions to antimalarial drugs. Recent Adv. Chemother. **2**, 187–269 (1951)

Foley, G.E., McCarthy, R.E., Binns, V.M., Snell, E.E., Girard, B.M., Kidder, G.W., Dewey, V.C., Theyer, P.S.: A comparative study of the use of microorganisms in the screening of potential antitumor agents. Ann. N.Y. Acad. Sci. **76**, 413–441 (1959)

Gerberg, E.J.: Evaluation of antimalarial compounds in mosquito test systems. Trans. R. Soc. Trop. Med. Hyg. **65**, 358–363 (1971)

Hahn, F.E.: Structure-activity rules and the receptor hypothesis. Top. Infect. Dis. **1**, 3–14 (1975)

Hahn, F.E., Ciak, J.: Elimination of bacterial episomes by DNA-complexing compounds. Ann. N.Y. Acad. Sci. **182**, 295–304 (1971)

Hahn, F.E., Ciak, J.: Elimination of resistance determinants from R-factor R1 by intercalative compounds. Antimicrob. Agents Chemother. **9**, 77–80 (1976)

Hahn, F.E., Krey, A.K.: Interaction of alkaloids with DNA. Prog. Mol. Subcell. Biol. **2**, 134–151 (1971)

Hahn, F.E., O'Brien, R.L., Ciak, J., Allison, J.L., Olenick, J.G.: Studies on modes of action of chloroquine, quinacrine and quinine and on chloroquine resistance. Mil. Med. **131**, 1071–1089 (1966)

Hill. J.: The schizontocidal effect of some antimalarials against *Plasmodium berghei*. Ann. Trop. Med. Parasitol. **44**, 291–297 (1950)

King, H., Work, T.S.: Antiplasmodial action and chemical constitution. V. Carbinolamines derived from 6-methoxyquinoline. J. Chem. Soc. **1942**, 401–404

Krey, A.K., Hahn, F.E.: Studies on the methyl green-DNA complex and its dissociation by drugs. Biochemistry **14**, 5061–5067 (1975)

Lambin, S., Bernard, J.: Sur les modalités d'action des substances alcaloîdiques. C. R. Soc. Biol. **149**, 492–495 (1955)

Lantz, C.H., Van Dyke, K.: Studies concerning the mechanism of action of antimalarial drugs – II. Inhibition of the incorporation of adenosine-5′-monophosphate-^{3}H into nucleic acids of erythrocyte-free malarial parasites. Biochem. Pharmacol. **20**, 1157–1166 (1971)

O'Brien, R.L., Olenick, J.G., Hahn, F.E.: Reactions of quinine, chloroquine and quinacrine with DNA and their effects on the DNA and RNA polymerase reactions. Proc. Natl. Acad. Sci. USA **55**, 1511–1517 (1966)

Peters, W.: Chemotherapy and drug resistance in malaria. New York: Academic Press 1970

Pinder, R.M.: Antimalarials. In: Medicinal chemistry, 3rd ed. Part I. Burger, A. (ed.) New York Wiley & Sons 1970

Polet, H., Barr, C.F.: Chloroquine and dihydroquinine. In vitro studies of their antimalarial effect upon *Plasmodium knowlesi*. J. Pharmacol. Exp. Ther. **164**, 380–386 (1968)

Powell, R.D., Tigertt, W.D.: Drug resistance of parasites causing human malaria. Ann. Rev. Med. **19**, 81–102 (1968)

Priselkov, M.M., Samsonova, M.N., Pushkar, E.G.: Utilization of quinine and ditaine by microorganisms for biochemical purposes. Aptechn. Delo **7**, 32 (1958), through Chem. Abstr. **54**, 1655 (1960)

Romanovsky, D.L.: Specific action of quinine in malaria. Vrach (St. Petersburg) **12**, 438–440 (1891), through Zbl. Bakteriol. Parasitenkd. **11**, 219 (1892)

Schellenberg, K.A., Coatney, G.R.: The influence of antimalarial drugs on nucleic acid synthesis in *Plasmodium gallinaceum* and *Plasmodium berghei*. Biochem. Pharmacol. **6**, 143–152 (1961)

Schulemann, W.: Synthetic anti-malarial preparations. Proc. R. Soc. Med. **25**, 897–905 (1932)

Silverman, M.: Metal antagonism of the antibacterial action of atabrine and other drugs. Arch. Biochem. **19**, 193–198 (1948)

Stollar, D., Grossman, L.: The reaction of formaldehyde with denatured DNA: spectrophotometric, immunologic and enzymic studies. J. Mol. Biol. **4**, 31–38 (1962)

Tigertt, W.D., Clyde, D.F.: Drug resistance in the human malarias. In: Acquired resistance of microorganisms to chemotherapeutic drugs. Antibiotics and chemotherapy. Hahn, F.E. (ed.), Vol. 20, pp. 246–272. Basel: Karger 1976

Turner, R.B., Woodward, R.B.: The chemistry of the cinchona alkaloids. In: The alkaloids, chemistry and physiology III. p. 1 New York: Academic Press 1953

Walsh, C.J., Sherman, I.W.: Isolation, characterization and synthesis of DNA from a malaria parasite. J. Protozool. **15**, 503–508 (1968)

Waring, M.: Variations of the supercoils in closed circular DNA by binding of antibiotics and drugs: evidence for molecular models involving intercalation. J. Mol. Biol. **54**, 247–279 (1970)

Wiselogle, F.Y. (ed.): A survey of antimalarial drugs 1941–1945. Vol. I, p. 142. Ann Arbor: J.W. Edwards 1946

Showdomycin

D.W. VISSER and S. ROY-BURMAN

Introduction

Summaries of showdomycin and its mode of action by ROY-BURMAN (1970), SUHADOLNIK (1970), and VISSER (1975) have appeared previously. This review will concern primarily the mode of action of showdomycin reported subsequent to the previous reviews.

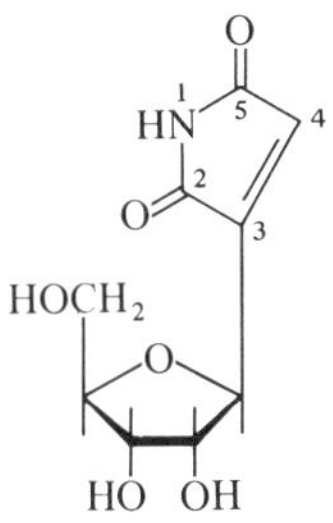

Fig. 1. Structure of showdomycin

Showdomycin was isolated from culture filtrates of *Streptomyces showdoensis* by NISHIMURA et al. (1964). Its isolation, physical and chemical properties, and activity as a broad spectrum inhibitor of gram-positive and gram-negative bacteria have been summarized by SUHADOLNIK (1970). The antibiotic is also active against cultured HeLa cells (MATSUURA et al., 1964) and Ehrlich ascites tumor in mice (MATSUURA et al., 1964; NISHIMURA et al., 1964).

The structure of showdomycin was shown to be 3-(β-D-ribofuranosyl)-maleimide (Chem. Abstr. 1 H-pyrrole-2,5-dione, 3 β-D-ribofuranosyl) based on spectroscopic studies, chemical transformations and x-ray chrystallographic examinations (DARNALL et al., 1967; NAKAGAWA et al., 1967). The chemical structure of the nucleoside antibiotic is related to uridine and pseudouridine. The maleimide moiety of showdomycin reacts in a manner similar to the sulfhydryl reagent, N-ethylmaleimide and its nucleoside-like structure is the basis for site-directed interactions with certain enzymes and transport sites.

Mechanism of Action

Recent publications have substantiated early experimental evidence (NISHIMURA and KOMATSU, 1968; ROY-BURMAN et al., 1968) that the inhibitory effects of showdomycin result from a rapid reaction of its maleimide moiety with accessible sulfhydryl groups of proteins. Several reports have also appeared which confirm the original observations (KOMATSU and TANAKA, 1968; NISHIMURA and KOMATSU, 1968) that the nucleoside structure of showdomycin may also be related to its biologic activity. Based on information from these recent studies it is probable that the random interaction of the antibiotic with sulfhydryl groups is the primary cause of its cytotoxic effects. The effects related to its nucleoside structure, however, are of considerable interest and are reviewed in a subsequent section of this review.

Thiotropic Nature of Showdomycin

The behavior of showdomycin is very similar to that of N-ethylmaleimide with respect to its mode of reaction with thiols (WATNABE, 1970), its ability to induce radiosensitization (TITANI and KATSUBE, 1969; TITANI and TSURUTA, 1974) and its synergism with alkylating agents (TITANI and KATSUBE, 1970). Recent studies have shown that reactivity of maleimides with sulfhydryl groups is greatly influenced by the nature and position of ring substituents particularly at the carbon-carbon double bond (MIYADERA and KOSOWER, 1972; TITANI and TSURUTA, 1974). For example, citraconimide (3-methylmaleimide) has a much closer structural relationship with showdomycin than with N-ethylmaleimide, but is considerably less active both in chemical and biologic reactions than showdomycin or N-ethylmaleimide (TITANI and TSURUTA, 1974). The extent to which substituted maleimides react with cellular sulfhydryl groups of *E. coli* does not correlate well with inhibitory effects on cell growth (TITANI and TSURUTA, 1974). Showdomycin triacetate, which reacts with cellular sulfhydryl groups faster and more completely than showdomycin, is much less active than showdomycin as an antimicrobial agent (TITANI and TSURUTA, 1974). The bicyclic maleimide antibiotic maleimycin (3-aza-6-hydroxybicyclo[3.3.0] oct-$\Delta^{1,5}$-ene-2,4-dione) which reacts with sulfhydryl groups more slowly than showdomycin, is 20 times more inhibitory than showdomycin against *Microbacterium phlei* (ELSTNER et al., 1973). These results may be attributed to differences in transport rates of the maleimide compounds and may also reflect interactions of showdomycin at the active sites of certain enzymes.

The usefulness of showdomycin as a therapeutic agent may be limited by its rapid and nonspecific interaction with sulfhydryl groups, resulting in its removal from circulation and limiting its ability to interact at specific enzyme and transport sites. Synthetic derivatives of showdomycin with a lower thiotropic character are therefore of considerable interest. Based on the evidence that substitution of a methyl group at the carbon–carbon double bond of the maleimide ring reduces markedly its thiotropic character. MIYADERA and KOSOWER

(1972) suggested 4-methyl showdomycin as a potentially interesting analog. It may be predicted that this derivative would have low reactivity with sulfhydryl groups while possibly retaining specificity for active sites of enzymes.

Several synthetic procedures for the synthesis of showdomycin and showdomycin derivatives have been reported recently (TRUMMLITZ and MOFFATT, 1973; TRONCHET, 1975; TRUMMLITZ et al., 1975; KALVODA, 1976), subsequent to the first synthetic procedure reported by KALVODA et al., 1970. These important contributions provide procedures for the synthesis of showdomycin derivatives, such as 4-methylshowdomycin (TRUMMLITZ et al., 1975), with low reactivity for sulfhydryl groups. Although retention of specificity for enzyme and transport sites by these derivatives is less predictable than reactivity towards sulfhydryl groups, such analogs are of particular interest because of their potential to produce covalent bonds at active site centers before they are removed from general circulation by nonspecific interactions with sulfhydryl groups.

Showdomycin as a Nonspecific Sulfhydryl Reagent

Showdomycin has been used as a convenient nonspecific sulfhydryl reagent in several recent studies. The induction of an ATP-energized mitochondrial volume change, which occurs when mitochondria are exposed to carcinogens or their metabolic products in the presence of showdomycin, has been reported in a number of recent publications (HADLER and DANIEL, 1972, 1973; HADLER and DEMETRIOU, 1975; HADLER et al., 1971). Neither showdomycin nor the carcinogen alone produces the mitochondrial volume changes. The authors suggest that the carcinogen results in exposure of mitochondrial sulfhydryl groups which then interact with showdomycin or other sulfhydryl reagents.

Showdomycin strongly inhibits the attachment of elongation factor EF-1 to ribosomes, and to a lesser extent impairs the binding of elongation factor EF-2 from Krebs II mouse ascites cells (NOLAN et al., 1975). Similar inhibitory effects on the binding of these elongation factors from Ehrlich ascites cells are also produced by N-ethylmaleimide. Showdomycin and a large number of other sulfhydryl reagents enhance the activity of peptidyl transferase of eukaryotic ribosomes (CARRASCO and VÁZQUEZ, 1975). Adenosine transport is irreversibly inhibited when freshly obtained rabbit lung macrophages are exposed to showdomycin (STRAUSS, 1974). This inhibitory effect on adenosine transport and the stimulatory effects of serum on cells treated with showdomycin can also be demonstrated using p-chloromercuribenzosulfonic acid instead of the antibiotic.

Specific Effects of Showdomycin in Biologic Systems

The observation that nucleosides reverse the inhibitory effects of showdomycin in *E. coli* was the first evidence indicating that the structure of the antibiotic may be related to its inhibitory effects (KOMATSU and TANAKA, 1968; NISHIMURA and KOMATSU, 1968). Several recent reports have confirmed and extended specific effects of showdomycin in biologic systems which may be related to its nucleoside-like structure.

The existence of a cysteine residue at or near the active site of the enzyme ($Na^+ + K^+$)-ATPase, prompted an investigation of showdomycin as a possible nucleotide-site-directed inhibitor of this enzyme (TOBIN and AKERA, 1975). It was found that showdomycin produces an irreversible time-dependent inhibition of ($Na^+ + K^+$)-ATPase from rat brain. Although inhibition of the enzyme showed the same general characteristics as N-ethylmaleimide, their data indicate some specificity of showdomycin for the active site, since N-ethylmaleimide is much less effective than showdomycin at low concentrations. In addition, micromolar concentrations of ATP protected against inhibition by showdomycin much more effectively than against inhibition by N-ethylmaleimide. It was suggested that the protective effect of ATP is due to direct shielding of the showdomycin binding site by ATP and that showdomycin inhibits ($Na^+ + K^+$)-ATPase by preferential interaction with sulfhydryl groups at the nucleotide binding site on this enzyme. The authors proposed that this behavior of showdomycin should afford specific labeling of the nucleotide-binding sites of this enzyme by either showdomycin or perhaps, even more effectively, by its 5′-phosphorylated derivative.

Inhibition of thymidylate synthetase by showdomycin is another interesting example of its selective affinity for active sites of enzymes (KALMAN, 1972). The antibiotic was found to produce a rapid and irreversible inactivation of thymidylate synthetase prepared from dichloromethotrexate resistant *Lactobacillus casei*. Pretreatment of the enzyme with dUMP protected against the inhibitory effect. Showdomycin-5′-phosphate is about ten times more effective than the unphosphorylated antibiotic, presumably because the nucleotide has a preferred substrate-like specificity. The results suggest that the maleimide moiety of showdomycin alkylates a reactive sulfhydryl group at the active site of thymidylate synthetase. This conclusion is consistent with the recent evidence (BELLISARIO et al., 1976; DANNENBERG and HEIDELBERGER, 1976) that the functional nucleophile is an enzymic sulfhydryl group which participates in the formation of a transient thioether linkage between thymidylate synthetase and position-6 of the nucleotide. The existence of an electrophilic carbon adjacent to the glycosyl bond of showdomycin which is analogous to carbon-6 of dUMP is also consistent with the above conclusion. If showdomycin-5′-phosphate is bound at the active site, the sulfhydryl group, which is presumably alkylated by carbon-4 of the maleimide ring, must be close to carbon-6 of dUMP when it is bound to the enzyme. Based on the above evidence it is predictable (KALMAN, 1972) that 2′-deoxyshowdomycin-5′-phosphate would be a much more potent inhibitor of thymidylate synthetase than is showdomycin-5′-phosphate, since the existence of a 2′-hydroxyl group is known to decrease the affinity of the substrate for the enzyme.

PINNEY et al. (1974) investigated the ability of showdomycin to induce thymineless conditions in *E. coli* by comparison of showdomycin with analogs such as 5-fluorodeoxyuridine and inhibitors of dihydrofolate reductase. 5-Fluorodeoxyuridine and antifolates are known to induce thymineless conditions which, like thymine starvation, result in the elimination of a plasmid (R factor 1818) in *E. coli*. The authors showed that, unlike 5-fluorodeoxyuridine, inhibition by showdomycin is only partially reversed by thymidine. In addition, showdomycin does not cause R factor elimination. They concluded that showdomycin does not produce thymineless conditions in vivo even though the antibiotic inhibits thymidylate synthetase in vitro (KALMAN, 1972). These results are consistent with the known ability of showdomycin to interact rapidly and nonspecifically with all accessible sulfhydryl groups and support the concept that these nonspecific effects are the predominant cause of its cytotoxic effects (see previous section). The ability of thymidine to reverse partially the inhibitory effect of showdomycin may be due to competition of thymidine for transport of showdomycin into the cells.

It has been reported that a showdomycin-resistant mutant of *E. coli* excretes RNA which induces a heritable change in *Agrobacterium tumefaciens* β_6, a bacterium which carries the oncogenic principle for tumor induction in plants (BELJANSKI et al., 1972a). The resulting transformants partially or completely lose their capacity for tumor induction in plants and synthesize new ribosomes whose components are "profoundly modified." Interpretation of these results is difficult, particularly since it has been demonstrated recently that a large plasmid DNA is required for virulence of *Agrobacterium tumefaciens* on dicotyledonous plants (CHILTON et al., 1977). Viable bacteria are required for tumor induction, but development of the tumor appears to be dependent upon incorporation of plasmid DNA into the plant cells. The extensive alteration in ribosomal RNA of *Agrobacterium tumefaciens* transformants reported by BELJANSKI et al. (1972a) is similar to previous reports by these authors that showdomycin-resistant mutants of *E. coli* have extensively modified RNA types. These earlier findings have been reviewed (VISSER, 1975). BELJANSKI et al. (1972b) also reported the isolation of showdomycin-resistant KB cells. The morphological appearance and growth rate of these transformed cells are similar to normal cells, but the transformed cells produce 28S and 18S RNA which were reported to be markedly different from those produced by normal cells.

Several recent studies have established that the entry of showdomycin into *E. coli* cells has an absolute requirement for nucleoside transport systems. KOMATSU (1971a) demonstrated that [^{14}C]-labeled showdomycin is rapidly transported into *E. coli* K-12 and that its transport is inhibited by several nucleosides but not by purines or pyrimidines. These results provide evidence that the antibiotic is transported by a system which is unique for nucleosides. Independent evidence in support of this conclusion was provided by ROY-BURMAN et al. (1971), who demonstrated that showdomycin inhibits uptake of sugars and amino acids in *E. coli* B and that this inhibition is reversed by preincubation with cysteine and common nucleosides except guanosine, deoxyguanosine, and pseudouridine.

The above investigations relate the nucleoside-like structure of showdomycin to its transport and provided the basis for subsequent studies on mechanisms of nucleoside and showdomycin transport. These transport studies were facilitated by the availability of showdomycin-resistant mutants which were shown to lack the capacity to transport the antibiotic (KOMATSU, 1971b; ROY-BURMAN and VISSER, 1972). These transport-defective mutants were isolated after exposure of *E. coli* K-12 to N-methyl-N′-nitro-N-nitrosoguanidine (KOMATSU, 1971b), or after exposure of *E. coli* B/r (TITANI and TSURUTA, 1974) or *E. coli* B to showdomycin (ROY-BURMAN and VISSER, 1972). The *E. coli* K-12 and *E. coli* B mutants are resistant to high concentrations of showdomycin, but retain their sensitivity to N-ethylmaleimide (KOMATSU, 1971b; ROY-BURMAN and VISSER, 1972; TITANI and TSURUTA, 1974). The mutant cells lack the ability to transport showdomycin (KOMATSU, 1971b; ROY-BURMAN and VISSER, 1972), and this defect is reflected in a diminished capacity to transport most of the commonly occurring nucleosides (KOMATSU, 1971b; KOMATSU and TANAKA, 1972; ROY-BURMAN and VISSER, 1972; KOMATSU, 1973; KOMATSU and TANAKA, 1973; VON DIPPE et al., 1973; ROY-BURMAN and VISSER, 1975; VON DIPPE et al., 1975; LEUNG and VISSER, 1977). The transport of purine and pyrimidine bases, sugars, and amino acids is identical in mutant and parent cells (KOMATSU, 1971b; ROY-BURMAN and VISSER, 1972; ROY-BURMAN and VISSER, 1975; LEUNG and VISSER, 1977).

Evidence that *E. coli* K-12 has two deoxyguanosine transport systems (KOMATSU and TANAKA, 1972), two deoxycytidine transport systems (KOMATSU and TANAKA, 1972, 1973), and three adenosine transport systems (KOMATSU, 1973), one each of which is defective in the showdomycin-resistant mutant, has been reported. The authors concluded that showdomycin is transported in *E. coli* K-12 by a system which is common for a wide variety of nucleosides, and that other transport systems for these nucleosides exist which are more specific for the individual nucleosides.

A showdomycin-resistant mutant of *E. coli* B exhibits nucleoside transport defects which are similar to those reported for the *E. coli* K-12 mutant except that guanosine and deoxyguanosine transport is unimpaired in the *E. coli* B mutant (ROY-BURMAN and VISSER, 1972). The apparent retention of a fraction of the nucleoside transport systems by the *E. coli* B and *E. coli* K-12 mutants has been questioned for the following reasons. It is known that nucleosides are rapidly degraded by nucleoside deaminase and phosphorylase enzymes in the periplasmic space of *E. coli.* The purines and pyrimidines produced in the medium by these enzymatic activities may be transported by systems which are separate from those involved in transport of intact nucleosides (VON DIPPE et al., 1973, 1975; ROY-BURMAN and VISSER, 1975; LEUNG and VISSER, 1977). Therefore, the observed uptake of radioactivity from [^{14}C]-labeled nucleosides is not an accurate measurement of nucleoside transport by either *E. coli* B or the mutants because total uptake of radioactivity reflects transport of intact nucleoside as well as transport of uracil, adenine, guanine, xanthine or hypoxanthine released into the medium by action of the periplasmic enzymes.

Ambiguities for uridine transport have been circumvented by comparisons of the uptake of [2-^{14}C]uridine and [U-^{14}C]uridine and by the use of mutants which lack the ability to transport uracil (VON DIPPE et al., 1973; LEUNG and VISSER, 1977). The results showed that the *E. coli* B showdomycin-resistant mutant completely lacks the ability to transport the intact nucleosides, but its ability to transport uracil is the same as that in *E. coli* B. Tetrahydrouridine, an inhibitor of cytidine and deoxycytidine deaminase, has also been used to limit degradation of these nucleosides in the periplasmic space. The results showed that deoxycytidine transport by *E. coli* B has the characteristics of a single transport system which is lost in the showdomycin-resistant mutant (VON DIPPE et al., 1975). Cytidine was reported to be transported by two systems in *E. coli* B, both of which are defective in the showdomycin-resistant mutant (LEUNG and VISSER, 1977). These studies also demonstrated the existence of a transport process in which only the ribose moiety of uridine is transported into the cell while uracil, in an approximate equimolar amount, is released into the medium. The showdomycin-resistant mutant lacks the ability to transport both intact uridine and the ribose moiety of uridine (LEUNG and VISSER, 1977).

Differences in nucleoside transport characteristics of the showdomycin-resistant mutants of *E. coli* B and *E. coli* K-12 may be due to the differences in strains used or ambiguities in the assay procedures. All of the studies, however, clearly show that showdomycin enters *E. coli* cells by specific nucleoside transport systems with a high degree of specificity. As discussed above, the antibiotic behaves predominantly as a sulfhydryl reagent after it is transported into the cell. It is of interest that transport-defective mutants may be selected in the presence of the antibiotic. Since showdomycin is not subject to enzymatic phosphorylation or phosphorolysis, its transport into the cell is the only apparent means by which resistance to its nonspecific interaction with a large number of sulfhydryl-containing enzymes and proteins can occur. Advantages in the use of showdomycin-resistant mutants and other transport-deficient mutants for studies of the complex processes involved in nucleoside transport have been demonstrated (LEUNG and VISSER, 1977). Additional studies of transport characteristics using showdomycin-resistant mutants which result from single gene mutations may provide more definitive information concerning the nature of these processes.

References

Beljanski, M., Beljanski, M., Manigault, P., Bourgarel, P.: Transformation of *Agrobacterium tumefaciens* into a non-oncogenic species by an *Escherichia coli* RNA. Proc. Natl. Acad. Sci. USA *69*, 191–195 (1972a)

Beljanski, M., Bonissol, C., Kona, P.: Showdomycin induced transformation of KB cells. C. R. Acad. Sci. Ser. D *274*, 3116–3119 (1972b) through Chem. Abstr. *77*, 97216a (1972b)

Bellisario, R.L., Maley, G.F., Galivan, J.H., Maley, F.: Amino acid sequence at the FdUMP binding site of thymidylate synthetase. Proc. Natl. Acad. Sci. USA *73*, 1848–1852 (1976)

Carrasco, L., Vázquez, D.: The involvement of SH groups in the peptidyl transferase center of eukaryotic ribosomes. Eur. J. Biochem. *50*, 317–323 (1975)

Chenon, M.T., Pugmire, R.J., Grant, D.M., Panzica, R.P., Townsend, L.B.: Carbon-13 NMR spectra of C-nucleosides: Showdomycin and β-pseudouridine. J. Heterocycl. Chem. *10*, 427–429 (1973)

Chilton, M.D., Merlo, D., Gordon, M.P., Drummond, M., Sciaky, D., Montoya, A., Nester, E.: Crown gall tumors. Stable incorporation of plasmid DNA into a eucaryotic genome. Abstr. Am. Soc. Microbiol. *38*, (1977)

Dannenberg, P.V., Heidelberger, C.: The effect of Raney nickel on the covalent thymidylate synthetase-5-fluoro-2′-deoxyuridylate-5,10-methylenetetrahydrofolate complex. Biochemistry *15*, 1331–1337 (1976)

Darnall, K.R., Townsend, L.B., Robins, R.K.: The structure of showdomycin, a novel carbon-linked nucleoside antibiotic related to uridine. Proc. Natl. Acad. Sci. USA *57*, 548–553 (1967)

Dippe, P.J. von, Roy-Burman, S., Visser, D.W.: Transport of uridine in *Escherichia coli* and a showdomycin-resistant mutant. Biochim. Biophys. Acta *318*, 105–112 (1973)

Dippe, P.J. von, Leung, K-K., Roy-Burman, S., Visser, D.W.: Deoxycytidine transport in the presence of a cytidine deaminase inhibitor and the transport of uracil in *Escherichia coli* B. J. Biol. Chem. *250*, 3666–3671 (1975)

Elstner, E.F., Carnes, D.M., Suhadolnik, R.J., Kreishman, G.P., Schweizer, M.P., Robins, R.K.: Isolation, structural elucidation, biological properties, and biosynthesis of maleimycin, a new bicyclic maleimide antibiotic isolated from the culture filtrates of *Streptomyces showdoensis*. Biochemistry *12*, 4992–4997 (1973)

Hadler, H.I., Daniel, B.G.: The *in vitro* interaction of a metabolite of N-acetyl-4-aminobiphenyl with rat liver mitochondria. Cancer Res. *32*, 1037–1041 (1972)

Hadler, H.I., Daniel, B.G.: A correlation between the carcinogenicity of isomeric N-hydroxy-N-acetylaminofluorenes and their *in vitro* effect on mitochondria. Cancer Res. *33*, 117–122 (1973)

Hadler, H.I., Demetriou, J.M.: The disturbance of oxidative phosphorylation by N-acetoxy-N-acetyl-2-aminofluorene, a model ultimate carcinogen. J. Antibiot. *28*, 809–818 (1975)

Hadler, H.I., Daniel, B.G., Pratt, R.D.: The induction of ATP energized mitochondrial volume changes by carcinogenic N-hydroxy-N-acetylaminofluorenes when combined with showdomycin. A unitary hypothesis for carcinogenesis. J. Antibiot. *24*, 405–417 (1971)

Kalman, T.I.: Inhibition of thymidylate synthetase by showdomycin and its 5′-phosphate. Biochem. Biophys. Res. Commun. *49*, 1007–1013 (1972)

Kalvoda, L.: Simple preparative synthesis of showdomycin. J. Carbohydrates Nucleosides Nucleotides *3*, 47–55 (1976)

Kalvoda, L., Farkaš, J., Šorm, F.: Synthesis of showdomycin. Tetrahedron Lett. *26*, 2297–2300 (1970)

Komatsu, Y.: Mechanism of action of showdomycin. Part IV. Interactions between the mechanisms for transport of showdomycin and of various nucleosides in *Escherichia coli*. Agric. Biol. Chem. *35*, 1328–1339 (1971 a)

Komatsu, Y.: Mechanism of action of showdomycin. V. Reduced ability of showdomycin-resistant mutants of *Escherichia coli* K-12 to take up showdomycin and nucleosides. J. Antibiot. *24*, 876–883 (1971 b)

Komatsu, Y.: Adenosine uptake by isolated membrane vesicles from *Escherichia coli* K-12. Biochim. Biophys. Acta *330*, 206–221 (1973)

Komatsu, Y., Tanaka, K.: Mechanism of action of showdomycin. Part I. Effect of showdomycin on the synthesis of nucleic acids and proteins in Escherichia coli K-12. Agric. Biol. Chem. *32*, 1021–1027 (1968)

Komatsu, Y., Tanaka, K.: A showdomycin-resistant mutant of *Escherichia coli* K-12 with altered nucleoside transport character. Biochim. Biophys. Acta *288*, 390–403 (1972)

Komatsu, Y., Tanaka, K.: Deoxycytidine uptake by isolated membrane vesicles from *Escherichia coli* K-12. Biochim. Biophys. Acta *311*, 496–506 (1973)

Leung, K-K., Visser, D.W.: Uridine and cytidine transport in *Escherichia coli* B and transport-deficient mutants. J. Biol Chem. *252*, 2492–2497 (1977)

Matsuura, S., Shiratori, O., Katagiri, K.: Antitumor activity of showdomycin. J. Antibiot. Ser. A *17*, 234–237 (1964)

Miyadera, T., Kosower, E.M.: Receptor site labeling through functional groups. II. Reactivity of maleimide groups. J. Med. Chem. *15*, 534–537 (1972)

Nakagawa, Y., Kano, H., Tsukuda, Y., Koyama, H.: Structure of a new class of C-nucleoside antibiotic, showdomycin. Tetrahedron Lett. *42*, 4105–4109 (1967)

Nishimura, H., Komatsu, Y.: Reversal of inhibiting action of showdomycin on the proliferation of *Escherichia coli* by nucleosides and thiol compounds. J. Antibiot. *21*, 250–254 (1968)

Nishimura, H., Mayama, M., Komatsu, Y., Kato, H., Shimaoka, N., Tanaka, Y.: Showdomycin, a new antibiotic from a *Streptomyces* Sp. J. Antibiot. Ser. A *17*, 148–155 (1964)

Nolan, R.D., Grasmuk, H., Drews, J.: The binding of tritiated elongation factors 1 and 2 to ribosomes from Krebs II mouse ascites tumor cells. Eur. J. Biochem. *50*, 391–402 (1975)

Pinney, R.J., Bremer, K., Smith, J.T.: R factor elimination by inhibitors of thymidylate synthetase (fluorodeoxyuridine and showdomycin) and the occurrence of single strand breaks in plasmid DNA. Mol. Gen. Genet. *133*, 163–174 (1974)

Roy-Burman, P.: Recent results in cancer research. Analogues of nucleic acid components. Mechanism of action, Vol. 25, p. 80. Berlin, Heidelberg, New York: Springer 1970

Roy-Burman, S., Visser, D.W.: Transport studies of showdomycin, nucleosides and sugars in *Escherichia coli* B and in showdomycin-resistant mutants. Biochim. Biophys. Acta *282*, 383–392 (1972)

Roy-Burman, S., Visser, D.W.: Transport of Purines and Deoxyadenosine in *Escherichia coli*. J. Biol. Chem. *250*, 9270–9275 (1975)

Roy-Burman, S., Roy-Burman, P., Visser, D.W.: Showdomycin, a new nucleoside antibiotic. Cancer Res. *28*, 1605–1610 (1968)

Roy-Burman, S., Huang, Y.H., Visser, D.W.: Inhibition of amino acid and sugar transport by showdomycin. Biochem. Biophys. Res. Commun. *42*, 445–453 (1971)

Strauss, P.R.: Effects of serum on membrane transport: II. Serum and the stimulation of adenosine transport, a possible mechanism. J. Cell Biol. *60*, 571–585 (1974)

Suhadolnik, R.J.: Nucleoside antibiotics: maleimide nucleosides, p. 393. New York: Wiley-Interscience of John Wiley & Sons, Inc. 1970

Titani, Y., Katsube, Y.: Radiosensitization of *Escherichia coli* B/r by showdomycin. Biochim. Biophys. Acta *192*, 376–369 (1969)

Titani, Y., Katsube, Y.: Enhancement of the lethal effect of 2,2′-dichlorodiethylamine on *Escherichia coli* by thiol-binding agents. Biochim. Biophys. Acta *208*, 310–316 (1970)

Titani, Y., Tsuruta, Y.: Some chemical and biological characteristics of showdomycin. J. Antibiot. *27*, 956–962 (1974)

Tobin, T., Akera, T.: Showdomycin, a nucleotide-site-directed inhibitor of $(Na^+ + K^+)$-ATPase. Biochim. Biophys. Acta *389*, 126–136 (1975)

Tronchet, J.M.J.: Synthesis of new types of C-nucleosides. Biol. Med. *4*, 83–104 (1975)

Trummlitz, G., Moffatt, J.G.: C-glycosyl nucleosides. III. A facile synthesis of the nucleoside antibiotic, showdomycin. J. Org. Chem. *38*, 1841–1845 (1973)

Trummlitz, G., Repke, D.B., Moffatt, J.G.: C-glycosyl nucleosides: VIII. Synthesis of 3-methylshowdomycin. J. Org. Chem. *40*, 3352–3356 (1975)

Visser, D.W.: Showdomycin, 5-hydroxyuridine and 5-aminouridine. In: Handbook of experimental pharmacology. Sartorelli, A.C., Johns, D.G. (eds.), Vol. 38, pp. 373–383. Berlin, Heidelberg, New York: Springer 1975

Watanabe, S.: Equimolecular reaction of showdomycin with thiols. J. Antibiot. *23*, 313–314 (1970)

Streptonigrin

N.S. MIZUNO

I. Biological Activity

Streptonigrin (Fig. 1), a metabolite produced by *Streptomyces flocculus*, was first isolated by RAO and CULLEN (1959–60). Its activity as a broad spectrum antibiotic was summarized in a previous review (BHUYAN, 1967). A method for the biological assay of streptonigrin in biological fluids based on its antibiotic activity against *Bacillus subtilis* ATCC6633 has been developed by PITTILLO and WOOLLEY (1974). Exposure to streptonigrin caused a first-order decline in the viability of bacteria, implying that only one hit per cell is required for lethality (LEVINE and BORTHWICK, 1963a). Streptonigrin is also an excellent inducer of bacteriophage production in lysogenic bacteria while inhibiting the net synthesis of host DNA (LEVINE and BORTHWICK, 1963a; MUSCHEL and SCHMOKER, 1966). A marked increase in genetic recombination was observed during a mixed bacteriophage infection in presence of the drug (LEVINE and BORTHWICK, 1963b).

Streptonigrin exhibited antitumor activity against Sarcoma 180, Adenocarcinoma 755, Lewis lung carcinoma, Ridgway osteogenic sarcoma, Walker 256 carcinosarcoma, spontaneous mouse mammary carcinoma (OLESON et al., 1961; REILLY and SIGIURA, 1961), and human tumor (HS No. 1) grown in rats (TELLER et al., 1961). The drug also inhibited viral tumors, such as Rauscher murine (MCBRIDE et al., 1966), Friend (EBERT et al., 1968) leukemia, and thymic lym-

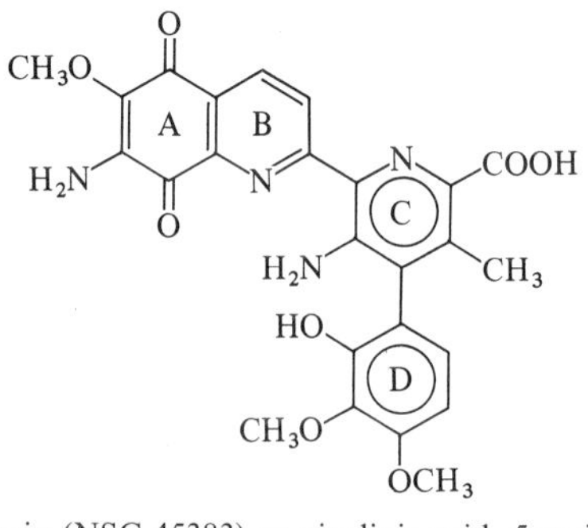

Fig. 1. Structure of streptonigrin (NSC-45383) or picolinic acid, 5-amino-6-(7-amino-5,8-dihydro-6-methoxy-5,8-dioxo-2-quinolyl)-4-(2-hydroxy-3,4-dimethoxyphenyl)-3-methyl

phoma (HAYS, 1974). It inhibited the replication of oncorna virus in vitro and in vivo (CHIRIGOS et al., 1965, 1973a, b; FURUSAWA et al., 1976). O'CONNER et al., (1975) showed that a concentration of streptonigrin which was not cytotoxic to cells inhibited the cell transformation with oncorna virus. The inhibition did not involve cellular polymerases, but the reverse transcriptase of the virus was found to be markedly inhibited (CHIRIGOS et al., 1973b), suggesting that this may be the mechanism whereby streptonigrin inhibited type C RNA virus expression. RNA synthesis in cells chronically infected with murine sarcoma or Moloney pseudotype virus was not inhibited by streptonigrin, but viral replication was diminished (WOODS et al., 1973). Streptonigrin was also shown to inhibit the in vitro transformation of high passage (>60) rat embryo cells by 3-methylcholanthrene (PRICE et al., 1974).

When streptonigrin was added to cultures of human leukocytes, it inhibited mitosis and caused the production of chromosomal breaks and other abnormalities (COHEN, 1963, 1969; COHEN et al., 1963). Streptonigrin-induced breaks were significantly increased in chromosome No. 1, and the distribution of the gaps was nonrandom. The centromeric segments of chromosomes No. 1 and No. 2 were highly susceptible to breakage in contrast to the corresponding region in chromosome No. 3. The telomer region of all chromosomes and the short arm of chromosome No. 2 were relatively resistant to the action of streptonigrin. NASJLETI and SPENCER (1967) also noted that there were frequently polyploidy and endo-reduplication of chromosomes. In the lateral roots of the broad bean, *Vicia faba*, streptonigrin induced subchromatid exchanges in early prophase cells, chromatid type aberrations in cells in late or middle interphase, and chromosome type exchange in early interphase (KIHLMAN, 1964; KIHLMAN and ODMARK, 1965). The effect of streptonigrin on chromosomes was not suppressed by anoxia or by inhibitors of oxidative phosphorylation (KIHLMAN, 1964). In chick embryos, streptonigrin inhibited prophase of mitosis in erythropoietic cells (GIRALDI et al., 1967). When streptonigrin was added to cells in meiosis (mouse ovum), it caused achromatic gaps, chromosome breaks at low concentrations and an agglutination of chromosomes at higher concentrations (JAGEILLO, 1967). PUCK (1964) reported that streptonigrin did not affect tissue culture cells when added after the completion of DNA synthesis, i.e., at late interphase or G_2 cycle. However cells which were synthesizing DNA at the time of drug addition showed chromosomal abnormalities and a large delay in reaching mitosis.

A single intraperitoneal injection of streptonigrin administered on the 5th–17th day of gestation produced malformation in the fetus which included exencephaly, encephalocele, cleft palate and lips, and deformed trunk, appendages, and tail (WARKANY and TAKACS, 1968; CHAUBE et al., 1969). Streptonigrin produced chromosomal breakage far more extensively in embryonic tissue culture cells than in vivo, leading SOUKUP et al., (1967) to speculate that chromosome protection and DNA repair mechanism may be more efficient in the intact animal. Streptonigrin inhibited chlorophyll synthesis and caused the production of irreversibly bleached organisms of *Euglena gracilis* (EBRINGER, 1972). It also produced back mutation when added to a hypoxanthine-less strain of the ascomycete *Ophiostoma multiannulatum* (ZETTERBERG and KIHLMAN, 1965).

When tritiated streptonigrin was added to tissue culture, and DNA, RNA and protein fractions extracted from the cells, the highest concentration of the label was associated with the DNA fraction (MIZUNO, 1965). Similar results were reported with the use of tritiated bruneomycin (streptonigrin) by PADRON et al. (1974). When an intravenous dose of tritiated methyl ester of streptonigrin was administered to human subjects, the half-time of the drug in circulation was 1.8 ± 0.23 h. At zero time the drug was distributed in a volume approaching total body water ($61 \pm 10\%$ body wt.). At the end of 24 h $18.5 \pm 0.7\%$ of the dose was excreted in the urine. Analysis of the tumor tissue obtained by biopsy showed that the drug was found in the highest concentration in the nuclear fraction (MIZUNO and HUMPHREY, 1964). After an intraperitoneal injection of tritiated methyl ester of streptonigrin to mice bearing sarcoma 180, 65% of the drug was excreted at the end of the first 24 h and 90% by the end of 48 h after the injection (MIZUNO, 1966). A study of tissue distribution of the label showed that the highest concentration occurred in the small intestine. The remainder of the organs were divided into three groups in the order of descending concentration: liver, spleen, sarcoma, large intestine > lung, kidney, stomach, muscle, skin, blood cells > plasma, heart, brain (MIZUNO, 1966).

II. Chemical Activity

Some of the chemical properties of streptonigrin were summarized in a previous review (BHUYAN, 1967). The structure (Fig. 1) assigned to streptonigrin by RAO et al., (1963) was confirmed by X-ray diffraction analysis (CHIU and LIPSCOMB, 1975). It is a monobasic acid and is readily susceptible to reversible two-electron reduction. Considerable interest has been paid to its aminoquinone moiety since this group is also present in other antitumor agents: mitomycin C, porfiromycin, rifamycin and geldanamycin. In order to gain insight into the relationship between the structure of streptonigrin and its antitumor activity, DRISCOLL et al. (1974) synthesized various derivatives of quinolinedione, a partial structure of streptonigrin, by altering substituents at C-2, C-6 and C-7 and assaying the compounds with a variety of experimental tumors (Table 1). It can be seen that no analog was as active as streptonigrin (Entry No. 1293). The 7-amino compound (Entry No. 1250) was active, while the 6-amino analog (entry No. 1249) was inactive. Acetylation or dialkylation of the 7-amino group reduced the activity. The 6,7-diamino derivative (Entry No. 1286) was completely inactive. The 7-amino-6-methoxy-5,8-quinolinequinone (Entry No. 1274) possessed low antitumor activity. However, LOWN and SIM (1976) reported that in presence of NADH and metal ions, it behaved quite similarly to streptonigrin by undergoing reduction followed by metal complex formation and autoxidation. Since the total activity of streptonigrin could not be duplicated by 7-amino-6-methoxy-5,8-quinolinequinone, other structural elements must be essential for its action.

RAO et al. (1974) have summarized the derivatives of streptonigrin which have been prepared (Fig. 2). Replacement of the amine group in ring A by

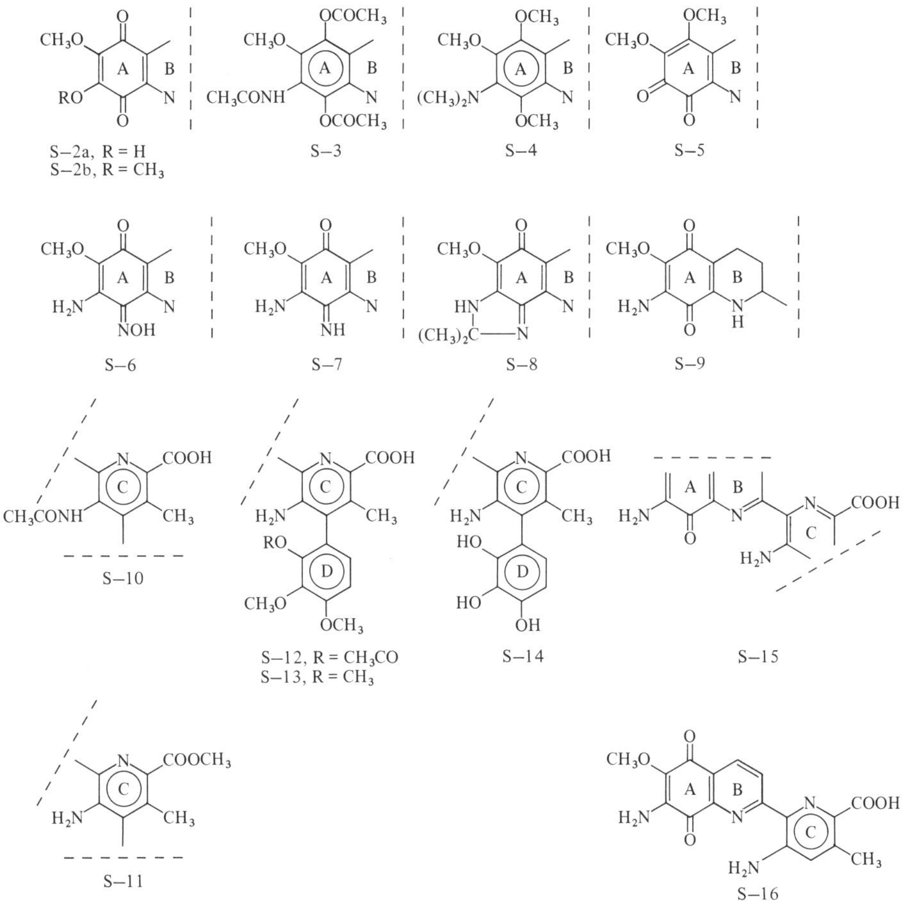

Fig. 2. Derivatives of streptonigrin (RAO, 1974)

OH (S-2a) or OCH_3 (S-2b), reductive acetylations (S-3) or reductive methylation (S-4) or the conversion of S-4 to S-5 all produced inactive compounds. The monoxime (S-6) was weakly active, and upon reduction and oxidation it formed azastreptonigrin (S-7) which had activity comparable to that of streptonigrin. Isopropylideneazastreptonigrin (S-8) had no activity in inhibiting the growth of bacteria, virus (CHIRIGOS et al., 1973b) and tissue culture cells (MIZUNO, 1967), however it had a low antitumor effect which was demonstrable after raising the dose to 100 times that of streptonigrin (KREMER and LASZLO, 1967). Its teratogenic activity was reduced to 1/53rd that of streptonigrin (CHAUBE et al., 1969). Since masking the aminoquinone structure greatly reduced the biological effect of streptonigrin, the presence of this group in streptonigrin appears to be essential for its maximum activity. In ring B, the hydrogenation to a tetrahydro derivative (S-9) resulted in a loss of activity. In ring C, acetylation of the amine group (S-10) gave an inactive compound. Esterification of the carboxy group produced the methyl ester of streptonigrin (S-11) which did

Table 1. Streptonigrin analogs[a]

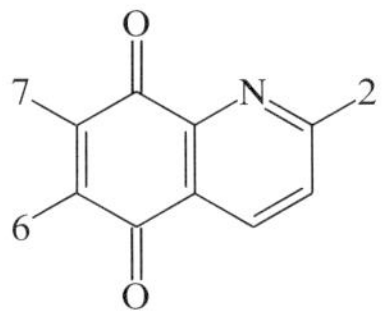

Entry No.	7	6	2	In vivo ILS or TWI (%)[b]				ED_{50} µg/ml[c]
				L1210	W-256	CA-755	S-180	
1247	H	H	H	toxic	24		30	
1249	H	NH_2	H	5	14		8	
1250	NH_2	H	H	0	55	13	29	2
1252	$NHCOCH_3$	H	H		26	12	45	
1253	H	$N(CH_3)_2$	H	0	0		0	
1254	$N(CH_3)_2$	H	H	3	25		0	
1257	H	OCH_3	H	0	29		0	
1260	Br	NH_2	H	0	35			
1261	Br	OCH_3	H	2	11			
1263	Cl	NH_2	H	0	16	0	40	0.36
1270	Cl	OCH_3	H		28	30	15	
1271	NH_2	NH_2	H		45	21	40	
1274	NH_2	OCH_3	H	0	18		0	
1276	OCH_3	$N(CH_3)_2$	H	0	25		0	
1277	$N(CH_3)_2$	OCH_3	H		15	23	28	
1278	N_3	OCH_3	H		45	35	13	
1279	OCH_3	$NHCOCH_3$	H	0	0		0	
1282	O^-	py[d]	H		45	4	49	
1283	SCH_3	NH_2	H	0	7		40	
1286	OCH_3	OCH_3	H	0	0		0	
1290	Br	OCH_3	CH_3		47			
1291	NH_2	OCH_3	CH_3		27			
1293[e]	NH_2	OCH_3	Het[f]	18	85	96		
1294[e]	NH_2	OCH_3	Het	15	60	95	70	
1295[e]	NH_2	OH	Het		47	36	toxic	
1296[e]	NH_2	OCH_3	Het		95	30	25	

[a] Table from DRISCOLL et al. (1974). For molecular formula corresponding to entry number, consult the original paper.

[b] ILS = increase of life span in leukemia-bearing mice. TWI = tumor weight inhibition of solid tumors.

[c] ED_{50} = µg/ml of drug which inhibits growth by 50%.

[d] Pyridinium.

[e] 1293 is streptonigrin; 1294 is streptonigrin methyl ester; 1295 is 6–OH analog of streptonigrin; 1296 is an isomeric form of streptonigrin.

[f] Heterocyclic ring.

not differ qualitatively from streptonigrin in biological activity. However in comparison to streptonigrin it had 1/100th the cytotoxic action (MIZUNO, 1967), 1/500th the antiviral activity (CHIRIGOS et al., 1973b), 1/3rd the activity in inhibiting DNA polymerase of C-type RNA virus (CHIRIGOS et al., 1973a), 1/55th the teratogenic activity (CHAUBE et al., 1969), and 1/2 the inhibitory effect on the energy metabolism of leukemic blood cells (KREMER and LASZLO, 1966). These results indicated that a carboxyl group in ring C was essential for maximum activity. The similarity of the effects of streptonigrin and streptonigrin methyl ester could not be explained on the basis of hydrolysis of the latter to the former since no free streptonigrin could be detected in cell extracts (MIZUNO, 1967) nor in the urine of individuals who received intravenous injections of streptonigrin methyl ester (MIZUNO and HUMPHREY, 1964). Acetylation (S-12) or methylation (S-13) of the phenolic hydroxyl of ring D did not abolish activity while complete demethylation of ring D (S-14) gave an inactive compound. Based on the above observations, RAO et al. (1974) proposed a molecular fragment which embodied the elements that are required for the biological activity of streptonigrin (S-15). A tricyclic analog which contained the S-15 structure (S-16) has been synthesized. It was shown to possess antibiotic activity against *Bacillus subtilis*. Data on its antitumor activity are not yet available.

The three dimensional structure of streptonigrin may be an important factor in the interaction of the drug with tissue constituents, and it may be of significance in the elucidation of the nature of its binding to DNA. CHIU and LIPSCOMB (1975) reported the existence of a large, nearly coplanar, region in the streptonigrin molecule which included rings A, B and C. This suggested intercalation as a possible mode of binding of streptonigrin to DNA, however the absence of hypochromic spectral shift, and lack of changes in T_m or viscosity rendered this unlikely (MIZUNO and GILBOE, 1970). ZEE-CHENG and CHENG (1970) observed among a number of non-alkylating antileukemic agents, including streptonigrin, a particular structural feature which was common to all. This consisted of an N atom with two O atoms with more or less definite interatomic distances between them. The N–O–O triangular region was suggested as a common receptor site for binding of the antitumor agents to macromolecules.

III. Mechanism of Action

The experimental data on the biochemical effects of streptonigrin in biological systems indicate interference with one of the following mechanisms: (1) DNA synthesis and (2) respiratory metabolism.

A. DNA Synthesis

Streptonigrin caused a rapid degradation of DNA which was attributed to single-strand breaks when added to cultures of *Salmonella typhimurium* (LEVINE and BORTHWICK, 1963a) or *B. subtilis* (SZYBALSKI, 1964). RADDING (1963) reported the breakdown of *Escherichia coli* DNA into acid-soluble material when the bacteria were grown in the presence of streptonigrin. When *E. coli* cells, in which the DNA was previously labeled with thymine, were exposed to streptonigrin, there was a large loss of radioactivity into the medium, mainly in the form of thymine or thymidine (WHITE and WHITE, 1968). Single-strand breaks were also induced in PM2 covalently-closed-circular DNA when it was exposed to streptonigrin reduced in situ (CONE et al., 1976). The dependence of this reaction on oxygen will be discussed later. Since 7-amino-6-methoxy-5, 8-quinolinequinone also cleaved PM2 covalently-closed-circular DNA, this moiety of streptonigrin was proposed to be responsible for DNA degradation in vivo (LOWN and SIM, 1976). MIKHAILOV and GAUSE (1974) reported that the mitochondria of unfertilized loach eggs incorporated negligible amounts of labeled deoxyribonucleoside triphosphates into DNA. However in presence of bruneomycin (streptonigrin), the uptake increased 30–50 fold. The uptake was exclusively by open ring molecules, i.e., molecules in which one strand is broken, indicating that activation of DNA synthesis was probably due to the induction of single-strand breaks. Streptonigrin did not affect the normal replication of mitochondrial DNA, but most likely stimulated DNA repair synthesis. Single-strand DNA breaks may also be invoked in the stimulation of phage production in lysogenic bacteria by streptonigrin (SZYBALSKI, 1964). Breaks in the DNA molecule will have to be postulated in order to explain the increased frequency of genetic recombination in streptonigrin-treated bacteriophage (LEVINE and BORTHWICK, 1963b).

Streptonigrin inhibited the uptake of labeled precursors by DNA, RNA and protein in tissue culture cells (MIZUNO, 1965; YOUNG and HODAS, 1965). The degree of depression was similar in DNA and RNA synthesis, and both were proportional to streptonigrin concentration. The decrease in protein synthesis appeared to be a secondary effect, occurring later and to a lesser extent than that of the nucleic acids. Streptonigrin also inhibited the incorporation of P^{32}-phosphate into DNA in excised *V. faba* roots (KIHLMAN and ODMARK, 1965). Uptake of P^{32}-phosphate by RNA was also affected but to a lesser extent.

IYER and SZYBALSKI (1964) and MIZUNO and GILBOE (1970) reported that the amount of binding of streptonigrin to DNA was not influenced by use of reducing conditions ($NaBH_4$ and N_2). There were at least two types of binding of streptonigrin to DNA in vitro: one, which was reversible by dialysis and the other, which was irreversible (MIZUNO and GILBOE, 1970). The stable bound streptonigrin was estimated to be 1 mol/2,000 mol deoxynucleotides. More streptonigrin was bound to denatured DNA, apurinic DNA and poly dC·poly dG than to native DNA. Intercalation was unlikely to be the mode of binding of streptonigrin to DNA because of lack of hyperchromic shift in the absorption spectrum of DNA-streptonigrin mixture, and the absence of changes in T_m and viscosity of DNA exposed to streptonigrin (MIZUNO and GILBOE, 1970). When DNA was treated with H^3-streptonigrin and the complex hydrolyzed enzymatically, the highest concentration of radioactivity was with the dCMP fraction. With synchronized tissue culture cells, streptonigrin was bound preferentially to DNA during the S (DNA synthesis) period of the cell cycle (MIZUNO and GILBOE, 1970). However WHITE and WHITE (1966) found that when salmon sperm or *Escherichia coli* DNA were exposed to streptonigrin under reducing conditions, there was an interaction which resulted in DNA with increased T_m and decreased sedimentation rate in sucrose density gradient centrifugation. No change in the viscosity of DNA was observed unless excess sodium borohydride was used. On the other hand, no change in T_m or bouyant density in CsCl density gradient centrifugation was found in DNA which was treated with reduced streptonigrin in vitro (MIZUNO and GILBOE, 1970) or in DNA which was isolated from streptonigrin-treated *E. coli* cells (MILLER et al., 1967).

Streptonigrin inhibited the incorporation of radioactive nucleoside triphosphates into RNA in vivo (OBERDISSE and NEUBERT, 1967) or in a cell-free RNA polymerase system (E.C. 2.7.7.6) in vitro (MIZUNO, 1965). The inhibition was reversible by the addition of undenatured DNA, but not by RNA or denatured DNA. Streptonigrin also inhibited the uptake of H^3-TTP by DNA in vitro.

B. Respiratory Metabolism

Streptonigrin catalyzed the oxidation of intra and extra-mitochondrial NADH and of extra-mitochondrial TPNH, with the concomitant formation of H_2O_2 (HOCHSTEIN et al., 1965). It was postulated that streptonigrin underwent a repeated cycle of reduction by NADH followed by metal complexation and auto-oxidation to the quinoid form with the production of H_2O_2. Its cytotoxic effect was attributed to the depletion of NADH and TPNH and to the formation of H_2O_2. While the production of H_2O_2 could be demonstrated in vitro, it could not be detected in vivo even when a lethal dose of streptonigrin was used (WHITE and WHITE, 1968). Therefore it is unlikely that H_2O_2 is the reactive species which was responsible for the degradation of DNA. Moreover, phenazine methosulfate which caused production of more H_2O_2 than streptonigrin in *E. coli* was not cytotoxic to the cells (WHITE and WHITE, 1968). Instead, phenazine methosulfate protected the cells against damage by streptonigrin by competing for electrons and preventing the reduction of the latter. Also it was shown that millimolar concentrations of hydrogen peroxide do not cause strand breaks in DNA (MORGAN et al., 1976), therefore it was assumed that a peroxy-free radical or a peroxide other than hydrogen peroxide was the cytotoxic species formed in vivo.

Intracellular streptonigrin can be reduced in the presence of an electron source, such as glucose (WHITE and DEARMAN, 1965). The presence of an electron source is essential for the antibacterial activity of streptonigrin. Cyanide, which facilitated the reduction of streptonigrin enhanced its lethality. Phenazine methosulfate, an auto-oxidizable electron scavenger which presumably would compete for electrons, antagonized the antibiotic action of streptonigrin. Oxygen was also necessary for the full lethal effect of streptonigrin. By electron spin resonance, WHITE and DEARMAN (1965) observed the spectra of free radicals in streptonigrin-treated cultures. The lifetime of these radicals was prolonged under anaerobic conditions. Recently it was shown that streptonigrin reduced in situ by NADH produced single-strand cleavage in covalently-closed-circular DNA. This reaction could be completely inhibited by superoxide dismutase (E.C. 1.15.1.1) (CONE et al., 1976). It was suggested that a more likely reactive species for degradation of DNA was the superoxide radical, or the hydroxyl radical.

The following reactions were proposed for the mechanism of reduction of streptonigrin (Cone et al., 1976):

$$SN + NADH + H^+ \rightarrow SNH_2 + NAD^+ \quad (1)$$

$$SNH_2 + O_2 \rightarrow SNH^{\cdot} + HO_2^{\cdot} \quad (2)$$

$$HO_2^{\cdot} \leftrightarrow O_2^{\cdot} + H^+ \quad (3)$$

$$2O_2^{\cdot} + 2H^+ \rightarrow H_2O_2 + O_2 \quad (4)$$

$$2H_2O_2 \rightarrow 2H_2O + O_2 \quad (5)$$

$$O_2^{\cdot} + H_2O_2 \rightarrow OH^{\cdot} + OH^- + O_2 \quad (6)$$

Streptonigrin which was reduced by NADH (reaction 1) is envisaged to be subsequently oxidized by O_2 to form semiquinone and hydroxyl-free radicals (reaction 2). When streptonigrin was added to cultures of *E. coli* or *Bacillus megaterium*, evidence for the semiquinone free radical formation was obtained (Ishizu et al., 1968). Both superoxide dismutase (E.C. 1.15.1.1) and catalase (E.C. 1.11.1.6) inhibited the DNA nicking effect by streptonigrin on covalently-closed-circular DNA and were suggested to be part of the cellular defense mechanism (Cone et al., 1976). The former catalyzed reaction 4 while the latter catalyzed reaction 5. Both enzymes would reduce the rate of reaction 6, and therefore decrease the formation of hydroxyl radical ($OH^{\cdot}$) which is a possible candidate for the damaging species which directly interacts with DNA. NADH oxidation and perioxide formation were inhibited by the addition of EDTA (Miller et al., 1967). The addition of Cu^{2+} and Fe^{2+}, but not Co^{2+} was found to stimulate the cleavage of covalently-closed-circular DNA by streptonigrin in presence of O_2 and NADH (Lown and Sim, 1976). The presence of O_2 enhanced the lethality of streptonigrin to *E. coli* (Gregory and Fridovich, 1973). Aerobically grown cells were more susceptible to the oxygen enhancement of streptonigrin toxicity than anaerobically grown cells in which superoxide dismutase synthesis had been induced (Hassan and Fridovich, 1977). In a mutant strain of green alga, resistance to the lethal effects of hyperbaric O_2 was correlated with resistance to streptonigrin and increased levels of superoxide dismutase (Pulich, 1974). It was possible to substitute 7-amino-6-methoxy-5, 8-quinolinequinone for streptonigrin in the cleavage reaction of covalently-closed-circular DNA (Lown and Sim, 1976), demonstrating the involvement of the aminoquinone moiety of the streptonigrin molecule in its activity. The bacteriocidal effect of streptonigrin is similar to that of mitomycin C, which also possesses an aminoquinone group (Iyer and Szybalski, 1964). Both antibiotics are synergized by agents such as cyanide, phenyl alcohol and carbonyl cyanide phenylhydrazone, all of which facilitate reduction. Both are antagonized by phenazine methosulfate. Both induce phage production in lysogenic bacteria. Mitomycin is also reduced intracellularly, and it has been shown to cause crosslinkage of DNA. No crosslinks have been observed in DNA with streptonigrin (Iyer and Szybalski, 1964; Miller et al., 1967; Mizuno and Gilboe, 1970).

The addition of streptonigrin to rat liver mitochondria resulted in a P/O of zero, and its oxidative phosphorylation was completely uncoupled (Hochstein et al., 1965). Levels of ATP as well as protein synthesis were decreased in leukemic leukocytes treated with streptonigrin (MILLER et al., 1967), however ATP was reported to be unchanged in *V. faba* which was exposed to the drug (KIHLMAN and ODMARK, 1965).

C. Bruneomycin (Streptonigrin)

Bruneomycin is an antibiotic which was isolated from the culture fluid of *Actinomycete albus var. bruneomycini* in USSR by BRAZHNIKOVA et al. in 1968. Its molecular weight, absorption and infra-red spectra, countercurrent distribution, and R_f in paper and thin-layer chromatography systems were found to be indistinguishable from those of streptonigrin, and bruneomycin was determined to be identical to streptonigrin. However, since the name "bruneomycin" continues to be used in Russian literature, studies reported on bruneomycin are summarized in this separate section. It is not a unique predicament to find that there is some discrepancy between the published work on bruneomycin and that on streptonigrin. The compound will be designated bruneomycin (streptonigrin) to indicate its interchangeability. Bruneomycin (streptonigrin) induced the development of phage in lysogenic *Micrococcus lysodeickticus* (DUDNIK, 1965), and caused marked degradation of DNA in vivo (DUDNIK and GAUSE, 1966). Since DNA degradation was prevented at a low temperature (2° C), it was suggested that the breakdown was mediated by the action of enzymes. Bruneomycin (streptonigrin) did not inhibit DNA or induce DNA degradation in vitro. *E. coli* B mutants with an impaired capacity for the repair of DNA damage by ultraviolet light had increased sensitivity to the action of bruneomycin (streptonigrin) according to DUDNIK et al. (1971). GAUSE and MIKHAILOV (1973) reported that mitochondria isolated from unfertilized loach eggs (*Misgurnus fossilis*) did not incorporate H^3-TTP into DNA, but when treated with bruneomycin (streptonigrin) there was a marked uptake. This was attributed to production in covalently closed-circular DNA of mitochondria of single-breaks which served as starting points for DNA synthesis. The radioactivity was found exclusively in the open circular molecules. Mitochondria of the mature loach oocyte are capable of DNA replicative synthesis (MIKHAILOV and GAUSE, 1976). When these oocytes were incubated with H^3-dATP in presence of 5-bromodeoxyuridine and the DNA isolated and separated by ethidium bromide-CsCl density gradient centrifugation, it was shown that the labeled DNA was covalently joined to unlabeled DNA fragments. The results indicated that bruneomycin (streptonigrin) did not induce DNA replication in the mitochondria, but stimulated the DNA repair process. After administration of bruneomycin (streptonigrin) to rats, glycogenolysis activity and ATP levels in the liver were found to be depressed (GOLDBERG and SALNIK, 1975). Bruneomycin (streptonigrin) had low activity on lymphatic leukosis tumor (SHORIN and BAZHANOV, 1974). It had a myelo-inhibitory effect in mice which received an LD_{50} dose of the drug (ANTIPOV et al., 1975). Decreased serotonin levels were found in blood, brain, liver and enterochromaffin cells of mice which were injected with bruneomycin (streptonigrin) (BAUMANIS et al., 1973). DUDNIK et al. (1973) could find no evidence of the binding of bruneomycin (streptonigrin) to DNA. The drug had no effect on the melting profiles of DNA or on the sedimentation rate in alkaline sucrose gradient. It was also not found to inhibit the activity of DNA-dependent RNA polymerase.

References

Antipov, I.G., Navitsky, V.V., Goldberg, E.D.: Myeloinhibitory effect of some antitumor antibiotics and its comparative estimation. Antibiotiki **20**, 897–902 (1975)

Baumanis, E.A., Elksnite, J.E., Liepinia, V.A.: Effect of antibiotic preparation on the enzymes of serotonin metabolism in the liver of mice. Vopr. Onkol. **19**, 36–39 (1973)

Bhuyan, B.K.: Phleomycin, xanthomycin, streptonigrin, nogalomycin and aurantin. In: Antibiotics, mechanism of action. Gottlieb, D., Shaw, P.D. (eds.), Vol. I, pp. 175–176. Berlin, Heidelberg, New York: Springer 1967

Brazhnikova, M.G., Ponomarenko, V.I., Kovsharova, I.N., Kruglyak, E.B., Proshlyakova, V.V.: Study of bruneomycin produced by *Act. Albus var. bruneomycini,* and its identification with streptonigrin. Antibiotiki **13**, 99–102 (1968)

Chaube, S., Kuffer, F.R., Murphy, M.L.: Comparative teratogenic effects of streptonigrin (NSC-45383) and its derivates in the rat. Cancer Chemother. Rep. **53**, 23–31 (1969)

Chirigos, M.A., Luber, E., March, R., Pettigrew, H.: Antiviral chemotherapeutic assay with Friend leukemia virus in mice. Cancer Chemother. Rep. **45**, 29–33 (1965)

Chirigos, M.A., Pearson, J.W., Papas, T.S., Woods, H.B., Jr., Spahn, G.: Effect of streptonigrin (NSC-45383) and analogs on oncorna replication and DNA polymerase. Cancer Chemother. Rep. **57**, 305–309 (1973a)

Chirigos, M.A., Pearson, J., Spahn, G., Rutman, R.: Current studies on oncorna virus therapy. Bibl. Haematol. **39**, 1208–1219 (1973b)

Chiu, Y.Y., Lipscomb, W.N.: Molecular and crystal structure of streptonigrin. J. Am. Chem. Soc. **97**, 2525–2530 (1975)

Cohen, M.M.: Thee specific effects of streptonigrin activity on human chromosomes in culture. Cytogenetics **2**, 271–279 (1963)

Cohen, M.M.L: The interaction of various drugs with human chromosomes. Can. J. Genet. Cytol. **11**, 1–24 (1969)

Cohen, M.M., Shaw, M.W., Craig, A.P.: The effects of streptonigrin on cultured human leukocytes. Proc. Natl. Acad. Sci. USA **50**, 16–24 (1963)

Cone, R., Hasan, S.K., Lowan, J.W., Morgan, A.R.: The mechanism of the degradation of DNA by streptonigrin. Can. J. Biochem. **54**, 219–223 (1976)

Driscoll, J.S., Hazard, G.F., Jr., Wood, H.B., Jr., Goldin, A.: Structure-antitumor activity relationships among quinone derivatives. Cancer Chemother. Rep. **4**, (Pt 2, No 2), 1–362 (1974)

Dudnik. J.V.: Induction of lysogenic *Micrococcus lysodiekticus* by antibiotics with the ability to affect DNA synthesis. Antibiotiki **2**, 112–117 (1965)

Dudnik, J.V., Gause, G.G.: Mechanism of bruneomycin action. Fed. Proc. **25**, 1109–1112 (1966)

Dudnik, J.V., Netyksa, E.M., Varik, O.Y.: Increased antibacterial effect of bruneomycin and sibiromycin in cultures with impaired reparation of DNA. Antibiotiki **16**, 487–491 (1971)

Dudnik, J.V., Gause, G.G., Karpov, V.L., Kozmyan, L.I., Padron, F.: On interaction in vitro of bruneomycin (streptomycin) with DNA. Antibiotiki **18**, 968–973 (1973)

Ebert, P.S., Chirigos, M.A., Ellsworth, P.A.: Differential response of Friend leukemia virus and lactate dehydrogenase virus to chemotherapy and in vitro neutralization. Cancer Res. **28**, 363–367 (1968)

Ebringer, L.: Are plastids derived from prokaryotic microorganisms? Action of antibiotics on chloroplasts of *Euglena gracilus*. J. Gen. Microbiol. **71**, 35–52 (1972)

Furusawa, E., Furusawa, S., Lee, J.V.B., Petanavanich, S.: Therapeutic activity of pretazettine, a narcissus alkaloid on Rauscher leukemia; comparison with tazettine and streptonigrin. Proc. Soc. Exp. Biol. Med. **152**, 186–191 (1976)

Gause, G.G., Jr., Mikhailov, V.S.: State of DNA synthesizing system in isolated mitochondria from the mature egg of the loach (*Misgurnus fossilis*). Biochem. Biophys. Acta **324**, 189–198 (1973)

Giraldi, A., Carco, F.P., Giraldi, M., Novati, M.: Antimitotic activity of streptonigrin. G. Ital. Chemioter. **14**, 13–19 (1967)

Goldberg, E.D., Salnik, G.A.: Bruneomycin effect on energy metabolism of liver tissue in experiment. Antibiotiki **20**, 66–71 (1975)
Gregory, E.M., Fridovich, I.: Oxygen toxicity and the superoxide dismutase. J. Bacteriol. **114**, 1193–1197 (1973)
Hassan, H.M., Fridovich, I.: Enzymatic defenses against the toxicity of oxygen and of streptonigrin in *E. coli.* J. Bacteriol. **129**, 1574–1583 (1977)
Hays, E.F.: Metabolic inhibitors and viral lymphomagenesis in thymic grafts. J. Natl. Cancer Inst. **53**, 561–566 (1974)
Hochstein, P., Laszlo, J., Miller, D.: A unique, dicumarol-sensitive, non-phosphorylating oxidation of DPNH and TPNH catalyzed by streptonigrin. Biochem. Biophys. Res. Commun. **19**, 289–295 (1965)
Ishizu, K., Dearman, H.H., Huang, M.T., White, J.R.: Electron paramagnetic resonance observation on biogenic semiquinone and 5-methyl phenylphenazinum radicals. Biochem. Biophys. Acta **165**, 283–285 (1968)
Iyer, V.N., Szybalski, W.: Mitomycins and porfiromycin: chemical mechanism of activation and cross-linkeng of DNA. Science **145**, 55–58 (1964)
Jagiello, G.: Streptonigrin effect on the first meiotic metaphase of the mouse egg. Science **157**, 453–454 (1967)
Kihlman, B.A.: The production of chromosomal aberrations by streptonigrin in *Vicia faba.* Mutat. Res. **1**, 54–62 (1964)
Kihlman, B.A., Odmark, G.: Deoxyribonucleic acid synthesis and the production of chromosomal aberrations by streptonigrin, 8-ethoxycaffeine and 1,3,7,9-tetramethyluric acid. Mutat. Res. **2**, 494–505 (1965)
Kremer, W.B., Laszlo, J.: Biochemical effects of the methyl ester of streptonigrin. Biochem. Pharmacol. **15**, 1111–1118 (1966)
Kremer, W.B., Laszlo, J.: Comparison of biochemical effects of isopropylidine azastreptonigrin (NSC-62709) with streptonigrin (NSC-45383). Cancer Chemother. Rep. 52, 19–24 (1967)
Levine, M., Borthwick, M.: The action of streptonigrin on bacterial DNA metabolism and on induction of phage production in lysogenic bacteria. Virology **21**, 568–574 (1963a)
Levine, M., Borthwick, M.: The action of streptonigrin on genetic recombination between bacteriophages. Proc. 11th Int. Congr. Genet., Netherlands: The Hague 1963b
Lown, J.W., Sim, S.K.: Studies related to antitumor antibiotics. Part VIII Cleavage of DNA by streptonigrin analogues and the relationship to antineoplastic activity. Can. J. Biochem. **54**, 446–452 (1976)
Mcbride, T.J., Oleson, J.J., Woolf, D.: The activity of streptonigrin against the Rauscher murine leukemia virus in vivo. Cancer Res. **26**, 727–732 (1966)
Mikhailov, V.S., Gause, G.G.: The DNA-synthesizing system of isolated mitochondria of unfertilized loach eggs and its artificial activation in vitro by the antibiotic bruneomycin. Mol. Biol. **8**, 108–118 (1974)
Mikhailov, V.S., Gause, G.G.: Repair of damage caused by bruneomycin to DNA in isolated mitochondria of mature loach oocytes. Dokl. Akad. Nauk. SSSR **229**, 1477–1480 (1976)
Miller, D.S., Laszlo, J., McCarty, K.S., Guild, W.R., Hochstein, P.: Mechanism of action of streptonigrin in leukemic cells. Cancer Res. **27**, 632–638 (1967)
Mizuno, N.S.: Effects of streptonigrin on nucleic acid metabolism of tissue culture cells. Biochim. Biophys. Acta **108**, 394–395 (1965)
Mizuno, N.S.: Distribution of tritiated methyl ester of streptonigrin in mice bearing sarcoma 180. Biochem. Pharmacol. **15**, 394–403 (1966)
Mizuno, N.S.: Comparative effects of streptonigrin derivatives on tissue culture cells. Biochem. Pharmacol. **16**, 933–940 (1967)
Mizuno, N.S., Gilboe, D.P.: Binding of streptonigrin to DNA. Biochim. Biophys. Acta **224**, 319–327 (1970)
Mizuno, N.S., Humphrey, E.W.: Metabolism of tritiated methyl ester of streptonigrin (NSC-45384) in humans with cancer. Cancer Chemother. Rep. **41**, 23–26 (1964)
Morgan, A.R., Cone, R.L., Elgert, T.M.: The mechanism of DNA strand breakage by vitamin C and superoxide and the protective roles of catalase and superoxide. Nucleic Acid Res. **3**, 1139–1149 (1976)
Muschel, L.H., Schmoker, K.: Activity of mitomycin C, other antibiotics, and serum against lysogenic bacteria. J. Bacteriol. **92**, 967–971 (1966)

Nasjleti, C.E., Spencer, H.H.: Chromosome polyploidization in human leukocyte culture treated with streptonigrin and cyclophosphamide. Cancer **20**, 31–35 (1967)

Oberdisse, E., Neubert, D.: Influence of several antibiotics, which can form complexes with DNA, on nucleic acid synthesis of warm-blooded animal cells in vivo. Nauyn-Schmiedebergs' Arch. Pharmakol. Exp. Pathol. **257**, 47–48 (1967)

O'Connor, T.E., Schoop-Stansly, P., Sethi, V.S., Hadidi, A., Okano, P.: Antibiotic control of infection of human or mouse cells with oncorna virus. Collect. Pap. Annu. Symp. Fundam. Cancer Res. **27**, 319 (1975)

Oleson, J.J., Calderella, L.A., Mjos, K.J., Peith, A.R., Thie, R.S., Toplin, I.: The effects of streptonigrin on experimental tumors. Antibiot. Chemother. **11**, 158–164 (1961)

Padron, E., Karpov, V.L., Gause, G.G., Dudnik, J.V.: Distribution of H^3-bruneomycin in tumor cell. Antibiotiki **19**, 387–389 (1974)

Pittillo, R.F., Woolley, C.: Biological assay of streptonigrin (NSC-45383) in body fluids and tissues of mice. Antimicrob. Agents Chemother. **5**, 82–85 (1974)

Price, P.J., Suk, Wa.A., Spah, G.J., Chirigos, M.A., Lane, J.A., Huebner, R.J.: Streptonigrin inhibition of 3-methylcholanthrene transformation in vitro. Proc. Soc. Exp. Biol. Med. **145**, 1197–1200 (1974)

Puck, T.T.: Phasing, mitotic delay and chromosomal aberration in mammalian cells. Science **144**, 565–566 (1964)

Pulich, W.M., Jr.: Resistance to high oxygen tension, streptonigrin and ultraviolet irradiation in the green alga *Chlorella Sorokiniana* strain ors. J. Cell Biol. **62**, 904–907 (1974)

Radding, C.M.: Incorporation of ^{3}H-thymidine by K12 (λ) induced by streptonigrin. In: Genetics today. Geerts, S.J. (ed.) p.22. Oxford: Pergamon Press 1963

Rao, K.V.: Quinone natural products; streptonigrin (NSC-45383) and lapachol (NSC-11905) structure-activity relationship. Cancer Chemother. Rep. **4** (Pt. 2, No 4), 11–17 (1974)

Rao, K.V., Cullen, W.P.: Streptonigrin, an antitumor substance, I. Isolation and characterization. Antibiot. Ann., 950–953 (1959–60)

Rao, K.V., Biemann, K., Woodward, R.B.: The structure of streptonigrin. J. Am. Chem. Soc. **85**, 2532–2533 (1963)

Reilly, H.C., Sigiura, K.: An antitumor spectrum of streptonigrin. Antibiot. Chemother. **11**, 174–177 (1961)

Shorin, V.A., Brazhanov, V.S.: Possibility of utilizing leukemia L1210 as a first screening model in the primary selection of new antitumor antibiotics. Antibiotiki **19**, 679–684 (1974)

Soukup, S., Takacs, E., Warkany, S.: Chromosome changes in embryos treated with various teratogens. J. Embryol. Exp. Morphol. **18**, 215–226 (1967)

Szybalski, W.: Structural modifications of DNA; crosslinking, circularization and single-strand interruptions. Abh. Dtsch. Akad. Berlin **4**, 1–19 (1964)

Teller, M.N., Wagshul, S.F., Woolley, G.S.: Transplantable human tumors in experimental chemotherapy: effects of streptonigrin on HS #1 and HEP3 in the rat. Antibiot. Chemother. **11**, 165–173 (1961)

Warkany, J., Takacs, E.: Changes of endocrine glands produced by teratogenic methods. The pituitary gland. Arch. Pathol. **85**, 101–113 (1968)

White, H.L., White, J.R.: Interaction of streptonigrin with DNA in vitro. Biochim. Biophys. Acta **123**, 648–651 (1966)

White, H.L., White, J.R.: Lethal action and metabolic effects of streptonigrin in *E. coli*. Mol. Pharmacol. **4**, 549–565 (1968)

White, J.R., Dearman, H.H.: Generation of free radicals from phenazine methosulfate, streptonigrin, and rubiflavin in bacterial suspensions. Proc. Natl. Acad. Sci. USA **54**, 887–891 (1965)

Woods, W.A., Massicot, J.G., Webb, J.H., Chirigos, M.A.: Inhibitory effect of streptonigrin on a murine sarcoma virus-induced tumor cell line (MSC) and selection of drug resistant clones. In Vitro **9**, 24–30 (1973)

Young, C.W., Hodas, S.: Acute effects of cytotoxic compounds on incorporation of precursors into DNA, RNA and protein of HeLa monolayers. Biochem. Pharmacol. **14**, 205–214 (1965)

Zee-Cheng, K.Y., Cheng, C.C.: Common receptor complement feature among some antileukemic compounds. J. Pharm. Sci. **59**, 1630–1634 (1970)

Zetterberg, G., Kihlman, B.A.: Production of mutation by streptonigrin in the ascomycete *Ophiostoma multiannulatum*. Mutat. Res. **2**, 470–471 (1965)

Tilorone Hydrochloride

P. CHANDRA, M. WOLTERSDORF, and G.J. WRIGHT

I. Introduction

Currently, great interest is taken in the search for antiviral drugs and their development. Broadly speaking, there are two strategic approaches to develop such drugs: (1) to search for compounds which offer protection against viruses by an indirect route, i.e., via production of interferon or similar antiviral proteins, (2) to look for compounds which interact directly with the virus or viral components, and in this way block the functional expression of the virus.

The first approach, though still in the experimental stage, has proved to be useful in developing compounds against infective, but nononcogenic viruses such as vaccinia, influenza, and others. The second approach, though one of the earliest approaches known to the chemist, has led in recent years to the development of some useful compounds against viruses; in particular against oncogenic DNA and RNA viruses (rev. by CHANDRA et al., 1977).

As the viral etiology of human cancer is gaining consideration (HAUSEN, 1975; GALLO, 1976; RAPP and REED 1976; SPIEGELMAN, 1976; CHANDRA and STEEL, 1977), the latter approach may prove to be of great importance for the future. However, the most important compounds will be those which possess a bifunctional "modus operandi", i.e., they exert their functional activity by both routes previously mentioned. Among the very few compounds which possess a bifunctional mode of action, tilorone hydrochloride (Fig. 1) has a distinguished place.

Tilorone derives its parentage from fluorene. Although one of its sister fluorene derivatives, the 2-acetylaminofluorene, is biologically hazardous through inducing malignant neoplasms (reviewed by MILLER, 1970), tilorone has become

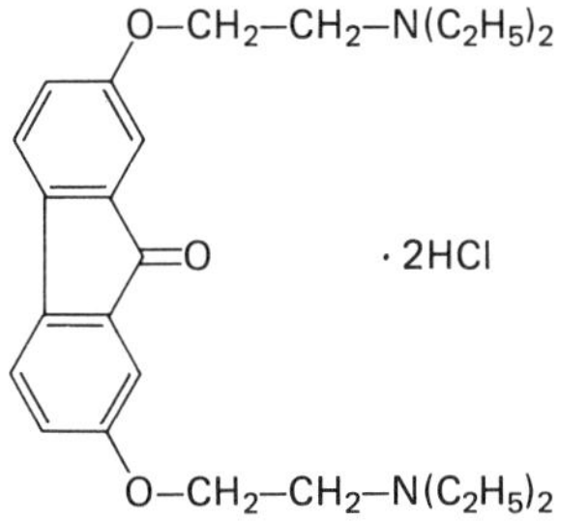

Fig. 1. Chemical structure of tilorone hydrochloride

established as a potent pharmacologic agent. It provides protection against a host of DNA and RNA viruses, including Semliki Forest virus, vesicular stomatitis virus, herpes simplex, and others (KRUEGER and MAYER, 1970).

This drug's additional properties of chemotherapeutic interest are:

1. Its ability to induce the antiviral principle, interferon: DECLERCQ and MERIGAN (1970, 1971); KRUEGER et al. (1970, 1971); MAYER and KRUEGER (1970b); MERIGAN (1970); BUCKLER et al. (1971); COLBY and MERIGAN (1971); FLEMING et al. (1971); GLASGOW (1971); KAUFMAN et al. (1971, 1972); NIBLACK (1971); CAMYRE and GROELKE (1972); DENNIS et al. (1972); GIRON et al. (1972a, b); SIEBER and ADAMSON (1972); STRINGFELLOW and GLASGOW (1972).

2. Its antineoplastic activity: ADAMSON (1971a, b); BARKER et al. (1971); MUNSON et al. (1971, 1972); RHEINS et al. (1971); RHOADS et al. (1971); ROYE et al. (1971); DENNIS et al. (1972); WAMPLER et al. (1972); CHANDRA et al. (1974).

3. Stimulation of humoral immune response: MUNSON et al. (1970); ROHOVSKY et al. (1970); HOFFMAN and RITTER (1971); GIRON et al. (1972); WAMPLER et al. (1972); ZBINDEN and EMCH (1972); DIAMANTSTEIN (1973); MEGEL et al. (1974).

4. Its ability to supress the cell-mediated immune responses directed against skin-allograft survivals and dermatotrophic inflammatory processes: GLASGOW (1971); MOBRAATEN et al. (1973); FRIENDLAENDER et al. (1974); MEGEL et al. (1974, 1975).

This review summarizes the information currently available in the literature or presented before numerous scientific forums. Since the literature is voluminous, the authors will not attempt to cite every paper, but will instead document the discussion to the extent that those who have a deeper interest can elaborate the information presented in this review.

II. Chemistry of Tilorone

The chemistry of tilorone hydrochloride and related compounds has been presented in a series of five papers by SILL et al. (1973); ALBRECHT et al. (1974); ANDREWS et al. (1974); GRISAR et al. (1974), and SILL et al. (1974).

The compounds found to have potent antiviral properties have two features in common (ALBRECHT, 1974):

1. Two side chains containing basic (amine) functions.
2. A lipophilic central ring system of an aromatic or heteroaromatic type.

Monobasic derivatives do not yield potent antiviral agents, nor do they induce interferon. Removal of the amine terminus results in loss of antiviral activity. Maximum activity is not observed with less than 3 rings in the central aromatic or heteroaromatic nucleus.

The central ring systems found to yield antiviral compounds have included fluorene (fluorenone), dibenzofuran, dibenzothiophene, fluoranthene, anthraquinone, acenaphthene, xanthene, thioxanthene, phenothiazine, carbazole, phenanthrene, and others. The side chains were represented by basic ethers, basic ketones, basic esters plus carboxymides, sulfonamides, alkanols, methylene, and others attached to the various ring systems. The amine function was usually substituted to the tertiary amine with various alkyl substituents although a few ring types (e.g., pyrrole or piperidino) were synthesized.

Tilorone hydrochloride, 2,7-bis(2-(diethylamine)ethoxy)-9H-fluorene-9-one dihydrochloride, is an orange-colored solid which is highly water-soluble at neutral and acidic pH. The compound is anhydrous and melts between 234–234.5° C with decomposition. The molecular weight is 483.47. Tilorone·HCl has an intense absorption band at 270 nm in water. The pKa of the amine functions are 8.64 and 9.27, respectively; the compound is stable in acid or base. The synthesis of tilorone hydrochloride was outlined by GAUR and WACKER (1973) and ANDREWS et al. (1974).

III. Toxicological Evaluation of Tilorone Hydrochloride

Preliminary toxicologic evaluation of tilorone hydrochloride has been reported by ROHOVSKY et al. (1971) in mice, rats, dogs, and monkeys. The 24 h oral LD_{50} was 959 mg/kg for mice and 852 mg/kg for rats. In subchronic studies oral doses up to 180 mg/kg/day in rats and mice produced a dose-related depression of body weight gain and food consumption. In dogs and monkeys oral administration of $\geqq 20$ mg/kg/day produced clinical signs of anorexia, emesis, ptosis, salivation, ataxia, and tremors. Oral doses of 3, 10 or 30 mg/kg/day in pregnant rabbits during days 9 through 16 of gestation produced no teratogenic effects.

ROHOVSKY et al. (1970) reported the appearance of vacuolization and granulation of peripheral leukocytes in the mouse, rat, dog and monkey. A concomitant alteration in the reticuloendothelial system also occurred, which consisted in intracytoplasmic accumulation of ovoid structures with vacuolated centers in Kupffer cells of the liver and mixed macrophages of the spleen and lymph nodes. Smears of bone marrow revealed abnormal granules in myeloid cells as primitive as neutrophilic myelocytes, but the myeloid:erythroid ratio was not altered. The post-treatment regression of these effects was species-dependent.

ZBINDEN and EMCH (1972) extended the observations of ROHOVSKY et al. (1970) of the effect of tilorone hydrochloride on the peripheral blood of laboratory animals. They described in rats a marked, but transient, lymphopenia after single oral doses of 100 mg/kg. Recovery from the lymphopenia started after 12 h and was accompanied by depletion of small lymphocytes in lymph follicles of the spleen and the appearance of young lymphocytes with vacuoles and basophile granules in smears of lymph nodes and spleen. Abnormal mononuclear cells whose protoplasm often contained vacuoles and basophilic granules appeared in the blood after 48 h and disappeared in the course of two to three weeks. Repeated dosing caused only minor hematologic changes and affected no other organs.

LEVINE et al. (1974) studied the depletion of the lymphocyte population caused by tilorone hydrochloride given orally or subcutaneously to rats and mice in spleen, lymph nodes, and Peyers patches. Although the thymus itself was not affected, thymus-dependent areas were affected in a manner similar to that caused by neonatal thymectomy, thymic aplasia, or antilymphocytic serum. The effects of tilorone were not dependent on the presence of adrenal, thymus, or spleen, and the depleted tissues were rapidly repopulated. The previously sensitive areas were resistant to further doses of the drug.

The effect of tilorone hydrochloride on the ability of platelets to aggregate was studied by MCKENZIE and SCHATZMAN (1975). In vitro, tilorone hydrochloride did not inhibit the first phase of human platelet aggregation induced by ADP, but was a potent inhibitor of the second phase of platelet aggregation (release reaction) caused by epinephrine. In rats, which received two doses of 100 mg/kg each 24 h apart, collagen-induced aggregation was inhibited in platelets obtained 24 h after the last dose. These results are consistent with inhibition of the second phase platelet aggregation (release reaction), similar to that seen with other nonsteroidal anti-inflammatory compounds. With the exception of aspirin, the effect of tilorone is of longer duration.

IV. Disposition and Pharmacokinetics of Tilorone Hydrochloride

WACKER et al. (1972) reported the distribution of ^{14}C-tilorone in mice 16 h after intraperitoneal injection of 1.5 mg in phosphate buffered saline. High concentrations of radioactivity were found in liver, followed by spleen, kidney, and lung. Relatively lower concentrations were found in thymus, heart, adipose tissue, skeletal muscle, and blood. A large proportion of the radioactivity isolated from liver homogenates and urine was unchanged tilorone. Two unidentified products were seen in addition to tilorone. A significant amount of the radioactivity was associated with the sediment following centrifugation. Since Triton X-100 was needed to release some of the radioactivity, binding to membrane particles was suggested. Nucleic acids extracted by phenol contained no radioactivity.

The metabolic disposition of ^{14}C-tilorone hydrochloride in mice, rats, and dogs has been studied by HOOK et al. (1974). In contrast to the studies reported by WACKER, all doses were administered orally. In the Long–Evans rat, elimination of a radioactive dose (100 mg/kg) of tilorone hydrochloride was about evenly divided between urine and feces. Elimination was biphasic with the $t_{1/2}$ of the first phase 1.3 days and the $t_{1/2}$ of the second phase 4.2 days.

Six days after dosing, 40%–45% of the dose remained in the rats. Tissue radioactivity was located principally in the liver (8%), lung (1%–2%), spleen (1%–2%), gastrointestinal tract and contents (4%–5%), and the carcass (20%–24%). Tissues having the highest concentrations of radioactivity six days post-dose were spleen, liver, lung, eyes, adrenals, and lymph nodes. Concentrations in heart, skeletal muscle, and brain were relatively low, while blood and plasma concentrations were very low. Concentrations of radioactivity in the liver reached a maximum at 3 h post-dose, in the lung at 4 h and went on increasing in the spleen at 6 h. These results imply rapid absorption with subsequent redistribution.

Elimination of radioactivity and of material with UV absorption properties similar to tilorone occurred with a half-life of 3.5–4 days in mice after a dose of 250 mg/kg.

In beagle dogs, urinary excretion accounted for 17%–21% of the dose (20 mg/kg) during 7 days following dosing. Excretion by way of feces accounted for 13%–14% of the dose. Only 8%–9% of the dose appeared in feces during the first 3 days, which suggested that absorption was at least 90%, if not 100%, complete. Seven days post-dose, radioactivity was located primarily in the liver (22%–24%), small intestine and contents (5%–6%), lung (2.7%–3.0%), and spleen (1.5%–1.7%). Highest concentrations of radioactivity were present in liver, spleen, and adrenals. Lower levels were found in heart, brain, and skeletal muscle. Low plasma concentrations of radioactivity, in comparison with tissue concentrations, resulted in extremely high tissue–plasma ratios. Ratios exceeding 1,000 to 1 were found for liver, spleen, adrenals, and pancreas. High concentrations of radioactivity occurred in the pigmented structures of the eye, the choroid and iris, and appreciable concentrations in the retina. Concentrations in all other eye substructures were quite low suggesting that binding to melanin-containing substructures had occurred.

Tissue metabolites from the rat were examined and identified. Thin-layer chromatography and autoradiography revealed the presence of six to eight radioactive compounds. Unchanged tilorone represented the major portion of the radioactivity in rat tissues, even at 6 days. Mono-de-ethylated tilorone was found in the highest quantities of any of the metabolites and represents the major metabolite. Di-de-ethylated tilorone with one ethyl group removed from each side chain was found in considerably lower amounts than the mono-de-ethylated product. Reduction of the carbonyl resulted in the fluorenol analog of tilorone. Polar metabolites were found to be the mono-N-oxide and di-N-oxide analogs of tilorone. Metabolism of tilorone proceeds by N-dealkylation, N-oxide formation, and carbonyl group reduction.

GAUR and CHANDRA (1976) extended their earlier studies in mice with ^{14}C-tilorone. Following an intraperitoneal injection of 20 mg/kg in male AKR-mice, the half-life of elimination was about 72 h with the major excretory route by way of the kidney. In confirmation of earlier findings, spleen and kidney had the highest specific activity. Distribution of radioactivity 24 h after the dose was: liver 25%, spleen 2.5%, kidney 2.3%, lungs and pancreas about 1.5% each, and less than 0.5% of the administered dose in each of the remaining tissues.

Subcellular distribution of tilorone hydrochloride has been examined. GAUR and CHANDRA (1973) studied the subcellular distribution of radioactivity in liver, spleen, brain, lungs, and kidney of mice; and liver, spleen, brain, kidney, and heart of rats, after a dose of 50 mg/kg of ^{14}C-tilorone by intraperitoneal injection. A substantial proportion of the radioactivity was found in the fraction which sediments at 700 *g* and contains, in addition to cell debris, the nuclei. The remaining radioactivity was distributed between the mitochondrial, microsomal, and supernatant fractions. The authors suggested that the primary target of tilorone hydrochloride may indeed be the molecular species localized in the nuclei, i.e., DNA.

The studies of GAUR and CHANDRA were extended by LEESON et al. (1975). Since CHANDRA et al. (1972b, c) had described the in vitro binding of tilorone to DNA, the studies of LEESON et al. were specifically designed to study the localization of tilorone and one of the metabolites in the nucleus of rat liver. Equilibrium dialysis studies showed that binding occurs in both plasma and tissue homogenates with stronger binding by the tissues. In confirmation of the findings reported by GAUR and CHANDRA (1973), the 700 *g* precipitate of rat liver homogenate contained the major fraction of drug-related material. However, intact nuclei isolated from the liver homogenate contained proportionately less drug-related material even though the DNA was relative concentrated. These in vivo findings suggest that tilorone does not selectively localize in the nuclei. Instead, the concentration of tilorone in the various subcellular fractions appeared to relate better to protein concentration, suggesting a relatively nonspecific binding throughout the cell.

V. Effect of Tilorone Hydrochloride on the Drug Metabolizing Enzymes of Rat Liver

In companion papers RENTON and MANNERING (1976), and LEESON et al. (1976) described the decrease in activity of the hepatic cytochrome P-450 mono-oxygenase system, following oral administration of tilorone hydrochloride (doses ranged from 20 to 250 mg/kg). Hexobarbital sleeping times were prolonged and blood levels of hexobarbital were elevated after doses of tilorone. Zoxazolamine paralysis times were prolonged after four doses of 100 mg/kg/day, but not after a single dose. Concentrations of cytochrome P-450 and NADPH-cytochrome reductase were reduced as were various enzyme activities related to the mono-oxygenase systems. Microsomal protein concentrations were initially reduced but had recovered to control levels with 21 days of continuing treatment with 100 mg/kg/day. Aminopyrine demethylase and hexobarbital oxidase remained decreased with 21 days of continuing treatment. Similarly, cytochrome P-450 concentrations remained decreased. Electron micrographs of rat liver, after treatment with tilorone hydrochloride 100 mg/kg/day for 21 days, revealed many membranous structures in the form of whorls in the cytoplasm of the cell. It was postulated that the whorls originated from the endoplasmatic reticulum in an attempt by the liver to restore full enzymatic capabilities upon continued drug administration.

Tilorone hydrochloride was not a direct inhibitor of the mono-oxygenase system of rat liver. In vitro addition of tilorone hydrochloride did not affect microsomal drug metabolism, nor did it affect cytochrome P-450 contents of the microsomes. The rate of incorporation of δ-amino (^{3}H) levulinic acid into cytochrome P-450 was not affected by tilorone·HCl.

VI. Antiviral Activity of Tilorone Hydrochloride

KRUEGER and MAYER (1970) first described tilorone as a broad-spectrum orally active antiviral agent. In the first publication activity against Semliki Forest, vesicular stomatitis, encephalo-myocarditis, Mengo, vaccinia, herpes simplex, and three strains of influenza viruses in mice was described. The authors (MAYER and KRUEGER, 1970) attributed the antiviral activity of tilorone largely to the induction of interferon in the treated mice. MAYER and KRUEGER (1970a) later described antiviral activity against Semliki Forest virus in rats, and eye lesions caused by herpes simplex in rabbits. Activity of tilorone against *Herpesvirus hominis*, type 1 and 2, in a rat and mouse tail-lesion test was described by YOSHIMURA et al. (1973).

In subsequent investigations, tilorone hydrochloride prolonged the survival time of mice infected with Friend leukemia virus (RHEINS and WILSON, 1971), protected Swiss mice against six intracerebral or six subcutaneous LD_{50}s of the CVS strain of rabies virus administered 19 h after treatment with the drug (FORNOSI et al., 1971), and prolonged the survival of mice infected subcutaneously by the "slow virus" scrapie (COCHRAN, 1972). HOFMANN and KUNZ (1972) described the protective effect of tilorone hydrochloride on experimental tick-borne encephalitis in mice. Mice infected with 80 LD_{50} foot-and-mouth disease virus, type O, were protected by 250 mg/kg of tilorone given orally (RICHMOND and CAMPBELL, 1973). Tilorone hydrochloride prevented the production of serum antibody to live Venezuelan equine encephalomyelitis vaccine in mice, presumably because of inhibition of viral replication through interferon production (MAYER et al., 1973). MAYER, et al. (1974) suggested, however, that not all of the activity against viruses can be attributed to the induction of interferon production. Direct virus inactivation was demonstrated and topical activity against herpes-induced lesions on mouse skin or in the rabbit eye was found.

VII. Induction of Interferon by Tilorone Hydrochloride

MAYER and KRUEGER (1970b) first described the appearance of an antiviral serum component in mice treated orally with tilorone hydrochloride, which fulfilled sufficient biologic criteria to be classified as an interferon. KRUEGER et al. (1971) described the interferon inducing properties of a number of analogs of tilorone and described the hyporesponsiveness which occurs with tilorone as well as with other antiviral agents. The interferon produced by treatment of mice and rats has been characterized by CAMYRE et al. (1971), and CAMYRE and GROELKE (1972). Serum from tilorone or poly I:C-treated mice was found to possess an interferon as a single molecular species with a molecular weight (by Sephadex G-100 chromatography) of 34,000. Serum interferon from tilorone-treated rats was associated with two distinct molecular species of 27,000 and 80,000. The interferons were resistant to ribonuclease and to heat. Some differences between rat and mouse interferons were described, e.g., sensitivity to pH 2.5.

Administration of cycloheximide (60 mg/kg) 1 h prior to tilorone administration inhibited the interferon response (DeClerq and Merigan, 1970; Mayer et al., 1971). The inhibition by cycloheximide suggested that protein synthesis was involved in the appearance of interferon in the serum. For a more complete discussion of interferon induction see the review on synthetic interferon inducers by DeClercq (1974).

In discussing the mechanism of antiviral protection and stimulation of interferon production in mice, DeClercq and Merigan (1971) concluded that there was a direct relationship between the extent of protection against vesicular stomatitis virus, the titers of interferon produced and the doses of tilorone. Giron et al. (1972a), however, found no correlation between interferon induction and protection against MM virus in mice. Protection was achieved at doses far below those at which detectable interferon was found in the serum. Both findings may be consistent with different mechanisms of viral inactivation of the two viruses under study.

Although interferon could be readily induced in mice and rats by tilorone, attempts to induce interferon in monkeys and humans have not been successful (Kaufman et al., 1971, 1972).

Interferon induction in normal and leukemic lymphocyte cultures with tilorone has been observed (Dennis et al., 1972). The interferon response observed in normal lymphocyte cultures appeared to be correlated with the toxic effect of tilorone. The effect observed in leukemic cultures required higher concentrations of tilorone but, similarly, appeared to be related to cell viability. Tiolorone has been reported to stimulate production of interferon by itself in mouse embryo fibroblasts and, in combination with poly rI: poly rC/DEAE-dextran, in mouse L929 cells (Groelke et al., 1974). Human foreskin fibroblasts were not stimulated. The degree of synergism between tilorone and the nucleotide-dextran complex was proportional to the concentrations of tilorone and poly rI:poly rC, and was influenced by the times of addition of the compounds relative to each other.

VIII. Effects of Tilorone Hydrochloride on Humoral and Cell-Mediated Immunity

Hoffman et al. (1972) presented evidence that a single oral dose of tilorone enhanced the primary immune response to sheep red blood cells (SRBC) in mice, as measured by the Jerne Plaque technique. They also reported an increase in hemolysin titer after tilorone administration. To evaluate further the action of tilorone on humoral antibody responses, Megel et al. (1974) have studied its effect on 19S and 7S production in the primary and secondary immune responses in mice. It was found that tilorone elevated 19S antibody titer on days 3 and 4 after immunization. After 9 days of continuous drug administration the 19S response for both groups was diminished as compared to days 3 and 4; however tilorone was found to cause a significant increase in the 7S antibody production as compared to controls. Tilorone also stimulated the 19S response to *E. coli* endotoxin, a thymus-independent antigen, on days 3 and 4 after immunization.

The effect of tilorone on 19S and 7S antibodies was also measured in the secondary immune response (MEGEL et al., 1974). In this study the mice were immunized with SRBC at day zero. Tilorone was administered at a dose of 50 mg/kg subcutaneously, starting on day 20. A second immunization was given at day 21 and tilorone was given daily until day 23 (3 days after challenging). Both 19S and 7S responses were significantly increased as compared to controls.

Besides IgG (7S) and IgM (19S) production tilorone was also found to elevate IgE levels. Using a parallel line assay, as described by FINNEY (1964), MEGEL et al. (1974) found that tilorone elevated IgE-like antibody levels 3.2 times with relation to saline controls.

The data show that the drug serves as an adjuvant for a variety of immunoglobin classes (IgG, IgM, and IgE antibody production). The effects on IgA responses to antigenic stimulation remain still to be determined.

In contrast to the effects of tilorone on humoral antibody production, the drug suppressed cell-mediated immune responses (MEGEL et al., 1974) as evidenced by the significant decrease in paralysis in the EAE (experimental allergic encephalomyelitis) model, the inhibition of the tuberculin skin reaction, and the reduction in the secondary swelling in adjuvant arthritis.

Tilorone appears to be selective in its action in that it enhances humoral antibody production while suppressing delayed hypersensitivity response. It differs from the well-known immunosuppressive compounds (e.g., glucocorticoids, antimetabolites, etc.), which are capable of suppressing both. More recently other synthetic compounds with selective effects on the immune systems have been reported. FREEDMAN et al. (1972), and FOX et al. (1973) have reported that oxisuran suppresses skin-graft rejections in mice, rats, and dogs but has no effect on antibody production. RENOUX and RENOUX (1972) have shown that levamisole enhances cell-mediated immunity as evidenced by its effect on graft vs host reactions. Thus, the results with tilorone and some other drugs suggest that the immune system can be modulated selectively by pharmacologic manipulating.

IX. Macromolecular Interactions and Their Biologic Consequences

A. Influence of Tilorone Hydrochloride on the Secondary Structure of DNA

The possibility that this compound may react directly with DNA was indicated by the cytogenetic studies of GREEN and WEST (1971). Tilorone was found to inhibit mitosis significantly at 3.0 µg/ml, and produced chromosomal abnormalities at 1.5 µg/ml. Soon it was discovered by CHANDRA et al. (1972a–c) that tilorone forms molecular complexes with DNA and polydeoxynucleotides.

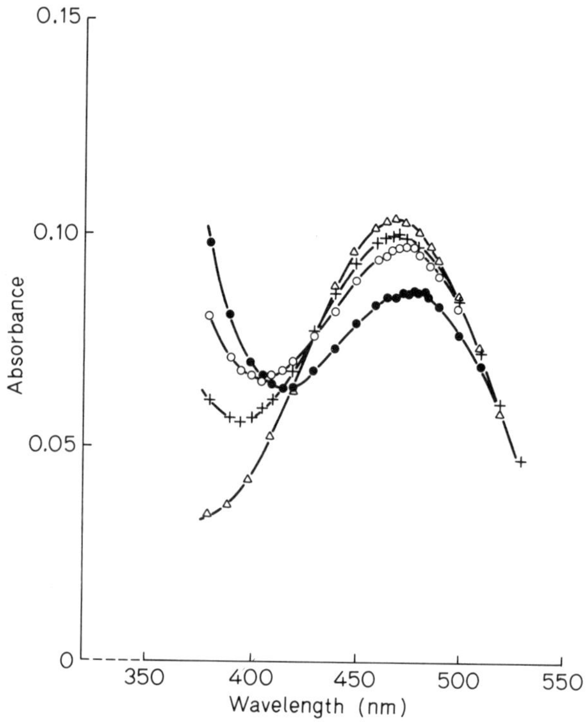

Fig. 2. Effect of calf thymus DNA on the visible absorption spectrum of tilorone hydrochloride. Samples contained 4.25×10^{-4} M of tilorone hydrochloride, 0.01 M Tris-HCl (pH 7.0), and DNA at 0.5×10^{-3} M (+ — +); at 1×10^{-3} M (○ — ○); at 2×10^{-3} M (● — ●). No DNA was added to the sample (△ — △)

Interaction between nucleic acids and biologically active compounds may induce changes in the electronic spectra of the components. Tilorone hydrochloride in water shows two absorption maxima, in the ultraviolet region around 271 nm, and in the visible region around 470 nm. Thus, the investigation of the long wavelength band, where DNA and RNA do not absorb, should provide some evidence whether or not the chromophore of tilorone hydrochloride is involved in the binding process.

Figure 2 depicts the absorption spectrum (350–500 nm) of tilorone hydrochloride alone (continuous line with triangles), or in the presence of various amounts of calf thymus DNA. There is a characteristic change in the tilorone spectrum in the presence of DNA. With calf thymus DNA the visible absorption spectrum of tilorone hydrochloride is depressed and red-shifted. The hypochromic effect of DNA on the absorption of the tilorone chromophore is dependent on DNA concentration. The largest hypochromic effect is observed at 2×10^{-3} M DNA-P in a 4.25×10^{-4}M solution of tilorone hydrochloride.

The concentration-dependent effect of calf thymus DNA on the visible absorption spectrum of tilorone hydrochloride indicates that the tilorone chromophore interacts with DNA. Figure 3 depicts the visible absorption spectra of tilorone alone (curve one), or in the presence of yeast RNA (curve two), dena-

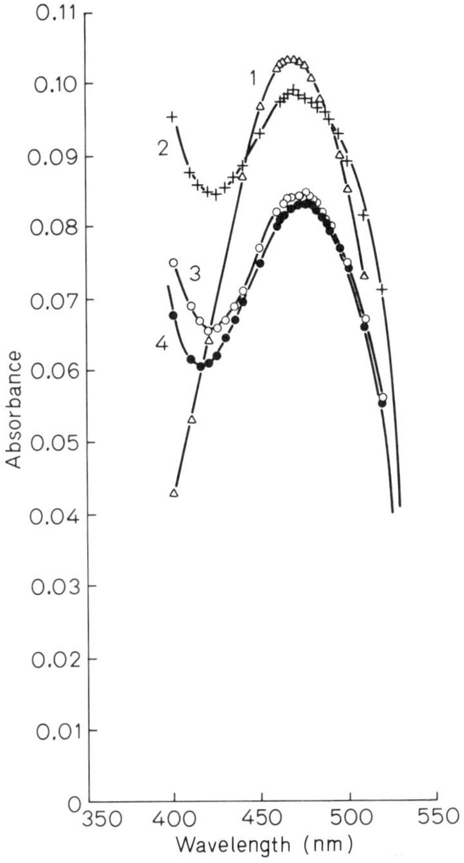

Fig. 3

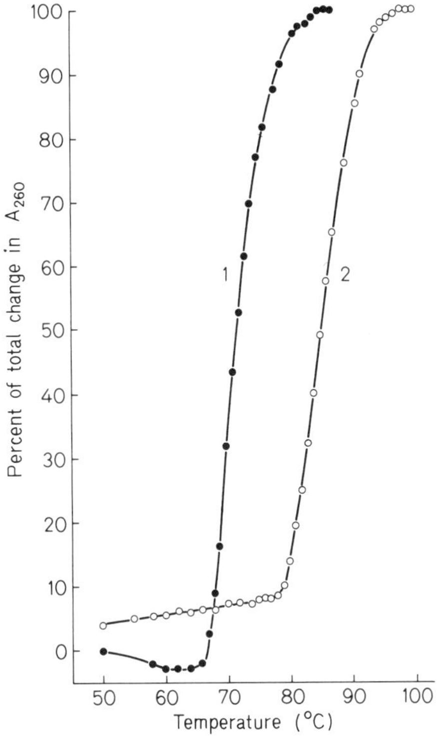

Fig. 4

Fig. 3. Effect of native calf thymus DNA, denatured calf thymus DNA, and yeast RNA on the visible absorption spectrum of tilorone in 0.01 M Tris-HCl (pH 7.0). Curve *1* is the spectrum of free tilorone (4.25×10^{-4} M). Other curves depict the spectra of tilorone in the presence of yeast RNA (*2*), denatured DNA (*3*), and native DNA (*4*). Molar concentrations of nucleic acids (2×10^{-3} M) refer to phosphorus content of the polymer

Fig. 4. Effect of tilorone on the thermal transition temperature (T_m) of calf thymus DNA. Solvent is 0.01 M Tris-HCl (pH 7.0), and the DNA concentration is 5×10^{-5} M in all experiments. Curve *1* represents the melting profile of DNA in the absence of tilorone, and *2* is the melting profile of DNA in the presence of 1×10^{-5} M tilorone hydrochloride

tured DNA (curve three), and native double-stranded DNA (curve four). The visible spectra indicate that at equimolar concentrations, DNA in its double helical state produced the largest changes in the absorption spectrum of tilorone, whereas the effect of single-stranded DNA was slightly weaker. In contrast, the yeast RNA exerts only a slight effect on the visible spectrum of tilorone hydrochloride. These data indicate a specificity of the tilorone chromophore for DNA.

Further information on the binding of tilorone with DNA was derived by studying the "melting" of the complex. In order to characterize the stability of DNA secondary structure in the presence of tilorone, temperature profiles were run at tilorone/DNA-P molar ratio of 1:5 (Fig. 4). Tilorone hydrochloride shows a large increase in the thermal transition temperature (T_m) of native DNA; the T_m of calf thymus DNA was raised from 71.6° to 85.2° C under these conditions.

B. Mode of Tilorone Hydrochloride Interaction to DNA

Hypochromic effect of native DNA on the absorption of tilorone chromophore is partially reversible by Mg^{+2} ions. Figure 5 depicts the absorption spectra (3350–550 nm) of tilorone hydrochloride alone, 4.25×10^{-4}M (curve one), in the presence of 4×10^{-3}M DNA-P (curve four), containing 0.01 M $MgCl_2$ (curve two), or 0.1 M NaCl (curve three). The effect of magnesium ions on tilorone binding to DNA was confirmed by density gradient studies using labeled tilorne hydrochloride.

Evidently, electrostatic forces contribute greatly to the binding process. The interaction between tilorone and DNA may, however, involve other kinds of forces. Tilorone forms a reversible complex with DNA, since the drug could be completely eluted from a DNA-cellulose column. Interaction of apurinic and apyrimidinic DNAs with tilorone hydrochloride also gave spectral changes. However, with the apyrimidinic DNA only, the spectrum of the bound drug was similar to that found with native DNA.

The absorption spectrum studies presented above merely reflect the electronic environment of the molecule and do not give specific information about the type of interaction. The data which must be accounted for in considering a physical mode for the binding process can be derived from several different approaches. Hydrodynamic measurements on the DNA-drug complex are of interest, since LERMAN (1961, 1964) has established that an increase in the intrinsic viscosity of DNA and a decrease in the sedimentation coefficient of the polymer are two criteria for intercalation of ring systems between base pairs of a double-helical DNA.

The relationship between the intrinsic viscosity of DNA and the amount ("r") of bound tilorone was studied. The intrinsic viscosity of the complex increases with r up to a limiting value of about 0.05. The maximum relative enhancement of viscosity was about 1.7. In addition, at the same ionic strength and at a ligand to DNA-P molar ratio of 0.1, the sedimentation rate of DNA was decreased to 78% of the value in the absence of ligand.

These observations are consistent with an intercalative mode of binding in the interaction of tilorone hydrochloride with double-helical DNA. These results were not extended to measurements of the length increase of sonicated DNA. For this reason, the intercalation model of the DNA complex remains tentative.

The interaction of tilorone hydrochloride with native DNA stabilizes the double-helical structure of the macromolecule towards thermal denaturation.

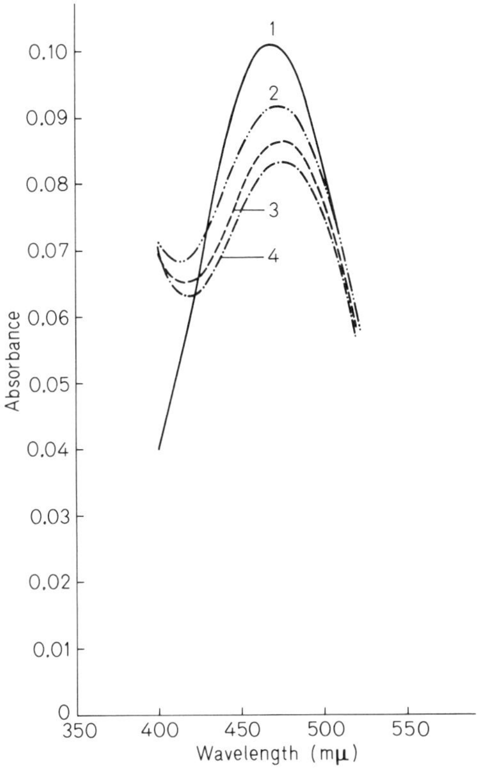

Fig. 5. Effect of Na^+ and Mg^{2+} on the visible absorption spectrum of the tilorone-DNA complex. Samples contained 4.25×10^{-4} M tilorone, 4×10^{-3} M DNA-P, 0.01 M Tris-HCl (pH 7.0), and 0.01 M $MgCl_2$ (*2*), or 0.1 M NaCl (*3*). Curve *1* is the spectrum of free tilorone; *4* is the spectrum of the tilorone-DNA complex in the absence of Na^+ and Mg^{2+}

The effect of tilorone hydrochloride on the thermal denaturation of DNAs with different base composition has been studied (Fig. 6). At a drug-to-DNA-P molar ratio of 0.21, ΔT_m increased with increasing A-T content of the DNA. This observation indicates that tilorone hydrochloride preferentially binds to the dAT portions of the DNA molecule. This is confirmed by the strong effect of tilorone hydrochloride on the thermal transition temperature of poly d(A-T), $\Delta T_m = 29°$ C.

The AT-specificity of the binding of tilorone to DNA was also observed in quantitative equilibrium binding measurements. The equilibrium binding data were plotted as r/(u) vs r, where r is the mol of bound tilorone divided by the DNA concentration in base pairs (CHANDRA et al., 1974), and (u) is the concentration of unbound tilorone. From this plot binding parameters were obtained appropriate to a model in which all DNA binding sites are considered to be independent of each other (CROTHERS, 1968). The equation from this model is:

$$r/(u) = K_{app}(B_{app} - r),$$

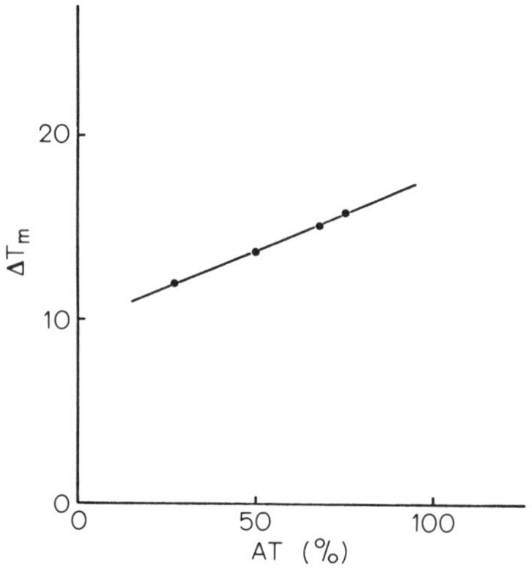

Fig. 6. Effect of tilorone on the T_m with DNA preparations of different base compositions. T_m values were obtained at a molar ratio of drug to DNA-P of 0.21. The T_m of DNA (5×10^{-5} M) with and without tilorone was determined in a medium of 0.01 M Tris-HCl (pH 7.0). AT-content of *B. cereus* DNA (65%), calf thymus DNA (58%), *E. coli* DNA (50%), and *M. lysodeikticus* DNA (28%); these DNA samples were used in these experiments

where K_{app} and B_{app} are the apparent binding constant and number of binding sites per base pair, respectively; K_{app} is the negative of the slope, and B_{app} the $r/(u)=0$ intercept of the linear region of the r/(u) vs r plot.

The Scatchard plots for the binding of tilorone to calf thymus DNA (Fig. 7a), *Mc. lys.* DNA (Fig. 7b), poly (dA-dT)·poly (dA-dT) (Fig. 7c), and poly (dG-dC)·poly (dG-dC) (Fig. 7d) are shown in Fig. 7. As follows from the Scatchard plots for natural DNAs (Fig. 7a, b), the independent site model does not fit for DNA-ligand interaction; however, we employed the binding parameters of this model to analyze the Scatchard plots. The binding parameters K_{app} and B_{app} derived from the Scatchard plots (Fig. 7a–d) are presented in Table 1.

As seen in Table 1, the apparent binding constants for both the natural DNAs are of the same magnitude, whereas the K_{app} for poly(dA-dT)·poly(dA-dT) is higher by a factor of 2. The K_{app} value for poly(dG-dC)·poly(dG-dC) is less by a factor of 10^{-2}, compared with those of natural DNAs and the synthetic polydeoxynucleotide poly(dA-dT)·poly(dA-dT). The data on the number of binding sites per base pair (B_{app}) for various DNAs show a strict correlation with the AT-content of the biopolymer. On the basis of the B_{app} data, the closest distance between bound tilorone molecules is four base pairs. The values shown in Table 1 give almost a linear correlation (Fig. 8), showing a direct dependency of B_{app} on the AT content of DNAs. The value for poly(dG-dG)·poly(dG-dC) has been extrapolated to zero (Fig. 8), since the Scatchard plot (cf. Fig. 7d) does not indicate any specific binding of tilorone to this polymer.

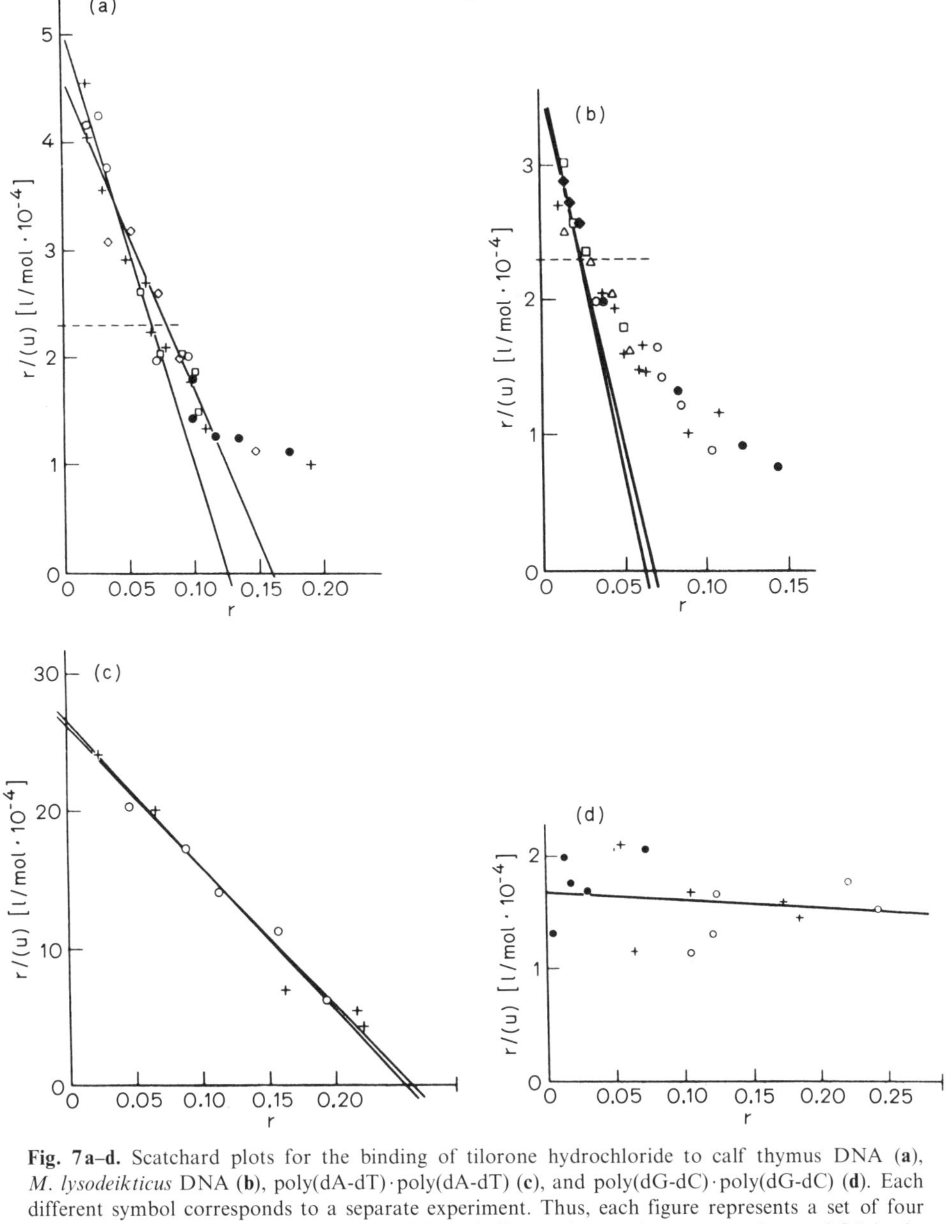

Fig. 7a–d. Scatchard plots for the binding of tilorone hydrochloride to calf thymus DNA (**a**), *M. lysodeikticus* DNA (**b**), poly(dA-dT)·poly(dA-dT) (**c**), and poly(dG-dC)·poly(dG-dC) (**d**). Each different symbol corresponds to a separate experiment. Thus, each figure represents a set of four or five separate experiments. *r* is mol of bound tilorone:base pair concentration and [*u*] is the concentration of unbound tilorone.

Equilibrium dialysis was carried out by a procedure and an apparatus (Dianorm, supplied by Dr. Virus KG, Bonn, Germany) described by WEDER et al. (1971). Dialysis membrane (0.025 mm thick) was sandwiched between two halves of a Teflon (round) macrocell (dialysable volume = 1 ml). The DNA, or labeled tilorone solutions, were introduced by separate microsyringes on either side of the membrane through the side valves. The valves closed airtight and the macrocells were fixed into a rotating machine. All equilibrium dialysis studies were carried out at 20° C, and at 10 rotations/min. Under these conditions, equilibrium was attained in 4–5 h. After the equilibrium was reached, 0.8 ml of the solution from either side of the membrane was withdrawn by microsyringes and the radioactivity was determined using dioxan scintillation fluid

Table 1. Binding constants for the interaction of tilorone hydrochloride with DNAs and synthetic polydeoxynucleotides

Source of DNA	B_{app} [a]	K_{app} [b] M^{-1}
A. Natural DNAs:		
Calf thymus	0.16	2.90×10^5
	0.12	4.10×10^5
Mic. Lysodeikticus	0.066	5.50×10^5
	0.062	6.00×10^5
B. Synthetic Polymers:		
Poly(dA-dT)·poly(dA-dT)	0.25	1.02×10^6
	0.25	1.04×10^6
Poly(dG-dC)·poly(dG-dC)	–	6.90×10^3

[a] Number of binding sites per base pair; [b] apparent binding constant.
All experiments were carried out at 20° C in 0.1 M Tris-HCl (pH 7.0). The binding parameters were derived from the Scatchard plots (Fig. 7a–d), and and the experiments carried out by equilibrium dialysis as described in Fig. 7.

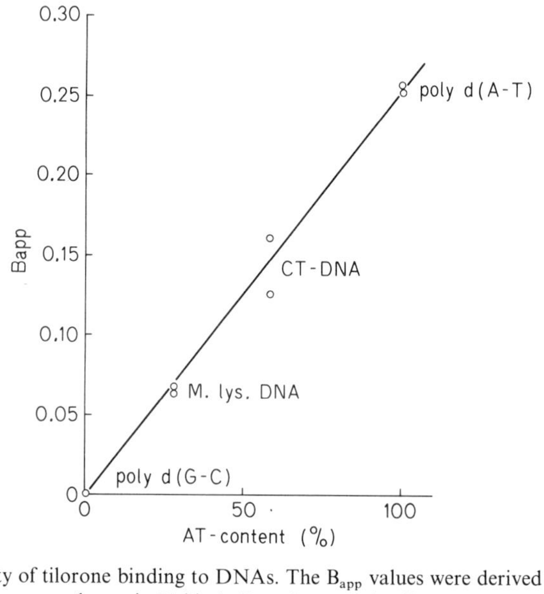

Fig. 8. A-T specificity of tilorone binding to DNAs. The B_{app} values were derived from the Scatchard plots of r/(u) vs r, as shown in Table 1. Experimental details are described under Fig. 7

C. Effect of Tilorone on the Template Activity of Nucleic Acids

The interaction of tilorone hydrochloride with DNA encouraged us to study the template activity of the complexes in DNA- and and RNA-polymerase systems from *E. coli*. Both activities were found to be inhibited by tilorone, the DNA polymerase reaction being more sensitive toward tilorone. The inhibi-

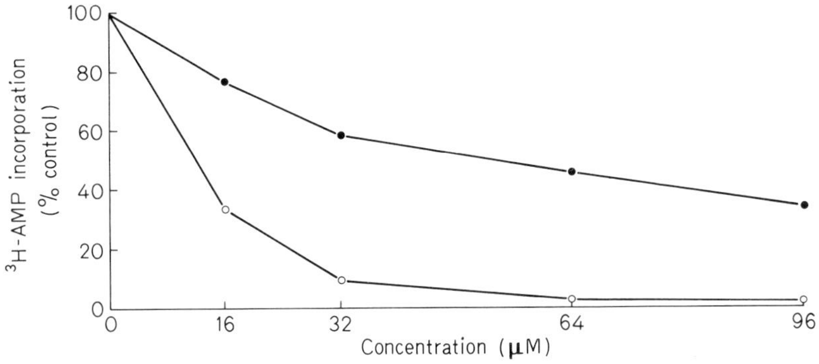

Fig. 9. Inhibition by tilorone of the RNA-polymerase reaction catalyzed by the templates: calf thymus DNA ●——●, and poly(dA-dT) ○——○. Regardless of the template, the reaction mixture (0.25 ml) contained 1 μg of the template. In the poly(dA-dT)-catalyzed reaction, GTP and CTP were omitted from the reaction mixture

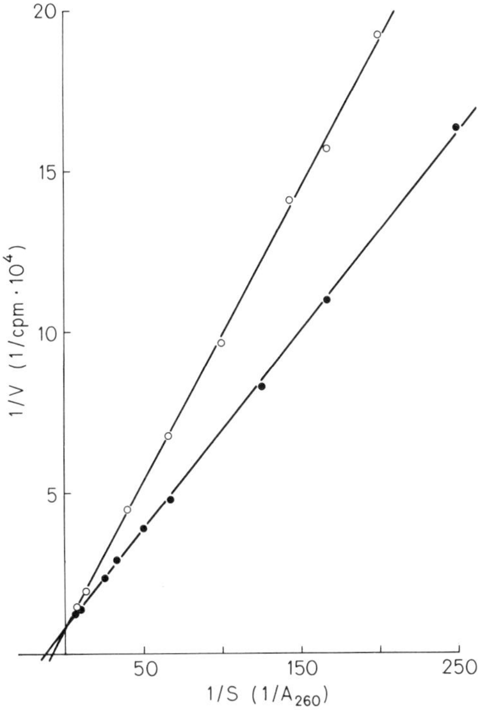

Fig. 10. Lineweaver-Burk plot of the effect of increasing concentrations of template DNA on the incorporation of ^{3}H-AMP into RNA by RNA polymerase of *E. coli* K-12, in the absence of tilorone (●——●), or in the presence of tilorone, 3.2×10^{-5} M (○——○). *Abscissa*: 1/S=(DNA template, A_{260} per reaction mixture)$^{-1}$. *Oridinate*: 1/V=(^{3}H-labeled AMP incorporated into RNA)$^{-1}$

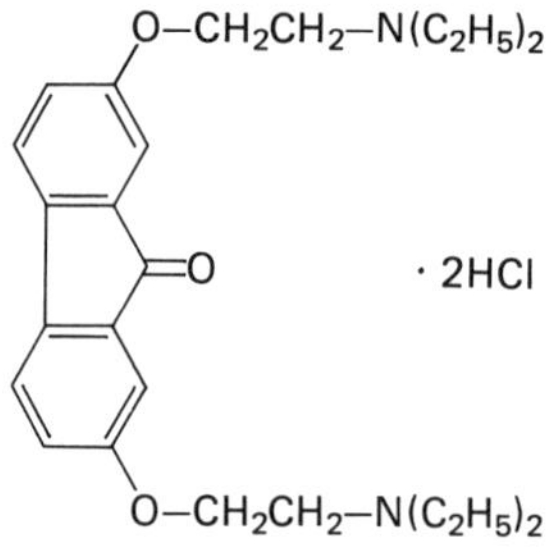

DEAE–fluorenone
Tilorone

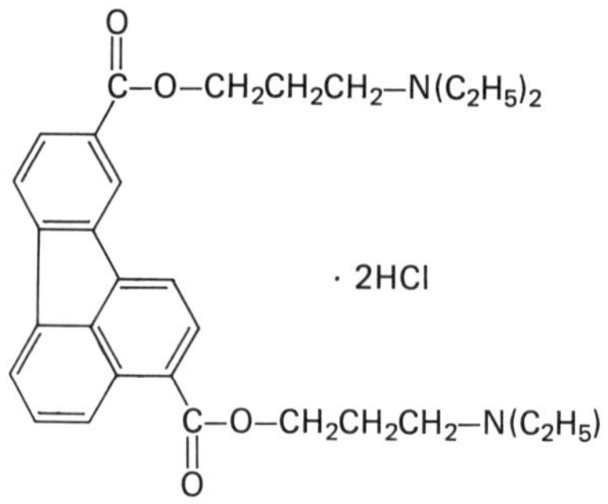

DEAP–fluoranthene
RMI–9563 DA

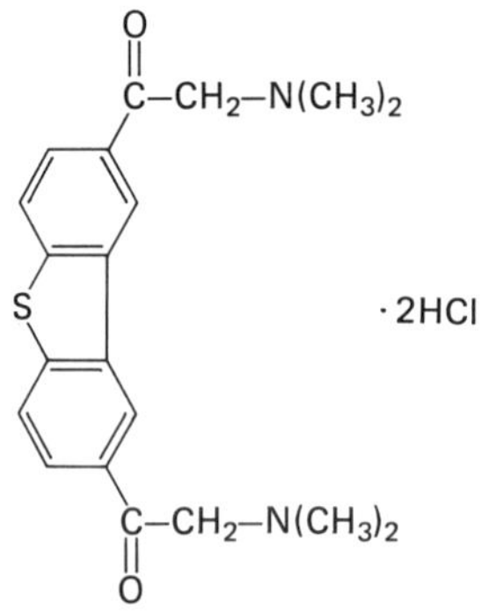

DMAA–dibenzothiophen
RMI–11877 DA

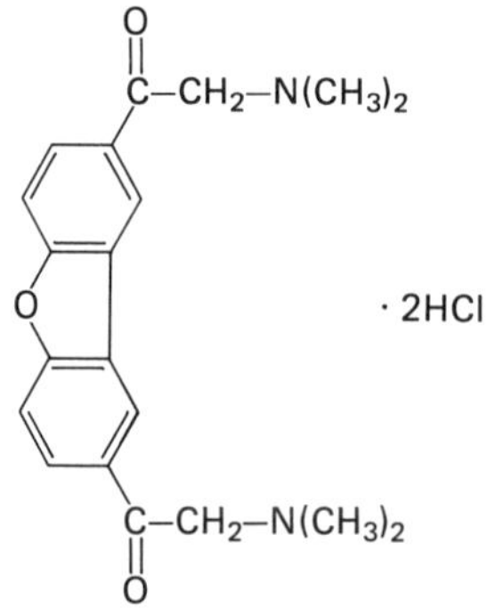

DMAA–dibenzofuran
RMI–11567 DA

Fig. 11. Chemical structures of tilorone and congeners

tion of the RNA-polymerase reaction by tilorone was dependent on the A-T content of the DNA template (Fig. 9).

The template activity of poly(dA-dT) (○ — ○) in the RNA-polymerase reaction is distinctly more sensitive toward tilorone than that of DNA (● — ●); particularly at low drug concentrations the poly(dA-dT)-catalyzed reaction is three times more sensitive than the DNA-catalyzed activity of RNA-polymerase reaction.

The nature of the inhibitory response is clearly shown in the Lineweaver-Burk plot of the kinetic data obtained by measuring the RNA-polymerase activity at various concentrations of template (Fig. 10). Figure 10 depicts the kinetic curves of the reactions in the absence of the inhibitor (○ — ●) and in the presence of 3.2×10^{-5}M tilorone (○ — ○). This shows that tilorone is a competitive inhibitor of DNA-template activity in the RNA-polymerase reaction.

D. Studies with Tilorone Congeners

The interaction of tilorone with DNA and synthetic polydeoxynucleotides can be influenced by modifying the tilorone structure. Such studies are indeed important to elucidate the role of structural entities in complex formation with DNA. Structure–activity relationship of tilorone derivatives (Fig. 11) has recently been studied in our laboratory (CHANDRA et al., 1974a, b).

The effect of tilorone and congeners (Fig. 11) on the DNA-dependent RNA-polymerase reaction is shown in Fig. 12. The template activity of native DNA is strongly inhibited by DEAE-fluoranthene, showing an 80% inhibition at a concentration of 8×10^{-6}M. Other derivatives at this concentration do not show any significant inhibition of the template activity of DNA. However, at higher concentrations one observes a dose-dependent inhibition of DNA-template activity by DEAE-fluorenone, DMAA-dibenzothiophene, DEAA-fluorene and DMAA-dibenzofuran. The mono-substituted derivative, MEAA-fluorene, does not show any activity, even at higher concentrations.

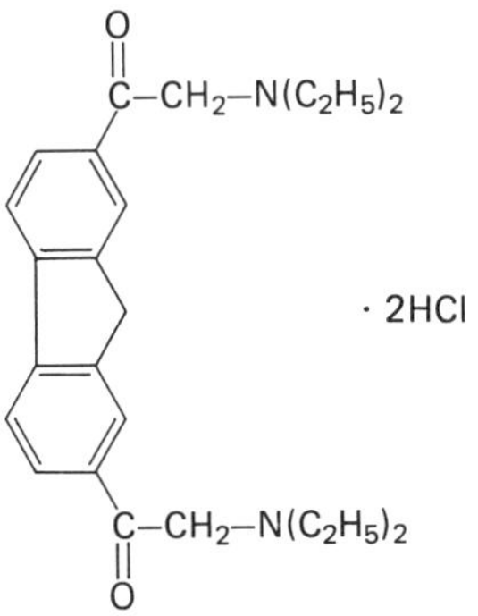

DEAA–fluorene
RMI–11002

MEAA–fluorene
RMI–11829 A
monosubstituted RMI 11002

Fig. 11 (continued)

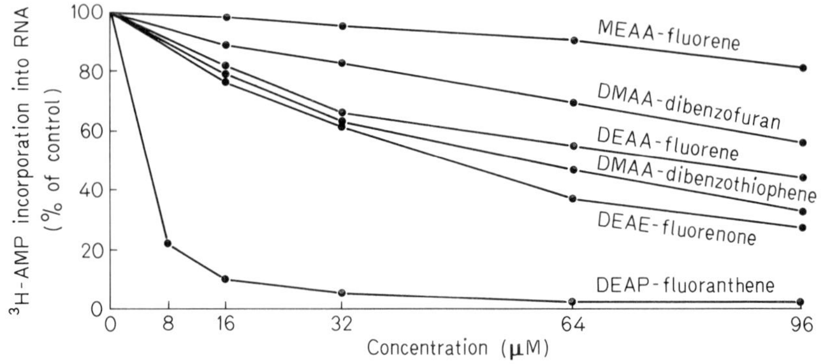

Fig. 12. Inhibition of the DNA-dependent RNA-polymerase reaction (*E. coli* K-12) by tilorone and congeners

The inhibition of DNA-template activity by tilorone and its congeners is strongly influenced by substitutions in the ring (e.g., thiophene, furan, etc.) as well as in the side chains. It was, therefore, of interest to study whether such substitutions influence their interaction to DNA. Figure 13 depicts the melting curves of calf thymus DNA alone (curve 1), or in the presence of MEAA-fluorene (curve 2), DEAA-fluorene (curve 3), DMAA-dibenzothiophene (curve 4), DMAA-dibenzofuran (curve 5), and DEAE-fluorenone (curve 6). These studies were carried out at a drug/DNA-P ratio (r) of 0.1. Tilorone hydrochloride (DEAE-fluorenone) shows a large increase in the thermal transition temperature (T_m) of native DNA (curve 6). The congener DEAE-fluoranthene, under these conditions, showed a very similar response (curve not shown). It is interesting to note that DMAA-dibenzofuran, though less active than DMAA-dibenzothiophene and DEAA-fluorene in the RNA-polymerase reaction, has a higher effect on the T_m of calf thymus DNA than exhibited by these two derivatives.

The structure–activity relationship observed in the RNA-polymerase reaction, is not reflected by the melting curves of DNA and congener complexes. The latter studies were done in the absence of magnesium ions, whereas the RNA-polymerase reaction requires magnesium ions for its enzymatic activity. The fact that compounds of tilorone type form complexes with Mg^{2+} may explain differences in the structure–activity relationships of congeners in the RNA-polymerase reaction, and their effects on the melting behavior of DNA. Thus the dibenzofuran congener, though less active than DEAA-fluorene in the RNA-polymerase reaction, has a higher affinity for DNA than DEAA-fluorene. The dibenzofuran derivative should have a higher tendency for chelating with magnesium ions, which leads to its partial inactivation in the RNA polymerase reaction.

To measure the effect of various tilorone congeners (Fig. 14) on the oncogenic activity of MSV(M), viral suspensions were incubated with 5×10^{-7} mol/ml of each compound at 37° C for 1 h. In the control group virus was preincubated with the solvent. Tris-buffer, 0.01 M, pH 7.4; 0.2 ml of this mixture containing 1×10^{-7} mol of the drug, was injected intraperitoneally. The amount of compound introduced this way had no direct physiologic effect in the host (unpub-

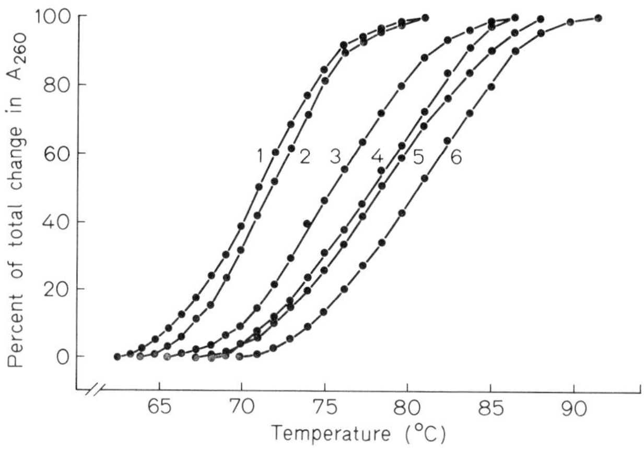

Fig. 13. Effect of tilorone and congeners on the thermal transition temperature (T_m) of calf thymus DNA. Solvent is 0.01 M Tris-HCl, pH 7.0, and the concentrations of DNA-P and congeners are 5×10^{-5} M and 5×10^{-6} M, respectively. Curve *1*, DNA; *2*, DNA + MEAA-fluorene; *3*, DNA + DEAA-fluorene; *4*, DNA + DMAA-dibenzothiophene; *5*, DNA + DMAA-dibenzofuran, and *6*, DNA + DEAE-fluorenone

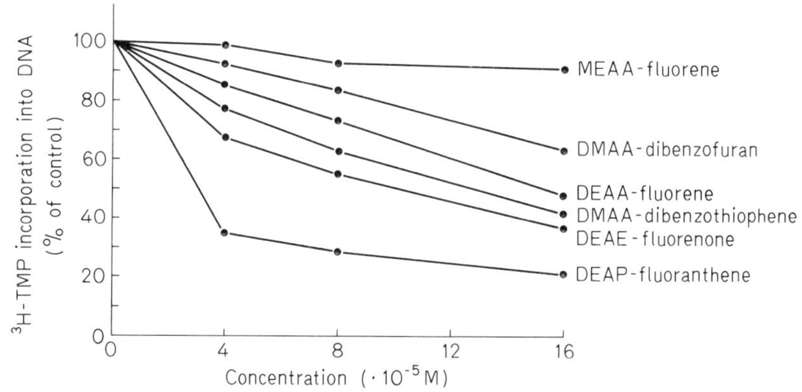

Fig. 14. Inhibition of endogenous RNase-sensitive FLV-DNA-polymerase activity by tilorone and congeners

lished results). The mortality and the survival time were significantly influenced by tilorone and two of its congeners, DEAE-fluoranthene showed a significant inhibition of splenomegaly induced by FLV, while DEAA-fluorene showed only slight activity. It is interesting to note that MEAA-fluorene does not show any activity in this system (CHANDRA et al., 1974).

Since none of the compounds at the concentrations used showed a complete suppression of splenomegaly, one would expect a residual viral activity in spleen extracts of mice that received FLV suspensions preincubated with these compounds. Studies are now in progress to evaluate the leukemogenic activity of cell-free spleen extracts, prepared from mice inoculated with pretreated suspensions. WU et al. (1973) have carried out such studies with RLV and rifamycin

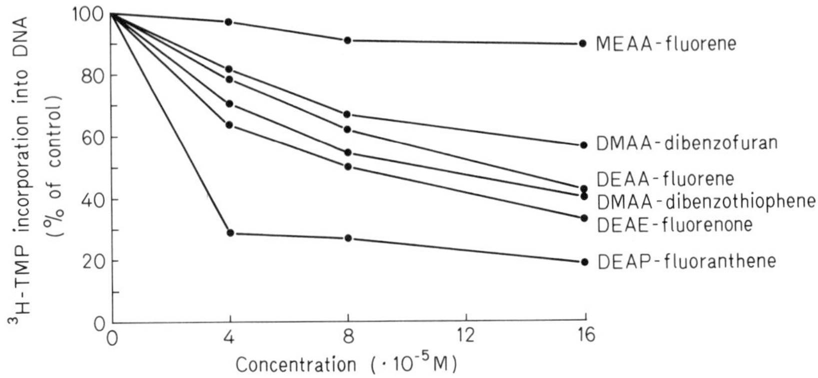

Fig. 15. Inhibition of the poly rA·$(dT)_{12}$-catalyzed FLV-DNA-polymerase activity by tilorone and congeners

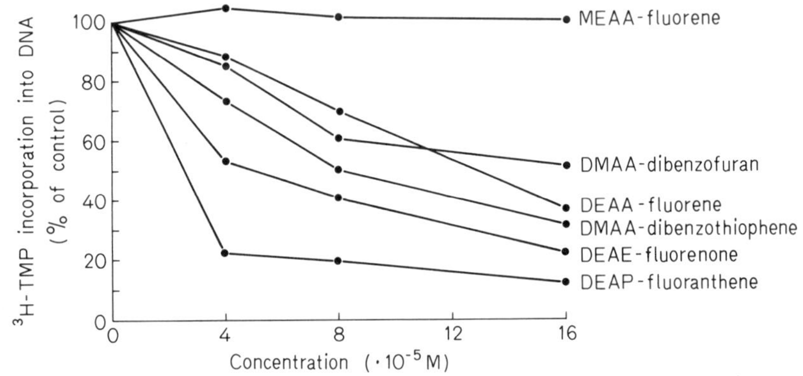

Fig. 16. Inhibition of the poly(dA-dT)-catalyzed FLV-DNA-polymerase activity by tilorone and congeners

derivatives. They reported that the inoculation of mice with inocula from mice infected with RLV pretreated with AF-ABDP and AF/DNF1 did not cause splenomegaly.

If the suppression of biologic activity of RNA tumor viruses is due to a block of some molecular event(s) involved in oncogenesis, one would expect an inhibition of DNA polymerases by these compounds. That tilorone does inhibit the DNA-polymerase activity of oncornaviruses has been shown by us earlier (CHANDRA et al., 1972a). An attempt was made to correlate the biologic response of various congeners with their inhibitory activity in the DNA-polymerase system of oncornaviruses. These studies were done using purified FLV, since in our hands this system showed a good endogenous activity.

The inhibition of the endogenous activity of FLV-DNA polymerase by tilorone and congeners is shown in Fig. 14. Maximum inhibition was obtained with DEAE-fluoranthene. The inhibitory responses of tilorone (DEAE-fluorenone), DMAA-dibenzothiophene and DEAA-fluorene were of the same magni-

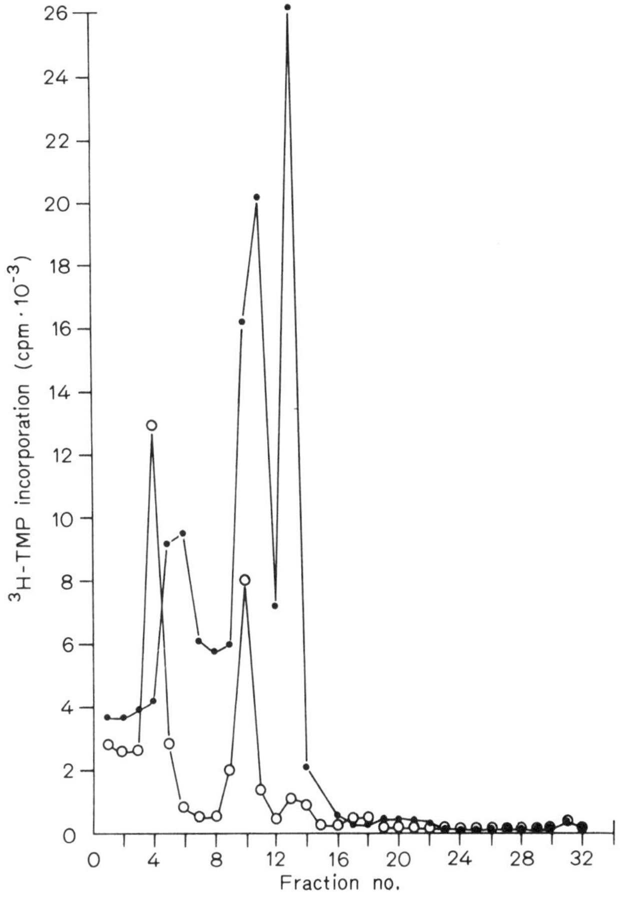

Fig. 17. Analysis of the DNA species synthesized by FLV-DNA polymerase by elution from hydroxylapatite column. Each column was filled with 1 g of hydroxylapatite and carefully washed with 0.05 M sodium phosphate (approx. 50 ml). The columns were loaded with the reaction products, as described in text, and washed with 0.05 M sodium phosphate buffer, pH 6.8, until equilibrium was reached. Macromolecules were eluted from the columns by a linear gradient of sodium phosphate (0.05–0.4 M). ●——● DNA species synthesized in the absence of tilorone; ○——○ DNA species synthesized in the presence of 10^{-4} M tilorone

tude; whereas DMAA-dibenzofuran showed a weak response. It is interesting to note that the monosubstituted congener MEAA-fluorene did not inhibit the endogenous reaction at any concentration tested.

A similar inhibitory response by the tilorone congeners was exhibited in the DNA-polymerase system of FLV, catalyzed by the template poly rA·$(dT)_{12}$, as shown in Fig. 15. The effect of tilorone and congeners on the FLV-DNA-polymerase reaction, catalyzed by poly(dA-dT), is shown in Fig. 16. This reaction was more sensitive to tilorone and its congeners than the endogenous, or poly rA·$(dT)_{12}$-catalyzed reactions. This is in accord with our findings on tilorone, reported earlier (CHANDRA et al., 1972a).

The data reported in Figs. 14–16 show that the poly(dA-dT)-catalyzed reaction of viral DNA polymerase is most sensitive to these compounds. It is possible that the biologic activity of these compounds is due to their interaction with the hybrid RNA-DNA (hy-DNA), single-stranded DNA (ss-DNA), or the DNA–DNA duplex (ds-DNA). It was therefore interesting to locate the site of action of tilorone in the viral DNA-polymerase system. It is still not clear whether a particular site or target in the DNA-polymerase system, other than the true RNA-dependent reaction, can be correlated with the biologic role of the oncornaviruses. The key role of the RNA-directed reaction in in vivo leukemogenesis using purified enzyme and rifamycin derivatives, has been convincingly demonstrated by WU et al. (1973)

We have conducted some model studies to analyze the products of the FLV-DNA-polymerase reaction under the influence of tilorone. The procedure was based on a report by KOTLER and BECKER (1972) on distamycin A, which has been shown by us to react with ss-DNA and ds-DNA (CHANDRA et al., 1970).

The product analysis of the DNA-polymerase reaction (FLV) in the absence and in the presence of tilorone (1×10^{-4} M) is depicted in Fig. 17. The products of the viral DNA-polymerase reaction were, under these conditions, eluted in three species. The first species to be eluted from the column contained ss-DNA, the second contained the RNA-DNA hybrid molecules (hy-DNA), and finally, the ds-DNA eluted in the last species. Analysis of products synthesized in the presence of tilorone showed that the ss-DNA and the hybrid species, but not the ds-DNA species were synthesized. This indicates that tilorone has a low affinity for viral RNA, but can block the synthesis of ds-DNA by interacting with ss-DNA or hy-DNA.

X. Biologic Implications of Tilorone Interaction with DNA

Following the discovery by HIROTA and IIJIMA (1957) that growing *E. coli* K-12F^{+} cells in the presence of acriflavin produced F^{-}-cells, considerable study has been devoted to search for compounds which eliminate resistance determinants from bacterial R factors. Most of the active eliminators of R factors are compounds that complex with DNA (reviewed by HAHN, 1976). Interestingly, the majority of these compounds complex with DNA by an intercalative mode of binding. HAHN and CIAK (1971) proposed, therefore, that intercalation binding into closed circular plasmid DNA is a general molecular mechanism through which the replication of plasmids can be selectively inhibited when plasmid-carrying bacteria are grown in the presence of subinhibitory concentrations of such compounds.

Based on the observations of CHANDRA et al. (1972a–c) that tilorone intercalates into DNA, HAHN (1976) has studied the effect of tilorone on the elimination of resistance determinants in *S. typhimurium*. He reported that tilorone at 10^{-4} M was able to eliminate 78%–85% resistance determinants tested against kanamycin, chloramphenicol, streptomycin *and* ampicillin. Similar observations were made by DE BARY (1976) who compared the elimination of four determi-

Table 2. Elimination of resistance determinants of an R-factor (R s-a) in *E. coli* K_{12} W3110 by tilorone and other DNA-complexing compounds

Compound used	Concentration (μg/ml)	% elimination of R Factors			
		C[a]	K[b]	S[c]	Su[d]
Acridine orange	32	0	0	0	0
Ethidium bromide	64	2	2	0	0
Tilorone hydrochloride	64	42	41	41	41
	128	55	54	54	54
	256	71	71	71	71

[a] Chloramphenicol; [b] kanamycin; [c] streptomycin; [d] sulfonamide. Bacterial Strain = *E. coli* K_{12} W 3110 rif. (Data from DeBary, 1976).

nants (chloramphenicol, kanamycin, streptomycin and sulfonamide) by tilorone and other DNA-complexing compounds (Table 2). Of all the compounds tested tilorone hydrochloride was reported to be the most effective eliminator of plasmids.

Another biologic effect of tilorone, based on its specific interaction with DNA, is a selective inhibition of sporulation of *B. subtilis* strains 60015 (RHAESE, 1977). At a drug concentration of 100 μg/ml the vegetative growth was not inhibited, but the sporulation was completely blocked. Tilorone-resistant mutants were asporogenous. The author has suggested that the selectivity in tilorone action may be due to the fact that A-T-rich regions are involved in the sporulating phase.

XI. Some Future Prospects

The data reported here show that tilorone, a compound endowed with many interesting biologic activities, requires very specific structural parameters for its biochemical action; and moreover, the same structural entities are also involved in its interaction with DNA. Using the molecular models of double-stranded helical DNA, one can examine the intercalation of tilorone at the same molecular dimensions. This approach could help to find out the groups or substitutions which will anchor best in A-T-rich sites of DNA, thus leading to active derivatives of tilorone.

References

Adamson, R.H.: Tilorone: A new antitumor drug. Proc. Am. Assoc. Cancer Res. *12*, 24 (1971a)

Adamson, R.H.: Antitumor activity of Tilorone hydrochloride against some rodent tumors: preliminary report. J. Natl. Cancer Inst. *46*, 431 (1971b)

Adamson, R.H., Ablashi, D.V., Armstrong, G.R., Ellmore, N.W.: Effect of Cytosine Arabinoside, Adenine Arabinoside, Tilorone and Rifamycin SV in multiplication of Herpesvirus samiri. In Vitro *1*, 82 (1972)

Albrecht, W.L.: Tilorone Analogues. In: Conf. modul. host immune resist. preven. treat. Induced neoplasias. Nat. Cancer Inst., Bethesda, Maryland. Fogarty Int. Center Proc. *28*, 83 (1974)
Albrecht, W.L., Fleming, R.W., Horgan, S.W., Kihm, J.C., Mayer, G.D.: J. Med. Chem. *17*, 886 (1974)
Andrews, E.R., Fleming, R.W., Grisar, J.W., Kihm, J.C., Wenstrup, D.L., Mayer, G.D.: J. Med. Chem. *17*, 882 (1974)
Barker, A.D.: The effect of Interferon-inducers on the progress of friend virus leukemia in mice. Diss. Abstr. Int. B. *32*, 2881 (1971)
Barker, A.D., Rheins, M.S., Wilson, H.E.: Amelioration of Friend virus leukemia by sequential administration of viral and nonviral interferon inducers. Proc. Soc. Exp. Biol. Med. *137*, 981 (1971)
Buckler, C.E., Du Buy, H.G., Rafajko, R.R., Baron, S.: Hyporesponsiveness: alterations by varying the inducer sequence. Int. Collq. Interferon and Interferon Inducers, Abstract. Belgium: Leuven 1971
Camyre, K.P., Groelke, J.W.: Characterization of the serum antiviral responses induced by Tilorone hydrochloride in rats and mice. Bacteriol. Proc. *22*, 187 (1972)
Camyre, K.P., Groelke, J.W., Mayer, G.D., Krueger, R.F.: Characterization of a Tilorone-induced antiviral response in rats. Bacteriol. Proc. *22*, 188 (1971)
Chandra, P.: Molecular approaches for designing antiviral and antitumor compounds. Invited chapter: Topics in current chemistry: medicinal chemistry, Vol. 52, p. 99. Berlin, Heidelberg, New York: Springer 1974
Chandra, P., Steel, L.K.: Purification, Biochemical and serological analysis of a reverse transcriptase from human spleen. Biochem. J. *167*, 513 (1977)
Chandra, P., Woltersdorf, M.: Influence of tilorone and congeners on the secondary structure and template activity of DNA. FEBS Lett. *41*, 169 (1974)
Chandra, P., Woltersdorf, M.: Tilorone Hydrochloride: a specific probe for AT-regions of duplex deoxyribonucleic acid. Biochem. Pharmacol. *25*, 877 (1976)
Chandra, P., Zimmer, Ch., Thrum, H.: Effect of distamycin A on the structure and template activity of DNA in RNA-polymerase system. FEBS Lett. *7*, 90 (1970)
Chandra, P., Zunino, F., Götz, A.: Bis-DEAE-fluorenone: a specific inhibitor of DNA polymerases from RNA tumor viruses. FEBS Lett. *22*, 161 (1972a)
Chandra, P., Zunino, F., Zaccara, Y.: Mode of tilorone hydrochloride on the secondary structure and template activity of DNA. FEBS Lett. *23*, 145 (1972b)
Chandra, P., Zunino, F., Gaur, V.P., Zaccara, Y.: Mode of tilorone hydrochloride interaction to DNA and polydeoxyribonucleotides. FEBS Lett. *28*, 5 (1972c)
Chandra, P., Will, G., Gericke, D., Götz, A.: Inhibition of DNA polymerases from RNA tumor viruses by tilorone and congeners: site of action. Biochem. Pharmacol. *23*, 3259 (1974)
Chandra, P., Steel, L.K., Ebener, U., Woltersdorf, M., Laube, H., Kornhuber, B., Mildner, B., Götz, A.: Chemical Inhibitors of oncornaviral DNA polymerases. Pharm. Ther. A. *1*, 231 (1977)
Cochran, K.W.: Chemprophylaxis with Tilorone hydrochloride of scrapie in mice. Am. Soc. Microbiol. 72nd. Meet. 23–23 April (1972)
Colby, C., Merigan, M.J.: Interferon induction and action. Annu. Rev. Microbiol. *25*, 333 (1971)
Crothers, D.M.: Calculation of binding isotherms for heterogeneous polymers. Biopolymers *6*, 575 (1968)
De Bary, E.: Eliminierung von Resistent-Plasmiden. M.D.-Thesis of Frankfurt Univ. (1976)
De Clercq, D.M.: Synthetic interferon inducers. Top. Curr. Chem. *52*, 173 (1974)
De Clercq, D.M., Merigan, T.C.: Stimulation or inhibition of interferon production depending on time of cycloheximide administration. Virology *42*, 799 (1970)
De Clercq, D.M., Merigan, T.C.: Bis-DEAE-fluorenone: mechanism of antiviral protection and stimulation of interferon production in the mouse. J. Infect. Dis. *123*, 190 (1971)
Dennis, A.J., Wilson, H.E., Barker, A.D., Rheins, M.S.: Interferon production in normal and leukemic human leukocyte cultures by tilorone hydrochloride. Proc. Soc. Exp. Biol. Med. *141*, 782 (1972)
Diamantstein, T.: Stimulation of humoral immune responses by tilorone hydrochloride. Immunology *24*, 771 (1973)
Finney, D.J.: Statistical methods in biological assay, p. 99. New York: Hafner Publishing Co. 1964

Fleming, R.W., Albrecht, W.L., Andrews, E.R., Grisar, J.M., Horgan, S.W., Sill, A.D., Wenstrup, B.L.: Bis-DEAE-fluorenone analogues: a new class of antiviral interferon inducers. Int. Colloq. Interferon and Interferon Inducers. Belgium: Leuven 1971

Fornosi, F., Talas, M., Weiszfeiler, G.: Acta Microbiol. Acad. Sci. Hung. *18*, 327 (1971)

Fox, A.E., Gawlak, D.L., Ballantyne, D.L., Jr., Freedman, M.M.: Transplantation *15*, 389 (1973)

Freedman, H.H., Fox, A., Shavel, J. Jr., Morrison, G.C.: Proc. Soc. Exp. Biol. Med. *139*, 909 (1972)

Friendlaender, G.E., Mosher, M.B., Mitchell, M.S.: Effect of tilorone hydrochloride upon cell-mediated immunity in mice. Cancer Res. *34*, 304 (1974)

Gallo, R.C.: RNA tumor viruses and leukemia: evaluation of present results supporting their presence in human leukemias. In: Modern trends in human leukemia II, p. 431. München: Lehmanns 1976

Gaur, V., Chandra, P.: Subcellular distribution of labeled tilorone hydrochloride in tissues of mice and rats. Naturwissenschaften *60*, 263 (1973)

Gaur, V., Chandra, P.: Tilorone hydrochloride: its pharmacokinetic parameters and its pharmacodynamic effects. Cancer chemotherapy II. Hellman, K., Conners, T. (eds.), Vol. 8, p. 43. New York: Plenum Press 1976

Gaur, V., Wacker, A.: Radiosynthesis of tilorone hydrochloride with carbon-14 at position 9 of the fluorene. J. Labelled Comp. IX, *2*, 282 (1973)

Giron, D.J., Schmidt, J.P., Pindak, R.: Tilorone hydrochloride: lack of correlation between interferon induction and antiviral protection. Antimicrob. Agents Chemother. *1*, 78 (1972)

Giron, D.J., Schmidt, J.P., Ball, R.J., Pindak, R.: Effect of interferon inducers and interferon on bacterial infections. Antimicrob. Agents Chemother. *1*, 80 (1972)

Glasgow, L.A.: Immunosuppression, interferon and viral infections. Fed Proc. *30*, 1846 (1971)

Green, S., West, W.L.: *In vitro* cytogenetic effects of tilorone·HCl. (Abstr.) Pharmacologist *13*, 260 (1971)

Grisar, J.M., Hickey, K.R., Fleming, R.W., Mayer, G.D.: J. Med. Chem. *17*, 890 (1974)

Groelke, J.W., Camyre, K.P.: The effect of tilorone hydrochloride on the *in vitro* induction of antiviral activity by Poly I:C. Am. Soc. Microbiol. Proc. Rep. Ohio. (1972)

Groelke, J.W., Camyre, K.P., Mayer, G.D.: Proc. Exp. Biol. Med. *148*, 1044 (1974)

Grossberg, S.E.: The interferons and their inducers: molecular and therapeutic considerations. N. Engl. J. Med. *287*, 13 (1972)

Hahn, F.: Experimental elimination of R factors. Antibiot. Chemother. *20*, 196 (1976)

Hahn, F., Ciak, J.: Elimination of bacterial episomes by DNA-complexing compounds. Ann. N.Y. Acad. Sci. *182*, 295 (1971)

Hausen, H. zur: Oncogenic herpesviruses. Biophys. Biochem. Acta *417*, 25 (1975)

Hirota, Y., Iijima, T.: Acriflavine as an effective agent for eliminating F-factor in *E. coli* K_{12}. Nature (London) *180*, 655 (1957)

Hoffman, P.F., Ritter, H.W.: The effect of tilorone hydrochloride on stimulation of the primary immune responses. J. Reticuloendothelial Soc. *9*, 638 (1971)

Hoffman, P.F., Ritter, H.W., Krueger, R.F.: In: Advances in antimicrobial and antineoplastic chemotherapy. Hejzlar, M., Semonsky, M., Masek, S. (eds.), p. 217. Munich: Urban and Schwarzenberg 1972

Hofmann, H., Kunz, C.: The protective effects of the interferon inducers tilorone hydrochloride and Poly IC on experimental tick-borne Encephalitis in mice. Arch. Ges. Virusforsch. *37*, 262 (1972)

Hook, R.H., Williams, J.M., Brunzie, G.F., Wright, G.J.: Toxicol. Appl. Pharmacol. *29*, 149 (1974)

Kaufman, H.E., Centifano, Y.M.: Species differences in interferon stimulation: minimal response in primates and man as compared to rodents. J. Clin. Invest. *50*, 53a (1971)

Kaufman, H.E., Centifanto, Y.M., Ellison, E.D., Brown, D.C.: Tilorone hydrochloride: human toxicity and interferon stimulation. Proc. Soc. Exp. Biol. Med. *137*, 357 (1971)

Kaufman, H.E., Ellison, E.D., Centifanto, Y.M.: Am. J. Ophthal. *74*, 89 (1972)

Kleinschmidt, W.J.: Biochemistry of interferon and its inducers. Annu. Rev. Biochem. *41*, 517 (1972)

Kotler, M., Becker, Y.: Effect of distamycin A and congocidine on DNA synthesis by RSV reverse transcriptase. FEBS Lett. *22*, 222 (1972)

Krueger, R.F., Mayer, G.D.: Tilorone hydrochloride: an orally active antiviral agent. Science *169*, 1213 (1970)
Krueger, R.F., Yoshimura, S.: Antiviral activity of tilorone hydrochloride, an oral interferon inducer. Fed. Proc. *29*, 29 (1970)
Krueger, R.F., Mayer, G.D., Yoshimura, S., Ludwig, H.: *In vivo* evaluations of tilorone hydrochloride against Semlike forest virus. Antimicrob. Agents Chemother. *1*, 486 (1970)
Krueger, R.F., Mayer, G.D., Camyre, K.P., Yoshimura, S.: Comparative interferon and antiviral responses of tilorone hydrochloride and other bis-basic substituted polycyclic aromatic compounds. Int. Colloq. on Interferon and Interferon Inducers. Belgium: Leuven 13–16 Sept. (1971)
Leeson, G.A., Biedenbach, S.A., Hook, R.H., Wright, G.J.: Proc. 9th Int. Congr. Chemotherap. (1975)
Leeson, G.A., Biedenbach, S.A., Chan, K.Y., Gibson, J.P., Wright, G.J.: Drug Metab. Dispos. *4*, 232 (1976)
Lerman, L.S.: Structural considerations in the interaction of DNA and acridines. J. Mol. Biol. *3*, 18 (1961)
Lerman, L.S.: Acridine mutagens and DNA structure. J. Cell Comp. Physiol. *64*, 1 (1964)
Levine, S., Gibson, J.P., Megel, H.: Selective depletion of thymus dependent areas in lymphoid tissue by tilorone. Proc. Soc. Exp. Biol. Med. *146*, 245 (1974)
Mayer, G.D., Fink, B.A.: Bis-DEAE-fluorenone, an oral inducer of interferon. Fed. Proc. *29*, 635 (1970)
Mayer, G.D., Krueger, R.F.: Proc. 5th Int. Congr. Infect. Dis. Vienna, 31 Aug–5 Sept. p. 245 (1970a)
Mayer, G.D., Krueger, R.F.: Tilorone hydrochloride: mode of action. Science *169*, 1214 (1970b)
Mayer, G.D., Krueger, R.F., Camyre, K.P., Bray, F., Hull, C.R.: Effects of cycloheximide on the *in vivo* responses of tilorone hydrochloride and polyinosinic:polycytidylic acid. Bacteriol. Proc. (Abstr.) p. 195 (1971)
Mayer, G.D., Hagan, A.C., Bray, F.: Abstr. Fed. Am. Soc. Biol., Atlantic City, 15–20 April (1973)
Mayer, G.D., Bray, F., Camyre, K.P.: In: 14th Intersci. Conf. Antimicrobiol. Agents and Chemother., San Francisco, 11–13 Sept. (1974)
McKenzie, R.D., Schatzman, G.L.: Scand. J. Haematol. *15*, 58 (1975)
Megel, H., Raychaudhuri, A., Goldstein, S., Kinsolving, C.R., Shemano, I., Michael, J.G.: Tilorone: its selective effects on humoral and cell-mediated immunity. Proc. Soc. Exp. Biol. Med. *145*, 513 (1974)
Megel, H., Raychaudhuri, A., Shemano, I., Beaver, T.H., Thomas, L.L.: Proc. Exp. Biol. Med. *148*, 89 (1975)
Merigan, T.C.: Boosting the body's interferon. New Sci. *48*, 498 (1970)
Miller, J.A.: Carcinogenesis by chemicals. Cancer Res. *30*, 559 (1970)
Mobraaten, L.E., De Maeyer, E., De Maeyer-guinard, J.: Prolongation of allograft survival in mice by inducers of interferon. Transplantation *16*, 415 (1973)
Munson, A.E., Munson, J.A., Regelson, W.: Tilorone and congeners: effect on host defense mechanisms. Int. Colloq. on Interferon Inducers. Belgium: Leuven, Abstr No. 27 (1971)
Munson, A.E., Munson, J.A., Regelson, W., Wampler, G.L.: Effect of tilorone hydrochloride and congeners on reticuloendothelial system, tumors and the immune responses. Cancer Res. *32*, 1397 (1972)
Niblack, J.F.: Interferon inducers in antiviral research. Int. Congr. Pure Appl. Chem. *3*, 111 (1971)
Portony, J., Merigan, T.C.: The effect of interferon stimulation on avian influenza. Clin. Res. *19*, 139 (1971a)
Portony, J., Merigan, T.C.: The effect of interferon and interferon inducers on avian influenzy. J. Infect. Dis. *124*, 545 (1971b)
Rapp, F., Reed, C.: Experimental evidence for the oncogenic potential of herpes simplex virus. Cancer Res. *36*, 800–806 (1976)
Renoux, G., Renoux, M.: Nature New Biol. *240*, 217 (1972)
Renton, K.W., Mannering, G.J.: Drug Metab. Dispos. *4*, 223 (1976)
Rhaese, M.J.: Personal communication (1977)
Rheins, M.S., Wilson, H.E.: The amelioration of Friend Virus leukemia by the sequential administration of a series of viral and non-viral interferon inducers. Bacteriol. Proc. p. 188 (1971)

Rheins, M.S., Barker, A.D., Wilson, H.E.: Therapeutical effects of non-viral interferon inducers on a viral-induced leukemia. Can. J. Microbiol. *17*, 1259 (1971)

Rhoads, A., Roye, D., West, W., Morris, H.P.: The effect of tilorone on the growth rate of Morris hepatomas 7777, 392A and Walker 256 carcinosarcoma. Amer. Chem Soc. 162nd Meeting (1971)

Richmond, J.Y., Campbell, C.H.: Arch. Gesamte Virusforsch. *42*, 102 (1973)

Rohovsky, M.W., Newberne, J.W., Gibson, J.P.: Effects of an oral interferon inducer on the hematopoietic and reticuloendothelial systems. Toxicol. Appl. Pharmacol. *17*, 556 (1970)

Rohovsky, M.W., Newberne, J.W., Gibson, J.P.: Preclinical toxicity studies with tilorone hydrochloride, an oral interferon inducer. Toxicol. Appl. Pharmacol. *19*, 415 (1971)

Roye, D., Rhoads, A., Morris, H.P., West, W.L.: Effect of tilorone on growth of tumors in rats. Pharmacologist *13*, 260 (1971)

Sieber, S.M., Adamson, R.H.: Embryotoxic activity of interferon and tilorone, a synthetic interferon inducer, in mice. Int. Congr. Pharmacol., San Fransisco, p. 231 (1972)

Sill, A.D., Albrecht, W.L., Andrews, E.R., Fleming, R.W., Horgan, S.W., Roberts, E.M., Sweet, F.W.: J. Med. Chem. *16*, 240 (1973)

Sill, A.D., Andrews, E.R., Sweet, F.W., Hoffman, J.W., Tiernan, P.L., Grisar, J.M., Fleming, R.W., Mayer, G.D.: J. Med. Chem. *17*, 965 (1974)

Spiegelman, S.: Molecular evidence for the association of RNA tumor viruses with human mesenchymal malignancies. In: Modern trends in human leukemia II. Neth, R., Gallo, R.C., Mannweiler, K., Moloney, W.C., (eds.), p. 391, München: Lehmanns 1976

Stringfellow, D.A., Glasgow, L.A.: Hyporeactivity of infection: potential limitation to therapeutic use of interferon-inducing agents. Infect. Immun. *6*, 743 (1972)

Wacker, A., Lodemann, E., Gaur, V., Diederich, J.: Distribution of labelled tilorone in mice. Naturwissenschaften *59*, 520 (1972)

Wampler, G.L., Munson, A.E., Regelson, W.: Tilorone and congeners: new antitumor agents with stimulating effects on host defense mechanisms. Proc. Am. Assoc. Cancer Res. *13*, 120 (1972)

Weder, H.G., Schildknecht, J., Kesselring, P.: Equilibrium dialysis. Am. Lab. *10*, 15 (1971)

Wu, A.M., Ting, R.C.Y., Gallo, R.C.: RNA-directed DNA-polymerase and virus-induced leukemia in mice. Proc. Natl. Acad. Sci. USA *70*, 1298 (1973)

Yoshimura, S., Christian, R.T., Camyre, K.P., Krueger, R.F.: Proc. 8th Int. Congr. Chemotherap., Athens, Greece, Sept. (1973)

Zbinden, G., Emch, E.: Effect of tilorone hydrochloride, an oral interferon-inducer, on leukopoiesis in rats. Acta Haematol. *47*, 49 (1972)

The Vinca Alkaloids

W.A. CREASEY

Introduction

History and Background

The vinca alkaloids are antineoplastic indole derivatives (Fig. 1) that are isolated from the leaves of the periwinkle plant, *Vinca rosea* L., or more correctly, *Catharanthus roseus* G. Don. This plant is of Madagascan origin, although its distribution is now pantropical (STEARN, 1975). Even in varieties selected for the highest alkaloid content, the concentrations of these antitumor agents are very low, as much as 1 kg of dried leaves being needed to obtain 3 mg of vincristine, for example.

The periwinkle plant has enjoyed a worldwide reputation as a medicinal herb. As early as 1653 CULPEPER mentioned the use of an infusion of the leaves to stop hemorrhage. This was also one of the applications described by PECKOLT (1910) in his study of Brazilian medicinal plants; other uses included the deadening of the pain of toothache, the treatment of scurvy, and the cleansing of wounds. It was, however, the use of the plant to treat diabetes (WHITE, 1925; GARCIA, 1954; WATT and BREYER-BRANDWIJK, 1962) in parts of the world as widely scattered as the Philippines, England, South Africa, and the British West Indies, that prompted the investigations which led to the isolation of antineoplastic alkaloids.

Two independent groups, one at the Collip Laboratories of the University of Western Ontario, the other at the Lilly Research Laboratories, studied the reputed hypoglycemic activity. No such activity was detected at that time, although subsequent studies have identified several hypoglycemic components whose activity is masked by the toxicity of the crude extracts (SVOBODA and BLAKE, 1975). Instead, the Canadian workers encountered granulocytopenia and depression of the bone marrow in rats treated with fractions derived from the plant extracts (BEER, 1955; CUTTS et al., 1957). From this material they isolated vinblastine sulfate (VLB), then called vincaleukoblastine (NOBLE et al., 1958; CUTTS et al., 1960). At about the same time the group at Lilly demonstrated that several fractions inhibited the growth of P-1534 leukemia carried in DBA/2 mice (JOHNSON et al., 1959).

These phytochemical studies of the antitumor activity continued with the isolation of vinleurosine (VLR), then termed leurosine, in addition to vinblastine (SVOBODA, 1958). It was noted that certain fractions that were free of both

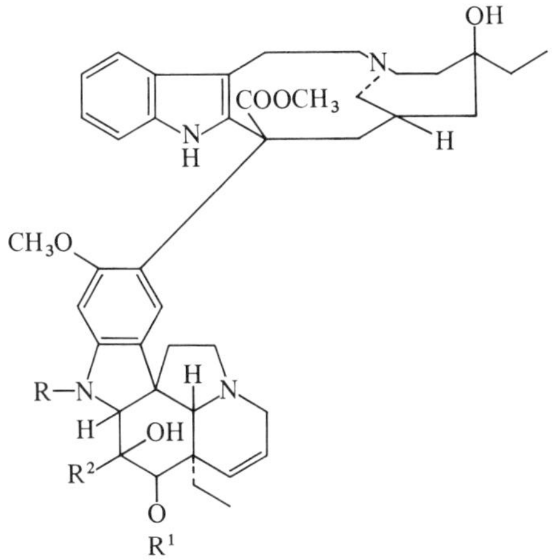

Vinblastine $-R = CH_3$, $R^1 = COCH_3$, $R^2 = COOCH_3$

Vincristine $-R = CHO$, $R^1 = COCH_3$, $R^2 = COOCH_3$

Vinglycinate $-R = CH_3$, $R^1 = COCH_2N(CH_3)_2$, $R^2 = COOCH_3$

Vindesine $-R = CH_3$, $R^1 = H$, $R^2 = CONH_2$

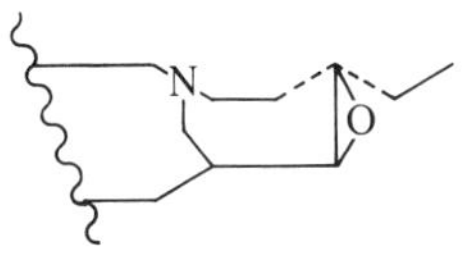

Vinleurosine $R = CH_3$, $R^1 = COCH_3$, $R^2 = COOCH_3$

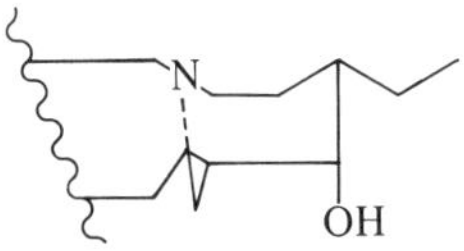

Vinrosidine $R = CH_3$, $R^1 = COCH_3$, $R^2 = COOCH_3$

Fig. 1. Structural formulas of vinca alkaloids

vinblastine and vinleurosine were more active than those containing the latter two alkaloids. From these highly active derivates, vincristine (VCR; leurocristine) and vinrosidine (VRD; leurosidine) were obtained (SVOBODA, 1961; JOHNSON et al., 1962). Four minor active dimeric alkaloids, leurosivine (SVOBODA, 1963), 4-desacetylvinblastine, rovidine (SVOBODA and BARNES, 1964), and leurocolombine (TAFUR et al., 1975) were isolated subsequently. A monomeric alkaloid, lochnerinine, also has relatively low antitumor activity (FARNSWORTH et al., 1967). 4-Desacetoxyvinblastine has been identified as a contaminant in some preparations of vinblastine (NEUSS et al., 1975), but there is no information as to whether it is cytotoxic. All the other alkaloids that have been isolated from the periwinkle plant, close to seventy in all, are not active antitumor agents. In clinical practice only vinblastine and vincristine, from among the naturally-occurring active alkaloids, are of proven value. Vinleurosine received quite extensive clinical trial, but offered no advantage over vinblastine.

Once the usefulness of the vinca alkaloids was established, attempts were made to synthesize derivatives by modifying one of the active alkaloids, usually vinblastine, which is more abundant than vincristine. Thus 6,7-dihydrovinblastine (NOBLE et al., 1967), vinglycinate, the 4-N, N-dimethylaminoacetyl derivative of desacetylvinblastine (ARMSTRONG, 1968), and vindesine, desacetylvinblastine amide, have been synthesized, and the latter two have reached clinical trial. 3′,4′-Dehydro derivatives of vinblastine, vincristine, and vindesine have been prepared by the action of sulfuric acid, and shown to possess cytotoxic activity (MILLER et al., 1977).

Structure

The anticancer alkaloids, with the exception of lochnericine and lochnerinine, which have only limited activity, all possess a dimeric indoledihydroindole structure (Fig. 1), with the indole group a part of the catharanthine nucleus, and the dihydroindole (indoline) moiety forming an element in the vindoline nucleus. Establishment of the structures of these compounds was based upon chemical fragmentation, circular dichroism, infrared and mass spectrometry, and X-ray crystallography (JOHNSON et al., 1963; ABRAHAM, 1975; KUTNEY et al., 1975b). The sheer complexity of the molecules led to much uncertainty regarding their detailed structures, especially in the case of vinleurosine.

A number of attempts have been made to synthesize dimeric compounds from the monomeric alkaloids. However, in most cases, these attempts have not produced active drugs, because of an inappropriate stereochemical orientation of the C18′ catharanthine-vindoline linkage (e.g., KUTNEY et al., 1975a). Recently products having the natural configuration were obtained by a modified

Table 1. Physical properties of antitumor vinca alkaloids

Alkaloid	Molecular weight	Melting point (°C)	pK_a	λ max (Et OH) nm.	$[\alpha]_D^{26}$ $CHCl_3$
4-Desacetylvin-blastine (sulfate)	867.0	>320 (decomp)	5.4, 6.9	214,266,294	
Leurocolombine	826.0		5.05, 6.3	217,265	
Leurosivine (sulfate)	831.0	>335 (decomp)	4.8, 5.8	214,265	
Rovidine (sulfate)		>320 (decomp)	4.82, 6.95	214,265,296	
Vinblastine	811.0 (base) 909.1 (sulfate)	201–211	5.4, 7.4	214,259	+42
Vincristine	825.0 (base) 923.1 (sulfate)	218–220 (decomp)	5.0, 7.4	220,255,296	+17
Vindesine	851.9 (sulfate)				
Vinleurosine	809.0	202–205 (decomp)	5.5, 7.5	214,259	+72
Vinrosidine	811.0	208–211 (decomp)	5.0, 8.8	214,265	+55.8

Polonovski reaction that involves skeletal fragmentation of ibogane derivatives in the presence of aspidospermane-type compounds. This presents analogies to the biosynthetic pathway (LANGLOIS et al., 1976).

As regards structure–activity relationships, certain requirements for activity have been defined:

1. Activity is associated mainly with the dimeric structure, monomeric alkaloids are generally inactive with very few exceptions.
2. The indole nitrogen of the catharanthine nucleus should retain its basic nature. Amidation of this nitrogen atom, for example, causes loss of activity.
3. The free hydroxyl functions should be unsubstituted. Total acetylation leads to loss of activity. It should be noted, however, that only one hydroxyl group is needed for activity, as in vinleurosine.
4. Complete reduction causes total loss of activity, but partial reduction, as in 6,7-dihydrovinblastine, leaves a less active product.

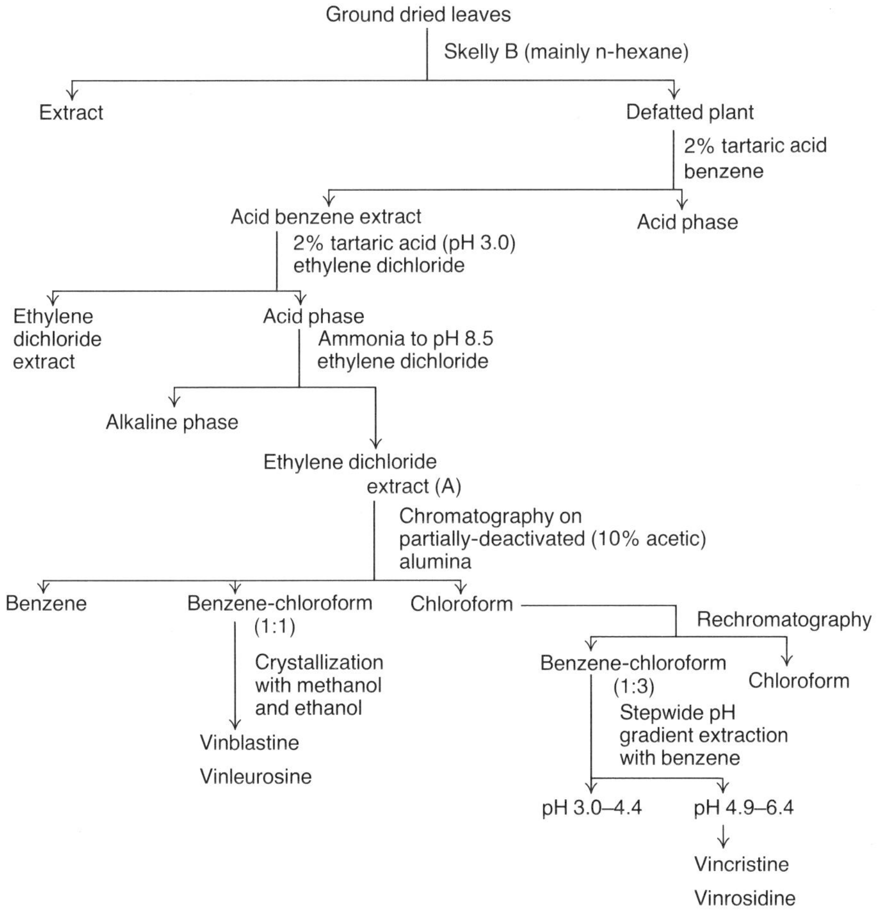

Fig. 2. Extraction schemata for the major active alkaloids

5. Replacement of the 4-acetyl group with other radicals may alter the activity significantly. Thus vinglycinate is less active than vinblastine, while 4-desacetylvinblastine is effective against different tumors. Removal of the 4-acetyl group coupled with change at the 3-position, as in vindesine, alters both antitumor activity and toxicity.
6. Dehydration at the C3′-4′ bond generally reduces the cytotoxic activity of the product, with the exception of Δ-3′,4′-dehydro-4-desacetyl vincristine, which is more active than the parent drug against melanoma B 16.

Some of the basic physical properties of the antitumor alkaloids appear in Table 1.

Isolation

Much of the detail concerning the procedures used for isolating and identifying the vinca alkaloids may be found in the reviews of JOHNSON et al. (1963), and SVOBODA and BLAKE (1975). Our concern here is to outline briefly the basic scheme that has been used to isolate the active alkaloids (Fig. 2). The principle behind the extraction procedures was termed selective or differential extraction, since a weak organic acid (tartaric acid) was used to bind the stronger bases, allowing the separation of alkaloids that complex only weakly with the acid, and in this form are soluble in benzene. Following chromatography on alumina, partially deactivated with 10% acetic acid, another form of differential extraction was employed. This involved stepwise adjustment of the pH, and extraction with benzene after each adjustment. In this way vincristine and vinrosidine were separated. Vinblastine and vinleurosine did not require this procedure, since they could be separated by crystallization rather readily. Vinleurosine only crystallized from methanol, whereas vinblastine could be crystallized from ethanol but not methanol.

Biologic Activity

Mitotic Arrest

The vinca alkaloids exert many biologic actions, of which the most characteristic is the arrest of mitosis at metaphase. This action is identical to that of colchicine or the derivatives of podophyllin, suggesting that there is a common underlying mechanism. Mitotic arrest is not simply the fixation of the mitotic apparatus in the metaphase configuration. Rather, there is an attack on the spindle itself, which undergoes dissolution, leaving the chromosomes that are initially in the metaphase orientation either to disperse within the cell, or to adopt unusual configurations such as ball mitoses (PALMER et al., 1963). Some idea of the order of drug concentrations needed to produce mitotic arrest of

Table 2. Concentrations of vinca alkaloids that produce significant mitotic arrest

Cell line	Effective concentration range (μg/ml)					
	Des VLB	VLB	VCR	VDS	VGL	VLR
L-Cells		0.01–0.05	0.05[a]			5×10^{-4} [a]
Chinese hamster (CHO)	0.001	0.01–0.02	0.001–0.02	0.001	0.2–2.0	0.2–2.0
HeLa		0.002–2.0	0.01–2.0		2–200	2–200
J96		0.001–10	0.01			0.001–10
KB		10^{-6} [a]	0.001[a]			10^{-5} [a]

[a] Values for the ED_{50}.
Abbreviations: DesVLB, desacetylvinblastine; VLB, vinblastine; VCR, vincristine; VDS, vindesine; VGL, vinglycinate; VLB, vinleurosine.
Concentration ranges within which partial or complete mitotic arrest occurs are listed.

cell lines growing in tissue culture may be gleaned from Table 2. Data for the minor alkaloids is sparse, but leurocolombine, for example, inhibits mitosis in KB cells at concentrations of about 0.02 μg/ml.

Mitotic arrest in vivo is generally observed at therapeutic dosage levels, for example after 1 or 0.1 mg/kg of vinblastine in mice or humans, respectively.

Although arrest of mitosis by vincristine may exhibit some degree of irreversibility (GEORGE et al., 1965; JOURNEY et al., 1968), a large proportion of arrested cells may resume proliferating after removal of all of the drugs. The sequence involved in this reversal, as described by KRISHAN (1968) using Earle's L cells treated with vinblastine, includes resumption of division by many micronucleate and metaphase-blocked cells in as little as 4 h after removal of the alkaloid. The oöcytes of starfish and of the marine worm *Pectinaria gouldi* provide excellent systems for studying the reversibility of spindle dissolution. Within minutes vinblastine provokes attrition and disappearance of the spindle, which reappears rapidly on washing away the drug with fresh sea water. Once again, recovery is not as complete after exposure to vincristine, followed by removal of drug (MALAWISTA et al., 1968, 1976).

A number of agents are known to antagonize the antimitotic action of the vinca alkaloids. This has been noted in Ehrlich ascites carcinoma growing in mice that received injection of both vinblastine and cortisone (DUSTIN, 1963), an effect known previously for colchicine and corticosteroids, and thought to result from facilitation of recovery of the damaged spindle (DE HARVEN, 1956). Tryptophan and glutamic acid also reduced the degree of mitotic arrest in Ehrlich ascites cells exposed to vinblastine (CUTTS, 1961). It was evident that the degree of arrest was less complete, and after 24 h there was no difference between cell populations exposed to drug alone, and those treated with alkaloid and antagonist. At least in the case of glutamic acid there is evidence for it acting as a competitive inhibitor of the uptake of vinblastine by cells (CREASEY et al., 1971); this could certainly explain the antagonism with respect to mitotic inhibition.

Experimental Antitumor Activity

The anticancer activity of periwinkle plant materials was first recognized in the P1534 leukemia. Although the sensitivity of the strain has changed over the years, the data reported in 1963 by JOHNSON et al. are reproduced in Table 3 to give some idea of the comparative efficacy and dosage levels of the four major naturally occurring alkaloids. The sensitivity of this tumor to the vinca alkaloids was fortunate, for had reliance been placed on what was at that time the major element in the conventional mouse tumor screen, the L1210 leukemia, the activity of these drugs might have escaped detection. Treatments in Table 3 were given daily. In Table 4 data from our laboratory indicate that daily doses of vinblastine are more effective than single doses; similar results are seen in sarcoma 180 ascites and with vincristine. On the other hand, data from the Eli Lilly Laboratories showed that this was true only over certain dose ranges for vindesine, and both schedules achieved similar results at their respective optimal dosage levels. Table 5 provides information on the spectra of activity of four natural and two semisynthetic alkaloids. It can be seen that the structural modifications that have been discussed earlier lead to significant alterations in the responses obtained with the six drugs, especially in adenocarcinoma 755, B 82A leukemia, Erhlich ascites carcinoma, Ridgeway osteogenic sarcoma, and sarcoma 180 ascites. As an accompaniment to this data, acute LD_{50} values for rats and mice are given in Table 6.

Table 3. Comparative efficacy of the four major natural alkaloids as inhibitors of P 1534 leukemia

Alkaloid (sulfate)	Dose mg/kg/day	Toxic deaths	% increase in survival	Indefinite survivors
Vinblastine	0.05	0	41	0
	0.01	0	53	0
	0.3	0	70	0
	0.45	0	131	0
	0.6	1	150	0
Vincristine	0.06	0	24	0
	0.09	0	55	2
	0.2	1	110	2
	0.25	0	226	3
	0.35	2	30	1
Vinleurosine	7.5	0	0	0
	10.0	0	32	0
	11.25	0	41	0
	20.0	1	76	1
Vinrosidine	2.0	0	21	0
	3.0	0	30	0
	4.0	0	70	0
	5.0	0	127	0
	10.0	1	?	4

The tumor was carried in DBA/2 mice, 5 animals to a group. Injections were given i.p. daily for 10 days. Data taken from JOHNSON et al. (1963).

Table 4. Comparison of the effects of consecutive and single doses of vinblastine (VLB) and vindesine (VDS) on ascites tumors

Tumor	Drug	Dosage mg/kg × day	% increase in life span	Survivors[a]
Ehrlich ascites carcinoma	VLB	0	–	0/37
		0.5 × 1	+ 22	0/10
		1.0 × 1	+ 31	0/10
		2.0 × 1	+ 8	0/26
		4.0 × 1	+ 1	0/11
		0.05 × 10	+ 29	1/10
		0.1 × 10	+136	9/24
		0.2 × 10	+165	6/14
		0.4 × 10	+ 36	5/12
P388 leukemia	VDS	0	–	0/20
		1.8 × 1	+ 54	0/10
		4.0 × 1	+ 77	0/10
		6.0 × 1	+109	1/10
		9.0 × 1	+190	3/10
		13.5 × 1	+231	4/10
		0.18 × 9	+109	0/10
		0.4 × 9	+172	3/10
		0.6 × 9	+213	4/10
		0.9 × 9	+177	4/10
		1.35 × 9	– 10	0/10

[a] This is the number surviving 50 days after VLB and 40 days after VDS. Data derived from CREASEY (1966) and ELI LILLY (1975).

There is less information available about the effects of these alkaloids on cells in culture. Inhibition of growth occurs at levels that arrest mitosis (Table 2), and cell death may follow prolonged exposure at these concentrations, or more rapidly at higher levels. KB cells, derived originally from a human nasopharyngeal carcinoma, are very sensitive to the vinca alkaloids, and thus have been used frequently as a bioassay system (FARNSWORTH et al., 1967; DIXON et al., 1969). Values for the ED_{50} in this cell line in $\mu g/ml$ are: vinblastine, 1×10^{-6}; vincristine, 1×10^{-3}; vinleurosine, 1×10^{-5}; lochnerinine, 1×10^{-2}; and lochnericine, 1.1.

An important finding of studies with cells in culture is that the vinca alkaloids are primarily lethal in the S phase of the cell cycle, with some enhanced sensitivity during late G_1 in the case of vinblastine (MADOC-JONES and MAURO, 1968), while they block the cycle in M phase.

Clinical Antitumor Activity

Various aspects of the early use of the vinca alkaloids have been reviewed by JOHNSON et al. (1963), and a later article has covered this area until the period of rapid proliferation of combination chemotherapy regimens (DE CONTI and CREASEY, 1975).

Table 5. The spectra of antitumor activity of the major natural and synthetic alkaloids

Tumor	Host	Alkaloids					
		VDS	VGL	VCR	VLB	VLR	VRD
Adenocarcinoma 755	C57BL/6	++	−	++	+	−	−
AKR leukemia	AKR	−	−	++	−	+	−
B 16 melanoma	C57BL/6	++		+	+++		
B 82A leukemia	C58		+	+++	++	+	++
C1498 leukemia	C57BL/6	−	−	−	−	−	−
Dunning	Rat			++	++		
Ehrlich ascites	Swiss	+++	−	+++	+++	+++	−
Freund ascites	CAF[1]		++	++	+++	+++	++
Gardner lymphosarcoma	C3H	++	−	−	−	−	+
L1210 leukemia	DBA/2	−	+	−	−	−	−
L5178Y leukemia	Swiss	−	−	−	−		
Lilly mammary	DBA/1	−	−	+	+	−	−
Lilly rhabdomyosarcoma	Rat		+	−	+	−	−
Mecca lymphosarcoma	AKR		−	+	−	−	+
P388 leukemia		+++		+++	+++		
P1534 leukemia	DBA/2	+++	+++	+++	++	++	+++
Ridgeway osteogenic sarcoma	AKR	+++	−	+++	−	−	+++
S91 melanoma	DBA/1		−	−	−	−	−
Sarcoma 180	CAF[1]		+	−	−	−	−
Sarcoma 180 ascites	CAF[1]	++	+++	+++	+++	−	+
Walker 256	Rat	−	−	−	+	+	+
Walker 256 ascites	Rat	+++		+++	+++		
X 5563 myeloma	C3H		−	+			+

Data derived from Johnson et al. (1963, 1966), Venditti and Abbott (1967), Eli Lilly (1975), and Miller et al. (1977). Abbreviations: VDS, vindesine; VGL, vinglycinate; VCR, vincristine; VLB, vinblastine; VLR, vinleurosine; VRD, vinrosidine. Antitumor data expressed as percent inhibition of solid tumor growth or percent prolongation of survival time for leukemias and ascitic tumors: −, <30%; +, 30%–50%; ++, 50%–100%; +++, >100%.

Table 6. Acute LD_{50} values for intravenously administered vinca alkaloids

Alkaloid (as sulfate)	Mouse mg/kg ± S.E.	Rat mg/kg ± S.E.
Vinblastine	10.0 ± 0.9 (3.2 ± 0.02 intraperitoneal)	2.9 ± 1.5
Vincristine	2.1 ± 0.1	1.0 ± 0.1
Vindesine	6.3 ± 0.6	2.0 ± 0.2
	Lethal dose in mouse mg/kg	
Desacetylvinblastine	5	
Vinleurosine	50	
Vinrosidine	100	

Table 7. Human toxicity of the vinca alkaloids

% incidence	Vinblastine	Vincristine	Vindesine
Above 50		Paresthesias	Leukopenia
30–50	Leukopenia	Loss of deep tendon reflex	
10–30	Nausea, vomiting, anorexia	Constipation, hoarseness	Thrombocytopenia, hair loss, paresthesias, loss of deep tendon reflex, weakness and lethargy
5–10	Hair loss, neurotoxicity (all forms total)	Weakness and lethargy, hair loss, slapping gait	Nausea, vomiting, anorexia constipation, jaw pain, phlebitis
Below 5	Stomatitis, diarrhea, constipation, lethargy, phlebitis, ileus	Abdominal pain, muscle cramps, depression, phlebitis, cranial nerve palsy	Cellulitis, chills and fever, abdominal cramps

Data derived from DE CONTI and CREASEY (1975), BLUM and DAWSON (1976), BODEY and FREIREICH (1976), and CURRIE et al. (1976).

Vincristine has proved most effective in the treatment of Hodgkin's disease, lymphosarcoma, acute lymphoblastic leukemia, reticulum cell sarcoma, and Burkitt's lymphoma. It has also been widely used for carcinomas of the breast, bronchus and cervix, Wilm's tumor, rhabdomyosarcoma, Ewing's sarcoma, testicular tumors, melanoma, neuroblastoma, acute myeloblastic leukemias, and some nonmalignant conditions such as Letterer-Siwe disease. Although initially used as a single agent for these diseases, vincristine is now seldom employed in this way, but rather forms an important component of many regimens of combination chemotherapy. This is based upon features of its action with respect to the cell cycle, and to its unique neurologic toxicity, which does not overlap the side effects of other drugs (SARTORELLI and CREASEY, 1973; CLARKSON, 1974; FREI and GOTTLIEB, 1974; GOLDIN et al., 1974; CREASEY, 1977a).

Vinblastine has a narrower spectrum of usefulness than vincristine, in part because its limiting toxicity, bone marrow depression, is common to many other antineoplastic agents, thus reducing the potential of this alkaloid for use in combination chemotherapy. Its major clinical applications have been for Hodgkin's disease, many lymphomas including Burkitt's lymphoma, choriocarcinoma, testicular tumors, and carcinoma of the ovary. This spectrum of activity is narrower and somewhat different from that of vincristine. Even more striking is the divergence in the range of toxic side effects (Table 7). Vincristine administration is limited by the severe neurotoxicity that intervenes before the dosage level that would lead to leukopenia can be reached. Similar neurologic effects may be exerted to some extent by vinblastine, but generally at dosage levels that cannot be tolerated. The neurologic toxicity, which will be discussed later, involves demyelination and degeneration of nerve fibers (GOTTSCHALK et al., 1968), and action on the muscle spindle (Tobin and Sandler, 1966; 1968). Another interesting reaction is hyponatremia with inappropriate antidiuretic hormone secretion (Fine et al., 1966; Slater et al., 1969). Phlebitis usually results from local irritation and extravasation during injection.

Vinleurosine has been employed as the methiodide (Hodes et al., 1963) and the sulfate (Mathé et al., 1965; Gailani et al., 1966). It resembles vinblastine in its activity, but is probably inferior. A shock-like syndrome accompanied rapid intravenous injection, but its toxicity otherwise is similar to that of vinblastine.

Vinglycinate has shown activity in Hodgkin's disease, lymphosarcoma, and bronchogenic carcinoma (Armstrong et al., 1967). In both the antitumor action and the toxicity it resembles vinblastine, but requires a tenfold higher molar dosage.

Vindesine is now being studied intensively (Todd et al., 1975; Blum and Dawson, 1976; Bodey and Freireich, 1976; Currie et al., 1976). Responses have occurred in patients with acute myelocytic and lymphoblastic leukemias, Ewing's sarcoma, lymphomas, and squamous and renal cell carcinomas. Toxicity includes (in man but not in some experimental animals) both the neurologic toxicity of vincristine, and the myelosuppressive action of vinblastine (Table 7). Unlike the other two drugs, a high incidence of thrombocytopenia has been noted in these early trials of vindesine. In contrast, both vinblastine and vincristine have been reported to induce thrombocytosis (Hwang et al., 1969; Robertson and McCarthy, 1969); this may be related to the induction of membrane-lined vesicles in human leukemic lymphoblasts exposed to these alkaloids, in a process that resembles platelet formation from megakaryocytes (Krishan and Frei, 1975).

Typical therapeutic dosages of these alkaloids in many combination schedules are: vinblastine, 6–8 mg/M^2; vincristine, adults 1.4 mg/M^2, children 2 mg/M^2; vindesine (Phase I), 0.5–6 mg/M^2, vinleurosine (not in use) 100–250 mg/M^2.

Antiviral Activity

The earliest observation of an antiviral effect of the vinca alkaloids was reported by Johnson (1965) who showed that vincristine, but not vinblastine, was active against Mengo virus in vivo. Subsequently a wide range of alkaloids derived from *Catharanthus* species was screened by an agar diffusion method using green monkey cells. In terms of protecting cells from damage caused by Vaccinia virus, the potency of the antitumor alkaloids declined in the order: vincristine, vinblastine, leurosivine, vinrosidine, and desacetyl vinblastine at concentrations of 125 to 1,000 μg/ml. Vinleurosine and lochnerinine were inactive. None of the alkaloids were antiviral in a Polio III Screen (Farnsworth et al., 1968). Of the non-antitumor alkaloids pericalline was the most active. Vindesine inhibits the spleen enlargement and increases in red blood cell volume that result from administration of Friend leukemia virus to mice (Eli Lilly, 1975).

Antiinflammatory Action

Vinblastine is able to exert an antiinflammatory action to relieve acute gouty episodes (KRAKOFF, 1965). This presents a strong analogy to colchicine, a traditional drug for this disease.

Neuromuscular Actions

Neurologic toxicity is the dose-limiting toxicity for vincristine, a major untoward effect of vindesine, and a comparatively infrequent side effect of vinblastine (Table 7). In humans, asymptomatic depression of the Achilles tendon reflex, paresthesias of the extremities, cranial and sensory nerve involvement, and slapping gait may occur (SANDLER et al., 1969). Other side effects with neurologic etiology include constipation, paralytic ileus, muscle weakness (CASEY et al., 1970), and reduced nerve conduction velocities (MCLEOD and PENNY, 1969).

Pathologic and biochemical studies have described axonal degeneration and demyelination (GOTTSCHALK et al., 1968), lysis of dorsal root ganglion cells and inhibition of Schwann cell proliferation (UY et al., 1967), and inhibition of rapid axonal transport of labeled materials (OCHS and WORTH, 1975), including norepinephrine storage granules, acetyl choline, and choline acetyl transferase (DAHLSTRÖM et al., 1975).

Behavioral changes have been studied in mice, where the sulfates of vincristine (1–2.5 mg/kg), desacetyl vinblastine (5 mg/kg), and vinrosidine (10–100 mg/kg) act as CNS depressants, while vinleurosine (5–25 mg/kg) acts as an adrenergic blocking agent (SVOBODA and BLAKE, 1975).

There appears to be a direct action of vincristine on muscle cells (TOBIN and SANDLER, 1966, 1968), reflected in degenerative changes in the motor end plates and the appearance of spheromembranous bodies (ANDERSON et al., 1967; BRADLEY et al., 1970). Reduction in calcium uptake and an altered profile of the phospholipids of rat skeletal muscle microsomes also have been associated with muscle damage produced by vincristine (YASIN et al., 1973).

Autonomic Actions

A hypertensive action has been ascribed to both vincristine and vindesine, which apparently is not due to enhanced response to sympathetic amines, but might have some autonomic basis (UEDA et al., 1969; ELI LILLY, 1975). Hypotension and an abnormal Valsalva response have also been attributed to vincristine (HANCOCK and NAYSMITH, 1975). Other workers have found that vinblastine and vincristine both reduced the effects of noradrenergic nerve stimulation and sensitized the myocardium to norepinephrine (BENNETT and GARDINER, 1975). The uptake of norepinephrine by rat brain synaptosomes (NOMURA and SEGAUA, 1975) and adrenergic fibers (COSTA and FILOGOMO, 1970) is inhibited by vinblastine, as is the release of histamine from rat peritoneal mast cells (GILLESPIE et al., 1968). Obviously, work needs to be done to clarify the situation regarding these autonomic effects, since the literature reports are rather conflicting.

Miscellaneous Biologic Actions

Although they are not among the most active immunosuppressive agents, the vinca alkaloids have long been known to inhibit both antibody synthesis and delayed hypersensitivity in rats (AISENBERG, 1963). Vincristine inhibits the secretion of IgM antibody (TEPLITZ et al., 1975), but does not cause lysis of antibody-coated target cells (GELFAND et al., 1975).

Apart from inappropriate secretion of antidiuretic hormone mentioned above, which can be corrected by rigorous fluid restriction (STUART et al., 1975), there are a number of other hormonal effects of the vinca alkaloids. Release of adrenal steroids is increased (CHUNG and GABOUREL, 1971), whereas mobilization of thyroid hormone (WOLFF and BHATTACHARYYA, 1975), secretion of insulin (LACY et al., 1968), the bethanechol-stimulated release of pancreatic amylase (WILLIAMS and LEE, 1976), and isoproterenol-mediated release of renin (CAPPONI and VALLOTTON, 1976), in vitro are reduced. Secretion of plasma lipoproteins is also reduced by the vinca alkaloids (ORCI et al., 1973; STEIN et al., 1974). Absorption may also be impaired after exposure to the vinca alkaloids. Reduced absorption of amino acids, accompanied by morphological changes, have been reported in studies using rat ileum (SHARMA and NAGCHAUDHURI, 1976). In the same system vincristine produces an early time-dependent decrease in glucose absorption V (ECKNAUER, 1976).

Vinblastine causes aggregation of ribosomes in *Escherichia coli* cells, which lack microtubules (KINGSBURY and VOELZ, 1969), in human leukemic lymphoblasts and mouse fibroblasts (KRISHAN and HSU, 1971), and also precipitates suspensions of ribosomes (WILSON et al., 1970). This effect may be related to the binding of the alkaloid by ribosomes (SWERDLOW and CREASEY, 1975).

Although no human fetal abnormalities have been described, the vinca alkaloids have been shown to be teratogenic in golden hamsters (FERM, 1963) and rats (COHLAN and KITAY, 1965).

Finally, the hypoglycemic activity for which the plant extracts were originally screened with negative results has been traced to a number of pure alkaloids. Of these the only one which belongs to the dimeric antitumor group is vinleurosine. This drug lowers blood sugar levels rather slowly, the onset being at two hours and the maximum effect at five to seven hours after administration (SVOBODA and BLAKE, 1975).

Mechanism of Action

The mechanisms by which the vinca alkaloids exert their antitumor and cytotoxic effects are complex. Furthermore, the various noncytotoxic biologic effects must also be considered. Basically, two major types of intervention can account for most of the biologic effects: interaction with the microtubule system and inhibition of biosynthetic pathways (CREASEY, 1975a, 1977b).

Microtubule Interactions

Microtubules are tubular elements with diameters of about 250 Å, often many microns in length, that occur in eukaryote but not prokaryote organisms. They may be found singly, but for the most part they occur in groups as loose aggregates near cell surfaces or intracellular organelles, as actual cell membrane components exposed at the surface of neurons (ESTRIDGE, 1977), or as constituents of structured entities such as the mitotic spindle and flagella. A number of reviews may be consulted that detail the nature and functions of the microtubule system (ADELMANN et al., 1968; OLMSTED and BORISY, 1973; BURNSIDE, 1975). Our concern here is to outline briefly some of the features of this system, and point out how the vinca alkaloids might intervene in it.

Microtubules are composed of a number of protofibrils, commonly 13, which are in dynamic equilibrium with the subunit protein, tubulin. This normally occurs as a heterodimer with each chain close to a molecular weight of 55,000 (FINE, 1971). Intracellular concentrations of tubulin reach a maximum during late S and G_2 phase of the cell cycle (KLEVECZ and FORREST, 1975). The process of assembly of microtubules is complex (KIRSCHNER et al., 1975; ENGELBORGHS et al., 1976), requiring not only the free (6S) tubulin, but also forms of tubulin of higher sedimentation coefficient (36S), such as double ring and spiral structures that may serve as nucleation centers. A high molecular weight protein is needed for these special forms to be produced from 6S tubulin (SCHMITT et al., 1977), whereas tubulin hoops, which show an arrangement of dimers like that in flagellar B tubules, form during poymerization of purified 6S material (MANDELKOW et al., 1977). The microtubules themselves may be associated with high molecular weight proteins (BORISY et al., 1975) and cyclic AMP-dependent protein kinases (SOIFFER et al., 1976).

Structures derived from the microtubule system are mainly involved in movement, or in maintaining shape or rigidity. The neurotubules may act as stationary or moving tracts associated for example with mitochondria or vesicles (SMITH et al., 1975), while microtubules may slide over one another or may lose subunits from the polar end to produce shrinkage of spindle fibers during mitosis (MCINTOSH et al., 1975).

Antimitotic drugs intervene in both the organization and function of the microtubule system (CREASEY, 1975a; WILSON, 1975a, b). The fundamental mechanism of the intervention takes the form of binding of drug by tubulin. However, beyond this point the situation becomes increasingly complex. Various antimitotic drugs are bound at different sites, with colchicine and podophyllin, derivatives and griseofulvin appearing to occupy a different type site from those with which the vinca alkaloids interact. Agents from the colchicine-site class will stabilize the binding of vinca alkaloids and vice versa, while within the same group competition for binding is evident. Disappearance of microtubules and microtubule-containing structures such as the mitotic spindle is the result

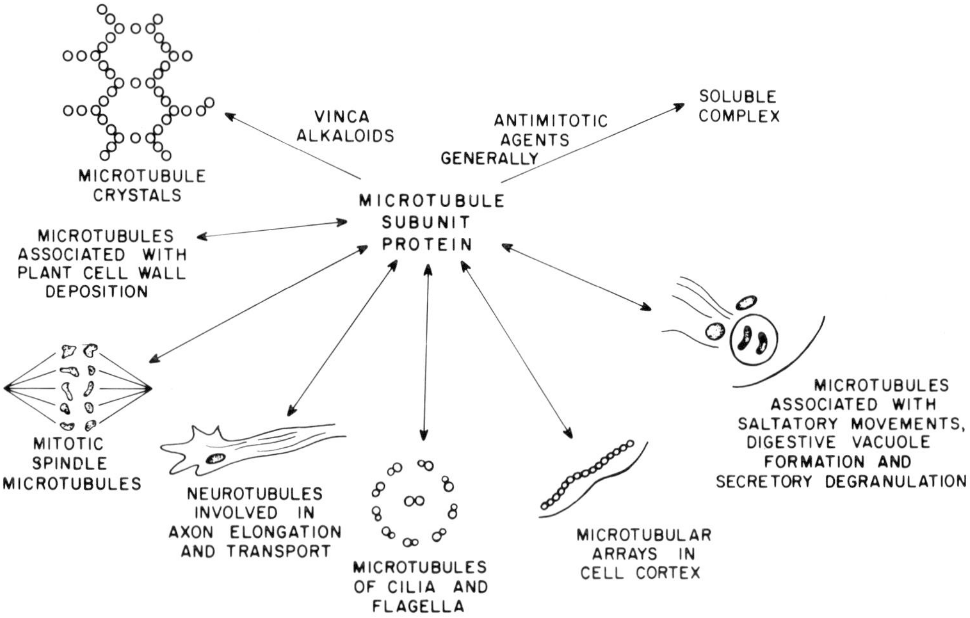

Fig. 3. The microtubule system and the interaction with vinca alkaloids. The binding phenomenon that yields soluble complex and microtubule crystals inhibits polymerization leading to dissolution of microtubules that are in equilibrium (with differing rate constants) with the subunit (tubulin) pool

of this interaction. This situation undoubtedly reflects the underlying equilibrium between tubulin and the microtubule-containing structures (Fig. 3). Complex formation removes subunits from the free pool which disturbs the equilibrium, causing dissociation of the formed elements. Rates of dissolution of these elements would reflect the kinetics of the specific equilibria. The microtubules of cilia and flagella, for example, are relatively stable (Behnke and Forer, 1967), whereas those of the mitotic spindle are labile. Damage to microtubules in the axons appears to be greatest with vinblastine despite the lesser neurotoxicity, suggesting that uptake into neuronal tissue is critical (Donoso et al., 1977).

After the disappearance of microtubules in cells exposed to vinca alkaloid, but not colchicine, cytoplasmic inclusion bodies may make their appearance, especially at high drug concentrations. These inclusions may take the form of uniaxial birefringent crystals consisting of regular aggregates of microtubules of somewhat larger diameter than normal, and sharing their walls in common in a hexagonal arrangement (Bensch and Malawista, 1969; Marantz and Shelanski, 1970). Similar crystals have been reported in a variety of tissues including starfish oocytes (Malawista and Sato, 1969), human (Schochet et al., 1968) and rabbit neurons (Kotorii et al., 1971), as well as in isolated tubulin preparations (Bensch et al., 1969; Olmsted et al., 1970).

It would seem that for each molecule of tubulin dimer there are two sites normally occupied by GTP, one site for the binding of colchicine, and two high affinity sites for vinblastine (Bryan, 1972). There are, in addition, as many as 10 to 20 low affinity sites at which vinblastine may bind to tubulin (WILSON, 1975a). From their kinetic properties, the high affinity sites seem to correspond to the depolymerization induced by the alkaloid which results from inhibition of polymerization (OWELLEN et al., 1976). The low affinity sites may be responsible for aggregation, which underlies the formation of microtubules and the precipitation of tubulin in vitro (BHATTACHARYYA and WOLFF, 1976).

These interactions with the microtubule system are sufficient to explain a wide range of biologic actions indicated in Fig. 3. Mitotic arrest is a fairly obvious result of microtubule dissolution, as is the inhibition of the regeneration of protozoan cilia (ROSENBAUM and CARLSON, 1969), since both mitotic spindles and cilia have tubules as an integral component. Changes in activity of phagocytes in joints might result from inhibition of saltatory motion, necessary for phagocytosis, and thus lead to relief of acute pain from gout. Secretion and absorption also may require microtubules for movement of granules, as also does axon transport. Thus, all these processes could be blocked by alkaloid-induced dissolution of the microtubules. Cytotoxicity, however, may require additional damage apart from the reversible attrition of tubules. This additional damage may result from the known effects of these alkaloids on many biosynthetic pathways (CREASEY, 1974, 1975b, 1977b).

Interference with Nucleic Acid Biosynthesis

Vinblastine and/or vincristine have been reported to inhibit the synthesis of DNA and RNA in a wide range of experimental systems. They include Ehrlich ascites carcinoma cells (CREASEY and MARKIW, 1964a, b), rat spleen, bone marrow (VAN LANCKER et al., 1966), thymus (JONES et al., 1966), and regenerating liver (LUCYCKX and VAN LANCKER, 1966), the protozoan *Tetrahymena pyriformis* (SLOTNICK et al., 1966), mouse brain (AGUSTIN and CREASEY, 1967), human leukocytes (CLINE, 1968; CREASEY, 1968), HEp-2 cells in culture (WAGNER and POIZMAN, 1968), and rat embryos in culture in vivo (KROWKE et al., 1970). There was considerable variation in the relative sensitivities of DNA and RNA synthesis, as well as of the RNA subfractions. Human leukemic lymphoblasts were extremely sensitive to vincristine, as regards RNA synthesis, which is in keeping with the response of these cells to treatment. Both vinrosidine (RICHARDS et al., 1966) and vinleurosine (CREASEY, 1969) inhibited nucleic acid biosynthesis in rat thymus and sarcoma 180 cells, respectively. In our laboratory we have found recently that vindesine inhibits the synthesis of nucleic acids by S180 cells in vitro, with DNA synthesis being most sensitive.

At the enzymatic level, vincristine inhibits isolated preparations of RNA polymerase (CLINE, 1968), while vinblastine prevents the increased activity of high molecular weight cytoplasmic DNA polymerase that accompanies stimulation of nucleated erythrocytes with erythropoietin (ROODMAN et al., 1975).

In contrast to these inhibitory effects there is a report that in dense cultures of mouse embryo fibroblasts, in which proliferation and DNA synthesis are inhibited, probably by cell surface changes, low levels (0.05–0.4 μg/ml) of vinblastine or colchicine initiate the incorporation of thymidine into DNA (VASILIEV et al., 1971).

Inhibition of Protein Synthesis

Reports of the inhibition of protein biosynthesis by the vinca alkaloids include studies on Ehrlich ascites cells (CREASEY and MARKIW, 1965; WARNECKE and SEEBER, 1968), human leukemic leukocytes (CLINE, 1968), and rat embryos in in vivo culture (KROWKE et al., 1970). These effects could depend upon inhibition of RNA synthesis, reduced amino acid transport (CREASEY, 1975a), or binding by ribosomes (SWERDLOW and CREASEY, 1975).

Effects on Lipid Biosynthesis and Respiration

In view of the demyelination of nerve fibers that accompanies neurotoxicity, it is no surprise that vinca alkaloids affect lipid biosynthesis. Inhibitory effects have been noted in the gastrocnemius muscle of rats treated with vincristine (GRAFF et al., 1967), in S180 cells exposed to vinleurosine (CREASEY, 1969) or vincristine (CREASEY, 1975b) and in rat embryos treated with vincristine (KROWKE et al., 1970). Phospholipid synthesis generally seemed to be the more sensitive parameter.

Inhibition of respiratory processes occurs in L1210 cells (HUNTER, 1963), leukocytes engaged in phagocytosis (GOLDFINGER et al., 1965), and in tumor cells (OBRECHT and FUSENIG, 1966), as a result of the action of vinca alkaloids.

Metabolism and Distribution

The general outlines of vinca alkaloid metabolism and distribution have now been fairly well established, although much detail still needs to be worked out.

When rats were given tritiated vinblastine, about 25% of the dose found its way into the intestine in 24 h, while urinary excretion was only about 6%; only 2% of biliary tritium was in the form of unchanged drug (BEER and RICHARDS, 1964). Of the radioactivity in rat blood, 60% was in the platelets, 15%, in the leukocytes, 10% in the red cells, and 15% in the plasma; all the platelet label was unchanged vinblastine (HEBDEN et al., 1970). The plasma half-lives of vinblastine in dogs were 17–38 min and 3 to 5 h. As much as 79% of plasma tritium was protein-bound, and drug levels in the leukocytes were 2 to 12 times those of the coincident plasma. Vinblastine was the major (47%–81%) biliary component, and 30%–36% of the dose was excreted in the feces in 9 days compared with 12%–17% in the urine (CREASEY et al., 1975). In humans, labeled vinblastine shows plasma half-lives of about 4 and 190 min. Platelets bound the drug avidly. Fecal excretion amounted to 25% to 41% in 72 h, compared to 19% to 23% in the urine. Between 17% and 50% of urinary tritium was present as vinblastine (OWELLEN and HARTKE, 1975).

Early bioassay procedures (DIXON et al., 1969) showed that after 1 mg/kg of vincristine serum levels fell from a range of 0.3 to 1 μg/mg down to 0.02

to 0.05 μg/ml in 6 h in dogs and monkeys, and to undetectable levels within 3 h in rats. Availability of tritiated vincristine enabled the secondary plasma half-life in rats to be estimated at 70 min, while the spleen, adrenal, small intestine and thyroid had unusually high drug levels (OWELLEN and DONIGIAN, 1972). In a comparative study of rats and dogs given tritiated vincristine both species showed a biphasic plasma clearance curve with initial and secondary half-lives of about 15 and 75 min. Vincristine appeared to undergo less metabolism than vinblastine, with less than 10% of biliary and urinary tritium as metabolites in the rat (CASTLE et al., 1976). It is of interest that a carrier-mediated mechanism for the transport of vincristine exists in many tumor cells (BLEYER et al., 1975). If vinblastine is transported by the same mechanism, this would make sense of the competitive relationship with glutamate uptake (CREASEY et al., 1971) and the generally high intracellular levels of this drug. Vincristine, like vinblastine and colchicine, undergoes extensive binding by serum proteins (75% at physiologic concentrations), especially the α- and β-globulins (DONIGIAN and OWELLEN, 1973).

A recent pharmacokinetic analysis of the fate of vinblastine, vincristine, and vindesine has been made in humans (OWELLEN et al., 1977a, b). Vinblastine and vindesine kinetics were fitted to a three-compartment model. Parameters for vinblastine were:

α phase, tl/2 = 3.9 min, V = 16.8 l; β phase, tl/2 = 53 min, V = 79 l; γ phase, tl/2 = 1173 min, V = 1656 l.

Corresponding parameters for vindesine were:

α phase, tl/2 = 3.2 min, V = 4.8 l; β phase, tl/2 = 99 min, V = 58.2 l; γ phase, tl/2 = 1213 min, V = 598 l.

The β phase here corresponds to the initial phase of NELSON et al. (1976), with a tl/2 of 0.1 to 0.9 h. Vincristine was only studied by OWELLEN over 4 h when it behaved as a two-compartment system with α phase, tl/2 = 3.4 min, V = 4.5 l and β phase, tl/2 = 155 min, V = 57.3 l. In the first 24 h 13.2% of vindesine and 9.5% of vincristine were eliminated in the urine. Such data reflect the primary biliary excretion of these compounds and the extensive binding within tissues and with serum proteins.

References

Abraham, D.J.: Structure elucidation and chemistry of the bis catharanthus alkaloids. In: The catharanthus alkaloids, botany, chemistry, pharmacology, and clinical use. Taylor, W.I., Farnsworth, N.R. (eds.), p. 125. New York: Marcel Dekker 1975

Adelmann, M.R., Borisy, G.G., Shelanski, M.L., Weisenberg, R.C., Taylor, E.W.: Cytoplasmic filaments and tubules. Fed. Proc. *27*, 1186–1193 (1968)

Agustin, B.M., Creasey, W.A.: Effects of vinca alkaloids on the synthesis of RNA in mouse brain. Nature (London) *215*, 965–966 (1967)

Aisenberg, A.C.: Suppression of immune response by "vincristine" and "vinblastine". Nature (London) *200*, 484 (1963)

Anderson, P.J., Song, S.K., Slotwiner, P.: The fine structure of spheromembranous degeneration of skeletal muscle induced by vincristine. J. Neuropathol. Exp. Neurol. *26*, 15–24 (1967)

Armstrong, J.G.: New derivatives of the *Vinca rosea* alkaloids. Acta Genet. Med. (Roma) *17*, 193–196 (1968)

Armstrong, J.G., Dyke, R.W., Fouts, P.J., Hawthorne, J.J., Jansen, C.J. Jr., Peabody, A.M.: Initial clinical experience with vinglycinate sulfate, a molecular modification of vinblastine. Cancer Res. *27*, 221–227 (1967)

Beer, C.T.: The leukopenic action of extracts of *Vinca rosea*. A.R. Br. Emp. Cancer Campaign *33*, 487–488 (1955)

Beer, C.T., Richards, J.R.: The metabolism of *Vinca* alkaloids part II. The fate of tritiated vinblastine in rats. Lloydia *27*, 352–360 (1964)

Behnke, O., Forer, A.: Evidence for four classes of microtubules in individual cells. J. Cell Sci. *2*, 169–192 (1967)

Bennett, T., Gardiner, S.M.: The effects of intravenous injections of vinblastine or vincristine on the response of the rat heart to nerve stimulation and to drugs. Br. J. Pharmacol. *53*, 444 P (1975)

Bensch, K.G., Malawista, S.E.: Microtubule crystals in mammalian cells. J. Cell. Biol. *40*, 95–107 (1969)

Bensch, K.G., Marantz, R., Wisniewski, H., Shelanski, M.: Induction *in vitro* of microtubular crystals by vinca alkaloids. Science *165*, 495–496 (1969)

Bhattacharyya, B., Wolff, J.: Tubulin aggregation and disaggregation: mediation by two distinct vinblastine binding sites. Proc. Natl. Acad. Sci. USA *73*, 2375–2378 (1976)

Bleyer, W.A., Frisby, S.A., Oliverio, V.T.: Uptake of vincristine by murine leukemia cells. Biochem. Pharmacol. *24*, 633–639 (1975)

Blum, R.H., Dawson, D.M.: Vindesine (V) – phase I study of a vinca alkaloid. Proc. Am. Assoc. Cancer Res. *17*, 108 (1976)

Bodey, G.P., Freireich, E.J.: Initial clinical studies of vindesine (desacetylvinblastine amide sulfate). Proc. Am. Assoc. Cancer Res. *17*, 128 (1976)

Borisy, G.G., Marcum, J.M., Olmsted, J.B., Murphy, D.B., Johnson, K.A.: Purification of tubulin and associated high molecular weight proteins from porcine brain and characterization of microtubule assembly *in vitro*. Ann. N.Y. Acad. Sci. *253*, 107–132 (1975)

Bradley, W.G., Lassman, L.P., Pearce, G.W., Walton, J.N.: The neuromyopathy of vincristine in man. Clinical, electrophysiological and pathological studies. J. Neurol. Sci. *10*, 107–131 (1970)

Bryan, J.: Definition of three classes of binding sites in isolated microtubule crystals. Biochemistry *11*, 2611–2616 (1972)

Burnside, B.: The form and arrangement of microtubules: an historical, primarily morphological review. Ann. N.Y. Acad. Sci. *253*, 14–26 (1975)

Capponi, A.M., Vallotton, M.B.: Renin release by rat kidney slices incubated *in vitro*. Role of sodium and of alpha- and beta-adrenergic receptors and effect of vincristine. Circ. Res. *39*, 200–203 (1976)

Casey, E.B., Fullerton, P.M., Jelliffe, A.W.: Vincristine neurotoxicity: a clinical and electrophysiological study of eighteen patients. Clin. Sci. *38*, 23P–24P (1970)

Castle, M.C., Margileth, D.A., Oliverio, V.T.: Distribution and excretion of [^{3}H] vincristine in the rat and the dog. Cancer Res. *36*, 3684–3689 (1976)

Chung, L.W.K., Gabourel, J.D.: Adrenal steroid release by vinblastine sulfate and its contributions to vinblastine sulfate effects on rat thymus. Biochem. Pharmacol. *20*, 1749–1756 (1971)

Clarkson, B.: Clinical applications of cell cycle kinetics. In: Handbook of experimental pharmacology, Part I. Sartorelli, A.C., Johns, D.G. (eds.), Vol. 38, pp. 156–193. Berlin, Heidelberg, New York: Springer 1974

Cline, M.J.: Effect of vincristine on synthesis of ribonucleic acid and protein in leukaemic leucocytes. Br. J. Haematol. *14*, 21–29 (1968)

Cohlan, S.Q., Kitay, D.: The teratogenic effect of vincaleukoblastine in the pregnant rat. J. Pediatr. *66*, 541–544 (1965)

Costa, M., Filogamo, G.: Effetti della colchicina nella fibre adrenergiche dei plessi nervosi intestinali. Boll. Soc. Ital. Biol. Sper. *46*, 865–867 (1970)

Creasey, W.A.: Tumor-inhibitory effects of combinations of the vinca alkaloids with actinomycin D. Biochem. Pharmacol. *15*, 367–375 (1966)

Creasey, W.A.: Modifications in biochemical pathways produced by the vinca alkaloids. Cancer Chemother. Rep. *52*, 501–507 (1968)

Creasey, W.A.: Biochemical effects of the vinca alkaloids-IV. Studies with vinleurosine. Biochem. Pharmacol. *18*, 227–232 (1969)

Creasey, W.A.: The vinca alkaloids. Biochem. Pharmacol. Suppl. 2, *23*, 217–223 (1974)
Creasey, W.A.: Vinca alkaloids and colchicine. In: Handbook of experimental pharmacology, part II. Sartorelli, A.C., Johns, D.G. (eds.), Vol. 38, pp. 670–694. Berlin, Heidelberg, New York: Springer 1975a
Creasey, W.A.: Biochemistry of dimeric *Catharanthus* alkaloids. In: The catharanthus alkaloids, botany, chemistry, pharmacology and clinical use. Taylor, W.I., Farnsworth, N.R. (eds.), pp. 209–236. New York: Marcel Dekker 1975b
Creasey, W.A.: Pharmacological considerations in combination chemotherapy. Pharmacol. Ther. *A 1*, 307–325 (1977a)
Creasey, W.A.: Plant alkaloids. In: Cancer: a comprehensive treatise. Becker, F.F. (ed.), Vol. 5, pp. 379–425. New York: Plenum Press 1977b
Creasey, W.A., Markiw, M.E.: Biochemical effects of the vinca alkaloids-I. Effects of vinblastine on nucleic acid synthesis in mouse tumor cells. Biochem. Pharmacol. *13*, 135–142 (1964a)
Creasey, W.A., Markiw, M.E.: Biochemical effects of the vinca alkaloids-II. A comparison of the effects of colchicine, vinblastine and vincristine on the synthesis of ribonucleic acids in Ehrlich ascites carcinoma cells. Biochim. Biophys. Acta *87*, 601–609 (1964b)
Creasey, W.A., Markiw, M.E.: Biochemical effects of the vinca alkaloids-III. The synthesis of ribonucleic acid and the incorporation of amino acids in Ehrlich ascites cells *in vitro*. Biochem. Biophys. Acta *103*, 635–645 (1965)
Creasey, W.A., Bensch, K.G., Malawista, S.E.: Colchicine, vinblastine and griseofulvin. Pharmacological studies with human leukocytes. Biochem. Pharmacol. *20*, 1579–1588 (1971)
Creasey, W.A., Scott, A.I., Wei, C.C., Kutcher, J., Schwartz, A., Marsh, J.C.: Pharmacological studies with vinblastine in the dog. Cancer Res. *35*, 1116–1120 (1975)
Culpeper, N.: The Complete herbal, 1653. Reprinted for Imperial Chemical Industries. Birmingham: Kynoch Press 1953
Currie, V., Wong, P., Tan, R., Tan, C., Krakoff, I.: Preliminary clinical studies of desacetyl vinblastine amide sulfate (DVA), a new vinca alkaloid. Proc. Am. Assoc. Cancer Res. *17*, 174 (1976)
Cutts, J.H.: Changes in mitosis in ascites tumors and normal bone marrow induced by vincaleukoblastine *in vitro*. Can. Cancer Conf. *4*, 363–372 (1961)
Cutts, J.H., Beer, C.T., Noble, R.L.: Effects on hematopoiesis in rats of extracts of *Vinca rosea*. Rev. Can. Biol. *16*, 487 (1957)
Cutts, J.H., Beer, C.T., Noble, R.L.: Biological properties of vincaleukoblastine, an alkaloid in *Vincarosea* Linn., with reference to its antitumor action. Cancer Res. *20*, 1023–1031 (1960)
Dahlström, A., Heiwall, P.O., Häggendal, J., Saunders, N.R.: Effect of antimitotic drugs on the intraaxonal transport of neurotransmitters in rat adrenergic and cholinergic nerves. Ann. N.Y. Acad. Sci. *253*, 507–516 (1975)
De Conti, R.C., Creasey, W.A.: Clinical aspects of the dimeric *Catharanthus* alkaloids. In: The *catharanthus* alkaloids, botany, chemistry, pharmacology and clinical use. Taylor, W.I., Farnsworth, N.R. (eds.), pp. 237–278. New York: Marcel Dekker 1975
De Harven, E.: Action de la colchicine et de certaines hormones corticosurrénaliennes sur les mitoses des follicules pileux du rat. Rev. Belge Pathol. *25*, 277 (1956)
Dixon, G.J., Dulmadge, E.A., Mulligan, L.T., Mellett, L.B.: Cell culture bioassay for vincristine sulfate in sera from mice, rats, dogs, and monkeys. Cancer Res. *29*, 1810–1813 (1969)
Donigian, D.W., Owellen, R.J.: Interaction of vinblastine, vincristine and colchicine with serum proteins. Biochem. Pharmacol. *22*, 2113–2119 (1973)
Donoso, J.A., Green, L.S., Heller-Bettinger, I.E., Samson, F.E.: Action of the *Vinca* alkaloids vincristine, vinblastine, and desacetyl vinblastine, amide on axonal fibrillar organelles *in vitro*. Cancer Res. *37*, 1401–1407 (1977)
Dustin, P., Jr.: New aspects of the pharmacology of antimitotic agents. Pharmacol. Rev. *15*, 449–480 (1963)
Ecknauer, R.: Intestinal absorption of glucose immediately after vincristine administration in rats. Experientia *32*, 709–711 (1976)
Eli Lilly & Co.: Compound 99094, desacetyl vinblastine amide sulfate, an investigational new drug. Information for clinical investigators. Indianapolis: Eli Lilly & Co. 1975
Engelborghs, Y., Heremans, K.A.H., De Maeyer, L.C.M., Hoebeke, J.: Effect of temperature and pressure on polymerization equilibrium of neuronal microtubules. Nature (London) *259*, 686–688 (1976)

Estridge, M.: Polypeptides similar to the α and β subunits of tubulin are exposed on the neuronal surface. Nature (London) *268*, 60–63 (1977)
Farnsworth, N.R., Blomster, R.N., Buckley, J.P.: Catharanthus alkaloids XIII. Antineoplastic and hypotensive activity of alkaloid fractions and certain alkaloids from *Catharanthus lanceus*. J. Pharm. Sci. *56*, 23–27 (1967)
Farnsworth, N.R., Svoboda, G.H., Blomster, R.N.: Antiviral activity of selected *Catharanthus* alkaloids. J. Pharm. Sci. *57*, 2174–2175 (1968)
Ferm, V.H.: Congenital malformations in hamster embryos after treatment with vinblastine and vincristine. Science *141*, 426 (1963)
Fine, R.E.: Heterogeneity of tubulin. Nature New Biol. *233*, 283–284 (1971)
Fine, R.N., Clarke, R.R., Shore, N.A.: Hyponatremia and vincristine therapy. Syndrome possibly resulting from inappropriate antidiuretic hormone secretion. Am. J. Dis. Child. *112*, 256–259 (1966)
Frei, E., III, Gottlieb, J.A.: Combination chemotherapy: Clinical considerations. In: Handbook of experimental pharmacology, part I. Sartorelli, A.C., Johns, D.G. (eds.), Vol. 38, pp. 449–467. Berlin, Heidelberg, New York: Springer 1974
Gailani, S.D., Armstrong, J.G., Carbone, P.P., Tan, C., Holland, J.F.: Clinical trial of vinleurosine sulfate (NSC-90636): a new drug derived from *Vinca rosea* Linn. Cancer Chemother. Rep. *50*, 95–103 (1966)
Garcia, F.A.: A botany symposium on medicinal plants. In: Proc. 8th Pacific Sci. Congr. of the Natl. Res. Council of the Philippines, IV[A, 182 (1954)
Gelfand, E.W., Morris, S.A., Resch, K.: Antibody-dependent cytotoxicity: modulation by the cytochalasins and microtubule-disruptive agents. J. Immunol. *114*, 919–924 (1975)
George, P., Journey, L.J., Goldstein, M.N.: Effect of vincristine on the fine structure of HeLa cells during mitosis. J. Natl. Cancer Inst. *35*, 355–375 (1965)
Gillespie, E., Levine, R.J., Malawista, S.E.: Histamine release from rat peritoneal mast cells: inhibition by colchicine and potentiation by deuterium oxide. J. Pharmacol. Exp. Ther. *164*, 158–165 (1968)
Goldfinger, S.E., Howell, R.R., Seegmiller, J.E.: Suppression of metabolic accompaniment of phagocytosis by colchicine. Arthritis Rheum. *8*, 1112–1122 (1965)
Goldin, A., Venditti, J.M., Mantel, N.: Combination chemotherapy; Basic considerations. In: Handbook of experimental pharmacology, Part I. Sartorelli, A.C., Johns, D.G. (eds.), Vol. 38, pp. 411–448. Berlin, Heidelberg, New York: Springer 1974
Gottschalk, P.G., Dyck, P.J., Kiely, J.M.: Vinca alkaloid neuropathy: nerve biopsy studies in rats and in man. Neurology *18*, 875–882 (1968)
Graff, G.L.A., Guening, C., Hildebrand, J.: Action du sulfate de vincristine sur le gastrocnémien de rat I. Mis en evidence de deux compartements, metaboliquement distincts, pour le phosphate inorganique; effets sur les phosphates organiques acidosolubles et les phospholipides. C.R. Soc. Biol. *161*, 2645–2651 (1967)
Hancock, B.W., Naysmith, A.: Vincristine-induced autonomic neuropathy. Br. Med. J. *3*, 207 (1975)
Hebden, H.F., Hadfield, J.R., Beer, C.T.: The binding of vinblastine by platelets in the rat. Cancer Res. *30*, 1417–1424 (1970)
Hodes, M.E., Rohn, R.J., Bond, W.H., Yardey, J.: Clinical trials with leurosine methiodide, an alkaloid from *Vinca rosea* Linn. Cancer Chemother. Rep. *28*, 53–55 (1963)
Hunter, J.C.: Effects of vincaleukoblastine sulfate on metabolism of thioguanine-resistant L1210 leukemia cells. Biochem. Pharmacol. *12*, 283–291 (1963)
Hwang, Y.F., Hamilton, H.E., Sheets, R.F.: Vinblastine-induced thrombocytosis. Lancet *1969 II*, 1075–1076
Johnson, I.S.: Observations on antiviral screening. Ann. N.Y. Acad. Sci. *130*, 52–55 (1965)
Johnson, I.S., Wright, H.F., Svoboda, G.H.: Experimental basis for clinical evaluation of anti-tumor principles derived from *Vinca rosea* Linn. J. Lab. Clin. Med. *54*, 830 (1959)
Johnson, I.S., Armstrong, J.G., Gorman, M., Burnett, J.P. Jr.: The vinca alkaloids: A new class of oncolytic agents. Cancer Res. *23*, 1390–1427 (1963)
Johnson, I.S., Hargrove, W.W., Harris, P.N., Wright, H.F., Boder, G.B.: Preclinical studies with vinglycinate, one of a series of chemically derived analogs of vinblastine. Cancer Res. *26*, 2431–2436 (1966)

Jones, R.G.W., Richards, J.F., Beer, C.T.: Biochemical studies with the vinca alkaloids II. Effect of vinblastine on the biosynthesis of nucleic acids and their precursors in rat thymus cells. Cancer Res. *26*, 882–887 (1966)
Journey, L.J., Burdman, J., George, P.: Ultrastructural studies on tissue culture cells treated with vincristine (NSC-67574). Cancer Chemother. Rep. *52*, 509–517 (1968)
Kingsbury, E.W., Voelz, H.: Induction of helical arrays of ribosomes by vinblastine sulfate in *Escherichia coli*. Science *166*, 768–769 (1969)
Kirschner, M.W., Suter, M., Weingarten, M., Littman, D.: The role of rings in the assembly of microtubules *in vitro*. Ann. N.Y. Acad. Sci. *253*, 90–106 (1975)
Klevecz, R.R., Forrest, G.L.: Regulation of tubulin expression through the cell cycle. Ann. N.Y. Acad. Sci. *253*, 292–303 (1975)
Kotorii, K., Mori, H., Yoshida, M.: A peculiar crystalline structure in neurons of rabbits treated with vincristine. Kurume Med. J. *18*, 57–63 (1971)
Krakoff, I.H.: Discussion of conference on gout and purine metabolism. Arthritis Rheum. *8*, 760 (1965)
Krishan, A.: Time lapse and ultrastructure studies on the reversal of mitotic arrest induced by vinblastine sulfate in Earle's L. cells. J. Natl. Cancer Inst. *41*, 581–595 (1968)
Krishan, A., Frei, E. III: Morphological basis for the cytolytic effect of vinblastine and vincristine on cultured human leukemic lymphoblasts. Cancer Res. *35*, 497–501 (1975)
Krishan, A., Hsu, D.: Vinblastine-induced ribosomal complexes. Effect of some metabolic inhibitors on their formation and structure. J. Cell Biol. *49*, 927–932 (1971)
Krowke, R., Zimmerman, B., Merker, H.J.: Biochemical and electron microscopic studies of rat embryos in *in vivo* culture. Naunyn Schmiedebergs Arch. Pharmakol. *266*, 382–383 (1970)
Kutney, J.P., Gregonis, D.E., Imhof, R., Itoh, I., Jahngen, E.: Absolute sterochemistry of the bisindole alkaloids of the vinblastine type. Circular dichroism studies. J. Am. Chem. Soc. *97*, 5013–5015 (1975a)
Kutney, J.P., Beck, J., Bylsma, F., Cook, J., Cretney, W.J., Fuji, K., Imhof, R., Tresurywala, A.M.: Total synthesis of indole and dihydroindole alkaloids. VIII. Studies on the synthesis of bisindole alkaloids in the vinblastine-vincristine series. The chloroindolenine approach. Helv. Chim. Acta *58*, 1690–1719 (1975b)
Lacy, P.E., Howell, S.L., Young, D.A., Fink, C.J.: New hypothesis on insulin secretion. Nature (London) *219*, 1177–1179 (1968)
Langlois, N., Gueritte, F., Langlois, Y., Potier, P.: Application of a modification of the Polonovski reaction to the synthesis of vinblastine-type alkaloids. J. Am. Chem. Soc. *98*, 7017 (1976)
Luyckx, A., Van Lancker, J.L.: Metabolic effects of vinblastine. II. The effect of vinblastine on deoxyribonucleic acid and ribonucleic acid synthesis of regenerating liver. Lab. Invest. *15*, 1301–1303 (1966)
Madoc-Jones, H., Mauro, F.: Interphase action of vinblastine and vincristine: differences in their lethal action through the mitotic cycle of cultured mammalian cells. J. Cell Physiol. *72*, 185–196 (1968)
Malawista, S.E., Sato, H.: Vinblastine produces uniaxial, birefringent crystals in starfish oocytes. J. Cell Biol. *42*, 596–599 (1969)
Malawista, S.E., Sato, H., Bensch, K.G.: Vinblastine and griseofulvin reversibly disrupt the living mitotic spindle. Science *160*, 770–772 (1968)
Malawista, S.E., Sato, H., Creasey, W.A.: Dissociation of the mitotic spindle in oocytes exposed to griseofulvin and vinblastine. Exp. Cell Res. *99*, 193–197 (1976)
Mandelkow, E.M., Mandelkow, E., Unwin, N., Cohen, C.: Tubulin hoops. Nature (London) *265*, 655–657 (1977)
Marantz, R., Shelanski, M.: Structure of microtubule crystals induced by vinblastine *in vitro*. J. Cell Biol. *44*, 234–238 (1970)
Mathé, G., Schneider, M., Band, P., Amiel, J.L., Schwarzenberg, L., Cattan, A., Schlumberger, J.R.: Leurosine sulfate (NSC-90636) in treatment of Hodgkin's disease, acute lymphoblastic leukemia, and lymphoblastic lymphosarcoma. Cancer Chemother. Rep. *49*, 47–49 (1965)
McIntosh, J.R., Cande, Z., Snyder, J., Vanderslice, K.: Studies on the mechanism of mitosis. Ann. N.Y. Acad. Sci. *253*, 407–427 (1975)
McLeod, J.G., Penny, R.: Vincristine neuropathy: an electrophysiological and histological study. J. Neurol. Neurosurg. Psychiatr. *32*, 297–304 (1969)

Miller, J.C., Gutowski, G.E., Poore, G.A., Boder, G.B.: Alkaloids of *Vinca rosea* L. (*Catharanthus roseus* G. Don). 38. 4′-Dehydrated derivatives. J. Med. Chem. *20*, 409–413 (1977)
Nelson, R.L., Root, M.A., Dyke, R.W., Ahmadzai, S.: Pharmacokinetics of desacetyl vinblastine amide (Vindesine) in man. Proc. Am. Assoc. Cancer Res. *17*, 30 (1976)
Neuss, N.A., Barnes, J., Huckstep, L.L.: Vinca alkaloids XXXV. Desacetoxy-vinblastine a new minor alkaloid from *Vincarosea* L. (*Catharanthus roseus* G. Don). Experientia *38*, 18–20 (1975)
Noble, R.L., Beer, C.T., Cutts, J.H.: Further biological activities of vincaleukoblastine – an alkaloid from *Vinca rosea* (L). Biochem. Pharmacol. *1*, 347–348 (1958)
Noble, R.L., Beer, C.T., McIntyre, R.W.: Biological effects of dihydrovinblastine. Cancer *20*, 885–890 (1967)
Nomura, Y., Segawa, T.: Influences of colchicine and vinblastine on the uptake of 5-hydroxytryptamine and norepinephrine by rat brain synaptosomes and small vesicle fractions. J. Neurochem. *24*, 1257–1259 (1975)
Obrecht, P., Fusening, N.E.: Die Wirkung von Vincaleukoblastin (Velbe®) auf die Glykolyse von Tumorzellen. Eur. J. Cancer *2*, 109–115 (1966)
Ochs, S., Worth, R.: Comparison of the block of fast axoplasmic transport in mammalian nerve by vincristine, vinblastine and desacetyl vinblastine amide (DVA). Proc. Am. Assoc. Cancer Res. *16*, 70 (1975)
Olmsted, J.B., Borisy, G.G.: Microtubules. Annu. Rev. Biochem. *42*, 507–540 (1973)
Olmsted, J.B., Carlson, K., Klebe, R., Ruddle, F., Rosenbaum, J.L.: Isolation of microtubule protein from cultured mouse neuroblastoma cells. Proc. Natl. Acad. Sci. USA *65*, 129–136 (1970)
Orci, L., Lemarchand, Y., Singh, A., Assimacopoulos-Jennet, F., Rouiller, C.H., Jeanrenaud, B.: Role of microtubules in lipoprotein secretion by the liver. Nature (London) *244*, 30–32 (1973)
Owellen, R.J., Donigian, D.W.: [^{3}H] Vincristine. Preparation and preliminary pharmacology. J. Med. Chem. *15*, 894–898 (1972)
Owellen, R.J., Hartke, C.A.: The pharmacokinetics of 4-acetyl tritium vinblastine in two patients. Cancer Res. *35*, 975–980 (1975)
Owellen, R.J., Hartke, C.A., Dickerson, R.M., Hains, F.O.: Inhibition of tubulin-microtubule polymerization by drugs of the *Vinca* alkaloid class. Cancer Res. *36*, 1499–1502 (1976)
Owellen, R.J., Hartke, C.A., Hains, F.O.: Pharmacokinetics and metabolism of vinblastine in humans. Cancer Res. *37*, 2597–2602 (1977a)
Owellen, R.J., Root, M.A., Hains, F.O.: Pharmacokinetics of vindesine and vincristine in humans. Cancer Res. *37*, 2603–2607 (1977b)
Palmer, C.G., Warren, A.K., Simpson, P.J.: A comparison of the cytologic effects of leurosine methiodide and vinblastine in tissue culture. Cancer Chemother. Rep. *31*, 1–2 (1963)
Peckolt, T.: Heil- und Nutzpflanzen Braziliens. Ber. Dtsch. Pharm. Ges. *20*, 36–58 (1910)
Richards, J.F., Jones, R.G.W., Beer, C.T.: Biochemical studies with the vinca alkaloids I. Effect on nucleic acid formation by isolated cell suspensions. Cancer Res. *26*, 876–881 (1966)
Robertson, J.H., McCarthy, G.M.: Periwinkle alkaloids and the platelet count. Lancet *1969II*, 353–355
Roodman, G.D., Hutton, J.J., Bollum, F.J.: DNA polymerase activities during erythropoiesis. Effects of erythropoietin, vinblastine, colcemid, and daunomycin. Exp. Cell Res. *91*, 269–278 (1975)
Rosenbaum, J.L., Carlson, K.: Cilia regeneration in *Tetrahymema* and its inhibition by colchicine. J. Cell Biol. *40*, 415–425 (1969)
Sandler, S.G., Tobin, W., Henderson, E.S.: Vincristine-induced neuropathy. A clinical study of fifty leukemia patients. Neurology *19*, 367–374 (1969)
Sartorelli, A.C., Creasey, W.A.: Combination chemotherapy. In: Cancer medicine. Holland, J.F., Frei, E. III (eds.), pp. 707–717. Philadelphia: Lea and Febiger 1973
Schmitt, H., Josephs, R., Reisler, E.: A search for *in vivo* factors in regulation of microtubule assembly. Nature (London) *265*, 653–655 (1977)
Schochet, S.S., Lampert, P.W., Earle, K.M.: Neuronal changes induced by intrathecal vincristine sulfate. J. Neuropathol. Exp. Neurol. *27*, 645–658 (1968)
Sharma, R.K., Nagchaudhuri, J.: A study of amino acid absorption from small intestines of vinblastine-treated rats with altered mucosal morphology. Indian J. Med. Res. *64*, 1225–1234 (1976)

Slater, L.M., Wainer, R.A., Serpick, A.A.: Vincristine neurotoxicity with hyponatremia. Cancer *23*, 122–125 (1969)
Slotnick, I.J., Dougherty, M., James, D.H. Jr.: Vincristine inhibition of DNA synthesis in *Tetrahymena pyriformis*. Cancer Res. *26*, 673–675 (1966)
Smith, D.S., Järlfors, V., Cameron, B.F.: Morphological evidence for the participation of microtubules in axonal transport. Ann. N.Y. Acad. Sci. *253*, 472–506 (1975)
Soifer, D., Laszlo, A., Mack, K., Scotto, J., Siconolfi, L.: The association of a cyclic AMP-dependent protein kinase activity with microtubule protein. Ann. N.Y. Acad. Sci. *253*, 598–610 (1975)
Stearn, W.T.: Synopsis of the genus *Catharanthus* (Apocynaceae). In: The catharanthus alkaloids, botany, chemistry, pharmacology, and clinical use. Taylor, W.I., Farnsworth, N.R. (eds.), pp. 9–44. New York: Marcel Dekker 1975
Stein, O., Sanger, L., Stein, Y.: Colchicine-induced inhibition of lipoprotein and protein secretion into the serum and lack of interference with secretion of biliary phospholipids and cholesterol by rat liver *in vivo*. J. Cell Biol. *62*, 90–103 (1974)
Stuart, M.J., Cuaso, C., Miler, M., Oski, F.A.: Syndrome of recurrent increased secretion of antidiuretic hormone following multiple doses of vincristine. Blood *45*, 315–320 (1975)
Svoboda, G.H.: A note on several alkaloids from *Vinca rosea* Linn. I. Leurosine, virosine and perivine. J. Am. Pharm. Ass. *47*, 834 (1958)
Svoboda, G.H.: Alkaloids of *Vinca rosea* Linn. IX. Extraction and characterization of leurosidine and leurocristine. Lloydia *24*, 173–178 (1961)
Svoboda, G.H., Barnes, A.J. Jr.: Alkaloids of *Vinca rosea* Linn. (*Catharanthus roseus* G. Don) XXIV. Vinaspine, vincathicine, rovidine, desacetyl VLB and vinaphamine. J. Pharm. Sci. *53*, 1227–1231 (1964)
Svoboda, G.H., Blake, D.A.: The phytochemistry and pharmacology of *Catharanthus roseus*. In: The catharanthus alkaloids, botany, chemistry, pharmacology, and clinical use. Taylor, W.I., Farnsworth, N.R. (eds.), pp. 45–83. New York: Marcel Dekker 1975
Swerdlow, B., Creasey, W.A.: Binding of vinblastine *in vitro* to ribosomes of sarcoma 180 cells. Biochem. Pharmacol. *24*, 1243–1245 (1975)
Tafur, S., Jones, W.E., Dorman, D.E., Logsdon, E.E., Svoboda, G.H.: Alkaloids of *Vinca rosea* L. (*Catharanthus roseus* G. Don) XXXVI. Isolation and characterization of new dimeric alkaloids. J. Pharm. Sci. *64*, 1953 (1975)
Teplitz, R.L., Mazie, J.C., Gerson, I., Barr, K.J.: The effects of microtubular binding agents on secretion of IgM antibody. Exp. Cell Res. *90*, 392–400 (1975)
Tobin, W.E., Sandler, S.G.: Depression of muscle spindle function with vincristine. Nature (London) *212*, 90–91 (1966)
Tobin, W.E., Sandler, S.G.: Neurophysiologic alterations induced by vincristine (NSC-67574). Cancer Chemother. Rep. *52*, 519–526 (1968)
Todd, G.C., Gibson, W.R., Griffing, W.J., Morton, D.M.: The preclinical study of desacetyl vinblastine amide (DVA). Proc. Am. Assoc. Cancer Res. *16*, 70 (1975)
Ueda, M., Sawadi, M., Kawakami, M., Minesita, T., Takeda, H.: Pressure mechanism of vincristine sulfate. Jpn. J. Pharmacol. *19*, 324–325 (1969)
Uy, Q.L., Moen, T.H., Johns, R.J., Owens, A.H. Jr.: Vincristine neurotoxicity in rodents. Johns Hopkins Med. J. *121*, 349–360 (1967)
Van Lancker, J.L., Flangas, A.L., Allen, J.: Metabolic effects of vinblastine. I. The effect of vinblastine on nucleic acid synthesis in spleen and bone marrow. Lab. Invest. *15*, 1291–1300 (1966)
Vasiliev, J.M., Gelfand, I.M., Guelstein, V.I.: Initiation of DNA synthesis in cell cultures by colcemid. Proc. Natl. Acad. Sci. USA *68*, 977–979 (1971)
Venditti, J.M., Abbott, B.J.: Studies on oncolytic agents from natural sources. Correlations of activity against animal tumors and clinical effectiveness. Lloydia *30*, 332–348 (1967)
Wagner, E.K., Roizman, B.: Effect of the vinca alkaloids on RNA synthesis in human cells *in vitro*. Science *162*, 569–570 (1968)
Warnecke, P., Seeber, S.: Angriffspunkte von Vinca-Alkaloiden im Protein und Nucleinsäurestoffwechsel. Z. Krebsforsch. *71*, 361–367 (1968)
Watt, J.M., Breyer-Brandwijk, M.G.: Medicinal and poisonous plants of Southern and Eastern Africa. p. 85. London: E. & S. Livingston 1962

White, C.T.: Queensl. Agric. J. *23*, 143 (1925). Quoted in: Svoboda, G.H., Blake, D.A.: The phytochemistry and pharmacology of *Catharanthus roseus*. In: The catharanthus alkaloids. Taylor, W.I., Farnsworth, N.R. (eds.), p. 47. New York: Marcel Dekker 1975

Williams, J.A., Lee, M.: Microtubules and pancreatic amylase release by mouse pancreas *in vitro*. J. Cell Biol. *71*, 795–806 (1976)

Wilson, L.: Action of drugs on microtubules. Life Sci. *17*, 303–309 (1975a)

Wilson, L.: Microtubules as drug receptors: pharmacological properties of microtubule protein. Ann. N.Y. Acad. Sci. *253*, 213–231 (1975b)

Wilson, L., Bryan, J., Ruby, A., Mazia, D.: Precipitation of proteins by vinblastine and calcium ions. Proc. Natl. Acad. Sci. USA *66*, 807–814 (1970)

Wolff, J., Bhattacharyya, B.: Microtubules and thyroid hormone mobilization. Ann. N.Y. Acad. Sci. *253*, 763–770 (1975)

Yasin, R., Hughes, B.P., Parker, J.A.: The effect of vincristine on the calcium transport and phospholipid composition of rat skeletal muscle microsomes. Lab. Invest. *29*, 207–215 (1973)

Virazole (Ribavirin)

F.E. HAHN

Virazole is a broad-spectrum antiviral agent. The compound (Fig. 1) is a nucleoside analogue; it was designed and synthesized by WITKOWSKI et al. (1972).

Virazole is active in cell cultures against 25 DNA and RNA viruses. In laboratory animals, the compound is active against 10 RNA virus infections and 6 DNA virus infections (SIDWELL et al., 1974). As discussed later, virazole has been clinically tried in man as a drug against influenza virus infections, viral hepatitis, herpes, and a number of other virus infections. The drug is licenced for clinical use in man in Brazil, Mexico and Nigeria.

A natural C-nucleoside analogue of virazole is the antibiotic pyrazomycin (pyrazofurin) (SUHADOLNIK, 1970). The structure of this antibiotic is shown in Fig. 2. The similarity to virazole is evident. Pyrazomycin is a highly potent broad-spectrum antiviral drug (DELONG et al., 1971; GUTKOWSKI et al., 1975; DESCAMPS and DECLERCQ, 1977). The latter authors reported that the antibiotic inhibited vaccinia, polio, Coxsackie, measles, Sindbis and vesicular stomatitis virus replications at concentrations which were 100- to 1000-fold lower than those required for virazole. Pyrazomycin inhibited plaque formation of Gross leukemia virus at an ED_{50} of 0.01 μg/ml and produced a significant inhibition of Rauscher MLV-induced splenomegaly in mice (SHANNON, 1977). In view of these exceptional activities and its low toxicity, pyrazomycin warrants a study of its in vivo chemotherapeutic activities.

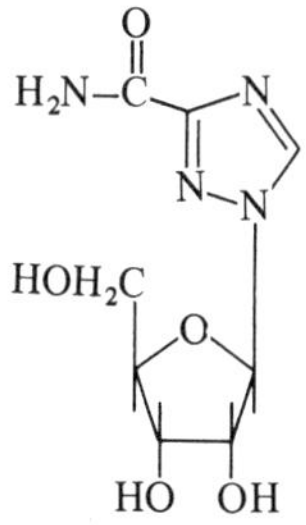

Fig. 1

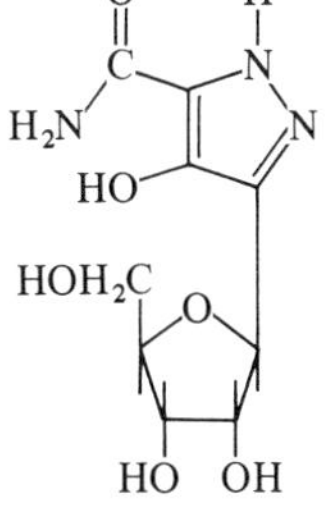

Fig. 2

Fig. 1. Structure of virazole. Molecular weight 244.21 daltons

Fig. 2. Structure of pyrazomycin (pyrazofurin [3(5)-ribofuranosyl-4-hydroxypyrazole-5(3)-carboxamide

Virazole as a Growth Inhibitor

The literature contains no data on the effects of virazole on the growth of microorganisms such as bacteria which can be propagated in lifeless media. According to SIDWELL et al. (1974), the 50% cytotoxic dose of virazole for mammalian cell cultures is approximately 320–1000 μg/ml.

A detailed study of the effects of virazole on the growth of L5178Y cells in Fisher's medium for leukemic cells has been reported by MÜLLER et al. (1977). The growth-inhibitory effect of virazole followed a classic log dosage/response correlation with an interpolated ID_{50} of 1.15 μg/ml, i.e., 4.7×10^{-6} M. The ID_{50} varied with the size of the cell inoculum. The inhibition of cell growth by three ID_{50}s was reversible (after 24 h incubation) but four or five ID_{50}s decreased cell viability by 24% or 57% respectively.

The same murine L5178Y cells were also studied by LOWE et al. (1977). By Coulter counting, 10^{-5} and 3.2×10^{-5} M virazole inhibited cell proliferation partly over a period of 45 h, while 10^{-4} M of the drug blocked cell proliferation almost entirely. No ID_{50} was given and no data on the viability of the experimental cultures were cited.

TOSHIO and NAKAO (1972) reported that 100–500 μg/ml inhibited the growth of HeLa cells. Inhibition of HeLa cell division by 100 μg/ml virazole for 24 h was reversed by removal of the drug (LARSSON et al., 1978).

Concerning non-neoplastic mammalian cells, virazole caused a decrease in viability of RK-13 cells at 500 and 1000 μg/ml (HUFFMAN et al., 1973; SIMON et al., 1973) and partially inhibited the growth of chick embryo cells (HUFFMAN et al., 1973). At 32 μg/ml, virazole reduced the viability of mouse embryo cells by one decadic logarithm during four days of incubation (SHANNON, 1977).

Toxicity and Safety Evaluation

The LD_{50} of virazole for mice is 2000 mg/kg given orally or 1200 mg/kg given intraperitoneally. When the drug was given twice daily for 9 days by either route, the LD_{50} was 250 mg/kg/day (SIDWELL et al., 1972). Lethal doses in rats caused diarrhea and decreases in hematocrit, erythrocyte count, and hemoglobin concentrations. Similar blood changes, reversible upon termination of treatment, were seen with high doses in monkeys (SIDWELL, et al., 1977). In rhesus monkeys, virazole was tolerated in single oral doses over 4000 mg/kg with a minor incidence of emesis and diarrhea as the only symptoms. No mortality was caused by single oral doses as high as 10,000 mg/kg (ICN Pharmaceuticals, Inc. undated).

In human volunteers, single oral doses of 100 mg–400 mg of virazole caused an occasional mild headache. One subject showed transient elevations in serum glutamic-oxaloacetic acid transaminase and serum lactic acid dehydrogenase. In chronic oral administration studies, virazole was administered at 600 mg/day to male volunteers for 28 consecutive days without significant adverse effects.

At doses higher than 600 mg/day, there occurred reductions in hemoglobin, hematocrit and erythrocyte count (ICN Pharmaceuticals, undated).

Teratogenicity in rats and hamsters and embryo lethality in rabbits was observed (SIDWELL et al., 1977). Virazole, given to pregnant rats from the 1st to the 6th day or 13th to the 20th day of gestation produced no teratogenic effects at levels of 150 mg/kg. There was a teratogenic effect if the drug was given from the 7th to the 12th day of gestation (SIMON, 1977). No significant teratogenic effects were seen in baboons treated with doses approximately ten times greater than the recommended human doses (SIDWELL et al., 1977).

Antiviral Effects in Cell Cultures

Early work on the suppression of the cytopathogenic effect of viruses by virazole was summarized by SIMON et al. (1973). Table 1 is reproduced from this summary. Experimental details of this work were published by HUFFMAN et al. (1973). The authors also investigated the reduction of the titer of type 1 herpes simplex virus in KB cells, the effects of virazole on hemagglutinin production by influenza and para-influenza viruses and on the virus titers in chick embryo cells and the effects of virazole on plaque formation by type 1 herpes virus in RK-13 cells. SUGANUMA and ISHIDA (1972, 1973) confirmed the effects of virazole on the growth of influenza A (PR-8 strain) in HeLa cells.

The effects of virazole on the formation of four influenza A structural antigens was studied in calf kidney cells, using an indirect immunofluorescence test (OXFORD, 1975). The production of all the virus-induced structural antigens (NP, MP, HA and NA) was inhibited to a similar degree. Whereas 90% of control cells were infected and showed the presence of all the different virus structural antigens, only 5–8% of cells were fluorescing in monolayers treated with 2×10^{-4} M virazole. The inhibition of fowl plague virus in chick embryo fibroblasts showed a classical log dosage/response curve of the decrease in plaque formation. The ED_{50} of virazole was 2×10^{-5} M; the plaques produced in the presence of the drug were significantly smaller than those in the untreated control plates (OXFORD, 1975).

The comparative sensitivity to virazole of five strains of type 2 herpes virus was investigated in KB cells. The drug inhibited these strains with MICs ranging from 10 to 100 μg/ml (ALLEN et al., 1977). In chick embryo fibroblasts, virazole at 10 μg/ml showed activity against Marek's disease herpes virus replication (EIDSON et al., 1974). The multiplication of adenovirus 19 in HeLa cells and the formation of its capsid proteins were inhibited by virazole; adenosine and guanosine were partially effective in antagonizing this action (SCHEFFLER et al., 1975). Virazole showed considerable activity on the growth of Gross murine leukemia virus in Swiss mouse embryo cells (SHANNON, 1977). The reduction in the number of plaques followed a classical log dosage/response curve with an ED_{50} of 3.2 μg/ml and an ED_{100} of 32 μg/ml.

Table 1. Summary of the viral CPE-inhibitory activity of virazole

DNA viruses					RNA viruses				
Virus[a]	Cells	No. of expts.	Avg. VR[b]	Median M.I.C.[c] (μg/ml)	Virus[a]	Cells	No. of expts.	Avg. VR[b]	Median M.I.C.[c] (Gg/ml)
AV/3	KB	7	0.7	32	RV/1A	KB	3	0.9	10
HSV/1	KB	21	1.1	1	RV/2	KB	1	0.4	100
HSV/1	RK-13	3	1.3	1	RV/8	KB	1	0.8	32
HSV/1	CE	2	1.4	0.32	RV/13	KB	15	0.7	32
HSV/1	VERO	2	0.4	100	RV/56	KB	3	0.9	10
HSV/1	WI-38	2	0.4	100	PIV/1	KB	1	0.9	10
HSV/1	HeLa	1	1.4	0.32	PIV/1	VERO	3	0.7	32
HSV/2	KB	2	1.1	1	PIV/1	CE	3	0.9	3.2
HSV/2	CE	1	0.4	100	PIV/3	KB	15	0.8	10
HSV/2	RK-13	1	0.8	3.2	CV/1	KB	5	0.4	100
HSV/2	VERO	2	0.0	–	PV/2	KB	6	0.2	1000
PRV	RK-13	3	0.0	–	VSV	KB	4	0.8	32
PRV	VERO	1	0.2	1000	VSV	RK-13	5	1.0	3.2
MV	RK-13	2	1.5	3.2	VSV	VERO	1	0.4	320
MCMV	ME	1	0.9	3.2	SSPEV	VERO	1	0.8	10
VV	KB	3	1.0	3.2	SFV	CE	2	0.6	32
VV	HeLa	1	0.6	32	NDV	CE	2	1.1	3.2
VV	VERO	1	0.4	320	MeV	VERO	2	0.6	32
VV	CE	1	0.8	3.2					
IBRV	EBTr	2	0.9	10					

[a] DNA Viruses: AV/3 Type 3 adenovirus, strain GB. HSV/1 Type 1 herpes simplex virus, strain HF. HSV/2 Type 2 herpes simplex virus, strain MS. PRV Pseudorabies virus, Aujeszky strain. MV Myxoma virus, strain Sanarelli. MCMV Murine cytomegalo virus, strain Smith. VV Vaccinia virus, strain Lederle CA. IBRV Infectious bovine rhinotracheitis virus, strain LA.
RNA Viruses: RV/1A Type 1A rhinovirus, strain 2060. RV/2 Type 2 rhinovirus, strain HGP. RV/8 Type 8 rhinovirus, strain CU-MRH. RV/13 Type 13 rhinovirus, strain 353. RV/56 Type 56 rhinovirus, strain CH82. PIV/1 Type 1 parainfluenza virus, strain Sendai. PIV/3 Type 3 parainfluenza virus, strain C243. CV/1 Type 1 coxsackie B virus, strain Conn-5. PV/2 Type 2 polio virus, strain MEF-1. VSV Vesicular stomatitis virus, strain Indiana. SSPEV SSPE measles virus, strain MUN-HT. SFV Semliki Forest virus, strain "Original". NDV Newcastle disease virus, strain L-Kansas. MeV Measles virus, strain Edmonston.
[b] Virus Rating. [c] Minimum Inhibitory Concentration.

Virazole did not eradicate potato X virus when administered to infected mesophyll protoplasts of tobacco or proliferating calli raised from protoplasts. However, treating the same calli with 10 mg/l of virazole in a medium that promoted the onset of shoot morphogenesis, resulted in the absence of potato virus X infection in 93% of the regenerated tobacco plants (SHEPARD, 1977).

The ability of herpes virus type 1 to develop resistance to virazole was studied in Vero cells (ALLEN and FINGAL, 1977) and in Vero and KB cells (HUFFMAN et al., 1977). In the presence of 10 μg/ml of virazole in the cell culture media 4–10 passages of the virus did not result in viral resistance to the drug.

A comparative study was carried out on the effects of virazole and amantadine HCl on the plaque reduction of four strains of influenza virus in calf kidney cells. The dosage response lines for virazole were similar for the four virus strains. Influenza A/Okuda/57 was the most sensitive strain. Three of the strains were more sensitive to amantadine HCl than to virazole but influenza A/NWS/33 was several hundred times less sensitive to amantadine than the other three strains (TISDALE and BAUER, 1977). A similar study, published earlier (TOGO, 1973), found virazole more active than amantadine HCl against influenza A and B strains.

Experimental Studies in Animals

There exists a large volume of literature on the treatment with virazole of experimental virus infections in animals. This author does not believe that a detailed review, publication by publication, of this literature would add much thought to the problem of the molecular biological mechanism of the action of the drug.

Table 2 presents a selection of results of virazole studies in virus-infected animals. In the tabulated results, the drug was administered for 7–12 days,

Table 2. Selected data on in vivo antiviral activity of virazole

DNA viruses	Animal host	Type of infection or disease symptom		Activity
Herpes virus type 1	Rabbit	Keratitis		++
Herpes virus type 1	Hamster	Keratitis-encephalitis		+
Herpes virus type 1	Mouse	Zoster-like lesions		++
Herpes virus type 1	Mouse	Encephalitis (death)		±
Vaccinia virus	Rabbit	Keratitis		++
Vaccinia virus	Mouse	Encephalitis (death)		–
Vaccinia virus	Mouse	Lesion		+
Marek's disease	Chicken	Visceral lesions		++
Shope fibroma	Rabbit	Fibroma		+
Adenovirus	Mouse	Antibody titer		–
RNA viruses				
Influenza virus type A_0	Mouse	Lung consolidation, death		+
Influenza virus type A_2	Mouse	Lung consolidation, death		++
Influenza virus type B	Mouse	Lung consolidation, death		++
Murine hepatitis	Mouse	Hepatitis, death		++
Semliki Forest virus	Mouse	Encephalitis, death		–
Western equine encephalitis	Mouse	Encephalitis, death		–
Vesicular stomatitis	Mouse	Lesion		±
Vesicular stomatitis	Mouse	Encephalitis, death		–
Friend leukemia	Mouse	Splenomegaly, hepatomegaly		++
Coxsackie A21	Mouse	Death	Single dose treatment	–
Polio type 1	Mouse	Death	Single dose treatment	–
Foot and mouth disease	Mouse	Death		+
Rauscher leukemia	Mouse	Spenomegaly		+
Newcastle disease	Chicken	Death		–
Encephalomyocarditis	Mouse	Death		–
Crapie	Mouse	Death		–

beginning 4 h pre- or post-virus inoculations. General references are by SIDWELL et al. (1974) and in an ICN Pharmaceuticals Product Monograph (undated). A review of Table 2 indicates that in DNA virus infections, virazole was markedly active against local lesions produced by vaccinia virus, herpes type 1 virus and in Marek's Disease. Among RNA virus infections, there was marked activity against types A and B influenza and type 1 para-influenza. The drug failed against infections with Semliki Forest, vesicular stomatitis, Coxsackie A, Newcastle Disease, encephalomyocarditis, scrapie and polio type 1 viruses.

Experimental and Clinical Studies in Man

Two double-blind studies on the effects of virazole in human volunteers, infected with influenza A virus (COHEN et al., 1976; MAGNUSSEN et al., 1977) and one such study of the drug's effect in influenza B-infected volunteers (TOGO and McCRACKEN, 1976) have been reported. Additionally, a clinical evaluation of virazole has been made in Mexico City during an outbreak of influenza A in a boarding school for girls (SALIDO-RENGELL et al., 1977).

In the first of the two experimental studies on influenza A infection in volunteers (COHEN et al., 1976), medication (200 mg three times daily) was begun two days before challenge with 2×10^4 50% tissue culture infective doses. Nine of the ten subjects who received virazole developed influenza. The prophylactic administration of virazole did not affect the development of the illness.

In the second experimental study (MAGNUSSEN et al., 1977), volunteers received 1000 mg/day in four divided doses, the first given 6 h after inoculation with $10^{3.4}$ 50% tissue culture infective doses. Virazole ameliorated symptoms and fever, indicative of moderate-to-severe illness, but had no effect on the manifestations of mild illness in response to influenza A challenge.

In the clinical study of 61 girls, aged 8 to 16 years, the results of double-blind treatment are listed in Table 3. Patients received 300 mg/day virazole. Influenza type A isolations were made in 22/24 of the placebo group but only in 3/21 of the virazole-treated group. Authors concluded that virazole therapy had a significant effect on the development of influenza in young patients (SALIDO-RENGELL et al., 1977).

In the influenza B studies in volunteers (TOGO and McCRACKEN, 1976), virazole suppressed signs and symptoms induced by influenza B challenge, but the effectiveness of the drug was "marginal."

A recent abstract (ELLENHORN et al., 1977) stated that "ribavirin in experimentally induced clinical influenza (double-blind placebo control) using up to 1000 mg/day for 5 days, and in natural infection (300 mg/day for 5 days) resulted in a significantly diminished quantity of virus shed in nasal wash specimens, and correlated with an amelioration of fever and symptoms."

AYROSA-GALVÃO and CASTRO (1977) treated 66 patients with a clinical diagnosis of acute viral hepatitis, 33 receiving a placebo and 33 receiving 100 mg of virazole every 6 h for a period of 10 consecutive days. There was a significant decrease in serum bilirubin, serum glutamic-oxaloacetic transaminase and serum

Table 3. Distribution of clinical signs of influenza in patients treated with disguised placebo or ribavirin

	Degree of severity[a] (no. of patients)					
	Mild		Moderate		Severe	
Clinical Sign	P[b]	R[c]	P	R	P	R
Fever	6	0	14	0	4	0
Malaise	6	2	14	2	4	0
Rhinitis (cough)	4	3	4	1	16	2
Pharyngitis	3	2	21	3	0	2
Gastroenteritis	0	0	0	0	0	0
Headache	3	1	19	2	2	0
Myalgia	15	0	0	3	0	0
Conjunctivitis	5	0	11	2	0	1

[a] Composite of determinations made beginning 24 h after initiation of therapy. [b] Placebo. [c] Ribavirin.

glutamic-pyruvic transaminase from the 5th to the 10th day of treatment in the virazole group. In the placebo group, such a decrease was also observed but was not statistically significant.

In an abstract, ELLENHORN et al. (1977) reported double-blind placebo controlled studies of a total of 195 patients with acute viral hepatitis at seven university medical centers, using 400–800 mg virazole/day for 10 days. The drug-treated patients showed significantly faster returns to normal levels of the two transaminases, of total bilirubin and of serum lactic acid dehydrogenase as well as a shorter duration of disease. Six studies on hepatitis B revealed 50% improvement in cases treated.

The results of a double-blind placebo controlled topical treatment of 14 patients with herpes zoster (ZERTUCHE and PERCHES, 1977) are shown in Table 4. Topically applied 5% virazole was definitely effective against this disease. In an abstract, ELLENHORN et al. (1977) reported that "placebo controlled studies in herpes zoster (400 mg/day for up to 18 days) in 18 patients disclosed significantly faster involution of lesions and decay of scabs with ribavirin. A double-blind placebo controlled study in herpes gingivo-stomatitis (400 mgday) with tablets dissolved in the mouth and then swallowed, for 4 days, resulted in significant reduction in duration and severity of pain, ulcers, difficulty in speaking and swallowing and adenopathy. Topical ribavirin 5% used twice daily for 8 days for herpes zoster in cancer patients (double-blind placebo) resulted in significant acceleration of recovery. In herpes zoster, intravenous ribavirin is effective in diminishing duration of pain, accelerating involution of lesions and beginning decay of scabs."

Finally, the results of uncontrolled clinical trials in 390 patients, suffering from a variety of virus infections (ZERTUCHE and PERCHES, 1977), are shown in Table 5. According to the clinical judgement of the attending physicians, a high percentage of the patients showed "definitive improvement" of their virus diseases upon treatment with virazole.

Table 4. Effect of topical treatment[a] with 5% ribavirin or placebo on herpes-zoster-infected Patients (Double-Blind Study)

Patient description				Type of treatment	Therapy results[b]	
No.	Sex	Age	Initial illness		Pain	Lesion
1	M	3	Lymphoblastic leukemia	Ribavirin	2	7
2	F	70	Mammary carcinoma	Placebo	7	7
3	F	35	Hodgkin's disease	Ribavirin	1	5
4	F	36	Hodgkin's disease + Mammary carcinoma	Placebo	5	> 10[c]
5	M	38	Seminoma	Ribavirin	3	6
6	F	46	Mammary carcinoma	Ribavirin	2	4
7	F	40	Mammary carcinoma	Ribavirin	4	4
8	M	56	Seminoma	Placebo	3	3
9	F	72	Bronchogenic carcinoma	Placebo	2	7
10	M	11	Lymphoblastic leukemia	Placebo	2	11
11	F	52	Mammary carcinoma	Placebo	7	7
12	F	58	Mammary carcinoma	Ribavirin	4	7
13	M	28	Hodgkin's disease	Placebo	> 10[c]	> 10[c]
14	F	32	Mammary carcinoma	Placebo	7	10

[a] b.i.d. × 8. [b] Final day any pain or discernible scabbing was observed. [c] Considered to be 11 for determination of mean.

Table 5. Summary of ribavirin therapy results in virus-infected patients in Mexico (noncontrolled studies)

Diseases treated	Total cases	Definitive improvement[a]	Moderate improvement[a]	No improvement[a]
Varicella	44	40	4	0
Mumps	55	48	7	0
Measles	10	8	2	0
Rubella	12	10	1	1
Hepatitis	58	41	17	0
Herpes simplex	32	26	6	0
Herpetic stomatitis	32	31	1	0
Herpes zoster	43	38	5	0
Influenza	72	70	1	1
Other resp. diseases	22	20	2	0
Contagious molluscum	5	2	3	0
Encephalitis	5	3	2	0

[a] As related to the natural history of the untreated disease in the specific population treated.

Virazole has only recently been introduced in Nigeria (ODELOLA, 1977) and clinical results are not yet available. The drug has been licenced by the U.S. Food and Drug Administration as a new investigative Drug, IND No. 9076, and more clinical results from investigative use can be expected.

Mode of Action of Virazole

The structure of virazole resembles the structures of guanosine and inosine. This is illustrated by the conventional projection formulas (Fig. 3). An X-ray crystallographic analysis of the drug (PRUSINER and SUNDARALINGAM, 1973) has furnished more precise evidence of these similarities. The carbonyl oxygen and the NH_2 group of the carboxamide moiety occupy stereochemically similar positions as the carbonyl oxygen and the ring nitrogen N(1) of guanosine or inosine. It is reasonable to assume that the drug interferes in some manner with nucleic acid metabolism.

The mammalian metabolism of virazole, orally administered to rats, has been studied in detail by analysis of urine, serum and internal organs, using chromatography and mass spectroscopy (MILLER et al., 1977). From that publication, the metabolic scheme (Fig. 4) is reproduced. Virazole can be mono-di- or tri-phosphorylated as shown at the bottom of Fig. 4. The free triazole base (T–$CONH_2$) is probably formed by the action of nucleosidase(s). This compound (T–$CONH_2$) possesses antiviral activity against both RNA and DNA viruses (SIDWELL et al., 1974).

The molecular biological mechanism of action of virazole is not yet fully understood. It can not even be stated with confidence whether there exists one single or several such mechanisms. Three hypotheses have been proposed to explain the action of virazole in molecular terms.

The first hypothesis has been advanced by MILLER et al. (1977) and by STREETER et al., (1977) and considers that virazole triphosphate may be utilized by RNA polymerase(s) and be incorporated as virazole monophosphate into viral RNA and virus messenger RNA.

This could render virus RNA incapable of being faithfully replicated and messenger RNA to be a faulty code for the translation of viral gene products (such as polymerases for viral nucleic acids). The hypothesis is supported by findings of MILLER et al. (1977) that lung > liver > kidney > spleen contained considerable quantities of virazole triphosphate 30–60 min after oral administration

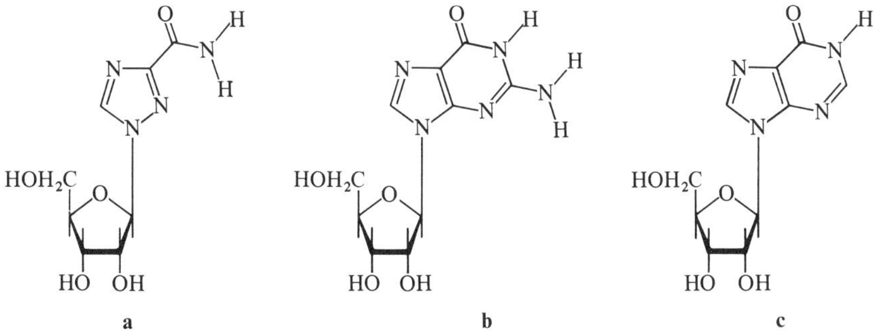

Fig. 3 a–c. Structures of **a** virazole, **b** guanosine, **c** inosine

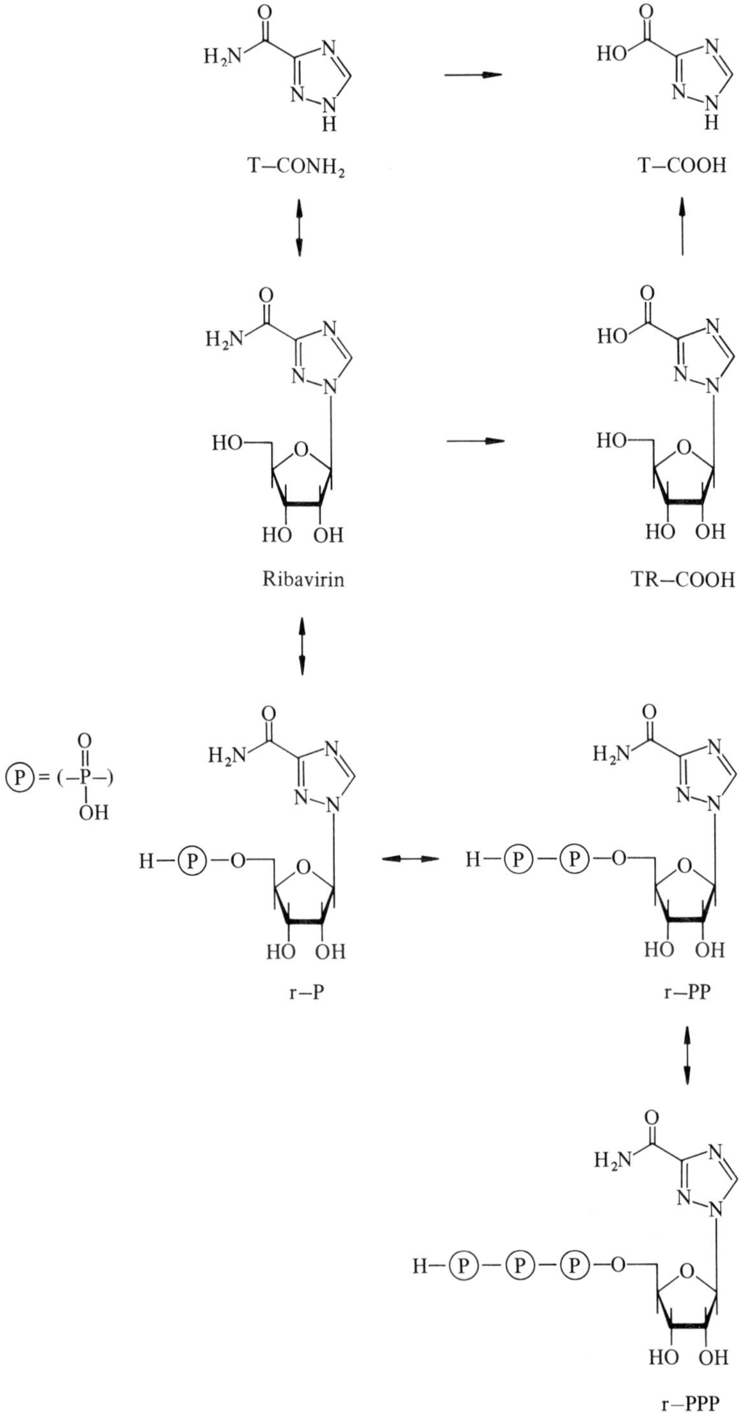

Fig. 4. Suggested scheme for the metabolism of virazole

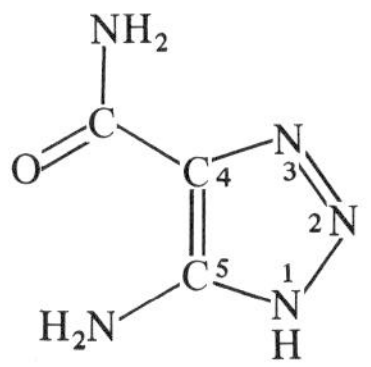

Fig. 5. Structure of 4-(5)-amino-1H-1,2,3, triazole-5-(4)-carboxamide

(rat). No virazole phosphates were detected in serum or urine. No experimental evidence exists of an incorporation of virazole monophosphate into any category of RNA and, in fact, virazole triphosphate has been shown to be an active inhibitor of influenza virus RNA polymerase in competition with adenosine and guanosine triphosphates (ERIKSSON et al., 1977).

When tobacco plants, infected with tobacco mosaic virus, were treated with the triazole, 4-(5)-amino-1H-1,2,3-triazole-5-(4)carboxamide (Fig. 5), the compound caused a delay in virus production and the virus RNA was found to contain a small amount of 8-azaguanylic acid (MATTHEWS and SMITH, 1955). It can be inferred that this triazole carboxamide was in vivo anabolized to become a substrate of RNA polymerase in the assembly of TMV RNA. The triazole inhibited the growth of *Escherichia coli* and became incorporated into the RNA of this bacterium as 8-azaguanine (MATTHEWS and SMITH, 1955). It should be noted that inhibitions of polymerase reactions by vicarious substrates and partial incorporation of such substrates are not necessarily contradictory conditions.

The second hypothesis is based upon precise experimental studies of ERIKSSON et al. (1977). The effects of virazole triphosphate on a variety of RNA polymerase systems was investigated. The triphosphate but not the 5′-monophosphate or the (unphosphorylated) drug virazole, inhibited in vitro the influenza virus type A RNA polymerase reaction in competition with the purines adenosine and guanosine triphosphates. The pyrimidine triphosphates of uridine and cytidine antagonized the inhibitory effect of virazole triphosphate in a non-competitive manner. RNA polymerases of calf thymus, *Escherichia coli* and vesicular stomatitis virus as well as DNA polymerases from calf thymus and *Micrococcus luteus* were not significantly inhibited by virazole triphosphate. Likewise, MÜLLER et al. (1977) reported that virazole triphosphate failed to inhibit in vitro eukaryotic DNA polymerases α and β, eukaryotic RNA polymerases I and II and eukaryotic poly-A polymerase.

The continued work of the team of ERIKSSON on the specific inhibitions of viral nucleic acid polymerases has so far only been reported in abstract form (ÖBERG and HELGSTRAND, 1977). Virazole triphosphate at 10^{-4} M also inhibited the DNA polymerase of herpes virus by 35%. Virazole itself was non-active against influenza RNA polymerase and herpes DNA polymerase. It is therefore possible that one mechanism of action of virazole is based upon the metabolic conversion of the drug to virazole triphosphate, followed by the selective inhibition of viral nucleic acid polymerase reactions in cells. Based upon the analytical studies of MILLER et al. (1977) one might then speculate that the effects of virazole on influenza and hepatitis virus infections could

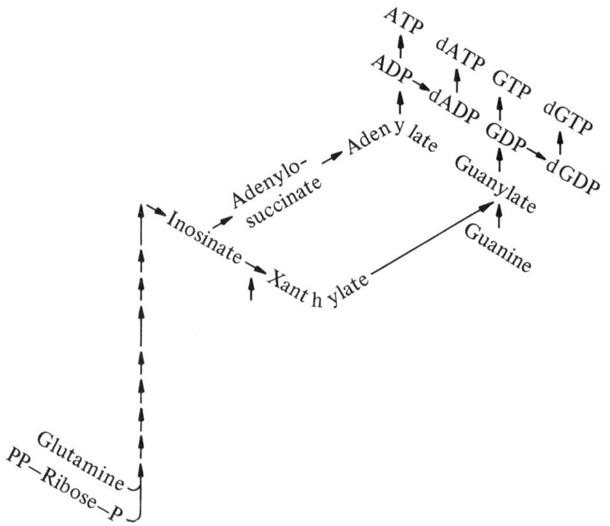

Fig. 6. Schematic pathways of purine nucleotide synthesis. *Arrow* points to the reaction, thought to be inhibited by virazole

be the results of the active conversion of the drug to virazole triphosphate in lung and liver tissues.

An across-the-board inhibition of the formation of influenza A structural antigens in calf kidney cells (OXFORD, 1975) may be considered circumstantial evidence in favor of the first or the second hypotheses.

The third hypothesis dates back to 1972 (SIMON et al., 1973). The inhibition of the proliferation of measles virus in Vero cell cultures was reversed by guanosine or xanthosine and to a slightly lesser extent by inosine (STREETER et al., 1973). These observations gave rise to the hypothesis that virazole inhibits the conversion of inosine-5′-phosphate to xanthosine-5′-phosphate by inhibiting the enzyme inosine-5′-phosphate dehydrogenase (STREETER et al., 1973), and hence blocks the biosynthetic pathway to guanylic acid, as shown schematically in Fig. 6. This idea gains plausibility by the similarities between virazole, guanosine, and inosine (PRUSINER and SUNDARALINGAM, 1973). Guanylic acid deficiency could explain the throttling of nucleic acid biosyntheses. The selective toxicity for virus replication might, accordingly, not depend upon qualitative differences between viral and cellular nucleic acid syntheses but rather on rate differences which would affect the faster processes more strongly.

In vitro, virazole inhibited preparations of inosinate dehydrogenase from *E. coli* and Ehrlich ascites tumor cells (STREETER et al., 1973). The effects of virazole on the intermediary metabolism of the guanylate pathway has been studied in Ehrlich ascites tumor cells (SMITH et al., 1974) and in murine lymphoma L5178Y cells (LOWE et al., 1977; MÜLLER et al., 1977).

SMITH et al. (1974) tested virazole against eight enzyme activities of the hypoxanthine metabolism. At 4×10^{-5} M the drug inhibited prominently inosinate dehydrogenase but the authors did not discuss this result in connection with virus chemotherapy.

LOWE et al. (1977) showed in L5178Y cells that a cytostatic concentration of 4×10^{-4} M virazole permitted significant production of dATP, had little influence on the cellular levels of dCTP and TTP but caused a significant drop in the intracellular concentration of dGTP. A shunt in purine nucleotide synthesis at the conversion of inosinate to xanthylate (Fig. 6) may perhaps result in an increased production of adenylate. Again, the work was not discussed in its relevance to virus chemotherapy.

MÜLLER et al. (1977) showed that supplying guanosine, inosine or xanthosine (but not adenosine) reversed to significant extents the effects of virazole on the proliferation rates of L5178Y cells. A concentration of virazole (7.6×10^{-5} M) which reduced the doubling rate of the cells to 18% of that of an untreated control culture, inhibited DNA synthesis by 72%, RNA synthesis by 55% but protein synthesis by only 17%. This last observation is difficult to bring into consonance with the interpretation that the putative inhibition of messenger RNA synthesis caused the concentration of polysomes to decrease by 82%. How did the cells manage to synthesize 83% of their normal proteins with only 18% of their normal polysome complement? The test concentration of 7.6×10^{-5} M virazole (in this experiment decreasing the doubling rate to 23% that of an untreated control culture) reduced the intracellular pool of dGTP by 60%, while reducing the GTP pool by 50%. It can be noted that the reduction in the rate of DNA biosynthesis (72%) is roughly commensurate to the reduction in the dGTP pool (60%). The same rough correlation exists for the reduction of the GTP pool (50%) and the decrease in RNA synthesis (55%). Cum grano salis, the deficiencies in dGTP and GTP might explain, therefore, the reduced rates of biosyntheses of both categories of nucleic acids. The authors emphasized that their cell cultures were not virus-infected and that they studied virazole for its activity as a cytostatic agent.

With reference to the second and third hypotheses, LARSSON et al. (1978) working with HeLa cells, showed that after one hour incubation with 2.5×10^{-4} M virazole, the rate of DNA synthesis had decreased by 84%, the rate of RNA synthesis by 28% and the rate of protein synthesis by <4%. After 24 h, a plateau was attained with 1×10^{-4} M virazole at which DNA synthesis had ceased, RNA synthesis was decreased by 80% and the rate of protein synthesis by 30%. Inhibitions of nucleic acid biosyntheses could be reversed by removing virazole after 18 h of exposure. Inhibition of cell proliferation could be reversed after 24 h exposure to virazole by removal of the drug. Clearly, virazole acted as a cytostatic agent for HeLa cells. The authors mentioned the fact that virazole has antiviral properties but stated their intention to characterize the effects of the drug on cellular metabolism.

Discussion

The mechanism of the selective antiviral action of virazole remains hypothetical. The drug is not virucidal and does not induce interferon (ALLEN et al., 1973; CAHN and LUBIN, 1973), nor does it appear to interfere with viral attachment to, or penetration into, the host cells (SIDWELL et al., 1974). Virazole is not a potent inhibitor of eukaryotic protein biosynthesis (MÜLLER et al., 1977; LARSSON et al., 1978). The immunofluorescence observations on influenza virus antigens (OXFORD, 1975) do not constitute evidence of a preferential and direct inhibition of the biosynthesis of virus proteins by virazole.

There can be no doubt that the mode of cytostatic action of virazole is an inhibition of nucleic acid biosyntheses, especially that of DNA (MÜLLER et al., 1977; LARSSON et al., 1978). Important information on the inhibition of viral nucleic acid synthesis comes from the work of SCHOLTISSEK (1976) and DRACH and SHIPMAN, Jr. (1977).

SCHOLTISSEK (1976) demonstrated a selective and total inhibition of the syntheses of fowl plague RNA, and of its "complementary" RNA at 4.1×10^{-4} M virazole, which did not inhibit the cytoplasmic RNA synthesis of the chick embryo host cells. The reported failures of hemagglutinin formation and of the appearance of the fowl plague RNA polymerase are observations to be expected in a condition in which the synthesis of viral RNAs is completely suppressed and, hence, little translation into viral gene products is possible.

Screening a series of antiviral compounds for their inhibitions of DNA biosyntheses in KB cells, either uninfected or infected with herpes simplex virus, DRACH and SHIPMAN, Jr. (1977) determined the following 50% inhibitory concentrations of virazole:

1. DNA synthesis in uninfected cells: 1.9×10^{-6} M.
2. Total DNA synthesis in infected cells: 1.84×10^{-4} M.
3. Cellular DNA synthesis in infected cells: $> 1.5 \times 10^{-3}$ M.
4. Viral DNA synthesis (in infected cells): 1.45×10^{-4} M.

The authors have commented on the "negative selectivity" inherent in the ID_{50} for DNA synthesis in uninfected cells (1.9×10^{-6} M) as compared to the ID_{50} for virus DNA synthesis (1.45×10^{-4} M). They also commented on the "positive selectivity" inherent in the ID_{50} for cellular DNA synthesis in infected cells ($> 1.5 \times 10^{-3}$ M) as compared to the ID_{50} for virus DNA synthesis (1.45×10^{-4} M). However they have not come to molecular biological terms with the dramatic difference between cellular DNA biosyntheses as concerns susceptibility to virazole, depending upon whether the KB cells were infected or not. In what manner does herpes virus infection condition KB cellular DNA synthesis to render it 1000 times less sensitive to virazole than DNA synthesis in uninfected cells? Yet, the decreased sensitivity of KB cellular DNA synthesis to virazole in infected cells constitutes the numerical basis of the selective anti-herpes virus action of the drug.

The central question is, of course, that of the molecular mechanism of the selective action of virazole against RNA and DNA virus nucleic acid synthesis. All three hypotheses, developed in the preceding section, could conceivably explain such effects.

1. If one assumes the first hypothesis, the incorporation of virazole-5′-monophosphate into RNA, there exists an analogy, viz, the antiviral activity of 5-iodo-5′-amino-2′-di-deoxyuridine (FISCHER et al., 1977) and its incorporation into herpes simplex virus DNA. There exists a direct parallelism between the incorporation of the thymidine analog into the viral DNA and the degree of inhibition of herpes virus replication. Furthermore, the work of MATTHEWS

and SMITH (1955), cited previously, has shown the incorporation of a triazolecarboxamide into viral and bacterial RNA. However, a serious consideration of the first hypothesis would minimally require an experimental demonstration that virazole-5′-monophosphate (or the ^{14}C-labelled triazole moiety) is indeed incorporated into a viral RNA.

2. The second hypothesis, viz, an inhibition of viral (not cellular) nucleic acid polymerases by virazole triphosphate seems possible because the triphosphate is formed in mammalian organs from orally administered virazole (MILLER et al., 1977). In vitro, virazole triphosphate specifically inhibits the RNA polymerase of influenza virus (ERIKSSON et al., 1977) and the DNA polymerase of herpes simplex virus (ÖBERG and HELGSTRAND, 1977). The triphosphate has no effect on a variety of non-viral RNA and DNA polymerases (MÜLLER et al., 1977; ÖBERG and HELGSTRAND, 1977).

3. The third hypothesis, the blockade of guanylate synthesis (STREETER et al., 1973) and the demonstrated depletion of the GTP and dGTP pool (MÜLLER et al.; LOWE et al., 1977), in conjunction with observations that supplying guanosine, xanthosine or inosine reverses the anti-measles effect of virazole in Vero cells (STREETER et al., 1973) as well as the cytostatic action of virazole in L5178Y cells (MÜLLER et al., 1977) invite comparison. The comparison can be made to an analogous situation in which partial depletion of the UTP pool caused a preferential inhibition of RNA virus replication but did not significantly impair RNA biosynthesis in non-infected control cells (SCHOLTISSEK et al., 1975). However, in order to explain a selective antiviral effect by the depletion of the guanylate pool, especially GTP and dGTP, one would need to introduce auxiliary assumptions such as: (1) a drastic difference in the rates of viral as compared to cellular nucleic acid syntheses, (2) a lesser affinity of viral nucleic acid polymerases as compared to the analogous cytoplasmic enzymes for guanosine or d-guanosine triphosphates, or (3) the operational existence of independent triphosphate "pools", one that would be used for viral nucleic acid synthesis and could be depleted, and the other used for cellular nucleic acid synthesis which would be depleted only partly.

Additional speculations concerning the modes of action of virazole (MILLER et al., 1977) are: (1) An interference by virazole triphosphate with the formation of adenylosuccinate from inosinate and L-aspartate, a reaction that uses GTP as an energy donor and produces adenylic acid. However, the formation of ATP is stimulated by virazole (LOWE et al., 1977). (2) An inhibition of protein synthesis by interfering with the functions of GTP at the ribosomal level. Virazole, however, has low effects on protein biosynthesis (MÜLLER et al., 1977; LARSSON et al., 1978). No experimental evidence, direct or circumstantial, exists at this time to support the two speculations of MILLER et al. (1977).

Structure/Activity Relationships

Data on the activities of synthetic relatives of virazole are limited in extent and numerical precision in addition to being heterogenous. They do not afford the formulation of structure/activity rules. Such rules can become important corollaries of the knowledge of mechanisms of drug action (e.g., HAHN and GUND, 1975) and, ideally, should guide the design of superior second-generation drugs. Thus far, no synthetic compound, related to virazole, has been found to surpass the activity of the drug.

DEA et al. (1974) concluded from NMR studies of virazole and related compounds that the major determinants of activity are not the solution conformation but are steric in nature, i.e., they reside "in a particular spatial distribution" of the substituents and of the site of glycosylation which, in turn, are governed by the location of the nitrogen atoms in the triazole moiety.

The carbohydrate moiety must be furanosyl ribose. Replacing it by arabinose or xylose produced non-active compounds. Of some importance for ideas concerning the mechanism of action of virazole, is the fact that the 2'deoxyribofuranosyl derivative also is devoid of activity. Apparently, this compound did not function as an analog of deoxyguanosine. Shifting the ribose substituent from N(1) to C(5) of the triazole ring system, produced a non-active compound (HUYNH-DINH and Igolen, 1977).

Deleting the ribose moiety of virazole entirely, resulted in 1,2,4-triazole-3-carboxamide which "retained activity". However, the few tabulated data indicate that antiviral activity in vivo (as well as mouse toxicity) were drastically reduced (SIDWELL et al., 1974). Changing the 1,2,4-triazole ring in virazole to

Table 6. Pyrazofurin, pyrazofurin isopropylidene, and ribavirin: effect on virus-induced cytopathogenicity in various cell cultures

Virus	Cell culture[a]	50% inhibitory dose (μg/ml)[b]		
		Pyrazofurin	Pyrazofurin isopropylidene	Ribavirin
Vaccinia	PRK	0.1	1	30
Herpes simplex-1 (KOS)	PRK	20	150	70
Herpes simplex-1 (KOS)	HSF	20	200	40
Herpes simplex-2 (333)	HSF	20	100	40
Vesicular stomatitis	PRK	0.01	2	40
Vesicular stomatitis	HSF	0.04	7	20
Vesicular stomatitis	HeLa	0.02	40	7
Newcastle disease	HSF	4	200	40
Measles	Vero	0.01	1	7
Sindbis	BHK	0.03	3	40
Polio-1	HeLa	0.02	4	20
Coxsackie B-4	HeLa	0.1	2	20
Coxsackie B-4	Vero	2	150	150

[a] Abbreviations: PRK, primary rabbit kidney; HSF, human skin fibroblast (VGS strain); Vero, a continuous line of green monkey kidney cells; BHK, a continuous line of baby hamster kidney cells (line 21). Cell cultures were used when confluent.

[b] Concentration required to reduce virus-induced cytopathogenicity by 50%. The compounds were added immediately after virus adsorption. Virus input: 100 $CCID_{50}$ (100 × virus dose that infects 50% of the cell cultures).

its isomeric 1,2,3-triazole resulted in a loss of activity (SIDWELL et al., 1974).[1] A tetrazole analogue of virazole in which the carboxamide is substituted to the ring carbon, adjacent to the ribosylated ring nitrogen, likewise was non-active in vivo (POONIAN et al., 1976).

As stated in the Introduction, the antibiotic, pyrazomycin (pyrazofurin) (Fig. 2), exhibits in cell cultures broad-spectrum antiviral activity superior to that of virazole. This is documented by the data in Table 6 from DESCAMPS and DECLERCQ (1977). The antibiotic possesses a pyrazole ring system (one ring nitrogen less than triazole) which is an isomer of imidazole. In contrast to virazole, pyrazofurin inhibited DNA and RNA syntheses only at concentrations which are 10^3 to 10^4-fold higher than those which inhibit virus replication; it is also not a potent inhibitor of protein synthesis. At the current state of knowledge, it is not clear if pyrazofurin can be included in the consideration of structure/activity relationships in the virazole series. Two ring-substituted ribofuranosyl-imidazole-4-carboxamides have been synthesized and compared with virazole as concerns activity against eight different viruses. Virazole was the superior drug (DECLERCQ et al., 1975).

To summarize, none of the structural changes of the virazole molecule, nor its tetrazole or imidazole analogs possessed antiviral activity superior to that of virazole. The results of molecular modifications do not offer any guidelines for designing a superior drug nor for the elucidation of virazole's molecular biological mechanism of action. The relationship between virazole and pyrazofurin remains an intriguing scientific question.

Addendum

Among publications on virazole which have appeared in print after the completion of this article, three have a bearing on the mode of action of the drug.

Virazole was without plaque-inhibiting activity on several bacterial DNA (λ, φ105) and RNA (f2, M12, Qβ) viruses The drug inhibited plaque formation of one DNA virus, LLP-1, which multiplies in a blue alga, *Plectonema boryanum*. The growth of *Escherichia coli* strains was only slightly inhibited in agar diffusion tests, employing an excessive concentration of 10^{-1} M virazole (MENZEL and STENZ, 1978).

Continued studies of the action of virazole in L5178Y cells (ZIMMERMAN and DEEPROSE, 1978) have shown that the drug was converted into its 5′-triphosphate but was not incorporated into RNA. A possible incorporation into viral RNAs remains to be investigated.

Concerning structure-activity relationships, it has been reported that the activity of the molecule depends upon its *anti* glycosidic conformation (MILES et al., 1978). The nonactive tetrazole analog of ribavirin (POONIAN et al., 1976) is unstable in the postulated high *anti* conformation.

1 However, compare this to the incorporation of the 1,2,3-triazole-carboxamide, Fig. 5, into TMV RNA (MATTHEWS and SMITH, 1955).

References

Allen, L.B., Fingal, C.M.: Failure of type 1 herpesvirus to develop resistance to ribavarin. Antimicrob. Agents Chemother. *12*, 120–121 (1977)

Allen, L.B., Huffman, J.H., Sidwell, R.W.: Failure of 1-β-D-ribofuranosyl-1,2,4-triazole-3-carboxamide to stimulate interferon. Antimicrob. Agents Chemother. *3*, 534–535 (1973)

Allen, L.B., Wolf, S.M., Hintz, C.J., Huffman, J.H., Sidwell, R.W.: Effect of ribavirin on type 2 herpesvirus hominis (HVH/2) *in vitro* and *in vivo*. Ann. N.Y. Acad. Sci. *284*, 247–253 (1977)

Ayrosa-Galvão, P.A., Castro, I.O.: The effect of 1-β-D-ribofuranosyl-1,2,4-triazole-3-carboxamide on acute viral hepatitis. Ann. N.Y. Acad. Sci. *284*, 278–283 (1977)

Cahn, F., Lubin, M.: Antiviral drugs and protein synthesis in reticulocyte lysates. Intervirology *1*, 376–385 (1973)

Cohen, A., Togo, Y., Khakoo, R., Waldman, R., Sigel, M.: Comparative clinical and laboratory evaluation of ribavirin, amantadine hydrochloride and placebo in induced human influenza type A. J. Infect. Dis. Suppl. *133*, A 114–A 120 (1976)

Dea, P., Schweizer, M.P., Kreishman, G.P.: Nuclear magnetic resonance studies of the solution properties of the antiviral nucleoside, 1-β-D-ribofuranosyl-1,2,4-triazole-3-carboxamide, the corresponding 5′-phosphate, and related triazole nucleosides. Biochemistry *13*, 1862–1867 (1974)

DeClercq, E., Luczak, M., Reepmeyer, J.C., Kirk, K.L., Cohen, L.A.: Fluoroimidazoles as antiviral agents and inhibitors of polynucleotide biosynthesis. Life Sci. *17*, 187–194 (1975)

DeLong, D.C., Baker, L.A., Gerzon, K., Gutkowski, G.E., Williams, R.H., Hamill, R.L.: Inhibition of Friend Leukemia virus-induced splenomegaly by pyrazomycin. Abstr. 7th Int. Congr. Chemother. A-5/35 (1971)

Descamps, J., DeClercq, E.: Broad-spectrum antiviral activity of pyrazofurin (pyrazomycin). Current Chemotherapy. Proc. 10th Int. Congr. Chemother., 354–357 (1977)

Drach, J.C., Shipman, C., Jr.: The selective inhibition of viral DNA synthesis by chemotherapeutic agents: an indicator of clinical usefulness. Ann. N.Y. Acad. Sci. *284*, 396–409 (1977)

Eidson, C.S., Than, V.T., Kleven, S.H.: The in vitro and in vivo effect of chemotherapeutic agents on the Marek's disease herpesvirus of chickens. Poult. Sci. *53*, 1533–1538 (1974)

Ellenhorn, M.J., Sidwell, R.W., Lima, J.M., Long, R., Allen, L.B., Fernandez, H.: Ribavirin (Virazole): review of clinical efficacy in human viral infections. Abstr. 10th Int. Congr. Chemother., 351 (1977)

Eriksson, B., Helgstrand, E., Johansson, N.G., Larsson, A., Misiorny, A., Noren, J.O., Philipson, L., Stenberg, K., Stening, G., Stridh, S., Öberg, B.: Inhibition of influenza virus ribonucleic acid polymerase by ribavirin triphosphate. Antimicrob. Agents Chemother. *11*, 946–951 (1977)

Fischer, P.H., Chen, M.S., Prusoff, W.H.: A relationship between the antiviral activity of 5-iodo-5′-amino-2′,5′-dideoxyuridine and its incorporation into herpes simplex virus DNA. Pharmacologist *19*, 209 (1977)

Gutkowski, G.E., Sweeney, M.J., DeLong, D.C., Hamill, R.L., Gerzon, K., Dyke, R.W.: Biochemistry and biological effects of the Pyrazofurins (pyrazomycins); initial clinical trial. Ann. N.Y. Acad. Sci. *255*, 544–551 (1975)

Hahn, F.E., Gund, P.: A structural model of the chloramphenicol receptor site. Top. Infect. Dis. *1*, 245–266 (1975)

Huffman, J.H., Sidwell, R.W., Khare, G.P., Witkowski, J.T., Allen, L.B., Robins, R.K.: In Vitro effect of 1-β-D-ribofuranosyl-1,2,4-triazole-3-carboxamide (Virazole, ICN 1229) on deoxyribonucleic acid and ribonucleic acid viruses. Antimicrob. Agents Chemother. *3*, 235–241 (1973)

Huffman, J.H., Allen, L.B., Sidwell, R.W.: Comparison of the development of resistant strains of type 1 herpes simplex virus to in vitro antiviral activity of 5-iodo-2′-deoxyuridine or ribavirin. Ann. N.Y. Acad. Sci. *284*, 233–238 (1977)

Huynh-Dinh, T., Igolen, J.: Synthesis of C-nucleosides. Part 14. 5(3)-glycosyl-1,2,4-triazole-3(5)-carboxamides and analogues of ribavarin. J. Chem. Soc. Perkin *I*, 761–764 (1977)

ICN Pharmaceuticals, Inc.: Virazole (ribavirin ICN) Product Monograph (undated)

Larsson, A., Stenberg, K., Öberg, B.: Reversible inhibition of cellular metabolism by ribavirin. Antimicrob. Agents Chemother. *13*, 154–158 (1978)

Lowe, J.K., Brox, L., Henderson, J.F.: Consequences of inhibition of guanine nucleotide synthesis by mycophenolic acid and virazole. Cancer Res. *37*, 736–743 (1977)

Magnussen, C.R., Douglas, R.G., Betts, R.F., Roth, F.K., Meagher, M.P.: Double-blind evaluation of oral ribavirin (Virazole) in experimental influenza A virus infection in volunteers. Antimicrob. Agents Chemother. *12*, 498–502 (1977)

Matthews, R.E.F., Smith, J.D.: The chemotherapy of viruses. Adv. Virus Res. *3*, 49–148 (1955)

Menzel, G., Stenz, E.: Wirkungen von Virazol (Ribavirin) in Virus/Prokaryonten-Systemen. Acta Microbiol. Acad. Sci. Hung. *25*, 11–15 (1978)

Miles, D.L., Miles, D.W., Eyring, H.: A conformational basis for the antiviral inactivity of tetrazole ribonucleosides. Biochim. Biophys. Acta *518*, 17–30 (1978)

Miller, J.P., Kigwana, L.J., Streeter, S.D., Robins, R.K., Simon, L.N., Roboz, J.: The relationship between the metabolism of ribavarin and its proposed mechanism of action. Ann. N.Y. Acad. Sci. *284*, 211–229 (1977)

Müller, W.E.G., Maidhof, A., Taschner, H., Zahn, R.K.: Virazole (1-β-D-ribofuranosyl-1,2,4-triazole-3-carboxamide) a cytostatic agent. Biochem. Pharmacol. *26*, 1071–1075 (1977)

Öberg, B., Helgstrand, E.: Selective inhibition of viral polymerases by ribavarin triphosphate. Current Chemotherapy. Proc. 10th Int. Congr. Chemother., 332–334 (1977)

Odelola, H.A.: Antiviral activity of virazole on replication of viruses isolated in Nigeria. Abstr. 10th Int. Congr. Chemother., 398 (1977)

Oxford, J.S.: Inhibition of the replication of influenza A and B viruses by a nucleoside analogue (ribavirin). J. Gen. Virol. *28*, 409–414 (1975)

Poonian, M.S., Nowoswiat, E.F., Blount, J.F., Williams, T.H., Pitcher, R.G., Kramer, M.J.: Synthesis of tetrazole ribonucleosides and their evaluation as antiviral agents. J. Med. Chem. *19*, 286–290 (1976)

Prusiner, P., Sundaralingam, M.: A new class of synthetic nucleoside analogues with broad-spectrum antiviral properties. Nature New Biol. *244*, 116–117 (1973)

Salido-Rengell, F., Nasser-Quinones, H., Briseno-Garcia, B.: Clinical evaluation of 1-β-D-ribofuranosyl-1,2,4-triazole-3-carboxamide (ribavirin) in a double-blind study during an outbreak of influenza. Ann. N.Y. Acad. Sci. *284*, 272–277 (1977)

Scheffler, P., Haghchenlas, D., Wigand, R.: The effect of purine and pyrimidine analogues and virazole on adenovirus replication. Acta Virol. (Prague) *19*, 106–115 (1975)

Scholtissek, C.: Inhibition of influenza RNA synthesis by virazole (ribavirin) Arch. Virol. *50*, 349–352 (1976)

Scholtissek, C., Rott, R., Klenk, H.-D.: Two different mechanisms of the inhibition of the multiplication of enveloped viruses by glucosamine. Virology *63*, 191–200 (1975)

Shannon, W.M.: Selective inhibition of RNA tumor virus replication *in vitro* and evaluation of candidate antiviral agents *in vivo*. Ann. N.Y. Acad. Sci. *284*, 472–507 (1977)

Shepard, J.F.: Regeneration of plants from protoplasts of potato virus X-infected tobacco leaves: influence of virazole on the frequency of infection. Virology *78*, 261–266 (1977)

Sidwell, R.W., Huffman, J.H., Khare, G.P., Allen, L.B., Witkowski, J.T., Robins, R.K.: Broad-spectrum antiviral activity of virazole: 1-β-D-ribofuranosyl-1,2,4-triazole-3-carboxymide. Science *177*, 705–706 (1972)

Sidwell, R.W., Simon, L.N., Witkowski, J.T., Robins, R.K.: Antiviral activity of virazole. Review and structure-activity relations. Prog. Chemother. Proc. 8th Int. Congr. Chemother, 1973, *2*, 889–903 (1974)

Sidwell, R.W., Ellenhorn, M.J., Hillyard, I.W., Lime, J.M.: Safety evaluation of the broad spectrum antiviral, Ribavirin (Virazole®). Abstr. 10th Int. Congr. Chemother., 399 (1977)

Simon, L.N.: Discussion. Ann. N.Y. Acad. Sci. *284*, 291 (1977)

Simon, L.N., Sidwell, R.W., Khare, G.P., Streeter, D.G., Miller, J.P., Witkowski, J.T., Huffman, J.H., Robins, R.K.: Molecular basis of antiviral chemotherapy: virazole a new broad spectrum antiviral agent. In: Virus research, ICN-UCLA Symp Mol. Biol. Proc., 2nd. ed. Fox, F.C. (ed.), pp. 415–436. New York: Academic Press 1973

Smith, C.M., Fontenelle, L.J., Muzik, H., Paterson, A.R.P., Unger, H., Brox, L.W., Henderson, J.F.: Inhibitors of inosinate dehydrogenase activity in Ehrlich ascites cells in vitro. Biochem. Pharmacol. *23*, 2727–2735 (1974)

Streeter, D.G., Witkowski, J.T., Khare, G.P., Sidwell, R.W., Bauer, R.J., Robins, R.K., Simon, L.N.: Mechanism of action of 1-β-D-ribofuranosyl-1,2,4-triazole-3-carboxamide (Virazole), a new broad spectrum antiviral agent. Proc. Natl. Acad. Sci. USA *70*, 1174–1178 (1973)

Streeter, D.G., Miller, J.P., Robins, R.K., Simon, L.N.: The enzymic conversion of 1,2,4-triazole-3-

carboxamide to ribavirin-5′-phosphate and its relationship to the proposed mechanism of action. Ann. N.Y. Acad. Sci. *284*, 201–210 (1977)

Suganuma, T., Ishida, N.: Antiviral effect of virazole [1-β-D-ribofuranosyl-1,2,4-triazole-3-carboxamide]. Chemotherapy (Tokyo) *20*, 795–796 (1972)

Suganuma, T., Ishida, N.: An evaluation of a new antiviral agent "Virazole" against influenza virus infections. Tohoku J. Exp. Med. *110*, 405–406 (1973)

Suhadolnik, R.J.: Pyrazole nucleosides. In: Nucleoside antibiotics, pp. 390–392. New York: Wiley-Interscience 1970

Tisdale, M., Bauer, D.J.: The relative potencies of anti-influenza compounds. Ann. N.Y. Acad. Sci. *284*, 254–263 (1977)

Togo, Y.: In vitro effect of virazole against influenza viruses. Antimicrob. Agents Chemother. *4*, 641–642 (1973)

Togo, Y., McCracken, E.A.: Double-blind assessment of ribavirin (Virazole) in the prevention of induced infection with Type B influenza virus. J. Infect. Dis. Suppl. *133*, A 109-A 113 (1976)

Toshio, S., Nakao, I.: Antiviral effect of virazole [1-β-D-ribofuranosyl-1,2,4-triazole-3-carboxamide]. Chemother. *20*, 795–796 (1972)

Witkowski, J.T., Robins, R.K., Sidwell, R.W., Simon, L.N.: Design, synthesis and broad spectrum antiviral activity of 1-β-D-ribofuranosyl-1,2,4-triazole-3-carboxamide and related nucleosides. J. Med. Chem. *15*, 1150–1154 (1972)

Zertuche, H.F., Perches, R.D.: Clinical experiences using the antiviral 1-β-D-ribofuranosyl-1,2,4-triazole-3-carboxamide (ribavirin) in Mexico. Ann. N.Y. Acad. Sci. *284*, 284–288 (1977)

Zimmerman, T.P., Deeprose, R.D.: Metabolism of 5-amino-1-β-D-ribofuranosyl-imidazole-4-carboxamide and related five-membered heterocycles to 5′-triphosphates in human blood and L5178Y cells. Biochem. Pharmacol. *27*, 709–716 (1978)

Subject Index